ANNALS OF THE NEW YORK ACADEMY OF SCIENCES

Volume 815

The New York Academy of Sciences
2 East 63rd Street
New York, New York 10021

B LYMPHOCYTES AND AUTOIMMUNITY

ANNALS OF THE NEW YORK ACADEMY OF SCIENCES
Volume 815

B LYMPHOCYTES AND AUTOIMMUNITY

Edited by Nicholas Chiorazzi, Robert G. Lahita, Karel Pavelka, and Manlio Ferrarini

The New York Academy of Sciences
New York, New York
1997

∞ *The paper used in this publication meets the minimum requirements of American National Standard for Information Sciences—Permanence of Paper for Printed Library Materials, ANSI Z39.48-1984.*

Cover: The illustration on the softcover edition of this volume depicts the labeling of myelin structures on ultrathin sections of rat cerebral tissues (see Kirschning et al., page 457).

Library of Congress Cataloging-in-Publication Data

B lymphocytes and autoimmunity/edited by Nicholas Chiorazzi . . . [*et al.*].
p. cm.—(Annals of the New York Academy of Sciences, ISSN 0077-8923; v. 815).
Includes bibliographical references and index.
ISBN 1-57331-076-X (cloth: alk. paper).—ISBN 1-57331-077-8 (pbk.: alk. paper).
1. B cells—Congresses. 2. Autoimmunity—Congresses. 3. Autoantibodies—Congresses. I. Chiorazzi, Nicholas. II. New York Academy of Sciences. III. Series.
[DNLM: 1. B-Lymphocytes—congresses. 2. Autoimmunity—congresses. 3. Autoimmune Diseases—congresses. W1 AN626YL v. 815 1997/WH 200 B11025 1997]
Q11N5 vol. 815
[QR185.8.B15]
500 s—dc21
[616.07′98]
DNLM/DLC
for Library of Congress 97-3680
CIP

SP
Printed in the United States of America
ISBN 1-57331-076-X (cloth)
ISBN 1-57331-077-8 (paper)
ISSN 0077-8923

ANNALS OF THE NEW YORK ACADEMY OF SCIENCES

Volume 815
April 5, 1997

B LYMPHOCYTES AND AUTOIMMUNITY[a]

Editors and Conference Organizers
NICHOLAS CHIORAZZI, ROBERT G. LAHITA, KAREL PAVELKA, and MANLIO FERRARINI

CONTENTS

[a]This volume is the result of a conference entitled B Lymphocytes and Autoimmunity, which was sponsored jointly by the Institute of Rheumatology of Prague and the New York Academy of Sciences, under the auspices of the Ministry of Health of the Czech Republic, and held on May 21–25, 1996, in Prague, the Czech Republic.

Part IV. Development, Activation, and Tolerance in Autoreactive B Cells

Part V. Induction of Autoreactive B Cells and Autoantibody Responses

Part VI. Anatomic, Phenotypic, and Functional Subsets of B Cells

Part VII. Pathophysiologic Aspects of Autoantibodies

Part VIII. Structural and Functional Properties of Autoantibodies in Various Disease States

Part IX. Roles of T-B Cell Collaboration and Cytokines in Autoantibody Responses

Part X. Novel Therapies of Autoantibody-mediated Diseases

Part XI. Poster Papers

Financial assistance was received from:

Major funders

- HARRY WINSTON FOUNDATION, INCORPORATED
- MUCOS PHARMA

Supporters

- BAXTER BIOTECH/HYLAND DIVISION
- COMMISSION OF THE EUROPEAN COMMUNITIES
- CZECH RHEUMATOLOGY INSTITUTE
- LEO PHARMACEUTICAL PRODUCTS
- THE ROCKEFELLER UNIVERSITY
- SANDOZ PHARMA, LIMITED
- SANOFI WINTHROP
- ZENECA PHARMACEUTICALS

Contributors

- BIOGEN, INCORPORATED
- BOEHRINGER INGELHEIM PHARMACEUTICALS, INCORPORATED
- BRISTOL-MYERS SQUIBB PHARMACEUTICAL RESEARCH INSTITUTE
- DAKO CORPORATION
- DNAX RESEARCH INSTITUTE OF MOLECULAR AND CELLULAR BIOLOGY, INCORPORATED
- GENELABS TECHNOLOGIES, INCORPORATED
- ISTITUTO NAZIONALE PER LA RICERCA SUL CANCRO (IST)

- LA JOLLA PHARMACEUTICAL COMPANY
- MEDICAL & BIOLOGICAL LABORATORIES COMPANY, LIMITED
- NOVO NORDISK A/S
- PFIZER, INCORPORATED
- PHARMINGEN
- SCHERING-PLOUGH LABORATORY FOR IMMUNOLOGICAL RESEARCH, FRANCE
- SCHERING-PLOUGH RESEARCH INSTITUTE
- SPECIALTY LABORATORIES, INCORPORATED
- THERAPEUTIC ANTIBODIES, INCORPORATED

Preface

Over the past decade, remarkable progress has been made in our understanding of the composition, triggering, and molecular genetics of lymphocyte subsets. Instrumental in these achievements has been the advent of several technical advances. These include more-sophisticated immunofluorescent technologies that permit the convenient definition and isolation of lymphocyte cell subpopulations and molecular techniques that allow the rapid identification, sequencing, transfer, and targeted deletion of relevant genes. This progress has been slowly and progressively making its way into the clinical arena, especially in the fields of B lymphocyte subsets and their relationship to autoimmune disease. For this reason, we felt that a meeting that would analyze human and animal B lymphocyte subsets, their function, and their signaling pathways in relationship to autoimmunity would be timely.

The site chosen for this meeting was Prague, the Czech Republic. This city, and the area of the world that it embodies, has a long tradition of excellence in science and culture. Although this tradition was interrupted significantly by the political environment that pervaded Central and Eastern Europe for many years, the politics of this region has now become more open, and it was the hope of this meeting to help celebrate the return of Central and Eastern Europeans to the mainstream of immunobiology and science.

The meeting comprised two types of presentations: those by a series of invited speakers and those selected from among the more than 100 abstracts submitted by conference attendees. In each case, novel and exciting data were presented that stimulated fertile discussions and interactions.

Among these exciting findings were certain concepts that deserve special mention and will be easily appreciated by reading the papers found in this volume. These included the following:

- the demonstration that autoreactivity plays a positive as well as a negative role in the selection of the evolving B cell antigen-receptor repertoire;
- data regarding the rescue and death of cells passing through the germinal center;
- the roles of antigen binding, the Bcl2 family of proteins, and the CD40–CD40 ligand and the Fas–Fas ligand triggering pathways in these processes;
- various peripheral tolerance pathways defined in transgenic mice that silence or eliminate autoantigen-binding B cells;
- the role of B cell presentation of autoantigen in the breaking of self-tolerance;
- evidence for both T cell–dependence and T cell–independence of autoantibody generation;
- methods for the separation of human B lymphocytes into marginal zone, follicular mantle, and germinal center B cells;
- novel insights into the effector pathways of autoimmunity and, in particular, the roles of autoantibodies, complement, and Fcγ receptors;

- new therapeutic approaches aimed either directly at B cells or at collaborating interactions of other cells of the immune system.

The presentations on these topics clearly showed the great progress made in a relatively short time in the field. The discussions that followed also indicated that while certain issues are settled, the majority of the topics still present a number of controversies. The different points of view expressed by the various scientists fostered new ideas for novel experimental approaches that are suitable for cooperative enterprises among the participants from both sides of the Atlantic Ocean.

This book collects most of the presentations of the meeting and provides a summary of the "state of the art" in the field of B lymphocytes and autoimmunity. We hope that this volume will serve as a durable reference work designed to assist the research immunologist, academic clinician, or student of biology to appreciate the progress of the past few years with regard to immune regulation. As with all books of this nature, in the long term it is not only what lies between the covers that will have a lasting effect on our area of investigation, but also the ideas that evolve from a careful reading of selected papers.

Nicholas Chiorazzi
Robert G. Lahita
Karel Pavelka
Manlio Ferrarini

Autoantibodies and Autoimmunity: A Three-Decade Perspective

A Tribute to Henry G. Kunkel[a]

ENG M. TAN

The Scripps Research Institute
La Jolla, California 92037

THE EARLY YEARS OF AUTOANTIBODIES

It is easy to appreciate the fact that some of the earliest studies on autoantibodies in human disease began with systemic lupus erythematosus (SLE), which has been considered a prototype autoimmune disease because of the abundance of autoantibodies and the demonstration that some autoantibodies participate in immune-mediated pathogenesis. In fact, before anything was known concerning autoantibodies in this disease, Hargraves *et al.*[1] discovered the LE cell phenomenon. This was a neutrophil that had ingested a large amorphous basophilic inclusion body and was demonstrable in smears made from bone marrow or clotted blood of SLE patients. The LE cell phenomenon was the reaction of an antinuclear antibody with autologous nuclear material. The discovery of this phenomenon led ten years later to the recognition of antibody reactive with DNA by several laboratories. The laboratories of Kunkel and Ceppellini[2,3] demonstrated this by complement fixation, whereas Seligmann[4] did so by immunoprecipitation and Miescher and Strassle[5] did so by hemagglutination. Many important biochemical and clinical observations concerning antibody to DNA followed these studies. Biochemical observations demonstrated the presence of antibodies reactive with "native" and "denatured" DNA, and clinical observations established the importance of antibody to native DNA in lupus and its significance in immune complex–mediated vasculitis. In a review of this subject in 1964,[6] Kunkel stated that there were separate antinuclear antibodies reacting with DNA, with histone, with nucleoprotein, and with "phosphate extract". Typical of his keen insight, he stated that this was a minimal number of autoantibodies because there was evidence for several types of antibodies to nucleoprotein and that multiple antigens were present in the phosphate extract of nuclei.

In the late 1950s and early 1960s, the extensive research into pathogenic mechanisms associated with immune complex vasculitis and the application of the immunofluorescence technique set the stage for the demonstration of the important role of antibodies to DNA in SLE. Immune complex glomerulonephritis and vasculitis had been produced in experimental models of serum sickness.[7] When tissues from patients with lupus were examined with the newly introduced immunofluorescence

[a]This work constitutes publication no. 10108-MEM and was supported by grants from the National Institutes of Health.

technique, deposits of immunoglobulin were found in the glomerular capillary loops of diseased kidneys and in vascular lesions of other organs.[8,9] Further investigations showed the presence of the C3 component of complement in association with the deposited immunoglobulin. These findings strongly suggested that immune complex–mediated mechanisms could be playing an important role in tissue injury in lupus.

The nature of the antigen or antigens participating in immune complex–mediated pathogenesis, however, was not known until a study showing the sequential appearance of DNA antigen and antibody in the blood of patients with lupus.[10] In one such patient (FIGURE 1), antibody to DNA had been detected on four successive occasions

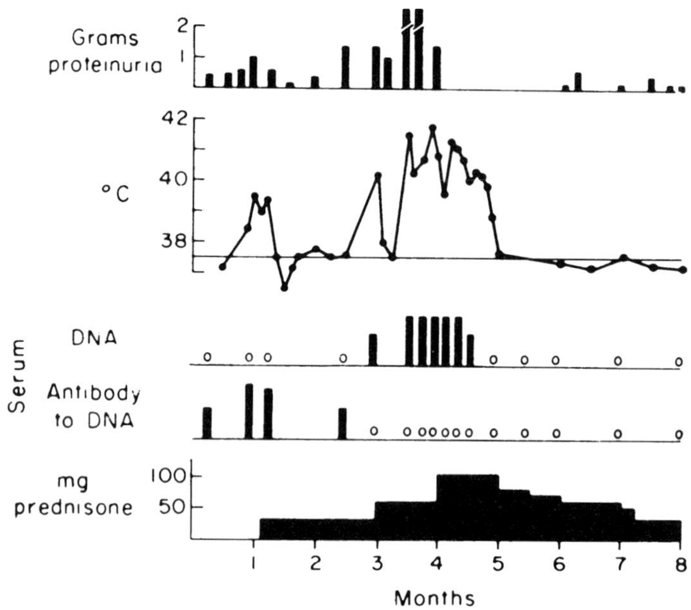

FIGURE 1. A patient with SLE initially showing DNA antibody in four consecutive serum samples. Exacerbation of illness with high fever and increased proteinuria coincided with appearance of DNA antigen in serum and with disappearance of antibody, a sequence of events highly suggestive of immune complex formation. The patient appeared to have a period of antibody excess, followed by equivalence and antigen excess.

in the serum prior to an acute exacerbation of his disease. During this exacerbation, the patient had prolonged high fever, generalized skin rash, and increased proteinuria. Antibody to DNA disappeared from the serum, to be replaced by DNA over a period of six weeks. It could be shown that serum taken from the earlier period of his illness, when DNA antibody was present, was autoreactive with DNA antigen present in later periods of his illness, when DNA was detected during the exacerbation phase. Subsequent studies by several other investigators have confirmed these findings and DNA antigen was demonstrated on the glomerular basement membrane of lupus kidneys. Elution of immunoglobulin from kidney homogenates showed enrichment of

DNA antibody manyfold over its concentration in serum.[9] Thus, the required conditions for autoimmunity causing disease pathogenesis were met with the demonstration of circulating autoantibodies complexing with autoantigens to cause immune complex–mediated tissue injury.

DIVERSITY OF ANTIBODY SPECIFICITIES

It soon became evident that autoantibodies of many different antigen-antibody specificities could be identified in the sera of patients with lupus, scleroderma, Sjögren's syndrome, and other systemic autoimmune diseases. This was facilitated by two assay systems. One was indirect immunofluorescence using cellular substrates, in which it could be shown that antibodies reacted in a highly specific manner with antigens localized to different compartments of the nucleus; thus, different patterns of nuclear immunofluorescence staining could be observed. The broad categories of antigen localization could be separated into those that showed homogeneous distribution of the antigens in the nucleus, a pattern largely related to antibodies reactive with DNA and histones. Another major pattern was one in which the antigens were distributed in a speckled fashion in the nucleoplasm. This has been shown to be related to numerous antibodies that react with different antigens, including those involved in precursor-mRNA splicing and transcription. In addition, many autoantigens were present in the nucleolus and in the cytoplasm, as well as antigens that varied in their distribution in the cell cycle. Another assay that helped in confirming that multiple antibodies were present in autoimmune sera was immunoprecipitation, using immunodiffusion as the assay system. With this method, immunoprecipitin lines of different antigen-antibody specificities could be demonstrated using soluble extracts of homogenized cells. In the 1970s, there was a great spurt of activity using serum antibodies for the screening of cDNA expression libraries and many cDNAs encoding autoantigens have been cloned. This has resulted in the definitive identification of many autoantigens at the molecular and functional levels (reviewed in reference 11). An example of some antigen-antibody systems in systemic lupus erythematosus is shown in TABLE 1. Antibodies to double-strand DNA, anti-Sm, anti-ribosomal P proteins, and anti-PCNA are antibodies that have high diagnostic specificity for lupus, whereas other antibodies such as anti-U1 RNP, anti-SS-A/Ro, and anti-SS-B/La are not specific for lupus because they are seen in other diseases such as mixed connective tissue disease (for anti-U1 RNP) and Sjögren's syndrome (anti-SS-A/Ro and anti-SS-B/La). What emerged from these studies was the understanding that some antigen-antibody specificities were more tightly related to a specific disease, whereas others could be related to two or three diseases. Autoantibodies have been extremely useful as adjuncts in the differentiation of autoimmune diseases and have an established place in diagnostic medicine.

NATURE OF AUTOANTIGENS

Steitz and her colleagues pioneered in the field of establishing the function of autoantigens.[12] In an elegant study, it was shown that anti-Sm antibodies were directed

TABLE 1. Diagnostically Relevant Autoantibodies in Systemic Lupus Erythematosus

Identity of Autoantibody	Nature of Autoantigen	Frequency of Autoantibody (%)	Specificity
anti-double-strand DNA	double-strand DNA	40–60	high
anti-DNA histone	all histone classes H1, H2A, H2B, H3, and H4	60–80	medium
anti-Sm	components (B and D) of small nuclear ribonucleoproteins (snRNP)—28/29-kDa and 19-kDa proteins	25–30	high
anti-U1 RNP	components (A and C) of U1 snRNP—32- and 23-kDa proteins and 70-kDa associated splicing factor	30–40	low
anti-SS-A/Ro	components of RNP particles—60-kDa protein and 52-kDa associated protein	40	low
anti-SS-B/La	components of RNP particles involved in precursor tRNA processing—48-kDa protein	20–25	low
anti-ribosomal P proteins	15-, 16-, and 38-kDa proteins (cytoplasmic in location) of ribosomes	15–20	high
anti-Ku	DNA-dependent protein kinase doublet of 70/80-kDa proteins	10–15	medium
anti-PCNA	DNA polymerase δ auxiliary factor—36-kDa protein	3	high

against the small nuclear ribonucleoprotein (snRNP) family of splicing factors. They showed that anti-Sm and anti-U1 RNP antibodies were capable of immunoprecipitating the small nuclear RNA components of snRNP. These small nuclear RNAs (snRNAs) were the uridine-rich RNAs (U1, U2, and U4–U6 snRNAs). However, the antigenic molecules were the protein and not the RNA components of the snRNP complexes. This new information concerning the molecular identity and function of the antigens recognized by anti-Sm and anti-U1 RNP autoantibodies provided one of the early challenging ideas about the nature of immunogens in autoimmune diseases and the concept that the immunogens are present in the form of multimolecular particles.

Another special feature of nuclear autoantigens was the observation that the antigens were proteins that were highly conserved in evolution. In addition, even the epitopes on antigens recognized by autoantibodies were highly conserved regions of these proteins. One example is proliferating cell nuclear antigen (PCNA), which is a nuclear protein involved in DNA replication and is an accessory protein in the DNA polymerase δ complex. The 36-kDa antigen is the target of autoantibodies in a small percentage of patients with lupus and, with the antibody as a tracer, it was shown early on that the antigen was cell-cycle-related and most highly expressed in late G1 and S phases of the cell cycle.[13,14] Studies with thymidine labeling showed that the nuclear domains staining with anti-PCNA antibodies were also those regions showing thymidine uptake, thereby confirming that these were the sites of DNA replication. The highly conserved nature of PCNA as well as the autoreactive epitope is shown in TABLE 2. Proteins with homology to PCNA have been shown to extend in species distribution from man to yeast and baculovirus. In addition, epitopes recognized by human autoantibody have been detected in birds, fish, protozoa, and plants (soybean). This remarkable phenomenon of epitope conservation is not limited to PCNA, but is a highly generalized characteristic of autoantigens in the autoimmune diseases.

A number of studies have shown that the determinants or epitopes recognized by autoantibodies are frequently conformation-dependent and composed of discontinuous regions of the primary sequence. This was illustrated in a study to determine the epitope on PCNA recognized by autoantibody.[15] Compound peptides of PCNA were synthesized from regions of this protein depicted in FIGURE 2. Of interest were peptides designated 10-12 and 16-12, which had a common 9-mer amino acid covering residues 127–135. Another compound peptide designated 15-25 consisted of the regions of PCNA as shown in the figure. Rabbits were immunized with these synthetic peptides and the resultant antisera were studied for their immunoreactivity. FIGURE 3 shows that preincubation of antisera to peptides 10-12 and 16-12 could be completely inhibited by either one or the other synthetic peptide, suggesting that possibly the common 9-mer sequence (127–135) was the common determinant recognized by the two antisera. On the other hand, antiserum to 15-25 was only inhibited by the homologous peptide. FIGURE 3B displays the key experimental evidence distinguishing the important differences between anti-10-12 and anti-16-12 on the one hand and anti-15-25 on the other. When primary continuous sequence peptides were used for inhibition studies, only the synthetic peptide of sequence 121–135 inhibited the anti-10-12 and anti-16-12 antisera. This supported the earlier assumption that the determinant was located in the 127–135 sequence. The interesting finding was that antiserum to 15-25 could not be inhibited by any of the primary continuous sequence peptides, suggesting that the determinant eliciting the immune

TABLE 2. Species Distribution of PCNA

Species	DNA Homology	Immunological Identity (Reactive with Human Autoantibody)[a]
man (protein of 261 aa)		
rat	98% nucleotide identity	yes
rabbit		yes
bovine		yes
bird		yes
fish		yes
drosophila	70% nucleotide identity	NT
rice	76% nucleotide homology	NT
soybean		yes (root tip nuclei)
protozoa		yes (replication band)
yeast	functional protein (26 kDa)	no (?)
baculovirus	40% nucleotide identity	NT

[a]NT = not tested.

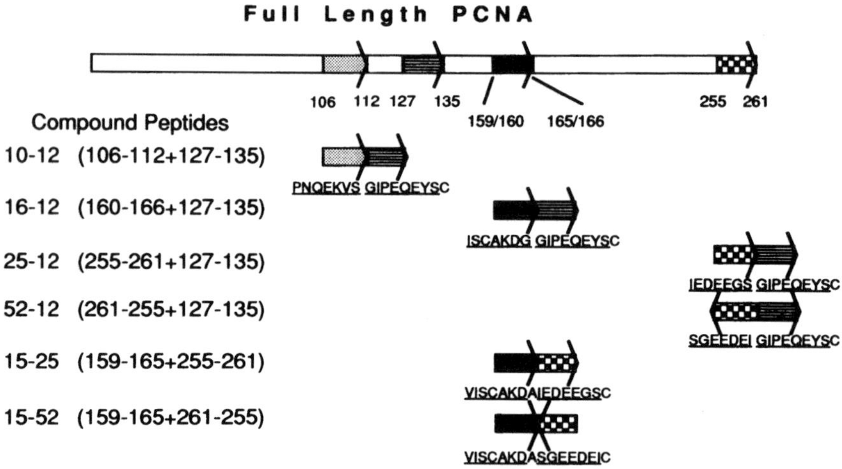

FIGURE 2. Construction of compound peptides of PCNA. The horizontal bar at the top represents full-length PCNA with 261 amino acid residues. The shaded portions of this bar represent the regions that were selected for making compound peptides, with the arrowhead indicating the C-terminus of each region. Compound peptide 10-12 was a combination of peptide 106–112 covalently linked to 127–135. Compound peptide 15-25 was a combination of peptide 159–165 covalently linked to 255–261. Compound peptide 16-12 has a similar region of 127–135 as compound peptide 10-12, but a separate N-terminal portion of 160–166.

response was a conformation-dependent epitope and not inherent in the primary continuous sequences. This was confirmed by showing that only antiserum to 15-25 gave immunofluorescence staining of late G1 and S phase cells and that the staining colocalized with that demonstrated by human anti-PCNA antibodies. The conformation-dependent property of antigenic determinants is a generalized property of many autoepitopes.

Epitopes recognized by autoimmune sera can be quite different from the epitopes recognized by sera raised with experimental immunization. SS-B/La is a ubiquitous nuclear protein of 46–48 kDa and is a target antigen of autoantibodies in lupus and Sjögren's syndrome. This protein is involved in the maturation of RNA polymerase III transcripts such as 5S RNA and tRNAs. Murine monoclonal antibodies raised against calf thymus SS-B/La antigen were analyzed for their immunoreactivities in comparison with human autoimmune serum.[16] The human serum Ze reacted strongly with the 48-kDa native SS-B/La and with a spontaneous 43-kDa degradation product, whereas the monoclonal antibodies that reacted strongly with the native protein were totally nonreactive with the 43-kDa fragment. SS-B/La could be digested by S.a.V8 protease to generate fragments X/X′/X″ (28/29/30 kDa) and Y/Y′ (23/24 kDa). FIGURE 4B shows that the monoclonal antibodies have completely different reactivities compared with human serum. The critical results that further elucidated the differences between autoimmune sera and experimentally induced antisera are shown in TABLE 3. When these sera were analyzed in immunofluorescence on tissue culture cells from many species, the human SS-B autoantibodies reacted with SS-B antigen from many species, whereas even the most-reactive monoclonal antibodies (A1, A2, and A3) reacted with SS-B antigen in a more species-restricted manner. Although monoclonal antibodies A1, A2, and A3 gave typical nuclear staining patterns with human, monkey, rabbit, and bovine cell lines, they gave no staining with hamster, rat, mouse, and rat-kangaroo cell lines. These studies provide further support for the view that autoimmune antibodies recognized very highly conserved epitopes.

The observations that human autoantibodies are reactive with highly conserved regions of proteins go hand in hand with the many studies that show that autoantibodies have the capability of inhibiting the functions of the cognate antigens. This is shown in TABLE 4. Autoantibodies to Sm and nuclear RNP inhibit precursor-mRNA splicing,[17] antibodies to PCNA inhibit DNA replication and repair directed by DNA polymerase δ,[18] and antibody to Scl-70 inhibits the function of DNA topoisomerase I.[19] Similar inhibitory capabilities have been demonstrated for autoantibodies to RNA polymerase I, to the centromere protein antigens CENP-A, -B, and -C, to DNA topoisomerase II, and to several tRNA synthetases.[20]

MECHANISMS THAT MIGHT BE INDUCING AN ANTIGEN-DRIVEN AUTOANTIBODY RESPONSE

Recently, there has been great interest in the relationship of apoptosis and autoimmunity, especially with the observation of Fas abnormalities in the MRL/lpr/lpr

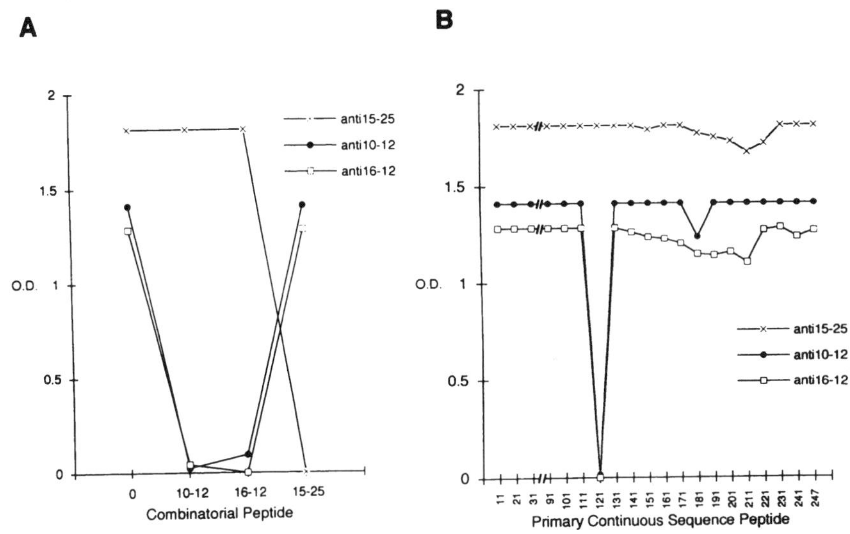

FIGURE 3. Inhibition of antibody binding to recombinant PCNA by peptides: (A) preincubation with compound peptides; (B) preincubation with 15-mer primary structure continuous sequence peptides. One hundred μL of recombinant PCNA fusion protein (5 μg/mL) was coated as antigen in wells of ELISA plates and reacted with 100 μL of rabbit antisera mixed with synthetic peptides (300 ng/mL). In part B, peptide nos. 11, 21, 31, . . . , represent 15-mer synthetic peptides, 11–25, 21–35, 31–45, . . . , of the continuous primary structure covering the total PCNA sequence from residue 11 to the C-terminal end residue 261.

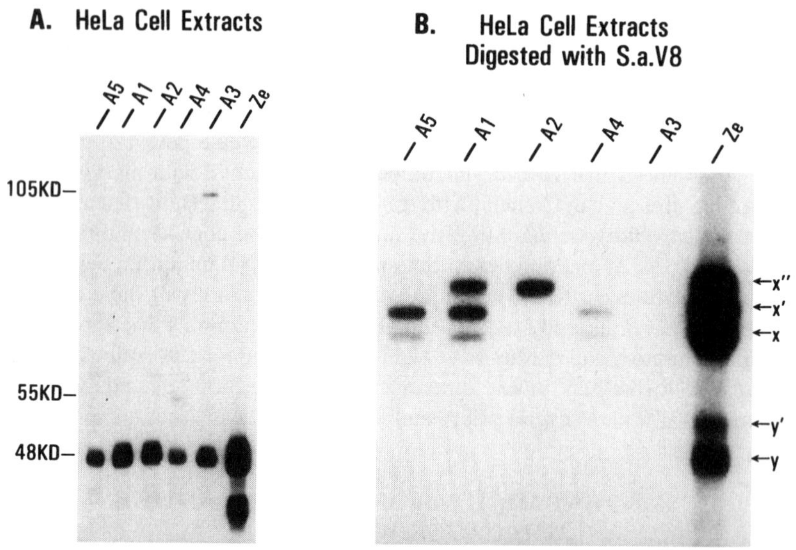

FIGURE 4. Murine monoclonal antibodies (A1–A5) were produced by immunization with purified calf thymus SS-B/La protein and were analyzed by immunoblotting against whole HeLa cell extract (A) and HeLa cell extract partially digested with S.a.V8 protease (B). Although all murine monoclonal antibodies blotted the native 48-kDa SS-B/La antigen, their other reactivities were clearly different from the human serum Ze.

TABLE 3. Species-specific Reactivities of Monoclonal Antibodies to SS-B/La Antigen as Detected by Immunofluorescence

		Immunofluorescence[a]					
		Murine Monoclonal Antibodies					Human Sera
Species	Cell Line Origin	A1	A2	A3	A4	A5	Ze[b]
human	HEp-2, larynx	+	+	+	–	–	+
human	HeLa, cervix	+	+	+	–	–	+
human	Raji, Burkitt lymphoma	+	+	+	–	–	+
monkey	Vero, kidney	+	+	+	–	–	+
rabbit	R9ab, lung	+	+	+	–	–	+
bovine	MDBK, kidney	+	+	+	–	–	+
hamster	BHK-21, kidney	–	–	–	–	–	+
rat	6m2, kidney	–	–	–	–	–	+
mouse	3T3, fibroblast	–	–	–	–	–	+
rat-kangaroo	Ptk2, kidney	–	–	–	–	–	+

[a]Cells were grown in Lab-Tek tissue culture chambers and fixed in a mixture of acetone and methanol (3:1) at −20 °C for 2 min.

[b]Ze serum is the CDC reference serum for anti-SS-B/La specificity.

strain of mice having lupus-like autoimmune disease.[21–23] Some of the cellular protein substrates that are cleaved early in apoptosis are poly-ADP ribose polymerase (PARP) and NuMA (nuclear mitotic apparatus) protein, both of which are known autoantigens. We have used Fas-mediated apoptosis in Jurkatt cell lines as the model for studying cleavage of autoantigens.[24] Monospecific autoimmune sera were used to monitor the presence or absence of proteolytic cleavage of 25 different autoantigens. FIGURE 5 shows that the autoantigens PARP, DNA topoisomerase I, U1 RNP–70-kDa protein, NuMA, lamin B, and NOR-90–UBF are autoantigens that are cleaved during Fas-mediated apoptosis. However, many other autoantigens such as PCNA, Ku, Sm antigens, fibrillarin, the nucleolar protein B23, Jo-1, ribosomal RNP, SS-A/Ro, and SS-B/La do not show any detectable cleavage products. Thus, only a select number of autoantigens are cleaved during Fas-mediated apoptosis. There appears to be a hierarchy in the order of substrate cleavage as shown in FIGURE 6, with PARP and NuMA appearing to be the earliest proteins that are degraded when the process was examined from zero time to 7 hours after monoclonal antibody to Fas was added to the Jurkatt cells. Other investigators have shown that autoantigens like SS-A/Ro and SS-B/La are displaced during apoptosis and appear in the cytoplasmic blebs of apoptotic cells.[25] The notions being entertained at this time are that cleavage products of certain substrates during apoptosis may be immunogens driving the autoantibody response and, in addition, displacement of certain cellular proteins during this form of cell death may be a factor conferring immunogenicity to certain proteins. These notions are waiting for experimental verification.

TABLE 4. Functions of Nuclear Autoantigens Inhibited by Autoantibodies

Autoantigen	Function	Presence of Autoantibody
Sm/nRNP (U1,2,4–6 snRNP)	pre-mRNA splicing	SLE
PCNA (DNA pol δ auxiliary protein)	DNA replication and repair	SLE
Scl-70 (DNA topoisomerase I)	DNA replication and transcription	scleroderma
RNA polymerase I	transcription of rRNA	scleroderma
centromere proteins CENP-A,B,C	microtubule-based chromosome movement during mitosis	CREST
DNA topoisomerase II	DNA replication	hepatocellular carcinoma
tRNA synthetases (histidyl, threonyl, alanyl)	amino acylation of tRNAs	dermatomyositis and polymyositis

Another interesting possibility as to how cellular proteins might be driving autoantibody formation comes from studies of the p53 tumor suppressor protein. Abnormalities of the p53 gene have been shown to be present in approximately 50% of patients with lung and breast cancer and, in this group, 20–30% have been found to have antibodies to p53. Cell lines from patients with small cell lung cancer (SCLC)

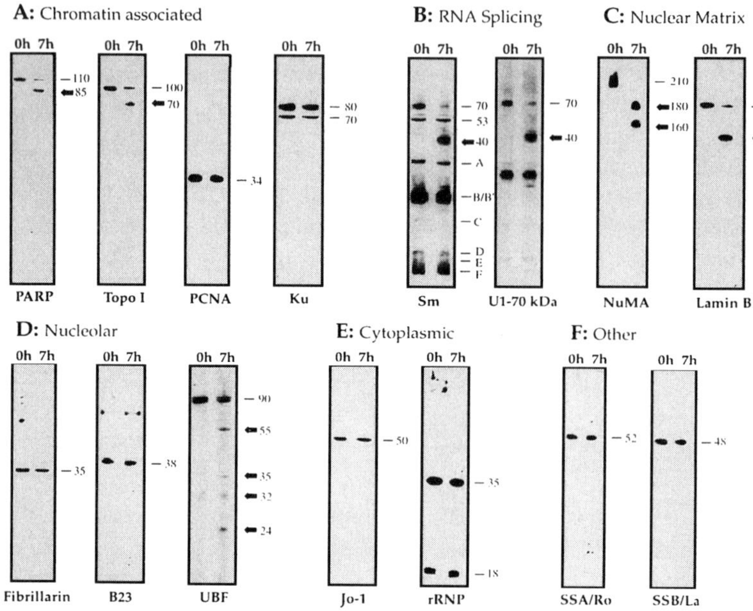

FIGURE 5. Proteolytic cleavage of a subset of autoantigens during CD95 (Fas)–mediated apoptosis of Jurkatt cells. Cells were induced to undergo apoptosis by exposure to anti-CD95 monoclonal antibody (100 ng/mL) for 7 h. Control and anti-CD95-treated cells were lysed and proteins were separated by SDS-PAGE and immunoblotted using highly specific human autoimmune sera. Representative blots of cleaved and noncleaved autoantigens are shown. Intact proteins are indicated by lines, whereas proteolytic fragments are indicated by arrows. Numbers to the right of each blot represent relative molecular weights in kDa. Autoantigens are grouped in categories according to their subcellular localization or functions—(A) chromatin-associated: PARP, DNA topo I, PCNA, and 70/80-kDa Ku doublet; (B) RNA splicing: Sm and U1/70 kDa; (C) nuclear matrix: NuMA and lamin B; (D) nucleolar proteins: fibrillarin, B23, and UBF; (E) cytoplasmic protein: Jo-1 (histidyl tRNA synthetase) and ribosomal proteins P0, P1/P2; (F) other: the 52-kDa component of the SS-A/Ro particle and the 48-kDa SS-B/La protein. (Reproduced from reference 24.)

and other forms of lung cancer have been established and the p53 mutations were identified and included point mutations, stop codon mutations, and frameshift mutations.[26] Patients with point mutations had single amino acid substitutions and detectable p53 protein in their cell lines. The detectable levels of p53 were related to increased stability of the protein, which in normal situations is rapidly degraded in the cell cycle. The majority of patients with autoantibodies to p53 had such point mutations that resulted in persistence of p53. These studies in lung cancer have been confirmed in another study on breast cancer where, in addition to mutations in p53 resulting in abnormally stabilized protein, there was complexing of the p53 to heat shock protein 70.[27] Antibodies to p53 have now been found to present in other forms of cancer including prostate, thyroid, and bladder cancers. Recent studies have shown that autoantibodies to p53 recognize both wild-type and mutant p53 and that the autoepitopes in p53 are the amino and carboxyl termini of the protein, outside the region of the mutational hot spots. Therefore, the evidence points to the fact that mutant p53 molecules do not possess novel antigenic epitopes that are driving the autoimmune response. Rather, it appears that the abnormal persistence of p53 and perhaps the complexing of mutant p53 molecules with other cellular proteins are factors driving the autoimmune reaction.

On the basis of the data accumulated over the past three decades of research by numerous investigators, it appears reasonable to make the following statements:

(1) The autoantibody response in systemic autoimmune diseases is antigen-driven.
(2) Autoantigens are components of multimolecular subcellular particles.
(3) Autoantigens are involved in important cell functions.
(4) Autoepitopes are frequently functional regions or catalytic domains of subcellular particles.

From these observations, it is appropriate to advance a couple of hypotheses for consideration:

(A) Autoantibodies may be clues to intracellular processing events (caused by mutations, viruses, toxins, chemicals, etc.) that cause perturbations in cell function and result in damage or abnormal accumulation of certain cellular proteins.

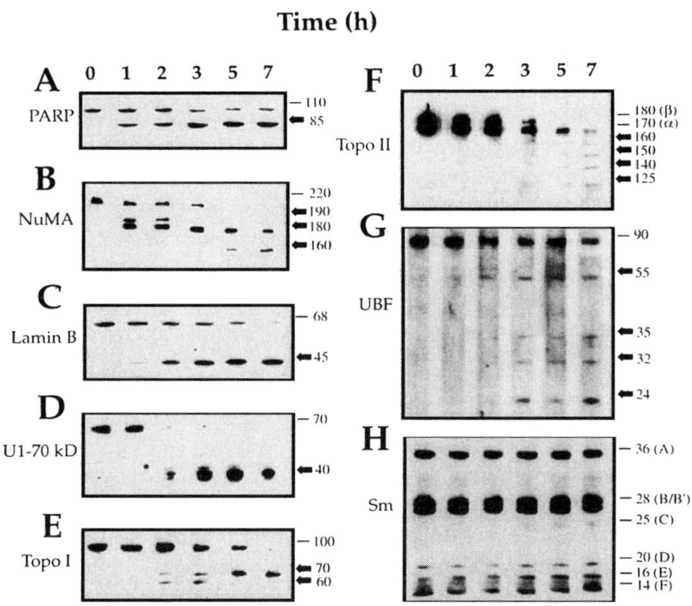

FIGURE 6. Kinetics of autoantigen cleavage after addition of anti-CD95 monoclonal antibody to Jurkatt T cells. The substrates are arranged in the order of early to late cleavage of the proteins. (Reproduced from reference 24.)

(B) Autoantibodies might be considered as "messengers" of these provoking events that induce an autoimmune response. These provoking events show disease specificity, but the resultant autoantibodies are not necessarily involved in pathogenesis.

Conceptually, this hypothesis says that the immune system is making a response to a self protein that has become abnormal because the protein has been altered by mutation, by atypical association with other proteins, by changes in its metabolism, or by ectopic localization. In other words, the immune system is functioning normally and is making a response to an abnormal cellular event. Lewis Thomas said that "the molecule of DNA was ordained from the beginning to make small mistakes".[28] This property of DNA allowed for all-important evolution to take place, but also for occasional unavoidable harmful consequences such as mutations, leading to carcinogenesis. An unfortunate side effect of immune system function might be the mounting of immune responses to dysregulated self proteins.

In all studies of human disease, it is of great importance to go back to the disease under study and ask how the laboratory observations fit with the clinical manifestations. If one looks at SLE, in which we have extensive clinical and pathological information, the hallmark of tissue pathology is the deposition of immunoglobulin and complement in the blood vessels of many different tissues. There is good evidence to show that this immunopathology is related to antigen-antibody reactions that either take place in the circulation and are subsequently deposited in the blood vessels or are due to antibody reacting with implanted or *in situ* antigens in various tissues, such as the kidney glomeruli. These immune complex reactions result in the activation of inflammatory pathways, including the complement system, the coagulation cascade, and the mobilization of many inflammatory cells such as neutrophils, eosinophils, mast cells, macrophages, and lymphocytes.[29] It is probably important to take into consideration that some of the T cell abnormalities that are reported in SLE and other autoimmune diseases might be related to an interplay of many inflammatory cytokines initiated by antigen-antibody immune complex reactions. Thus, in many autoimmune diseases where antibodies have been detected, it might be the B cell that is playing a pivotal role in initiating inflammation and leading to a host of downstream events such as participation of T cells introducing new inflammatory pathways and further escalating pathogenic mechanisms.

DEDICATION

This symposium on B Lymphocytes and Autoimmunity would have delighted the heart of a great scientist and teacher, the late Henry G. Kunkel, of the Rockefeller University. He was a scientist whose laboratory observations were profound in their elucidation of basic biological mechanisms, but he was at the same time always mindful of what contributions they would make to the understanding of disease. There are many participants at this meeting who have felt his touch and I for one would like to dedicate this presentation as a tribute to his wisdom and vision.

REFERENCES

1. HARGRAVES, M. M., H. RICHMOND & R. MORTON. 1948. Presentation of two bone marrow elements: the "tart" cells and the "L.E." cell. Mayo Clin. Proc. **27:** 25–28.
2. ROBBINS, W. C., H. R. HOLMAN, H. DEICHER & H. G. KUNKEL. 1957. Complement fixation with cell nuclei and DNA in lupus erythematosus. Proc. Soc. Exp. Biol. Med. **96:** 575–579.
3. CEPPELLINI, R., E. POLLI & F. COLADA. 1957. A DNA-reacting factor in serum of a patient with lupus erythematosus diffusus. Proc. Soc. Exp. Biol. Med. **96:** 572–575.
4. SELIGMANN, M. 1957. Mise en evidence dans le serum de malade atteints de lupus d'une substance determinant une reaction de precipitation avec l'acide desoxyribonucleique. C. R. Acad. Sci. (Paris) **245:** 243–247.
5. MIESCHER, P. & R. STRASSLE. 1957. New serological methods for the detection of the L.E. factor. Vox Sang. **2:** 283–288.
6. KUNKEL, H. G. & E. M. TAN. 1964. Autoantibodies and disease. Adv. Immunol. **4:** 351–395.
7. DIXON, F. J., J. D. FELDMAN & J. VAZGUEZ. 1961. Experimental glomerulonephritis: the pathogenesis of a laboratory model resembling the spectrum of human glomerulonephritis. J. Exp. Med. **113:** 899–909.
8. LACHMANN, P., H. J. MULLER-EBERHARD, H. G. KUNKEL & F. PARONETTO. 1962. The localization of *in vivo* bound complement in tissue sections. J. Exp. Med. **115:** 63–82.
9. KOFFLER, D., P. H. SCHUR & H. G. KUNKEL. 1967. Immunological studies concerning the nephritis of systemic lupus erythematosus. J. Exp. Med. **126:** 607–619.
10. TAN, E. M., R. I. CARR, P. H. SCHUR & H. G. KUNKEL. 1966. DNA and antibody to DNA in the serum of patients with systemic lupus erythematosus. J. Clin. Invest. **45:** 1732–1740.
11. TAN, E. M. 1989. Antinuclear antibodies: diagnostic markers for autoimmune diseases and probes for cell biology. Adv. Immunol. **44:** 93–151.
12. LERNER, M. R. & J. A. STEITZ. 1979. Antibodies to small nuclear RNAs complexed with proteins are produced by patients with systemic lupus erythematosus. Proc. Natl. Acad. Sci. U.S.A. **76:** 5495–5497.
13. MIYACHI, K., M. J. FRITZLER & E. M. TAN. 1978. Autoantibody to a nuclear antigen in proliferating cells. J. Immunol. **121:** 228–234.
14. BRAVO, R., S. J. FEY, J. BELLATIN, P. M. LARSON, J. ARVELO & J. E. CELIS. 1981. Identification of a nuclear and of a cytoplasmic polypeptide whose reactive proportions are sensitive to changes in the rate of cell proliferation. Exp. Cell Res. **136:** 311–317.
15. MURO, Y., W-M. TSAI, R. HOUGHTEN & E. M. TAN. 1994. Synthetic compound peptide simulating antigenicity of conformation-dependent autoepitope. J. Biol. Chem. **269:** 18529–18534.
16. CHAN, E. K. L. & E. M. TAN. 1987. Human autoantibody-reactive epitopes of SS-B/La are highly conserved in comparison with epitopes recognized by murine monoclonal antibodies. J. Exp. Med. **166:** 1627–1640.
17. YANG, V. W., M. R. LERNER, J. A. STEITZ & S. J. FLINT. 1981. A small nuclear ribonucleoprotein is required for splicing of adenoviral early RNA sequences. Proc. Natl. Acad. Sci. U.S.A. **78:** 1371–1375.
18. TAN, C-K., K. SULLIVAN, X. LI, E. M. TAN, K. W. DOWNEY & A. G. SO. 1987. Autoantibody to the proliferating cell nuclear antigen neutralizes the activity of the auxiliary protein for DNA polymerase δ. Nucleic Acids Res. **15:** 9299–9308.
19. SHERO, J. H., B. BORDWELL, N. F. ROTHFIELD & W. C. EARNSHAW. 1986. Autoantibodies to topoisomerase I are found in sera from scleroderma patients. Science **231:** 737–740.
20. TAN, E. M. 1991. Autoantibodies in pathology and cell biology. Cell **67:** 841–842.
21. ADACHI, M., R. WATANABE-FUKUNAGA & S. NAGATA. 1993. Aberrant transcription caused by the insertion of an early transposable element in an intron of the Fas antigen gene of lpr mice. Proc. Natl. Acad. Sci. U.S.A. **90:** 1756.
22. WU, J., T. ZHOU, J. HE & J. D. MOUNTZ. 1993. Autoimmune disease in mice due to the integration of an endogenous retrovirus in an apoptosis gene. J. Exp. Med. **178:** 461.

23. CHU, J-L., J. DAPPA, A. PARNASSA & K. B. ELKON. 1993. The defect in Fas mRNA expression in MRL/lpr mice is associated with insertion of the retrotransposon, Etn. J. Exp. Med. **178:** 723.
24. CASIANO, C. A., S. J. MARTIN, D. R. GREEN & E. M. TAN. 1996. Cleavage of a subset of nuclear autoantigens associated with different functions during CD95 (Fas/Apo-1)–mediated T cell apoptosis. J. Exp. Med. In press.
25. CASIOLA-ROSEN, L. A., G. ANHALT & A. ROSEN. 1994. Autoantigens targeted in systemic lupus erythematosus are clustered in two populations of surface structures on apoptotic keratinocytes. J. Exp. Med. **179:** 1317–1330.
26. WINTER, S. J., J. D. MINNA, B. E. JOHNSON, T. TAKAHASHI, A. F. GAZDOR & D. P. CARBONE. 1992. Development of antibodies against p53 in lung cancer patients appears to be dependent on the type of p53 mutation. Cancer Res. **52:** 4168–4174.
27. DAVIDOFF, A. M., J. D. INGLEHART & J. R. MARKS. 1992. Immune response to p53 is dependent upon p53/HSP70 complexes in breast cancers. Proc. Natl. Acad. Sci. U.S.A. **89:** 3439–3442.
28. THOMAS, L. 1980. The wonderful mistake. *In* The Medusa and the Snail, p. 22–24. Bantam Books. New York.
29. GALLIN, J. I. 1993. Inflammation. *In* Fundamental Immunology. W. E. Paul, Ed.: 1015–1030. Raven Press. New York.

B Lymphocyte Developmental Lineages

KYOKO HAYAKAWA, YUE-SHENG LI,
ROBERT WASSERMAN, SUSAN SAUDER, SUSAN SHINTON,
AND RICHARD R. HARDY

Institute for Cancer Research
Fox Chase Cancer Center
Philadelphia, Pennsylvania 19111

The mechanisms of central and peripheral tolerance and the activation signals involved in tolerance for autoreactive lymphocytes have been extensively investigated in recent years. In contrast, the reasons why some autoreactive lymphocytes appear to be generated as a normal physiological process ("natural" autoreactive lymphocytes) and why some such autoreactive lymphocytes even show preferential survival remain vexing questions. An infrequent B cell population recognized by surface expression of CD5 exhibits an enrichment of autoreactive B cells[1–3] and has provided a good case for studying the development of natural autoreactive lymphocytes. The most-intriguing outcome arising from these studies is that the generation of a spectrum of autoreactive B cells may be a feature of B cell development that occurs early in ontogeny; that is, the process of repertoire generation and selection during B cell development may not be identical during fetal and adult stages.[4–6]

B CELL DEVELOPMENT AND REPERTOIRE ESTABLISHMENT IN THE ADULT

The development of B lymphocytes involves several critical stages for cells to survive and differentiate, finally establishing the mature B cell repertoire. This process has been characterized in mouse bone marrow, where the majority of B lymphopoiesis occurs in the adult (FIGURE 1),[7,8] and each step provides a possible controlling point for regulating cells with the potential to encode autoreactivity. The earliest stage of B-lineage commitment can be recognized by chromatin reorganization at the immunoglobulin (Ig) μ heavy-chain locus, prior to rearrangement, allowing generation of a germline μ transcript, known as sterile μ (μ_o).[9,10] As production of recombinase-activating proteins, Rag-1 and Rag-2,[11,12] increases, rearrangement of Ig DNA is initiated first between D and J segments of the μ heavy chain (D-J_H) on both chromosomes, at the Pro-B cell stage. Subsequently, V_H-D rearrangement is initiated, which, if in-frame, results in production of μ protein. After μ expression, rapid cell proliferation occurs during the early Pre-B cell stage. The surrogate light chain (SLC), comprising λ5 and VpreB,[13,14] is produced at the highest levels during the Pro-B cell stage and can form a μ/SLC protein complex[15] at this transitional Pro-B to Pre-B cycling stage. SLC levels diminish during the cycling stage and germline light-chain transcripts (κ_o) become detectable, indicating locus accessibility.[9,16] After exiting from the cycles, Rag-1,2 is reinduced,[17] whereupon light-chain rearrangement occurs

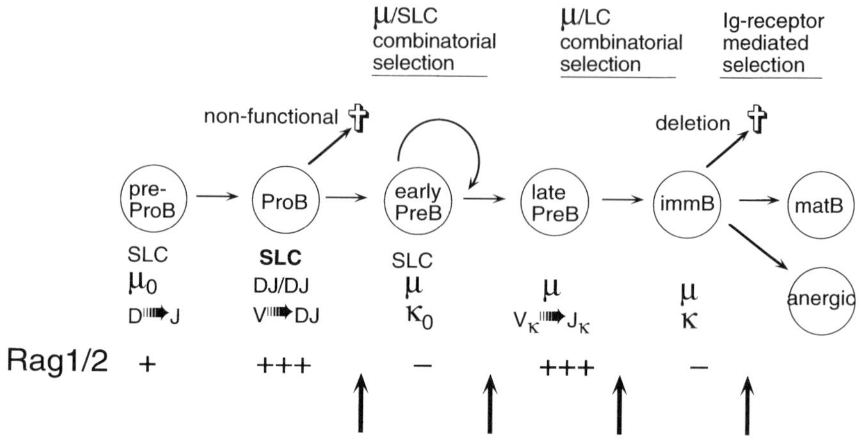

FIGURE 1. B cell development in adult mouse bone marrow. Arrows indicate the critical checkpoints for cells to further differentiate and mature.

during the late Pre-B cell stage. Finally, cells begin to express μ and light chain on the cell surface at low levels as immature B cells and eventually progress into the mature B cell stage, mostly after exiting from the bone marrow (BM).

During B-lineage cell development, expression of signal-transducing molecules, Igα and Igβ, is important as a part of the B cell receptor complex.[18] Igα/β is expressed from the earliest B-lineage stages and the fate of B-lineage cells during this process is critically dependent on expression of both immunoglobulin gene products and Igα/β.[19] Another potential player to determine cell fate is the enzyme, terminal deoxynucleotidyl transferase (TdT). There is a high production of TdT at the Pro-B cell stage in adult B cell development.[8] TdT catalyzes template-independent nucleotide addition at the heavy-chain VD and DJ junctions, thereby increasing the structural diversity of the heavy chain.[20,21] Cells with nonfunctional rearrangement at this Pro-B stage are presumed to die and early B cells should express an appropriate μ: that is, failure of proliferation or even cell death may occur at this early Pre-B transitional stage by poor μ/SLC interaction. Cells permitted to progress finally express IgM on the surface, by which stage the second critical decision is made. Thus, strong signals at the immature B cell stage resulting from interaction with self-ligands lead to either cell death or an anergic state, eliminating or silencing autoreactive B cells.[22–25] It is possible that some cells may escape cell death by Ig gene editing, as demonstrated in several transgenic systems.[26]

ONTOGENIC DIFFERENCES IN B CELL DEVELOPMENT (B-1 VERSUS B-2)

A difference in B cell development occurring during the fetal stage compared with the adult has been suggested previously by several observations, including phenotypic distinctions in the B cells generated.[27,28] A higher frequency of CD5-expressing B cells is one such characteristic associated with B cells early in ontogeny, as observed *in situ* and also by stem cell transfer experiments.[4] Subsequently, cell transfer using Pro-B cells as a B-lineage committed progenitor population demonstrated ontogeny-dependent generation of distinctive B cells. Transfer of the Pro-B cells present in fetus when compared with transfer of a comparable population present in adult bone marrow revealed a dichotomy in B cell progeny: preferential $CD5^{+}IgM^{hi}IgD^{lo}$ B cell generation versus the more-typical $CD5^{-}IgM^{lo}IgD^{hi}$ phenotype as characteristic of fetal versus adult development, respectively. The most-important point, which was not evident from stem cell transfer results, is that fetal B cell development does not give rise to cells with $IgM^{lo}IgD^{hi}$ expression, the predominant B cell compartment in adult. This difference was found regardless of the sites of B cells analyzed in recipient mice, including PBL, spleen, and peritoneal cavity; that is, the ontogenic difference in B cell generation is already programmed at least by the Pro-B cell stage.

An ontogenic difference in hematopoietic cell development has been demonstrated by studies with at least two types of cell lineages, erythroid[29,30] and T lymphocyte,[31,32] by probing hemoglobin and TCR, respectively. Distinct waves of T cells are observed during ontogeny, with TCRγδ cell development prominent during the fetal stage after day 13–14 gestation in mice (FIGURE 2) and TCRαβ cells increasing by the perinatal stage.[33] B cells also begin to appear around a similar time in gestation. Because development of these cells presumably occurs from the same pluripotent hematopoietic stem cell via a lymphoid progenitor stage, it is not unreasonable to expect that B cells generated during the fetal stage might also possess features that distinguish them as fetal B cells. However, unlike T cells, B cells do not express a different Ig receptor locus early in ontogeny. Because Ig serves as a hallmark of B cells, this fact has made

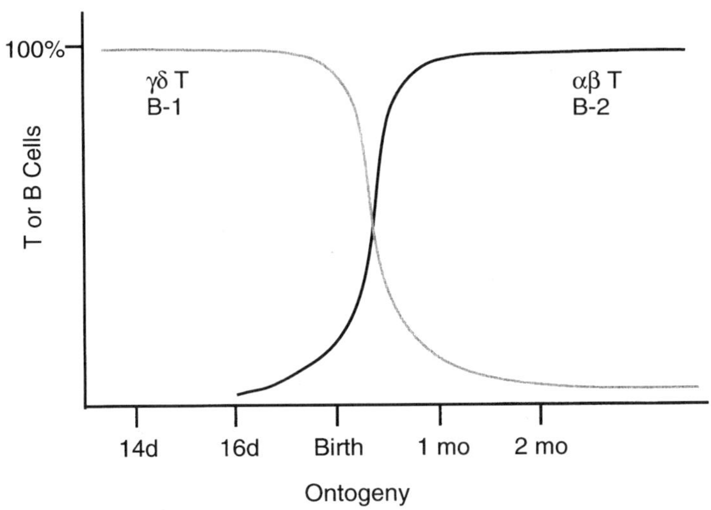

FIGURE 2. Developmental transition of the immune system.

it difficult to unambiguously distinguish fetal B cells from adult B cells. In this regard, cell transfer data with Pro-B cells are probably the strongest evidence to date suggesting that fetal B cell development differs in general from that of the adult. Accordingly, the nomenclature of "B-1" for B cells generated early in ontogeny (fetal/perinatal period) versus "B-2" for cells generated in the adult has been proposed (FIGURE 2).[34] By utilizing characteristic differences in the cell surface phenotype of B cells generated ($CD5^+$ B versus $CD5^-IgM^{lo}IgD^{hi}$), we found that exclusive B-1-type generation from Pro-B cells in day-16 fetal liver gradually declines afterwards, concomitant with an increase in B-2-type generation, suggesting a developmental transition in the immune system.

PROGRESSIVE B CELL MATURATION AND SURFACE PHENOTYPE CHANGE

The Pro-B cell transfer experiment has a significant advantage over stem cell transfer to trace ontogenically restricted B cell development. Pro-B cells are already restricted to the B-lineage and shortly differentiate into B cells, both *in vivo* and *in vitro*. Because most cells begin to differentiate, the transfer of Pro-B cells into mice allows recapitulation of B lymphopoiesis occurring at the specific time in ontogeny when the cells were harvested. The progressive cell differentiation occurring in recipients can be monitored by examining the surface phenotype of peripheral blood lymphocytes (PBL).

FIGURE 3 represents such data with fetal (gestation day 16) Pro-B cells and adult (3 month) Pro-B cells. SCID mouse recipients at 7 days after receiving either fetal or adult Pro-B cells begin to show a small, but significant, frequency of surface IgM^+ B cells in PBL at similar levels. B cells in both kinds of recipients progress to a high surface IgM–expressing cell stage (IgM^{hi}) and begin to upregulate IgD (FIGURE 3, left of BM Pro-B data). All similarly retain expression of high HSA levels, already upregulated at the Pre-B cell stage (not shown). A distinction between the recipients was first noticeable based on expression of CD5. Only fetal Pro-B cell progeny began to show surface CD5 expression, detectable by surface staining, albeit at low levels. After further cell differentiation, on day 14, the distinction was more clear: although most adult Pro-B cell progeny became IgM^{lo} (and downregulated HSA) with retention of high IgD, a large fraction of the fetal Pro-B progeny did not. Rather than becoming IgM^{lo}, most fetal Pro-B progeny became, or remained to be, IgD^{lo} cells with the retention of high levels of IgM, and a fraction showed further upregulation of CD5, typical of the $CD5^+$ B cell phenotype (FIGURE 3, middle). Finally, by 3 weeks after cell transfer, the B cells established in spleen (and peritoneal cavity) showed contrasting phenotypes, predominantly IgM^{hi}/IgD^{lo} cells (with or without CD5) as fetal B (B-1) and IgM^{lo}/IgD^{hi} cells (without CD5) as adult B (B-2), as described previously.[35]

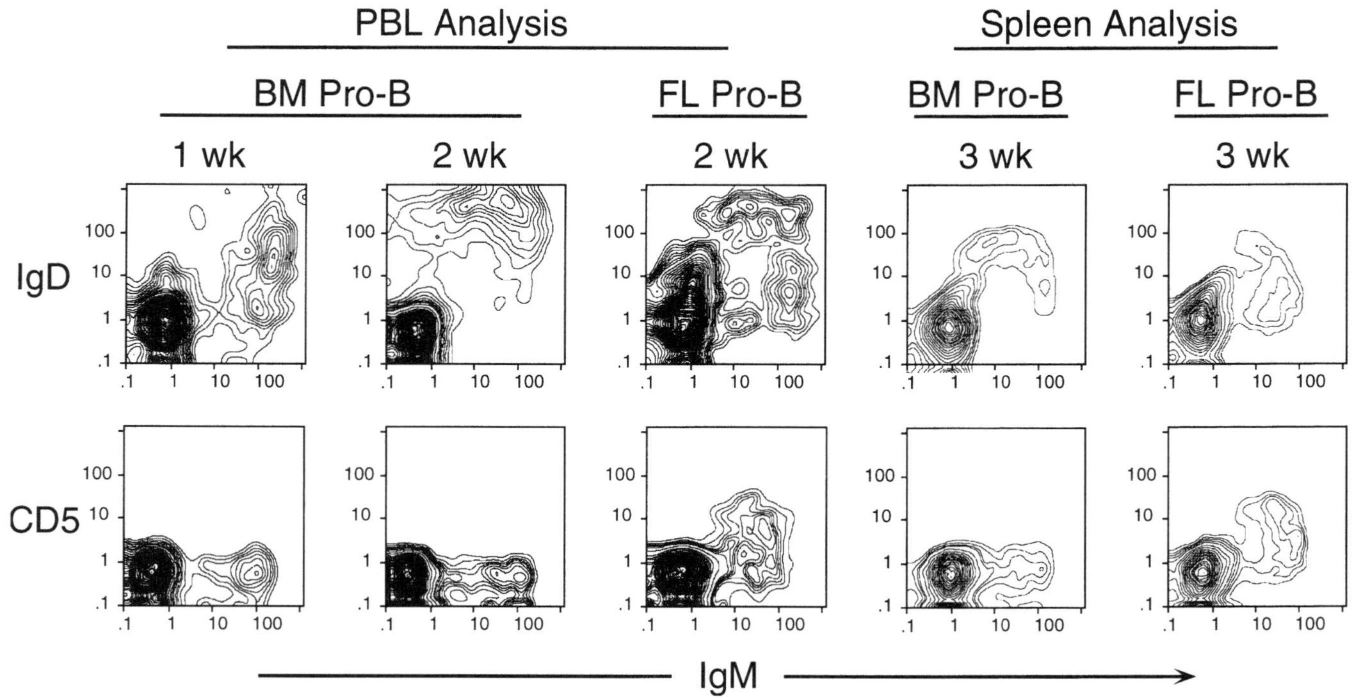

FIGURE 3. Progression of B cell development after transfer of Pro-B cells in adult bone marrow (BM) or fetal liver (FL): 1×10^5 Pro-B cells present in day-16 FL or adult (3-month) BM of BALB/c mice were injected into C.B-17 SCID mice. B cell development was followed by analysis of peripheral blood (PBL) at 1 and 2 weeks after transfer and by spleen analysis at 3 weeks after transfer.

AUTOREACTIVE B CELL GENERATION IN B-1 DEVELOPMENT AND ITS MECHANISM

The most-interesting feature of B-1 B cells is their production of autoantibody to senescent red blood cells (mimicked by bromelain enzyme treatment, BrMRBC; anti-BrMRBC), which recognizes the cell membrane component phosphatidylcholine as a part of the antigenic determinant.[36–38] Anti-BrMRBC is a long-recognized natural autoantibody present in normal healthy individuals.[39] Fetal stem cell or Pro-B transfer efficiently generates anti-BrMRBC-specific B cells in association with the $CD5^+$ phenotype and such cells persist through life (TABLE 1).[4,5] Because another well-recognized autoantibody, antithymocyte autoantibody, is also enriched in $CD5^+$ B cells, the question has arisen why fetal/neonatal B cell development preferentially generates such autoreactive B cells. As suggested from the scheme in FIGURE 1, the cell-fate decision may be determined by Ig gene components, by molecules involved in signal transduction, or by the environment where B cell development proceeds. The peripheral environment could also influence the shape of the final B cell repertoire. Thus, we have begun to investigate which element most critically determines the distinctive B-1 versus B-2 repertoires and the related issue of their fate.

TABLE 1. Anti-BrMRBC B Cell Generation in Association with Fetal B Cell Development

Transferred Cells	IgM^{lo} IgD^{hi} $CD5^-$ B-2	IgM^{hi} IgD^{lo} $CD5^+$ B-1a	Anti-PtC or Anti-BrMRBC
fetal liver stem	++	+	+
adult BM stem	++	− or +/−	−
fetal liver Pro-B	−	+	+
adult BM Pro-B	+	−	−

Differences in cell environment do not appear to be a principal factor for B-1 cell characteristics because cell transfers were performed in an adult environment.[4,5] Thus, possible reasons reside in the difference of B-lineage cell development per se, that is, due to the differences in Ig gene rearrangement (V_H usage, V_H-DJ μ and IgM proteins), selection mechanism (signal transduction and susceptibility to cell death), or a combination of both. In comparison to adult BM B-lineage cell studies, the details of early B cell development are far less clear at present. Fetal Pro-B cells express high levels of Rag-1/2 and SLC, and Ig gene rearrangement is dependent on Rag, as in adult BM B cell development.[8] However, because $CD5^+$ B cells can be generated in λ5-deficient mice, the importance of SLC for fetal B cell development is not clear (although B-2 cells could also be leaky).[40] Considering that γδ T cell development appears to be relatively independent of pre-T cell receptor interaction, in contrast with αβ T cells,[41] it is reasonable to suppose that B-1 and B-2 development may differ in terms of their utilization of SLC.

One clear-cut difference that we found between fetal and adult Pro-B cells is a difference in TdT level. Whereas TdT is expressed at the highest level by adult Pro-B cells, it is very low in fetal Pro-B cells,[8] suggesting a difference of Ig diversity between B-1 and B-2. The majority of anti-BrMRBC B cells utilize V_H11 and some V_H12, both of which show little TdT-mediated N-region addition, consistent with a TdT-deficient fetal repertoire.[35,42–45] This difference in TdT, possibly combined with preferential usage of certain V_H genes in V_H-DJ rearrangement, leading to potential differences in μ chain diversity, may provide a key reason to understand autoreactive B cell generation. Upregulation of CD5 (along with the IgD^{lo} phenotype) as seen in $CD5^+$ B cell generation may result from self-ligand-mediated cell activation due to increased numbers of autoreactive B cells in the fetal B cell pool. However, it is unlikely that the difference in TdT alone determines the B-1 versus B-2 dichotomy because TdT-deficient mice[46] do not show an exclusive B-1 B population; transfer of adult BM from $TdT^{-/-}$ mice predominantly generates $IgM^{lo}IgD^{hi}$ B-2 cells, rather than all B-1 cell phenotype (unpublished). Nonetheless, the potential difference in V_H-DJ μ is one important factor affecting the early B-lineage cell progression as well as immature B cell selection.

Even though bearing identical μ chains, cell fate could still differ depending on the precise mechanism of signal. This consists of signal(s) from the upstream surface receptor (if expressed), an intermediate cascade of signal transduction, and then downstream nuclear events. Expression of apoptosis-related molecules will also be important, influencing the outcome of this process. During early B-lineage development, the expression of several surface antigens changes coordinately.[7] In adult B cell development, CD43 is downregulated at the late Pre-B cell stage; in turn, class II and one of the class I molecules, Qa-2, are upregulated at this stage, before surface IgM expression.[47] CD40 is also expressed from the late Pre-B cell stage. After production of surface IgM, the expression of some of these antigens, such as class II, increases further, concomitant with peripheral maturation. Interestingly, fetal Pre-B and immature B cells express very low levels of class II,[47] Qa-2,[47–49] and CD40 (detected by anti-CD40, provided by M. Howard) when compared to the adult. In particular, class II is not expressed fetally even at the immature B cell stage, but is expressed increasingly after surface IgM. Precise roles for such surface antigens in B cell development are not established as yet. However, considering that a number of these surface molecules can transduce signals, or can affect cell activation through IgM, it is not unreasonable to assume that they may participate in cell-fate decisions. This delayed expression during fetal B cell development at the time of critical cell selection may have significant implications for determining the fate of potentially autoreactive cells, altering the strength of a cell activation signal. Expression of B220/CD45R is also low in fetal B cell development.[5] Whether or not this results in lower CD45 tyrosine phosphatase activity is not clear yet; however, this is potentially another parameter influencing the threshold for programmed cell death induced by surface IgM cross-linking.[50] A combination of these factors may favor the generation of certain autoreactive B cells during B-1 cell development.

In terms of information on the intermediate signal transduction events, our data are limited at present. In adult B cell development, there are specific changes in the message levels of several protein kinase genes associated with early B-lineage development: *fgr, flk2/flt3, tsk, blk,* and *ret.*[51] When Pro-B cells are compared, there is no apparent difference in constitutive expression of these protein kinases (RNA message) between fetal and adult. However, the question as to comparison of later events remains to be addressed. Interestingly, we found some suggestive data from the point of apoptotic cell death. The participation of apoptosis-related molecules differs depending on the B developmental stage and possibly also ontogenically. FIGURE 4 shows the relative expression of Bcl-2 family genes, Bcl-2, Bcl-x_L, and BAX, in addition to Fas during adult B-lineage development and in germinal center B cells (PNA^{hi}) induced by immunization, representing the activated mature B cells where selection is also proceeding.[52] In the course of early B-lineage cell development, Bcl-2 becomes downregulated, whereas another antiapoptotic molecule, Bcl-x_L, is upregulated, reminiscent of their pattern during T cell development in the thymus.[53] Interestingly, there is a time lag to finally reach the Bcl-2^{hi} Bcl-x_L^{lo} mature B cell stage, where early immature B cells are low for both the Bcl-2 and Bcl-x_L. Unlike T cell development, where Fas expression is quite high at the immature T cell stage, Fas message (as well as Fas protein) is maintained at a constant low level unless cells are activated after reaching the mature stage, such as germinal center B cells.

The patterns of Bcl-2, Bcl-x_L, BAX, and Fas expression during fetal B-lineage cell development appear similar to or not strikingly different from those in adult as far as message level analysis reveals. However, we have found that the expression of ICE (interleukin-l-converting enzyme) does differ significantly (FIGURE 5). ICE is an asparagine-specific cysteine protease with homology to *ced-3*, a gene that plays an essential role in apoptosis in *C. elegans.*[54,55] Transfection of ICE promotes apoptosis,[56] and an increased expression of asparagine-specific cysteine protease activity has been found in a number of cell types undergoing apoptosis or in experimental systems inducing apoptosis. Compared with almost uniform ICE message levels expressed during early B-lineage cell development in adult bone marrow, fetal Pro-B cells express fivefold lower levels of ICE. A potential reason due to differences in ongoing cell dynamics of B cell development appears unlikely because Pre-B and immature B cells (fractions D and E) generated after sublethal irradiation of adult mice (where essentially all mature B cells are eliminated and demand is very high) also showed the higher adult ICE level. How critically ICE (or other ICE homologues such as CPP32[57]) directly participates in cell selection during B cell development is not clear; however, these data may suggest less apoptotic events during fetal B-lineage cell development when compared to the adult.

SUMMARY OF B-1 AND B-2 CELL DEVELOPMENT AND B CELL POPULATIONS IN THE ADULT

FIGURE 6 presents a summary of several differences between B cell development occurring during the fetal (B-1) and adult (B-2) periods. The program to produce the B-1-type cell appears to be determined at a very early stage, before B-lineage cell

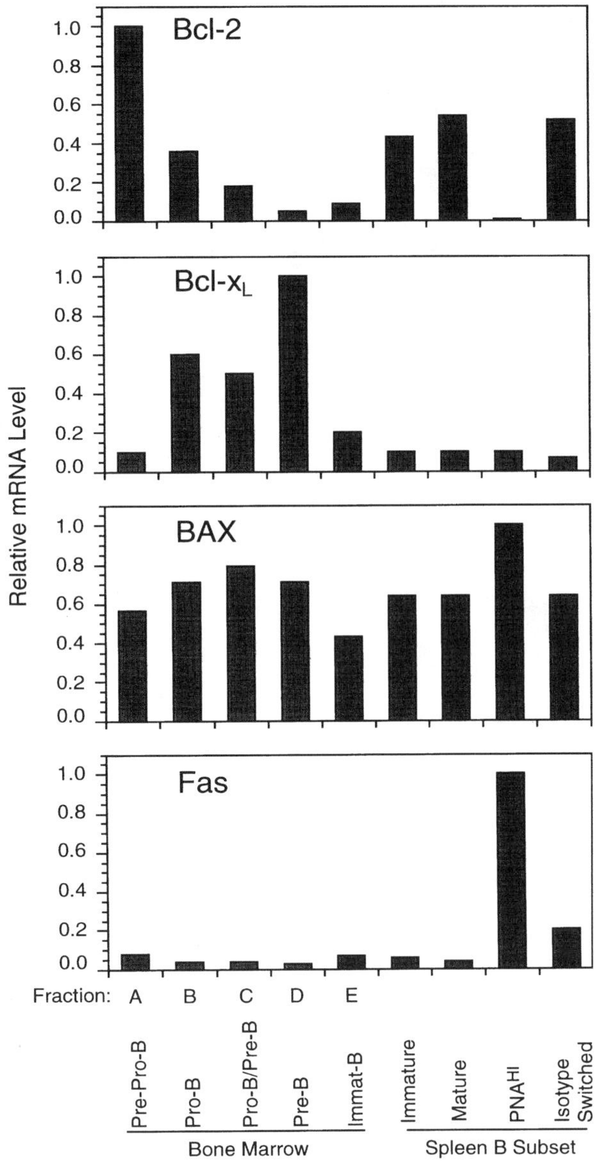

FIGURE 4. Altered Bcl-2 gene family representation and Fas expression during B cell development and by cell activation. Bone marrow early B-lineage cell fractions are as described in FIGURE 1. In spleen, immature and mature B cells were purified as $HSA^{hi}IgM^{hi}IgD^{lo}CD5^{-}$ cells and $HSA^{lo}IgM^{lo}IgD^{hi}CD5^{-}$ cells, respectively, from unimmunized mice. $B220^{+}PNA^{hi}IgD^{lo}$ germinal center B cells were purified from mice at 12 days after KLH antigen immunization. An isotype-switched memory B cell pool was purified from mice at >3 months after KLH immunization as $B220^{+}IgM^{-}IgD^{-}Ig\kappa^{+}$ B cells. Semiquantitative RT-PCR data are shown.

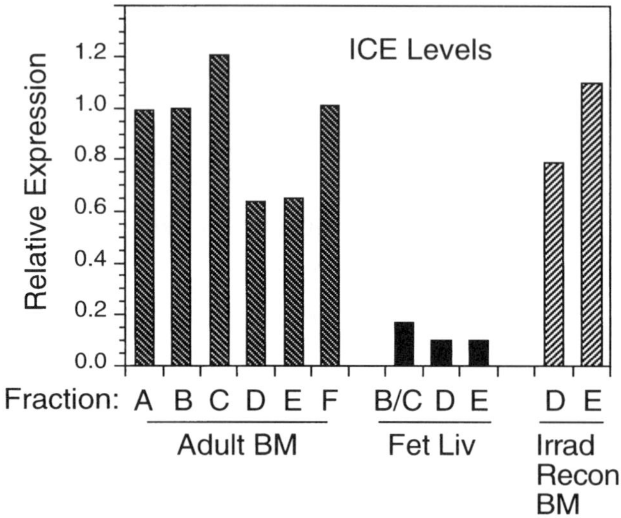

FIGURE 5. Lower ICE message levels by fetal B-lineage cells compared to adult. Fractions A–D represent Pre-Pro-B to late Pre-B cell stages as in FIGURE 4. Fractions E and F correspond to $IgM^{lo}IgD^{-}$ immature B cells and $IgM^{lo}IgD^{hi}$ mature B cells in the BM, respectively. The last two columns show data from BM Pre-B and immature B cell fractions of adult mice recovering after sublethal irradiation.

commitment, because transfer of a purified stem cell–enriched fraction into adult hosts also showed preferential generation of $CD5^{+}$ B cells, one of the characteristic features of B-1.[35] Restriction to B-1 versus B-2 appears to occur at least by the Pro-B cell stage, presumably as a normal part of fetal and adult hematopoietic cell development. The preferential generation of certain autoreactive B cells in B-1 appears to be due to a combination of factors that operate at several critical checkpoints. A potential difference in IgV_{H}-DJ μ products due to a paucity of TdT-mediated N-regions is one important consideration. Another consideration derives from observed differences in the timing of expression of cell surface molecules, particularly at the stage when the surface IgM B cell antigen receptor has just been expressed. Some of these differences might result in a difference in the strength of a signal generated by antigen cross-linking, determining the autoreactive cell's fate. Strong signal delivery at the immature stage results in cell death regardless of B-1 or B-2, as shown by the lack of B-1 (as well as B-2) in autoreactive transgenic mouse models. However, for B cells expressing certain autoreactive specificities, such as anti-BrMRBC or other natural autoantibodies (presumably delivering lesser signals), such differences in surface molecule expression may influence the signaling threshold. Autoreactive B-1 cells, such as anti-BrMRBC, generated during the fetal stage do not fall in the anergic/deletion range, whereas for B-2 anti-BrMRBC may. Eventual upregulation of CD5 occurring on a fraction of B-1 cells may reflect subsequent cell activation after further cell maturation proceeds. Once mature B cells are generated, the presence of appropriate self-ligands appears to promote B-1 cell survival, explaining in part an enrichment of autoreactive B cells among B-1 cells that persist in the adult and contributing to natural autoantibody production.

Some B-1 cells generated early in ontogeny can self-renew through life, coexisting with newly generated B cells from ongoing adult B cell development, resulting in a complex B cell population profile in adult mice (FIGURE 6). For the B cells generated early, environmental factors appear to influence their survival and further differentiation. The peritoneal cavity environment appears to provide a preferential site for B-1 cell survival. Thus, in adult mice, whereas $CD5^+$ B cells are rare in spleen, lymph

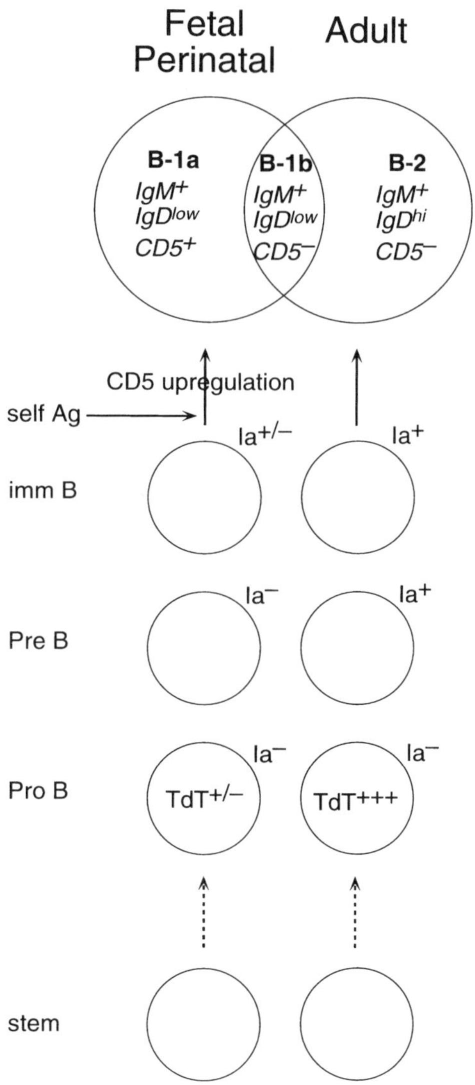

FIGURE 6. Distinctive fetal and adult B cell development in relation to B cell populations in adult mice.

nodes, and peripheral blood, they comprise a significant proportion of B cells in the peritoneal cavity.[28,58] Because $CD5^+$ B cell generation greatly declines with ontogeny, the majority of such $CD5^+$ B cells (and some $CD5^-$ B cells as well) appear to be fetal/neonatally generated. Due to the association between fetal/neonatal B cells, the $CD5^+$ B cell phenotype, and peritoneal cavity localization, the nomenclature "B-1" has often been used interchangeably based on one of these three (potentially segregated) criteria.[59] FIGURE 6 incorporates a proposed nomenclature for B cell populations found in the adult. However, assessing the exact ontogenic history for these populations in the adult from the point of surface phenotype carries a risk because surface phenotype may change due to different secondary activation. Certainly, "B-1b" used for peritoneal $CD5^-IgM^{hi}IgD^{lo}$ cells is a complex population that can be generated during both fetal and adult B cell development, likely by different mechanisms. Thus, we should always keep in mind the possible segregation between an induced surface phenotype versus one arising due to an ontogenic difference. At present, the B-1 versus B-2 B-lineage categories can be used to describe the ontogenic transitional change of B cell development. However, because the differences that we observe may be based on a number of parameters, each of which may be altering with ontogeny, it is difficult to single out a definitive marker. Whether or not it is possible to find a specific molecule restricted to a certain ontogenic timing is an interesting question and such investigations are in progress.

CONCLUSIONS

The developmental mechanism for fetal B cells allows the generation of certain autoreactive B cells, as well as other nonautoreactive B cells, as functional mature B cells. Survival and maintenance of such a B cell pool generated early in life are aided by self-reactivity and positive selection of autoreactive cells, resulting in the enrichment of certain autoreactive cells among CD5 B cells in the adult. Generation of such cells may be important for animals to sustain a fundamental immune system. As the mouse develops and the immune system matures to make more diverse specificities for potential encounters with dangerous foreign antigens, it simultaneously evolves a more intricate control system to select out autoreactive cells, resulting in increased sensitivity to negatively select autoreactive cells. Thus, the positive selection of autoreactive B cells is no longer tolerated and such cells will be either silenced or eliminated, unless rescuing signals are provided from other cell types. We would suggest that the immune system in the adult comprises such a mixture of lymphocytes with different ontogenic origins, serving distinct functional roles.

REFERENCES

1. HAYAKAWA, K., R. R. HARDY, D. R. PARKS & L. A. HERZENBERG. 1983. The "Ly-1 B" cell subpopulation in normal, immunodefective, and autoimmune mice. J. Exp. Med. **157:** 202–218.
2. HAYAKAWA, K., R. R. HARDY, M. HONDA, L. A. HERZENBERG, A. D. STEINBERG & L. A. HERZENBERG. 1984. Ly-1 B cells: functionally distinct lymphocytes that secrete IgM autoantibodies. Proc. Natl. Acad. Sci. U.S.A. **81:** 2494–2498.

3. HAYAKAWA, K., C. E. CARMACK, R. HYMAN & R. R. HARDY. 1990. Natural autoantibodies to thymocytes: origin, VH genes, fine specificities, and the role of Thy-1 glycoprotein. J. Exp. Med. **172:** 869–878.
4. HAYAKAWA, K., R. R. HARDY, L. A. HERZENBERG & L. A. HERZENBERG. 1985. Progenitors for Ly-1 B cells are distinct from progenitors for other B cells. J. Exp. Med. **161:** 1554–1568.
5. HARDY, R. R. & K. HAYAKAWA. 1991. A developmental switch in B lymphopoiesis. Proc. Natl. Acad. Sci. U.S.A. **88:** 11550–11554.
6. HARDY, R. R. & K. HAYAKAWA. 1994. CD5 B cells, a fetal B cell lineage. Adv. Immunol. **55:** 297–339.
7. HARDY, R. R., C. E. CARMACK, S. A. SHINTON, J. D. KEMP & K. HAYAKAWA. 1991. Resolution and characterization of pro-B and pre-pro-B cell stages in normal mouse bone marrow. J. Exp. Med. **173:** 1213–1225.
8. LI, Y-S., K. HAYAKAWA & R. R. HARDY. 1993. The regulated expression of B lineage associated genes during B cell differentiation in bone marrow and fetal liver. J. Exp. Med. **178:** 951–960.
9. SCHLISSEL, M. S., L. M. CORCORAN & D. BALTIMORE. 1991. Virus-transformed pre-B cells show ordered activation, but not inactivation of immunoglobulin gene rearrangement and transcription. J. Exp. Med. **173:** 711–720.
10. ALESSANDRINI, A. & S. DESIDERIO. 1991. Coordination of immunoglobulin DJ_H transcription and D-to-J_H rearrangement by promoter-enhancer approximation. Mol. Cell. Biol. **11:** 2096–2107.
11. SCHATZ, D. G., M. A. OETTINGER & D. BALTIMORE. 1989. The V(D)J recombination activating gene, RAG-1. Cell **59:** 1035.
12. OETTINGER, M. A., D. G. SCHATZ, C. GORKA & D. BALTIMORE. 1990. RAG-1 and RAG-2, adjacent genes that synergistically activate V(D)J recombination. Science **248:** 1517.
13. SAKAGUCHI, N. & F. MELCHERS. 1986. λ*5*, a new light-chain-related locus selectively expressed in pre-B lymphocytes. Nature **324:** 579.
14. KUDO, A. & F. MELCHERS. 1987. A second gene, *VpreB* in the λ*5* locus of the mouse, which appears to be selectively expressed in pre-B lymphocytes. EMBO J. **6:** 2267.
15. KARASUYAMA, H., A. KUDO & F. MELCHERS. 1990. The proteins encoded by the *VpreB* and λ*5* pre-B-cell-specific genes can associate with each other and with μ heavy chain. J. Exp. Med. **172:** 969.
16. LI, Y-S., R. WASSERMAN, K. HAYAKAWA & R. R. HARDY. 1996. An early stage of B lineage differentiation in mouse bone marrow characterized by sterile immunoglobulin heavy chain transcription prior to Rag-1 and Rag-2 expression. Immunity. In press.
17. GRAWUNDER, U., T. M. LEU, D. G. SCHATZ, A. WERNER, A. G. ROLINK, F. MELCHERS & T. H. WINKLER. 1995. Down-regulation of RAG1 and RAG2 gene expression in pre-B cells after functional immunoglobulin heavy chain rearrangement. Immunity **3:** 601–608.
18. RETH, M. 1992. Antigen receptors on B lymphocytes. Annu. Rev. Immunol. **10:** 97–121.
19. GONG, S. & M. C. NUSSENZWEIG. 1996. Regulation of an early developmental checkpoint in the B cell pathway by Igβ. Science **272**: 411–414.
20. DESIDERIO, S. V., G. D. YANCOPOULOS, M. PASKIND, E. THOMAS, M. A. BOSS, N. LANDAU, F. W. ALT & D. BALTIMORE. 1984. Insertion of *N* regions into heavy-chain genes is correlated with expression of terminal deoxytransferase in B cells. Nature **311:** 752–755.
21. YANCOPOULOS, G., T. K. BLACKWELL, H. SUH, L. HOOD & F. W. ALT. 1986. Introduced T cell receptor variable region gene segments recombine in pre-B cells: evidence that B and T cells use a common recombinase. Cell **44:** 251–259.
22. NEMAZEE, D. A. & K. BÜRKI. 1989. Clonal deletion of B lymphocytes in a transgenic mouse bearing anti-MHC class I antibody genes. Nature **337:** 562–566.
23. RUSSELL, D. M., Z. DEMBIC, G. MORAHAN, J. F. MILLER, K. BÜRKI & D. NEMAZEE. 1991. Peripheral deletion of self-reactive B cells. Nature **354:** 308–311.
24. HARTLEY, S. B., M. P. COOKE, D. A. FULCHER, A. W. HARRIS, S. CORY, A. BASTEN & C. C. GOODNOW. 1993. Elimination of self-reactive B lymphocytes proceeds in two stages: arrested development and cell death. Cell **72:** 325–335.
25. CHEN, C., M. Z. RADIC, R. R. HARDY, D. HUSZAR, S. A. CAMPER & M. WEIGERT. 1995. The site and stage of anti-DNA B-cell deletion. Nature **373:** 252–255.

26. TIEGS, S., D. M. RUSSELL & D. NEMAZEE. 1993. Receptor editing in self-reactive bone marrow B cells. J. Exp. Med. **177:** 1009–1020.
27. KINCADE, P. W. 1987. Experimental models for understanding B lymphocyte formation. Adv. Immunol. **41:** 181–267.
28. HAYAKAWA, K. & R. R. HARDY. 1988. Normal, autoimmune, and malignant $CD5^+$ B cells: the Ly-1 B lineage? Annu. Rev. Immunol. **6:** 197–218.
29. ZANJANI, E. D., G. LIM, P. B. MCGLAVE, J. F. CLAPP, L. I. MANN, T. H. NORWOOD & G. STAMATOYANNOPOULOS. 1982. Adult haemopoietic cells transplanted to sheep fetuses continue to produce adult globins. Nature **295:** 244.
30. WOOD, W. G., C. BUNCH, S. KELLY, Y. GUNN & G. BECKON. 1985. Control of haemoglobin switching by a developmental clock? Nature **313:** 320–323.
31. HAVRAN, W. L. & J. P. ALLISON. 1988. Developmentally ordered appearance of thymocytes expressing different T-cell antigen receptors. Nature **335:** 443–445.
32. IKUTA, K., T. KINA, I. MACNEIL, N. UCHIDA, B. PEAULT, Y. CHIEN & I. L. WEISSMAN. 1990. A developmental switch in thymic lymphocyte maturation potential occurs at the level of hematopoietic stem cells. Cell **62:** 863–874.
33. ALLISON, J. P. & W. L. HAVRAN. 1991. The immunobiology of T cells with invariant $\gamma\delta$ antigen. Annu. Rev. Immunol. **9:** 679–705.
34. KANTOR, A. 1991. A new nomenclature for B cells. Immunol. Today **12:** 392.
35. HARDY, R. R., C. E. CARMACK, Y-S. LI & K. HAYAKAWA. 1994. Distinctive developmental origins and specificities of murine $CD5^+$ B cells. Immunol. Rev. **137:** 91–118.
36. KAWAGUCHI, S. 1987. Phospholipid epitopes for mouse antibodies against bromelain-treated mouse erythrocytes. Immunology **62:** 11.
37. MERCOLINO, T. J., L. W. ARNOLD & G. HAUGHTON. 1986. Phosphatidylcholine is recognized by a series of $Ly\text{-}1^+$ murine B cell lymphomas specific for erythrocyte membranes. J. Exp. Med. **163:** 155–165.
38. MERCOLINO, T. J., L. W. ARNOLD, L. A. HAWKINS & G. HAUGHTON. 1988. Normal mouse peritoneum contains a large population of $Ly\text{-}1^+$ (CD5) B cells that recognize phosphatidylcholine: relationship to cells that secrete hemolytic antibody specific for autologous erythrocytes. J. Exp. Med. **168:** 687–698.
39. CUNNINGHAM, A. J. 1974. Large numbers of cells in normal mice produce antibody components of isologous erythrocytes. Nature **252:** 749–751.
40. KITAMURA, D., A. KUDO, S. SCHAAL, W. MULLER, F. MELCHERS & K. RAJEWSKY. 1992. A critical role of $\lambda5$ protein in B cell development. Cell **69:** 823–831.
41. FEHLING, H. J., A. KROTKOVA, C. SAINT-RUF & H. VON BOEHMER. 1995. Crucial role of the pre-T-cell receptor α gene in development of $\alpha\beta$ but not $\gamma\delta$ T cells. Nature **375:** 795–798.
42. REININGER, L., A. KAUSHIK, S. IZUI & J. C. JATON. 1988. A member of a new VH gene family encodes antibromelinized mouse red blood cell autoantibodies. Eur. J. Immunol. **18:** 1521–1526.
43. HARDY, R. R., C. E. CARMACK, S. A. SHINTON, R. J. RIBLET & K. HAYAKAWA. 1989. A single VH gene is utilized predominantly in anti-BrMRBC hybridomas derived from purified Ly-1 B cells: definition of the VH11 family. J. Immunol. **142:** 3643–3651.
44. PENNELL, C. A., K. M. SHEEHAN, P. H. BRODEUR & S. H. CLARKE. 1989. Organization and expression of V_H gene families preferentially expressed by $Ly\text{-}1^+$ (CD5) B cells. Eur. J. Immunol. **19:** 2115.
45. MERCOLINO, T. J., A. L. LOCKE, A. AFSHARI, D. SASSER, W. W. TRAVIS, L. W. ARNOLD & G. HAUGHTON. 1989. Restricted immunoglobulin variable region gene usage by normal $Ly\text{-}1^+$ (CD5) B cells that recognize phosphatidylcholine. J. Exp. Med. **169:** 1869–1877.
46. GILFILLAN, S., A. DIERICH, M. LEMEUR, C. BENOIST & D. MATHIS. 1993. Mice lacking TdT: mature animals with an immature lymphocyte repertoire. Science **261:** 1175–1178.
47. HAYAKAWA, K., D. TARLINTON & R. R. HARDY. 1994. Absence of MHC class II expression distinguishes fetal from adult B lymphopoiesis in mice. J. Immunol. **152:** 4801–4807.
48. KINCADE, P. W., L. FLAHERTY, G. LEE, T. WATANABE & J. MICHAELSON. 1980. Qa antigen expression on functional lymphoid, myeloid, and stem cells in adult mice. J. Immunol. **124:** 2879–2885.

49. KINCADE, P. W., G. LEE, T. WATANABE, L. SUN & M. P. SCHEID. 1981. Antigens displayed on murine B lymphocyte precursors. J. Immunol. **127:** 2262–2268.
50. CYSTER, J. G., J. I. HEALY, K. KISHIHARA, T. W. MAK, W. L. THOMAS & C. C. GOODNOW. 1996. Regulation of B-lymphocyte negative and positive selection by tyrosine phosphatase CD45. Nature **381:** 325–328.
51. WASSERMAN, R., Y-S. LI & R. R. HARDY. 1995. Differential expression of the Blk and Ret tyrosine kinases during B lineage development is dependent on Ig rearrangement. J. Immunol. **155:** 644–651.
52. SHOKAT, K. M. & C. C. GOODNOW. 1995. Antigen-induced B-cell death and elimination during germinal-centre immune responses. Nature **375:** 334–338.
53. NÚÑEZ, G., R. MERINO, D. GRILLOT & M. GONZÁLEZ-GARCÍA. 1994. Bcl-2 and Bcl-x: regulatory switches for lymphoid death and survival. Immunol. Today **15:** 582–588.
54. WILSON, K. P., J. F. BLACK, J. A. THOMSON, J. P. GRIFFITH, M. A. NAVIA, M. A. MURCKO, S. P. CHAMBERS, R. A. ALDAPE, S. A. RAYBUCK & D. J. LIVINGSTON. 1994. Structure and mechanism of interleukin-1b-converting enzyme. Nature **370:** 270–274.
55. YUAN, J., S. SHAHAM, S. LEDOUX, H. M. ELLIS & H. R. HORVITZ. 1993. The *C. elegans* cell death gene ced-3 encodes a protein similar to mammalian interleukin-1β-converting enzyme. Cell **75:** 641–652.
56. MIURA, M., H. ZHU, R. ROTELLO, E. A. HARTWIEG & J. YUAN. 1993. Induction of apoptosis in fibroblasts by IL-1β-converting enzyme, a mammalian homolog of the *C. elegans* cell death gene *ced-3*. Cell **75:** 653–660.
57. NICHOLSON, D. W., A. ALI, N. A. THORNBERRY, J. P. VAILLANCOURT, C. K. DING, M. GALLANT, Y. GAREAU, P. R. GRIFFIN, M. LABELLE, Y. A. LAZEBNIK, N. A. MUNDAY, S. M. RAJU, M. E. SMULSON, T-T. YAMIN, V. L. YU & D. K. MILLER. 1995. Identification and inhibition of the ICE/CED-3 protease necessary for mammalian apoptosis. Nature **376:** 37–43.
58. CARMACK, C. E., S. A. SHINTON, K. HAYAKAWA & R. R. HARDY. 1990. Rearrangement and selection of V_H11 in the Ly-1 B cell lineage. J. Exp. Med. **172:** 371–374.
59. HERZENBERG, L. A. & A. B. KANTOR. 1993. B-cell lineages exist in the mouse. Immunol. Today **14:** 79–83.

The Role of Autoreactivity in B Cell Selection[a]

B. DAVID STOLLAR, JEAN-MICHEL LECERF, AND YASUHIKO HIRABAYASHI[b]

Department of Biochemistry
Tufts University School of Medicine
Boston, Massachusetts 02111

Knowledge of Ig gene organization, rearrangement, and somatic modifications has provided insight into the diversity of antibody responses.[1–3] Given the number of possible gene segment reassortments, junctional variations, additions of untemplated nucleotides, and somatic mutations, the calculated potential for diversity is far greater than the numbers of B cells in an animal. Thus, the expressed repertoire is only a subset of all the potential sequence variants and it is especially limited in fetal and neonatal life.[4] Mechanisms for restricting and shaping the naive repertoire have been studied intensively. Autoreactivity can restrict and shape it through negative selection, with inactivation or elimination of emerging B cells that have sIg receptors with high affinity for autoantigens,[5–7] and through secondary rearrangements (receptor editing) that yield nonautoreactive Ig.[8,9] Further narrowing of the repertoire occurs if emerging cells that have no ligand interaction at all are short-lived.[10]

Some interaction with a cell surface Ig receptor that includes the μ-chain V region and the ψL chain is required for progression of B cells through pre-B cell development, particularly between pre-BI and pre-BII stages.[11–14] The ligands for these receptors are not known. Perhaps they are endogenous (i.e., self) ligands. Whether a positive or negative signal is triggered by self ligands could depend on the physical form or affinity of interacting components[15,16] or on the cooperating signals and signaling pathways available at various stages of development.[17] Cross-linking of receptors on immature B cells leads to apoptosis;[18] however, the occurrence of self-interactions that might yield positive effects at some stage of development would help to explain recurring nonrandom features of the primary Ig V gene repertoire.[19] The possibility that both positive and negative selection may be based on self-recognition is an issue for development of the T cell as well as the B cell repertoire.[20]

[a]This research was supported by Grant Nos. AI33180 and GM32375 from the National Institutes of Health.

[b]Present address: The Second Department of Internal Medicine, Tohoku University School of Medicine, Sendai, Migayi 980, Japan.

SUGGESTIONS THAT AUTOREACTIVITY MAY PROVIDE POSITIVE SELECTION OF THE B CELL REPERTOIRE

Natural Autoantibodies Are Produced by Healthy Individuals

In spite of a role for autoreactivity in negative selection, some cells that produce autoreactive Ig do survive and secrete their products in normal subjects. At a time when autoantibodies were generally considered only in terms of disease, Grabar proposed that they serve a physiological function.[21] Fournié *et al.* reported that injection of bacterial lipopolysaccharide into normal animals causes release of DNA into the circulation and the appearance of anti-DNA antibodies,[22] and Rubin and Carr reported that normal human sera contain a small amount of anti-DNA autoantibodies, mainly reactive with ssDNA.[23] Avrameas and colleagues presented a more extensive documentation of autoantibodies in the serum of normal animal and human subjects[24,25] and among myeloma proteins.[26,27] These natural autoantibodies are mainly IgM molecules and they react with several autoantigens, including actin, tubulin, and albumin, as well as ssDNA.[28] Some also cross-react with bacterial or viral antigens. In addition, many fetal immunoglobulins interact with each other.[29,30] The abundance of natural autoantibodies in adults may be higher than generally assumed because some that are undetected in serum can be unmasked in Ig purified from serum with ion exchange or affinity columns.[31–33] Natural autoantibodies are produced by a significant fraction of hybridomas from newborn mice[34] and from unimmunized adult mice.[35] The fact that a significant fraction of these IgM antibodies display autoreactivity could simply reflect promiscuous polyreactivity of proteins coded by randomly associated gene segments. On the other hand, it could reflect selection by interactions with self ligands at some stage in development.

Natural Autoantibodies Are Coded by Germline Genes

Autoreactive potential is inherent in germline genes and their rearrangements. There are many examples in which rearrangements of unmutated germline gene segments code for V_H domains of antibodies that react with other Ig molecules (rheumatoid factors), DNA, phospholipid, Sm ribonucleoprotein, pyruvate dehydrogenase, or erythrocyte i antigen (TABLE 1). In spite of the lack of mutations in their V gene segments, indirect evidence suggests that natural autoantibodies have been subjected to selection during their development. Selection could account for the overrepresentation of certain V_H and V_L gene segments among immunoglobulins with demonstrated autoreactivity.[36] Consistent with a high frequency of autoantibodies in a primary repertoire, the same sets of V_H, D_H, and J_H gene segments are overrepresented in germline-coded IgM cDNA libraries from B cells of fetal,[4] neonatal,[37] and adult origin;[38] clones in these libraries represent a general population not chosen for study on the basis of autoreactivity. The combination of recurrent use of particular gene segments and frequent expression of autoreactivity would be difficult to explain if subtraction of highly autoreactive clones from the universe of rearrangements, that is, negative selection, were the only operative process. Ligand-based positive selection may also be reflected in the finding that autoantigen binding and polyreactivity depend on residues in CDR3H segments,[39–42] in which unmutated portions of D_H and J_H segments may be combined with diverse junctions that are formed at the time of rearrangement.

Features of Autoantigens and Autoantibodies Are Highly Conserved

A system in which highly conserved autoantigens provide positive signals for emerging B cells may help to shape and stabilize the repertoire in the evolution of

TABLE 1. Germline V_H Segments of Each Family Occur in Diverse Human Autoantibodies[a]

Antibody	Reference	Germline Gene		V_H Mutations	Autoantibody Activity
21/28	77	1-3b	DP-25	1	ssDNA
8815	81	1-3b	DP-25	0	ssDNA
SMI	82	1-69	DP-10	0	RF
C10	83	2-	FL1-19	0	pyruvate dehydrogenase E-2
4B4	84	3-15	DP-38	0	Sm ribonucleoprotein
18/2	77	3-23	DP-47	0	ssDNA
8807	81	3-23	DP-47	0	ssDNA
10.2.3	85	3-23	DP-47	1	myosin, actin, vimentin, keratin, streptococcal M protein
Kim4.6	86	3-30	DP-49	0	ssDNA
F6	83	3-30	DP-49	0	pyruvate dehydrogenase E-2
9500	81	3-33	DP-50	0	ssDNA, platelet
C471	83	3-64	DP-61	1	ssDNA, platelet, DOPE
D9	83	4-30.2	DP-64	1	pyruvate dehydrogenase E-2
LES-C	87	4-34	DP-63	0	RF
PR-TS2	52	4-34	DP-63	0	RF, polyreactive
15A	88	4-34	4.21	0	i antigen (cold agglutinin)
TMC	52	4-34	DP-63	0	RF
STO 103	89	4-61	DP-66	0	platelet, phospholipid
AB37	52	5-	V_H32	0	acetylcholine receptor
B5	83	5-51	DP-73	0	pyruvate dehydrogenase E-2
SMA-1	52	5-51	DP-73	0	striated muscle
L16	90	6-1	DP-74	0	ssDNA, cardiolipin
ML1	90	6-1	DP-74	0	ssDNA

[a]Literature was surveyed to identify reported autoantibodies with unmutated V_H segments. Four examples of a larger population of Ig's with a single V_H segment mutation were also included.

species as well as in an individual.[43] Many autoantigens are highly conserved structures. Thus, anti-DNA autoantibodies react with DNA from any source.[44] Antihistone autoantibodies react with both invertebrate and mammalian histones, as do many autoantibodies to ribonucleoprotein antigens, topoisomerase, actin, tubulin, or vimentin.[43] Furthermore, natural autoantibodies of both humans and mice bind to the same autoantigens,[43] autoantibodies to ribosomal P protein autoantigen occur with the same frequency in human and mouse lupus,[45] and the same epitopes on ribosomal P protein or U1RNP 70-kDa protein are recognized by autoantibodies from both species.[45,46] Germline V_H gene segments, including those found in natural autoantibodies, are also conserved during evolution, as reflected, for example, in primary structures[43,47–49] and by the occurrence of cross-species idiotype recognition.[50,51] Sequence identity is also strikingly conserved among human germline V_H gene segments from people of diverse ethnic origin.[52] Parallel conservation of structure and patterns of autoreactivity and polyreactivity (including the ability to react with bacterial antigens) would imply that these are functionally important properties of the gene products,[49] and development of a stable primary repertoire may be such a function.

The data summarized above suggest that B cells making natural autoantibodies may arise through initial selection for both autoreactivity and polyreactivity, the latter encompassing bacterial and viral antigens. Such cells, in turn, may be precursors of cells that make antibodies of higher affinity and narrower selectivity after mutation and selection by foreign antigen or, in certain subjects, by autoantigens that drive formation of disease-related IgG autoantibodies. A possible example of such a progression was seen in responses of mice to the arsonate hapten.[53] A V_H gene segment associated with antiarsonate antibodies after immunization was found, before immunization, to code anti-ssDNA autoantibodies that did not bind arsonate; and after a single immunization, the same gene segment coded antibodies that bound both ssDNA and arsonate. As another possible example, in naive BALB/c mice B lymphocytes that recognize a particular epitope on mouse cytochrome c outnumber those that recognize a distinguishable epitope at the same site on foreign (pigeon) cytochrome c.[54] Furthermore, the anti-self B cells are activated early in the response to immunization of mice with the pigeon cytochrome c, to be followed by activation of more cells reactive with the foreign epitope.[55]

EXPLORATION OF RECEPTOR COMPONENTS OF DEVELOPING B CELLS

Positive selective signals for B cell survival and progression could be provided at varying points in B cell ontogeny, before and after assembly of the μL chain receptor, and could involve intracellular or cell surface interactions with Ig chains. If selection occurs before μL assembly, then the autoreactive potential of the H chain would be particularly important. The H chain is produced in pre-B cells, a stage of B cell development at which the L chain is not yet rearranged.[11] At that time, much of the μ chain product is retained in the Golgi network, bound to heavy-chain binding protein Bip,[56] but some μ chain is expressed on the cell surface, in a complex that includes components of the ψL chain—$V_{pre\text{-}B}$ and λ5 protein in mice or $V_{pre\text{-}B}$ and protein 14.1 in humans.[11,57] Expression of this μ-ψL complex on the cell surface is required for normal B cell development through pre-B cell stages, as demonstrated by targeted disruption of either the λ5 protein[13] or the membrane anchoring segment of the μ chain.[12] Consistent with these experiments, the lack of expression of the V_H81X gene segment in adult mice is correlated with its inability to form a full complex in pre-B cells.[58] Expression of the ψL chain is also required for H chain allelic exclusion.[59] The μ-ψL chain complex can serve as a receptor that triggers intracellular signaling events,[60,61] but the physiological ligands for this receptor are not known.

We have used bacterial expression of recombinant Fv domains, separate V_H or V_L domains, and $V_{pre\text{-}B}$ protein to explore the potential for antigen binding by various kinds of B cell products and receptors. The bacterial expression vector yields soluble Ig or $V_{pre\text{-}B}$ domains fused to a single B domain of staphylococcal protein A.[62–64] These products are affinity-purified from bacterial culture medium with an IgG-Sepharose column and a step of cation exchange chromatography.[64] In currently used versions of the vector (pIg20 or pIg203), a thrombin-sensitive site allows cleavage of the Ig portion from the protein A domain.

Exploring the Role of the V_H Domain

Although both H and L chains contribute to binding of anti-DNA antibodies,[65,66] as they do for virtually all antibodies,[67] there are several anti-DNA antibodies for which the V_H domain alone can bind the potential autoantigen. For example, the V_H domain of an IgG autoantibody, 2C10, binds ssDNA, dsDNA, and Z-DNA.[68] The 2C10 L chain alone does not bind DNA, but within the Fab it helps to define the more selective binding of dsDNA with AT-rich sequences. Barry and Lee also found that a V_H domain alone of a mouse anti-DNA autoantibody could bind ssDNA,[69] and Kieber-Emmons *et al.* observed DNA binding by a human H-chain V domain.[70]

Antigen can be bound by the V_H domain of immunization-induced anti-DNA antibodies as well as anti-DNA autoantibodies. Although a particular V_H-V_L combination is required for Z-DNA binding by mouse mAb Z22, the V_H domain alone binds Z-DNA with about the same affinity as the parent Fab or the Fv.[63] Amino acids in CDR3H are particularly critical for antigen binding.[71] The L chain alone does not bind DNA, but is important in permitting or vetoing Z-DNA binding by the H chain.[63] The V_H domain of another anti-Z-DNA mAb, Z44, differs by only one framework amino acid from germline V_H and J_H segments. This domain binds Z-DNA and ssDNA. The scFv, combining both V_H and V_L domains, binds Z-DNA selectively (H-I. Kim and B. D. Stollar, unpublished). A similar pattern occurs with an immunization-induced antibody to the nucleotide GMP: V_H alone can bind a nucleotide-protein conjugate or ssDNA; selectivity is modulated by the L chain, as the Fv shows a great increase in affinity for the GMP-protein and little change in ssDNA binding (A. Gebremichael and B. D. Stollar, unpublished data).

These results are similar to those that Weigert and colleagues observed with the H chain of the lupus mouse pathogenic IgG autoantibody 3H9.[72,73] The 3H9 H chain plays a dominant role in DNA binding, yielding a DNA-binding antibody even when paired with diverse L chains.[73] Some L chains modify the affinity and selectivity of the antibody and some do prevent DNA-binding activity.[74] In nonlupus animals transgenic for the 3H9 H chain, expression of this transgene is suppressed if the H/L combination is autoreactive,[7] but secondary rearrangement producing an L chain that prohibits autoreactivity (receptor editing) can rescue the expression of Ig with the 3H9 H chain.[75]

The disease-related or immunization-induced anti-DNA antibodies described above had mutated V_H domains. V_H domains expressed in pre-B cells are diverse in both rearrangements and junctions of the V, D, and J segments, but have not undergone mutation. A substantial number of IgM cDNA molecules cloned from unstimulated peripheral blood lymphocytes of two healthy human adults also had V gene segments without mutations.[38] Thus, we cloned and expressed, in bacteria, several variously mutated V_H domains from cDNA libraries of healthy human adults

TABLE 2. V_H Domains from Healthy Adult PBL, Expressed as V_H–Protein A Fusion Proteins

Clone[a]	V_H Family	V_H Mutations	V_H Gene	D_H	J_H	poly(dT) ELISA[b] ($A_{410\ nm}$)
TC69	3	0	3-7; DP-54	NA	6	0.215
AM1F6.3	3	0	3-9; DP-31	DQ52	4	0.355
18/2	3	0	3-23; DP-47	Dxp′1	5	0.209
AM1D11.3	3	0	3-23; DP-47	Dxp1	4	0.394
AM35.2	3	1	3-23; DP-47	DK4	6	0.412
AG6.3	3	1	3-23; DP-47	DA1	6	1.293
AM10.2	3	1	3-23; DP-47	Dxp4	6	1.341
AM1G5.3	3	3	3-23; DP-47	Dxp′1	6	0.624
AG34-1	3	5	3-23; DP-47	NA	6	0.229
AG21.3	3	15	3-23; DP-47	Dxp′1	5	2.224
AM1D4.3	3	0	3-53; DP-42	NA	4	0.982
AM6.3	4	0	4.18	DM1/5	3	0.547

[a]cDNA clones were obtained from unstimulated peripheral blood B cells of two healthy adult human subjects. They are among the clones described in reference 38 and were prepared as described earlier.[91]

[b]ELISA was performed with UV-irradiated polystyrene microtiter plates (Immunlon 1, Dynatech) coated with poly(dT) at 2 μg/mL and incubated with 1 μM recombinant V_H–protein A fusion product. Bound V_H–protein A was detected with normal rabbit IgG and alkaline phosphatase–labeled anti-rabbit IgG. Values were corrected for controls, in which recombinant protein was incubated in BSA-blocked wells with no poly(dT).

in order to test whether they react with autoantigens. We compared their V_H domains with that of mAb18/2, a human IgM autoantibody originally chosen for study because it bound ssDNA.[76] mAb18/2 has unmutated V_H3-23, Dxp′1, and J_H4-coded sequences, along with some amino acids coded by untemplated bases.[77] Its V_L domain has two differences from the κA30 germline gene.

We cloned and expressed the V_H domains of 12 human Ig cDNA's (TABLE 2). Eleven were V_H3 family members and 8 of those, including 18/2, had V_H segments identical to or derived from V_H3-23 (DP47), a frequently expressed Ig gene element.[78] Except for 18/2, these V_H domains were not chosen for study on the basis of any antigen-binding activity; they were initially picked at random from clones in IgM V-region cDNA libraries of normal adults. Six of these V_H domains reacted strongly with poly(dT) (TABLE 2), a polynucleotide that has been prominent in reactions of serum and hybridoma anti-ssDNA autoantibodies.[65,79,80] This reaction was measured with a micromolar concentration of V_H domain.

We also expressed the V_L domain of antibody 18/2 and measured its binding to the V_H domain. The 18/2 V_H-V_L domain association had a much lower affinity ($K_d = 1.7 \times 10^{-6}$ M^{-1})[64] than the association between V_H and V_L domains of an immunization-induced mouse IgG anti-Z-DNA mAb, Z22 ($K_d = 5.5 \times 10^{-8}$ M^{-1}).[63] Antibody 18/2 is a human polyreactive natural autoantibody, whereas Z22 is a highly selective immunization-induced mouse antibody. Further experiments will be required to determine whether a lower affinity of V_H-V_L association is generally characteristic of less-differentiated natural autoantibodies and whether it is a basis for flexibility and polyreactivity.

Molecular Interactions of $V_{pre\text{-}B}$ Protein

Models propose that, in pre-B cells, the V_H domain interacts with $V_{pre\text{-}B}$ protein and the J_H-like second exon of protein 14.1/λ5 and that the μCH1 domain interacts with the third exon of the 14.1/λ5 protein. We have begun to assemble the components for *in vitro* study of these interactions and of the potential for binding of self ligands by these assemblies. The human $V_{pre\text{-}B}$ gene was cloned and expressed in *E. coli.* The protein was purified from bacterial growth medium and cleaved from the protein A domain with which it was fused.[64] Recombinant $V_{pre\text{-}B}$ resembled native protein, as rabbit antibodies induced by the recombinant protein precipitated $V_{pre\text{-}B}$-containing complexes from cell lysates of pre-B cells (Y. Hirabayashi and B. D. Stollar, unpublished).

Purified $V_{pre\text{-}B}$ dimerized with itself and it bound to both V_H and V_L domains. As expected, $V_{pre\text{-}B}$ did not bind to the Fc fragment of IgG, but it did bind unexpectedly to Fab and intact IgG.[64] Thus, $V_{pre\text{-}B}$ can bind to V_H at a site other than where V_L binds, as evidenced also by formation of a trimolecular complex between V_H, V_L, and $V_{pre\text{-}B}$. These results show the potential for receptor cross-linking to occur via Ig-$V_{pre\text{-}B}$ interactions. However, experiments that include the 14.1/λ5 protein are required for further evaluation of both ligand binding and cross-linking of these complexes.

CONCLUSIONS

Although negative selection is the best documented consequence of autoreactivity, certain features of the primary Ig repertoire could be accounted for if binding of self ligands also had a positive selective effect at some stage of emerging B cell development. These features are the general occurrence of natural autoantibodies, especially in fetal and neonatal repertoires; the coding of natural autoantibodies by unmutated V gene segments; and the conservation of autoantigen structure and autoantibody function. Cloning and expression of Ig V_H domains from healthy adults reveals their potential for binding to poly(dT), a prominent *in vitro* reactant for anti-ssDNA antibodies. Similar cloning and expression of $V_{pre\text{-}B}$ and other components of pre-B cell surface Ig assemblies will permit detailed analysis of ligand binding by these receptors.

REFERENCES

1. TONEGAWA, S. 1983. Nature **302:** 575–581.
2. ALT, F. W., G. D. YANCOPOULOS, T. K. BLACKWELL, C. WOOD, E. THOMAS, M. BOSS, R. COFFMAN, N. ROSENBERG, S. TONEGAWA & D. BALTIMORE. 1984. EMBO J. **3:** 1209–1219.
3. ALT, F. W., T. K. BLACKWELL & G. D. YANCOPOULOS. 1987. Science **238:** 1079–1087.
4. SCHROEDER, H. W., JR., J. L. HILLSON & R. M. PERLMUTTER. 1987. Science **238:** 791–793.
5. HARTLEY, S. B., J. CROSBIE, R. BRINK, A. B. KANTOR, A. BASTEN & C. C. GOODNOW. 1991. Nature **353:** 765–769.
6. RUSSELL, D. M., Z. DEMBIC, G. MORAHAN, J. F. A. P. MILLER, K. BÜRKI & D. NEMAZEE. 1991. Nature **354:** 308–311.
7. ERIKSON, J., M. Z. RADIC, S. A. CAMPER, R. R. HARDY, C. CARMACK & M. WEIGERT. 1991. Nature **349:** 331–334.
8. GAY, D., T. SAUNDERS, S. CAMPER & M. WEIGERT. 1993. J. Exp. Med. **177:** 999–1008.
9. TIEGS, S. L., D. M. RUSSELL & D. NEMAZEE. 1993. J. Exp. Med. **177:** 1009.
10. OSMOND, D. G. 1986. Immunol. Rev. **93:** 103–124.
11. MELCHERS, F., D. HAASNER, U. GRAWUNDER, C. KALBERER, H. KARASUYAMA, T. WINKLER & A. G. ROLINK. 1994. Annu. Rev. Immunol. **12:** 209–225.
12. KITAMURA, D., N. ROES, R. KUHN & K. RAJEWSKY. 1991. Nature **350:** 423–426.
13. KITAMURA, D., A. KUDO, S. SCHAAL, W. MÜLLER, F. MELCHERS & K. RAJEWSKY. 1992. Cell **69:** 823–831.
14. YE, J., S. K. MCCRAY & S. H. CLARKE. 1996. EMBO J. **15:** 1524–1533.
15. GOODNOW, C. C. 1992. Annu. Rev. Immunol. **10:** 489–518.
16. RADIC, M. Z., S. M. IBRAHIM, J. RAUCH, S. A. CAMPER & M. WEIGERT. 1995. J. Immunol. **155:** 3213–3222.
17. WECHSLER, R. J. & J. G. MONROE. 1995. J. Immunol. **154:** 1919–1929.
18. NORVELL, A., L. MANDIK & J. G. MONROE. 1995. J. Immunol. **154:** 4404–4413.
19. SCHWARTZ, R. S. & B. D. STOLLAR. 1994. Immunol. Today **15:** 27–32.
20. ROBEY, E. & B. J. FOWLKES. 1994. Annu. Rev. Immunol. **12:** 675–705.
21. GRABAR, P. 1975. Clin. Immunol. Immunopathol. **4:** 453.
22. FOURNIÉ, G. J., P. H. LAMBERT & P. A. MIESCHER. 1974. J. Exp. Med. **140:** 1189–1206.
23. RUBIN, R. L. & R. I. CARR. 1979. J. Immunol. **122:** 1604–1607.
24. KARSENTI, E., B. GUILBERT, M. BORNENS & S. AVRAMEAS. 1977. Proc. Natl. Acad. Sci. U.S.A. **74:** 3997.
25. GUILBERT, B., G. DIGHIERO & S. AVRAMEAS. 1982. J. Immunol. **128:** 2779–2787.
26. DIGHIERO, G., B. GUILBERT & S. AVRAMEAS. 1982. J. Immunol. **128:** 2788–2797.
27. DIGHIERO, G., B. GUILBERT, J. P. FERMAND, P. LYMBERI, F. DANON & S. AVRAMEAS. 1983. Blood **62:** 264–270.
28. TERNYNCK, T. & S. AVRAMEAS. 1986. Immunol. Rev. **94:** 99.
29. FREITAS, A. A., O. BURLEN & A. COUTINHO. 1988. J. Immunol. **140:** 4097–4102.
30. KEARNEY, J. F. & M. VAKIL. 1986. Immunol. Rev. **94:** 39–50.
31. MUNNS, T. W., M. K. LISZEWSKI & S. K. FREEMAN. 1986. Biochem. Biophys. Res. Commun. **136:** 145.
32. SAENKO, V. A., A. E. KABAKOV & A. M. POVERENNY. 1992. Immunol. Lett. **34:** 1–6.
33. STAFFORD, H. A., C. J. ANDERSON & M. REICHLIN. 1995. J. Immunol. **155:** 2754–2761.
34. DIGHIERO, G., P. LYMBERI, D. HOLMBERG, I. LUNDQUIST, A. COUTINHO & S. AVRAMEAS. 1985. J. Immunol. **134:** 765–771.

35. SOUROUJON, M., M. E. WHITE-SCHARF, J. ANDRÉ-SCHWARTZ, M. L. GEFTER & R. S. SCHWARTZ. 1988. J. Immunol. **140:** 4173–4179.
36. DERSIMONIAN, H., A. LONG, D. RUBINSTEIN, B. D. STOLLAR & R. S. SCHWARTZ. 1990. Int. Rev. Immunol. **5:** 253–264.
37. MORTARI, F., J. A. NEWTON, J. Y. WANG & H. W. SCHROEDER, JR. 1992. Eur. J. Immunol. **22:** 241–245.
38. HUANG, C. & B. D. STOLLAR. 1993. J. Immunol. **151:** 5290–5300.
39. MARTIN, T., S. F. DUFFY, D. A. CARSON & T. J. KIPPS. 1992. J. Exp. Med. **175:** 983–991.
40. IKEMATSU, H., M. T. KASAIAN, E. W. SCHETTINO & P. CASALI. 1993. J. Immunol. **151:** 3604–3616.
41. MARTIN, T., R. CROUZIER, J-C. WEBER, T. J. KIPPS & J-L. PASQUALI. 1994. J. Immunol. **152:** 5988–5996.
42. ICHIYOSHI, Y. & P. CASALI. 1994. J. Exp. Med. **180:** 885–895.
43. STOLLAR, B. D. 1991. Mol. Immunol. **28:** 1399–1412.
44. STOLLAR, D., L. LEVINE & J. MARMUR. 1962. Biochim. Biophys. Acta **61:** 7–18.
45. BONFA, E., A. MARSHAK-ROTHSTEIN, H. WEISSBACH, N. BROT & K. ELKON. 1988. J. Immunol. **140:** 3434–3437.
46. TAKEDA, Y., U. NYMAN, A. WINKLER, K. S. WISE, S. O. HOCH, I. PETTERSSON, S. K. ANDERSON, R. J. WANG, G. S. WANG & G. C. SHARP. 1991. Clin. Immunol. Immunopathol. **61:** 55–68.
47. SCHROEDER, H. W., JR., J. L. HILLSON & R. M. PERLMUTTER. 1990. Int. Immunol. **2:** 41–50.
48. MEEK, K., T. EVERSOLE & J. D. CAPRA. 1991. J. Immunol. **146:** 2434–2438.
49. BOOKER, J. K. & G. HAUGHTON. 1994. Int. Immunol. **6:** 1427–1436.
50. WATTS, R. A., C. T. RAVIRAJAN, N. A. STAINES & D. A. ISENBERG. 1990. Immunology **69:** 348–354.
51. TAKEI, M., H. DANG, R. J. WANG & N. TALAL. 1988. J. Immunol. **140:** 3108–3113.
52. PASCUAL, V. & J. D. CAPRA. 1991. Adv. Immunol. **49:** 1–74.
53. NAPARSTEK, Y., J. ANDRÉ-SCHWARTZ, T. MANSER, T. WYSOCKI, L. BREITMAN, B. D. STOLLAR, M. GEFTER & R. S. SCHWARTZ. 1986. J. Exp. Med. **164:** 614–626.
54. MINNERATH, J. M., C. M. MUELLER, S. BURON & R. JEMMERSON. 1995. Eur. J. Immunol. **25:** 784–791.
55. MINNERATH, J. M., L. P. WAKEM, L. L. COMFORT, F. SHERMAN & R. JEMMERSON. 1995. Proc. Natl. Acad. Sci. U.S.A. **92:** 12379–12383.
56. BOLE, D. G., L. M. HENDERSHOT & J. F. KEARNEY. 1986. J. Cell Biol. **102:** 1558–1566.
57. GUELPA-FONLUPT, V., C. TONNELLE, D. BLAISE, M. FOUGEREAU & F. FUMOUX. 1994. Eur. J. Immunol. **24:** 257–264.
58. KEYNA, U., G. B. BECK-ENGESER, J. JONGSTRA, S. E. APPLEQUIST & H-M. JÄCK. 1995. J. Immunol. **155:** 5536–5542.
59. LÖFFERT, D., A. EHLICH, W. MÜLLER & K. RAJEWSKY. 1996. Immunity **4:** 133–144.
60. MISENER, V., G. P. DOWNEY & J. JONGSTRA. 1991. Int. Immunol. **3:** 1129.
61. BOSSY, D., M. MILILI, J. ZUCMAN, G. THOMAS, M. FOUGEREAU & C. SCHIFF. 1991. Int. Immunol. **3:** 1081.
62. BRIGIDO, M. M., M. POLYMENIS & B. D. STOLLAR. 1993. J. Immunol. **150:** 469–479.
63. POLYMENIS, M. & B. D. STOLLAR. 1995. J. Immunol. **154:** 2198–2208.
64. HIRABAYASHI, Y., J-M. LECERF, Z. DONG & B. D. STOLLAR. 1995. J. Immunol. **155:** 1218–1228.
65. HERRON, J. N., X. M. HE, D. W. BALLARD, P. R. BLIER, P. E. PACE, A. L. M. BOTHWELL, E. W. VOSS, JR. & A. B. EDMUNDSON. 1991. Proteins **11:** 159–175.
66. BARRY, M. M., C. D. MOL, W. F. ANDERSON & J. S. LEE. 1994. J. Biol. Chem. **269:** 3623–3632.
67. PADLAN, E. A. 1994. Mol. Immunol. **31:** 169–217.
68. JANG, Y. J. & B. D. STOLLAR. 1996. Mol. Immunol. **33:** 197–210.
69. BARRY, M. M. & J. S. LEE. 1993. Mol. Immunol. **30:** 833–840.
70. KIEBER-EMMONS, T., J. M. VON FELDT, A. P. GODILLOT, D. MCCALLUS, D. SRIKANTAN, D. B. WEINER & W. V. WILLIAMS. 1994. Lupus **3:** 379–392.

71. Polymenis, M. & B. D. Stollar. 1994. J. Immunol. **152:** 5319–5329.
72. Radic, M. Z., J. Mackle, J. Erikson, C. Mol, W. F. Anderson & M. Weigert. 1993. J. Immunol. **150:** 4966–4977.
73. Radic, M. Z., M. A. Mascelli, J. Erikson, H. Shan & M. Weigert. 1991. J. Immunol. **146:** 176–182.
74. Ibrahim, S. M., M. Weigert, C. Basu, J. Erikson & M. Z. Radic. 1995. J. Immunol. **155:** 3223–3233.
75. Radic, M. Z., J. Erikson, S. Litwin & M. Weigert. 1993. J. Exp. Med. **177:** 1165–1173.
76. Shoenfeld, Y., S. C. Hsu-Lin, J. E. Gabriels, L. E. Silberstein, B. C. Furie, B. Furie, B. D. Stollar & R. S. Schwartz. 1982. J. Clin. Invest. **70:** 205–208.
77. Dersimonian, H., R. S. Schwartz, K. J. Barrett & B. D. Stollar. 1987. J. Immunol. **139:** 2496–2501.
78. Stollar, B. D. 1995. Ann. N.Y. Acad. Sci. **764:** 265–274.
79. Stollar, D., L. Levine, H. I. Lehrer & H. van Vunakis. 1962. Proc. Natl. Acad. Sci. U.S.A. **48:** 874–880.
80. Lee, J. S., D. F. Dombroski & T. R. Mosmann. 1982. Biochemistry **21:** 4940–4945.
81. Rioux, J. D., E. Zdarsky, M. M. Newkirk & J. Rauch. 1995. Mol. Immunol. **32:** 683–696.
82. Crouzier, R., T. Martin & J. L. Pasquali. 1995. J. Immunol. **154:** 4526–4535.
83. Pascual, V., S. Cha, M. E. Gershwin, J. D. Capra & P. S. C. Leung. 1994. J. Immunol. **152:** 2577–2585.
84. Sanz, I., H. Y. Dang, M. Takai, N. Talal & J. D. Capra. 1989. J. Immunol. **142:** 883–887.
85. Quinn, A., E. E. Adderson, P. G. Shackelford, W. L. Carroll & M. W. Cunningham. 1995. J. Immunol. **154:** 4203–4212.
86. Cairns, E., P. C. Kwong, V. Misener, P. Ip, D. A. Bell & K. A. Siminovitch. 1989. J. Immunol. **143:** 685–691.
87. Roudier, J., G. J. Silverman, P. P. Chen, D. A. Carson & T. J. Kipps. 1990. J. Immunol. **144:** 1526–1530.
88. Silberstein, L. E., L. C. Jefferies, J. Goldman, D. Friedman, J. S. Moore, P. C. Nowell, D. Roelcke, W. Pruzanski, J. Roudier & G. J. Silverman. 1991. Blood **78:** 2372–2386.
89. Denomme, G. A., M. Mahmoudi, E. Cairns & D. A. Bell. 1994. J. Autoimmun. **7:** 521–535.
90. Logtenberg, T., F. M. Young, J. H. Van Es, F. H. J. Gmelig-Meyling & F. W. Alt. 1989. J. Exp. Med. **170:** 1347–1355.
91. Huang, C. & B. D. Stollar. 1991. J. Immunol. Methods **141:** 227–236.

Effects of Altered Bcl-2 Expression on B Lymphocyte Selection[a]

LAURA MANDIK,[b] MAKOTO KATSUMATA,[c]
AND JAN ERIKSON[b]

[b]*The Wistar Institute*
Philadelphia, Pennsylvania 19104

[c]*Department of Pathology and Laboratory Medicine*
University of Pennsylvania School of Medicine
Philadelphia, Pennsylvania 19104

INTRODUCTION

How autoreactive lymphocytes are regulated in healthy individuals and what factors affect their dysregulation in autoimmunity is the subject of a great deal of study. In this report, we will discuss the role of two regulators of cell death, Fas receptor (FasR) and bcl-2, whose altered expression has been associated with the occurrence of SLE-associated autoantibodies.

SLE and the MRL-*lpr/lpr* murine model for lupus are characterized by high titers of antinuclear antibodies (ANAs) and severe renal pathology.[1–3] *Lpr/lpr* crossed onto different nonautoimmune genetic backgrounds (BALB/c, C57BL/6, C3H) leads to the production of anti-DNA antibodies, suggesting that this autosomal recessive gene defect plays a role in autoantibody production.[1,4] The *lpr* defect has been shown to be a mutation in the FasR, a protein implicated in inducing programmed cell death (apoptosis).[5–7] To understand the molecular mechanisms for the B cell abnormalities observed in *lpr/lpr* mice, we and others have defined cell surface expression of FasR on various B cell populations isolated from normal and *lpr/lpr* mice, with particular emphasis on the stages of B cell maturation that are thought to be checkpoints in B cell selection.[8–10] In agreement with most other reports, we found that FasR is absent from *lpr/lpr* cells. We found that FasR is expressed at various cell surface densities on B cells throughout their development both in the bone marrow and in the periphery, with germinal center (GC) B cells displaying the highest FasR surface density.[8]

Recent studies have begun to assess the susceptibility of B cells to FasR-mediated apoptosis. Rothstein *et al.* showed that sensitivity to FasR/Fas ligand–induced apoptosis was acquired by activation through CD40 in the absence of a protective signal delivered through the Ig receptor.[11] These data were used to explain in part why B cells are not generally activated through "bystander" T cell help in the absence of Ig engagement. Additional studies by Wang *et al.* have confirmed this observation and

[a]Support for this work was provided by grants (to J. Erikson) from the National Institutes of Health (No. AI-32137), the PEW Charitable Trust, and the American Cancer Society (No. RJFA-460), as well as by N.C.I. Training Grant No. CA-09171 (to L. Mandik).

extended it to show the kinetics involved in the susceptibility process. Resting B cells are resistant to FasR-mediated death and remain so until 2–3 days postactivation.[12]

In contrast to that of FasR, the expression pattern of bcl-2 is tightly regulated: bcl-2 is not expressed in B cells during times of B cell selection, including pre-B and immature B cells in the bone marrow[13] and GC B cells.[14,15] Bcl-2 was originally identified as a participant in the t(14;18) translocation that characterizes follicular B cell lymphomas.[16,17] This translocation places the bcl-2 gene under the control of the Ig heavy-chain enhancer, leading to high constitutive levels of bcl-2 expression. Bcl-2 has been shown to protect cells from many triggers of cell death, including growth factor withdrawal, γ-irradiation, and dexamethasone (reviewed in reference 18). Consistent with the ability of bcl-2 to repress a number of apoptotic death programs, *in vitro* experiments have suggested that bcl-2 may block FasR-mediated apoptosis. These data are controversial, however, and seem to depend on properties of the individual cell lines used.[19–21] A number of studies have used bcl-2 as a transgene (tg) to study its role *in vivo*. Two recent reports used this approach to determine if bcl-2 is capable of protecting mice from the lethal fulminant hepatic failure observed after anti-FasR antibody treatment. Tg's that targeted bcl-2 expression to hepatocytes were able to block the majority of hepatocyte apoptosis, suggesting that bcl-2 is able to block FasR-mediated death *in vivo*.[22,23]

Several groups have generated bcl-2 tg's under the control of the Ig enhancer with the intent of targeting expression to lymphocytes.[24–26] These studies have shown that constitutive expression of bcl-2 leads to an increase in B and/or T cell number, an increase in serum Ig levels, a prolonged immune response *in vivo*, and increased lymphocyte survival *in vitro*. In one lineage of bcl-2 tg mice, most of the animals developed a fatal autoimmune disease. This disease was reported to resemble SLE in that the mice developed serum Ab to nuclear antigens such as snRNPs, histones, and dsDNA, and their kidneys showed evidence of immune complex glomerulonephritis.[24] However, autoimmune disease was only evident on certain genetic backgrounds and other bcl-2 lineages did not show this phenomenon.[25,26]

The effect of inappropriate bcl-2 expression on the selection of the immune repertoire is not clear. Teale's group has reported that deregulated bcl-2 expression alters the V_H gene repertoire. The D-proximal V_H families 7183 and Q52 were preferentially expressed in adult bcl-2 tg mice as compared to non-tg animals.[27] Why deregulated bcl-2 results in a dominance of these V_H segments that are preferentially expressed during fetal development is not clear. Two studies on negative selection of B cells in the context of the bcl-2 tg have been reported. The first was with the HEL model system, in which it was found that the presence of the bcl-2 tg resulted in a marked accumulation of anti-HEL tg B cells in the bone marrow, peripheral blood, and spleen of mice expressing membrane-HEL as a neo-self antigen. In the absence of the bcl-2 tg, anti-HEL B cells were shown to be deleted in the bone marrow. The cells that did persist in the context of the bcl-2 tg had an immature phenotype. The conclusion from this study was that bcl-2 did not interfere with tolerance as measured by maturational arrest, but did interfere with the death of tolerized cells.[28] In the second model system, bcl-2 tg mice were bred to mice tg for an antierythrocyte Ig. The presence of the bcl-2 tg did not interfere with clonal deletion of self-reactive antierythrocyte B cells in the bone marrow. The bcl-2 tg did have an effect, however, on the CD5 (B-1) B cells in the peritoneal cavity, which in the context of bcl-2 were resistant to activation-induced cell death (AICD).[29] Clearly, the roles that bcl-2 and blocking cell death play in the production of autoantibodies need to be addressed further.

The enormous cell death that occurs as B cells develop in the bone marrow is thought to include B cells that have undergone faulty Ig rearrangements as well as autoreactive B cells and possibly B cells that have not been positively selected on some yet to be identified ligand. The relative contribution of these factors to B cell death in the bone marrow is not known. Importantly, the studies described above suggest that we may be able to use bcl-2 tg mice to keep alive cells that would otherwise die, so we can study them experimentally. In the present study, we have used a tg that inappropriately expresses bcl-2 in the bone marrow and periphery to rescue cells that were destined to die. Here, we report the presence of unique populations of B cells that accumulate in these mice.

METHODS

Mice

BALB/cJ mice were purchased from Charles River (Wilmington, Massachusetts). Bcl-2 tg line 6 mice[26] and V_H3H9 tg mice[30] have been backcrossed onto the BALB/c background for at least three and nine generations, respectively. The mice have been bred and maintained in the animal facility at The Wistar Institute. In all cases, age-matched BALB/c mice or non-tg littermates were used as controls. The presence of the bcl-2 and V_H3H9 tg's was determined by PCR amplification of tail DNA with primers specific for human bcl-2[26] and V_H3H9,[30] respectively. At least four mice ($n = 4$) were used for each experiment.

Cell Preparations

BM (bone marrow), spleen, and LN (lymph node) cells were removed from bcl-2 tg and non-tg mice. Single-cell suspensions were prepared and, where necessary, the erythrocytes were removed by hypotonic lysis. Total cell numbers were determined by counting the number of cells that excluded trypan blue under a light microscope.

Flow Cytometry Analysis

Cells (5×10^5) were surface-stained according to standard protocol.[31] The following Ab's were used: 2C11-PE or -FITC (anti-CD3), RA3-6B2-biotin, -FITC, or -PE (anti-B220), Jo2-PE (anti-FasR), 53-7.3-PE (anti-CD5), R8-140 (anti-mouse Igκ), 6C8 (anti-human bcl-2), and 3F11 (anti-murine bcl-2), all purchased from Pharmingen; SBA-1-biotin (anti-IgD) from Southern Biotechnology; goat anti-mouse IgM-

FITC or -PE from Fisher; goat anti-mouse IgG-FITC from Sigma; PNA-FITC from Vector; JC5-biotin (anti-Igλ), a gift of J. Kearney; GK1.5 (anti-CD4) and 53.6.72 (anti-CD8) grown as supernatants; and KM201-FITC (anti-CD44), a gift from Ellen Pure. Secondary Ab's were streptavidin-Red670 purchased from GIBCO-BRL and goat anti-hamster Ig-FITC or -PE from Caltag.

All samples were analyzed on a FACScan flow cytometer (Becton Dickinson) using Cellquest software. At least 15,000 events were collected for each sample and gated for live cells based on forward and side scatter.

Intracellular Staining

Cells were stained intracellularly for bcl-2 according to the protocol described in reference 13. Briefly, cells were harvested and surface-stained. The cells were then fixed in 1% paraformaldehyde for 10 min at room temperature, washed twice in saponin wash buffer (0.03% saponin), and stained with anti-bcl-2 Ab in staining buffer (0.3% saponin) for 30 min. After washing twice in saponin wash buffer, the cells were stained with the goat anti-hamster Ig secondary Ab. The cells were then analyzed as described above.

RESULTS AND DISCUSSION

Bcl-2 tg Is Inappropriately Expressed in B Cells and a Subpopulation of T Cells

To assess the effect of bcl-2, it was first important to determine where the tg is expressed. We examined populations of lymphocytes from the bone marrow, spleen, lymph node, peritoneal cavity, and thymus of tg mice for expression of the bcl-2 tg. In all tissues examined, the expression of the tg bcl-2 did not have an apparent effect on the expression of endogenous bcl-2 (data not shown).

BM cells were stained with antibodies to distinguish B cell subpopulations, and levels of the bcl-2 tg within these populations were measured by flow cytometry. FIGURE 1A shows that the bcl-2 tg is expressed in all B cells in the BM from the pro- and pre-B ($B220^{low}/IgM^-$) stage, through the immature B ($B220^{low}/IgM^+$) stage, to the mature B ($B220^{high}/IgM^+$) cell stage. The bcl-2 tg is expressed both at stages where endogenous bcl-2 is expressed and, more importantly, at the pre-B and immature B cell stages where endogenous bcl-2 has been downregulated. The functional significance of the variable density of bcl-2 tg expression is not clear. To determine if the tg is expressed in peripheral B cells, we stained spleen, LN, and peritoneal cavity B cells. The bcl-2 tg continues to be expressed in B cells in the spleen (FIGURE 1B) and the LN (FIGURE 1C), and in B-1 and B-2 cells in the peritoneum (data not shown). In contrast to its expression pattern in peripheral resting B cells, endogenous bcl-2 is not expressed in germinal center B cells. To increase the frequency of germinal center B cells (defined as being PNA^{high}), we immunized mice with influenza (virus strain PR8). We found that the bcl-2 tg is expressed on PNA^{high} splenic B cells, in contrast to endogenous bcl-2 (data not shown).[26]

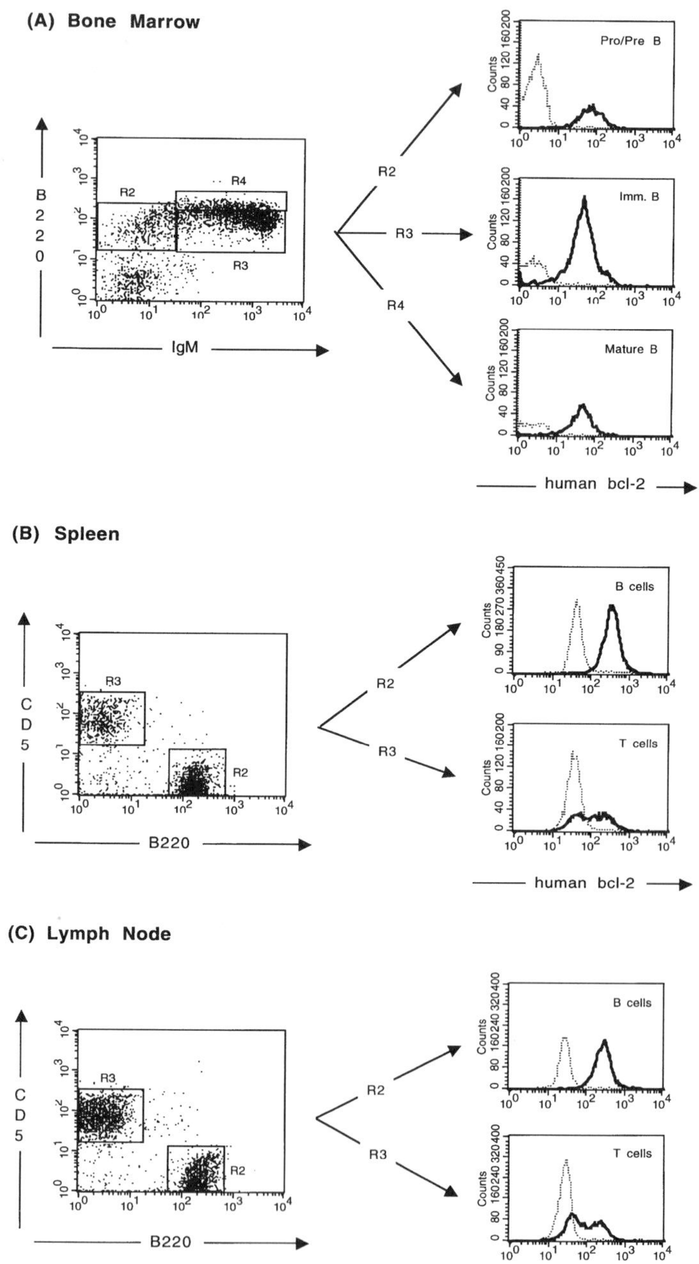
(A) Bone Marrow
B220
IgM
R2
R3
R4
Pro/Pre B
Imm. B
Mature B
Counts
human bcl-2
(B) Spleen
CD5
B220
B cells
T cells
(C) Lymph Node

FIGURE 1

TABLE 1. FasR and Bcl-2 Expression Patterns on B Cells

	FasR[8]	Bcl-2[13–15]	Bcl-2 tg
pro-B	+	+	++
pre-B	+	−	+
immature B	+	−	+
mature B	++	+	++
peripheral B	++	+	++
GC B	++++	−	+

To look at expression of the bcl-2 tg in T cells, we stained spleen, LN, and thymus with T cell specific markers (CD4, CD5, and CD8). As can be seen from FIGURE 1, only a fraction of the T cells in the spleen and LN expressed the tg. The majority of the T cells in the thymus were also negative for tg expression (data not shown). The percentage of T cells that stain positive for the bcl-2 tg varies from mouse to mouse (20–60%) and does not correlate with CD4/CD8 status or the activation marker CD44 (data not shown). At this point, it is unclear why only a fraction of the T cells express the bcl-2 tg. However, other tg's under the control of the IgH enhancer also show variable expression in T cells.[24,25,32]

The pattern of bcl-2 tg expression in these bcl-2 line 6 tg mice is different from that reported for other bcl-2 tg mice using similar constructs. The bcl-2-22 mice from Cory's group are reported to express the tg in all B cells in the BM as well as in peripheral B cells, but not in T cells.[33,34] Cory also describes lines of mice (bcl-2-25 and bcl-2-36) where the tg is expressed mainly in T cells.[33,35] Korsmeyer's bcl-2 tg mice are also reported to express the tg in BM B cells.[13] Reports on the tg expression in the periphery have been conflicting. Via mRNA, the thymus and spleen are tg(+).[36] However, by flow cytometry, levels of bcl-2 tg were only detectable on a fraction of peripheral T cells and on a small percentage of B cells.[32] The different expression patterns could be explained by the regulatory sequences that are part of the construct or the integration site of the transgene. This clearly shows that, for the same construct, different founders can have drastically different expression patterns.

Bcl-2 tg Mice Have Accumulated Populations of Cells with Distinct Phenotypes in the BM and Periphery

The intent of studying tg mice that inappropriately express bcl-2 during periods associated with B cell selection (see TABLE 1) is to rescue cells normally destined to

←

FIGURE 1. Bcl-2 tg mice express bcl-2 primarily in B cells. (A) Bone marrow, (B) spleen, and (C) lymph node cells were stained with anti-B220-biotin/streptavidin-Red670, anti-IgM-FITC, and/or anti-CD5-PE; then, they were fixed, permeabilized, and stained intracellularly with anti-human bcl-2 followed by anti-hamster Ig-PE or -FITC. The histograms show bcl-2 staining on bcl-2 tg (—) versus non-tg (···) B cells within the regions indicated on the dot plots. Note: the higher background staining in the spleen and LN plots is due to the difference in secondary Ab used (anti-hamster Ig-FITC in spleen and LN versus anti-hamster Ig-PE in BM).

die so that, by examining them, we can begin to understand the rules governing B cell selection. One prediction for inappropriately expressed bcl-2 in B cells is that there will be an accumulation of B cell populations eliminated in normal mice. As shown in TABLE 2, total cell number is increased in both the BM (1.5- to 2-fold) and spleen (2- to 10-fold) of bcl-2 tg mice when compared to tg(−) littermates. The relative frequency of B and T cells is not altered, but the absolute number of both is elevated. This is in contrast to the bcl-2 tg mice studied by Cory's and Korsmeyer's groups, where B cell, but not T cell, numbers are increased.[24,36]

Previous studies looking at other bcl-2 tg mouse strains have reported that the expanded populations of B cells are small and resting, and that they express normal levels of IgM, IgD, and Igκ (IgG and Igλ were not reported).[24,25,36] To characterize the expanded cell populations in the bcl-2 line 6 tg mice, we stained cells for B and T cell specific surface markers. As can be seen in FIGURE 2, the bcl-2 tg mouse has an increased percentage of B220$^+$/IgM^{low} B cells. Upon further analysis, these cells were shown to be IgG$^+$. Using flow cytometry, we cannot conclusively say whether these cells coexpress IgM and IgG. Additional studies are under way to look at heavy-chain isotype expression in individual B cells. As described below, we do find other evidence of a defect in allelic exclusion in the bcl-2 tg mice.

Coexpression of κ and λ Light Chains

To assess the consequences of deregulated bcl-2 expression on the B cell repertoire, we have looked at light-chain isotype expression. As shown in FIGURE 2, the majority of B cells in mice express the Igκ light chain, with only about 5% of the B cells being Igλ$^+$. The bcl-2 tg mice, in contrast, have a higher percentage (approximately 8%) of Igλ$^+$ B cells than non-tg B cells (FIGURE 2 and TABLE 1). One possibility for the increased number of Igλ$^+$ cells is that they are the result of a protracted period of light-chain recombination activity in the bone marrow. If this is the case, then we would predict that Igλ$^+$ B cells would also coexpress an Igκ light chain. In fact, when examined by three-color flow cytometry, all of the Igλ$^+$ B cells in the bcl-2 tg, but not the majority of Igλ$^+$ B cells in non-tg mice, coexpress a κ light chain (FIGURE 3A). This is the case for B cells in the BM, spleen, and LN. A previous report from Storb's group has shown that κ/λ-coexpressing B cells exist in BALB/c spleens, where they comprise approximately 20% of the Igλ$^+$ B cells.[37] When we gate

TABLE 2. Percentage of Lymphocyte Populations in Bcl-2 tg Mice

	Fold-Increase of Cell Number	Total Lymphocytes		Total B Cells	
		% B220$^+$	% CD3$^+$	% IgG$^+$	% Igλ$^+$
Bcl-2 tg					
spleen	2–10×	72.1 ± 10.3	19.9 ± 9.1	8.8 ± 1.1	7.6 ± 1.8
bone marrow	1.5–2×	86.9 ± 3.4	3.1 ± 1.7	2.7 ± 0.4	8.8 ± 2.2
Non-tg					
spleen	1×	57.0 ± 5.7	31.7 ± 4.6	1.6 ± 0.6	5.0 ± 1.2
bone marrow	1×	71.0 ± 8.9	3.5 ± 0.5	0.5 ± 0.2	3.2 ± 2.1

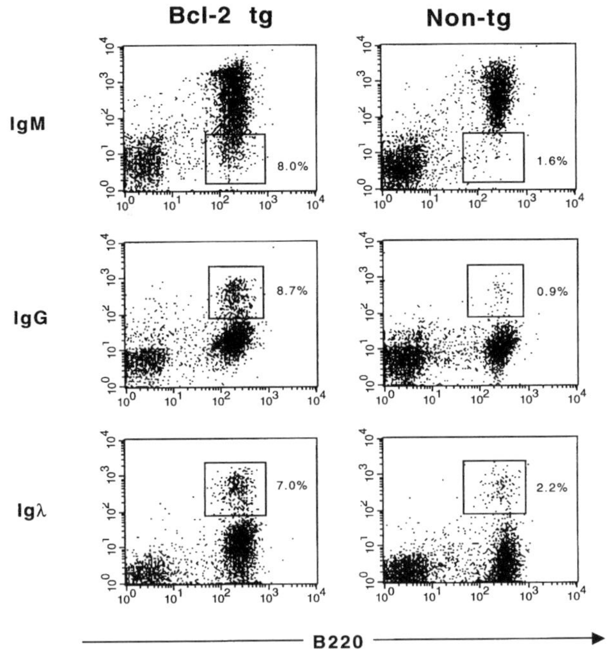

FIGURE 2. Bcl-2 tg mice accumulate distinct populations of IgM^{low}, IgG$^+$, and Igλ^+ B cells. Spleen cells were stained with anti-B220-PE or -biotin/streptavidin-Red670, anti-IgM-FITC, anti-IgG-FITC, and/or anti-Igλ-biotin/streptavidin-Red670. The dot plots compare lymphocyte populations from bcl-2 tg (left) versus non-tg (right) mice. Percentages are shown for the boxed regions.

on Igλ^+ cells and then look at κ versus λ, we also detect κ/λ coexpressers in the non-tg spleen cells, although at a much lower frequency than in the bcl-2 tg cells (FIGURE 3B). The remainder of Igκ^+ B cells in the bcl-2 tg mouse also appear to express a low level of Igλ (denoted R3 in FIGURE 3B). The existence of low levels of receptor is difficult to distinguish at the detection level of flow cytometry. We are in the process of confirming the κ/λ coexpression at the single cell level by the generation of hybridomas.

If indeed there is a protracted period of recombinase activity in the bone marrow of the bcl-2 tg mice, then one might predict that the period of heavy-chain rearrangement might also be extended. To test this possibility, we made use of an Ig tg mouse, namely, the V_H3H9 IgM heavy-chain tg mouse. This heavy chain efficiently excludes endogenous Ig rearrangement (see references 30 and 38; FIGURE 4). By crossing the V_H3H9 tg with our bcl-2 tg mice, we are able to distinguish endogenous Ig rearrangement by the presence of IgD. Non-tg splenic B cells are primarily IgM$^+$/IgD$^+$, whereas V_H3H9 tg B cells are IgM$^+$/IgD$^-$. However, spleens from V_H3H9/bcl-2 tg mice have a subpopulation of IgM$^+$/IgD$^+$ B cells (FIGURE 4). Failure of tg's to inhibit endogenous Ig gene expression is not an uncommon feature of Ig tg's.[39–41] The

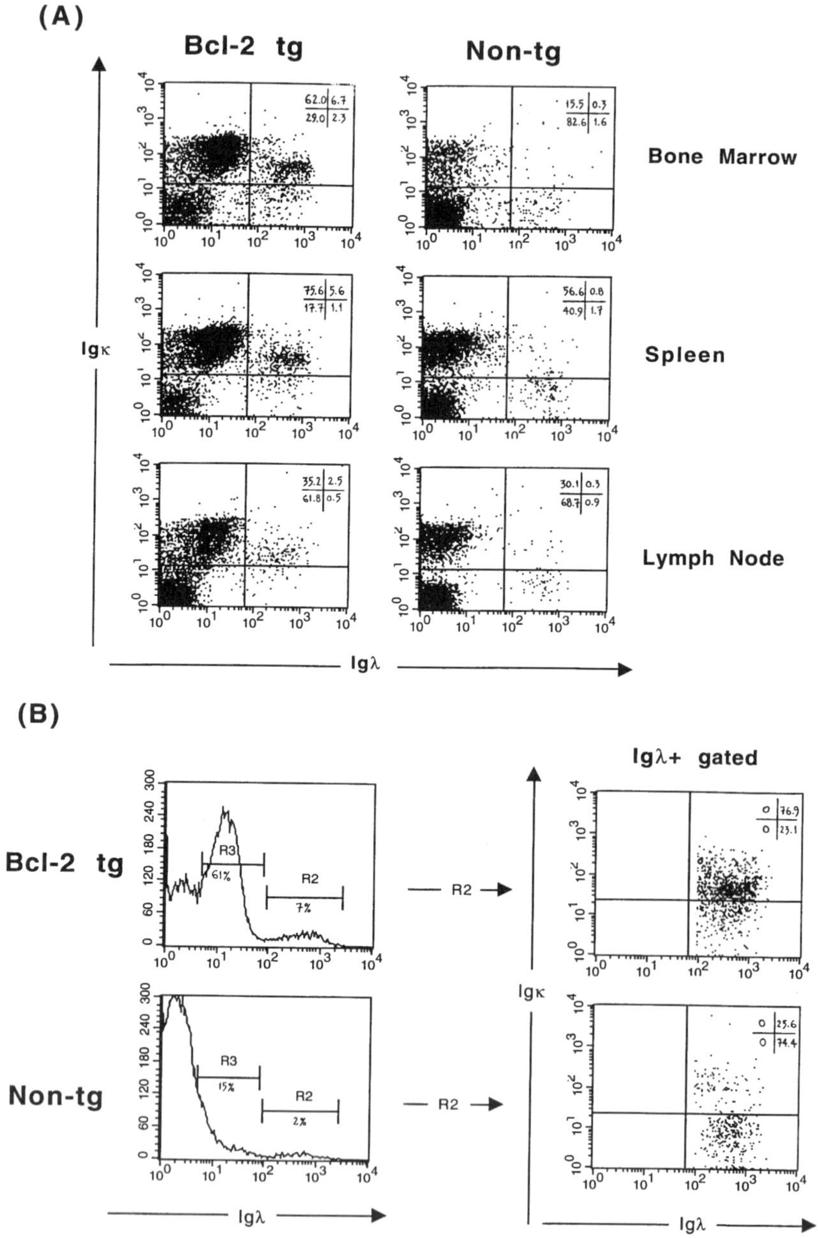
(A)
Bcl-2 tg
Non-tg
Bone Marrow
Spleen
Lymph Node
Igκ
Igλ
(B)
Bcl-2 tg
Non-tg
R3
R2
61%
7%
15%
2%
Igλ+ gated
Igκ
Igλ

FIGURE 3

present example is unusual, however, in that the same lineage excludes well in non-bcl-2 tg littermates, but not in the context of the bcl-2 tg. It will be important to extend this observation to B cells from bcl-2 tg mice without the Ig tg. To do this, we are crossing the bcl-2 tg onto ($IgH^a \times IgH^b$) F_1 mice to look for heavy-chain coexpression using Ig-allotype specific markers.

A Population of Bcl-2 tg B Cells Expressing High Levels of FasR

Interestingly, a subpopulation of B cells (approximately 16% of the splenic lymphocytes) in these mice (as compared to 1% in non-tg mice) expresses high levels of FasR (FIGURE 5A). These $FasR^{high}$ cells include both IgG^+ and IgM^+ B cells (FIGURE 5B). This leads to the intriguing suggestion that bcl-2 may be protecting these cells from FasR-mediated death. The ability of bcl-2 to block FasR-mediated death has been controversial. Studies using bcl-2 transfected cell lines have given conflicting results, and susceptibility versus protection appears to depend upon the particular cell line used.[19–21] One group using bcl-2 as a transgene expressed predominantly in T cells demonstrated partial protection from death signals initiated *in vitro.*[42] Others have used bcl-2 as a tg to examine its protective effect *in vivo.* Two recent reports used this approach to determine if bcl-2 is capable of protecting mice from the lethal fulminant hepatic failure observed after anti-FasR Ab treatment. By constructing tg's that targeted bcl-2 expression to hepatocytes, these investigators were able to block most of the hepatocyte apoptosis.[22,23] A different approach was used by Strasser's group. They crossed bcl-2 tg mice onto the *lpr/lpr* background to examine the effect of bcl-2 expression in the absence of FasR. Because the mice exhibited a more dramatic effect in terms of lymphadenopathy and were able to block cell death triggered by additional stimuli (e.g., SEB), they concluded that FasR and bcl-2 regulate distinct pathways to lymphocyte apoptosis.[42] The presence of a population of $FasR^{high}$ B cells in the bcl-2 tg mice analyzed in our studies suggests that bcl-2 may protect these cells from FasR-mediated death. Currently, we are directly testing this hypothesis by triggering bcl-2 tg B cells, after appropriate stimulation, with Fas ligand *in vitro.*

Serum

Antibodies that stain nuclei and mitotic figures in a homogeneous fashion in the antinuclear antibody (ANA) assay are one of the diagnostic criteria for SLE.[43] One line of bcl-2 tg mice (bcl-2-22 from Cory's group) was reported to have ANA^+ specificities in the serum and to go on to develop lupuslike symptoms by one year of

←

FIGURE 3. The $Ig\lambda^+$ B cells in bcl-2 tg mice coexpress an $Ig\kappa$ light chain. Bone marrow, spleen, and lymph node cells were stained with anti-B220-FITC, anti-$Ig\kappa$-PE, and $Ig\lambda$-biotin/streptavidin-Red670. (A) The dot plots show $Ig\kappa$ versus $Ig\lambda$ staining in the whole spleen for (left) bcl-2 tg versus (right) non-tg mice. (B) (left) Histograms show $Ig\lambda$ staining in the total spleen; (right) dot plots show $Ig\kappa$ versus $Ig\lambda$ staining within the $Ig\lambda^+$ gate (R2) on bcl-2 tg (top) versus non-tg (bottom) mice. Note: the region marked R3 is greatly expanded in the bcl-2 tg mice as compared to non-tg mice.

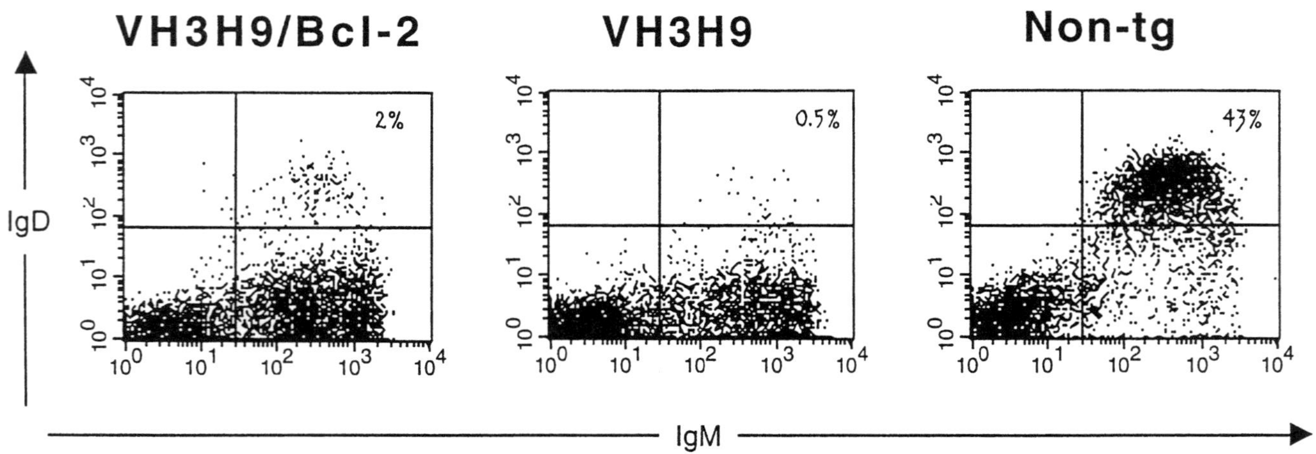

FIGURE 4. Endogenous heavy-chain expression in bcl-2 tg mice bearing an Ig tg. Spleen cells were stained with anti-IgD-biotin/streptavidin-Red670, anti-IgM-FITC, and anti-B220-PE. The dot plots show IgM versus IgD staining for non-tg (right), V_H3H9 tg (middle), or V_H3H9/bcl-2 tg (left) mice. Percentages are given for IgD^+ cells.

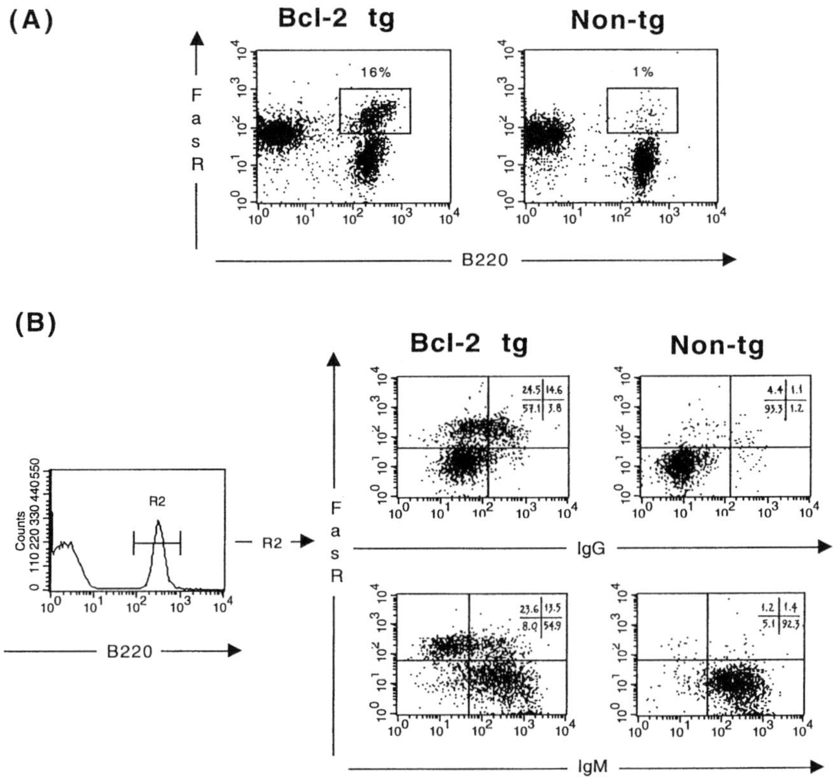

FIGURE 5. A subpopulation of B cells in the bcl-2 tg mouse expresses high levels of the Fas receptor. Lymph node cells were stained with anti-B220-biotin/streptavidin-Red670, anti-FasR-PE, anti-IgM-FITC, and/or anti-IgG-FITC. (A) Dot plots showing B220 versus FasR staining on lymphocytes from bcl-2 tg (left) versus non-tg mice (right). Percentages are shown for the boxed regions. (B) FasR levels on IgG$^+$ (upper plots) and IgM$^+$ (lower plots) B cells from bcl-2 tg (left) and non-tg (right) mice. The dot plots are gated on B220$^+$ cells.

age.[24] Preliminary data show evidence of ANA$^+$ specificities also in the serum of some bcl-2 tg mice in our study (n = 11; ages, 2–8 months). This is in contrast to the findings of Korsmeyer's group.[25,36]

CONCLUSIONS

We have shown in bcl-2 tg mice that the tg is expressed in all B cell developmental stages where endogenous bcl-2 is expressed. Importantly, the bcl-2 tg is also expressed at the pre-B, immature B, and GC B cell stages where endogenous bcl-2 is downregulated. These mice may be valuable sources of B cells at these critical checkpoints in selection, whose analysis can help us to understand the factors that dictate selection. Notably, there are FasR^{high} B cells present in bcl-2 tg mice that are not evident in non-tg mice. This is consistent with the ability of this bcl-2 tg to block FasR-mediated death *in vivo.* Another striking effect of the bcl-2 tg is the lack of light-chain isotype exclusion and possibly heavy-chain allelic exclusion. Currently, we are examining whether the presence of bcl-2 alters the expression of the recombinase genes, rag-1 and rag-2.

ACKNOWLEDGMENTS

We thank Anh Bui, Deepa Kurian, and Eden Haverfield for technical assistance.

REFERENCES

1. Izui, S., V. E. Kelley, K. Masuda, H. Yoshida, J. B. Roths & E. D. Murphy. 1984. Induction of various autoantibodies by mutant gene lpr in several strains of mice. J. Immunol. **133:** 227–233.
2. Cohen, P. L. & R. A. Eisenberg. 1991. Lpr and gld: single gene models of systemic autoimmunity and lymphoproliferative disease. Annu. Rev. Immunol. **9:** 243–269.
3. Theofilopoulos, A. N. & F. J. Dixon. 1985. Murine models of systemic lupus erythematosus. Adv. Immunol. **37:** 269–390.
4. Pisetsky, D. S., S. A. Caster, J. B. Roths & E. D. Murphy. 1982. *Lpr* gene control of the anti-DNA antibody response. J. Immunol. **128:** 2322–2325.
5. Watanabe-Fukunaga, R., C. I. Brannan, N. G. Copeland, N. A. Jenkins & S. Nagata. 1992. Lymphoproliferation disorder in mice explained by defects in Fas antigen that mediates apoptosis. Nature **356:** 314–317.
6. Chu, J-L., J. Drappa, A. Parnassa & K. B. Elkon. 1993. The defect in Fas mRNA expression in MRL/lpr mice is associated with insertion of the retrotransposon, Etn. J. Exp. Med. **178:** 723–730.
7. Wu, J., T. Zhou, J. He & J. D. Mountz. 1993. Autoimmune disease in mice due to integration of an endogenous retrovirus in an apoptosis gene. J. Exp. Med. **178:** 461–468.
8. Mandik, L., K-A. T. Nguyen & J. Erikson. 1995. Fas receptor expression on B-lineage cells. Eur. J. Immunol. **25:** 3148–3154.
9. Onel, K. B., C. L. Tucek-Szabo, D. Ashany, E. Lacy, J. Nikolic-Zugic & K. B. Elkon. 1995. Expression and function of the murine CD95/FasR/APO-1 receptor in relation to B cell ontogeny. Eur. J. Immunol. **25:** 2940–2947.
10. Drappa, J., N. Brot & K. B. Elkon. 1993. The Fas protein is expressed at high levels on CD4+CD8+ thymocytes and activated mature lymphocytes in normal mice, but not in the lupus-prone strain MRL-lpr/lpr. Proc. Natl. Acad. Sci. U.S.A. **90:** 10340–10344.
11. Rothstein, T. L., J. K. M. Wang, D. J. Panka, L. C. Foote, Z. Wang, B. Stanger, H. Cui, S-T. Ju & A. Marshak-Rothstein. 1995. Protection against Fas-dependent Th1-mediated apoptosis by antigen receptor engagement in B cells. Nature **374:** 163–165.
12. Wang, J., I. Tanuchi, Y. Maekawa, M. Howard, M. D. Cooper & T. Watanabe. 1996. Expression and function of Fas antigen on activated murine B cells. Eur. J. Immunol. **26:** 92–96.
13. Merino, R., L. Ding, D. J. Veis, S. J. Korsmeyer & G. Nunez. 1994. Developmental regulation of the bcl-2 protein and susceptibility to cell death in B lymphocytes. EMBO J. **13:** 683–691.
14. Hockenberry, D. M., M. Zutter, W. Hickey, M. Nahm & S. J. Korsmeyer. 1991. Bcl-2 protein is topographically restricted in tissues characterized by apoptotic cell death. Proc. Natl. Acad. Sci. U.S.A. **88:** 6961–6965.
15. Liu, Y-J., D. Y. Mason, G. D. Johnson, S. Abbot, C. D. Gregory, D. L. Hardie, J. Gordon & I. M. MacLennan. 1991. Germinal center B cells express bcl-2 protein after activation signals which prevent their entry into apoptosis. Eur. J. Immunol. **21:** 1905–1910.

16. TSUJIMOTO, Y., L. R. FINGER, J. YUNIS, P. C. NOWELL & C. M. CROCE. 1984. Cloning of the chromosome breakpoint of neoplastic B cells with the t(14;18) translocation. Science **226:** 1097–1099.
17. BAKHSHI, A., J. P. JENSEN, P. GOLDMAN, J. J. WRIGHT, O. W. MCBRIDE, A. L. EPSTEIN & S. J. KORSMEYER. 1985. Cloning the chromosomal breakpoint of t(14;18) human lymphomas: clustering around J_H on chromosome 14 and near a transcriptional unit of 18. Cell **41:** 899–906.
18. CORY, S. 1995. Regulation of lymphocyte survival by the bcl-2 gene family. Annu. Rev. Immunol. **13:** 513–543.
19. ITOH, N., Y. TSUJIMOTO & S. NAGATA. 1993. Effect of bcl-2 on Fas antigen-mediated cell death. J. Immunol. **151:** 621–627.
20. ENARI, M., A. HASE & S. NAGATA. 1995. Apoptosis by a cytosolic extract from Fas-activated cells. EMBO J. **14:** 5201–5208.
21. CHIU, V. K., C. M. WALSH, C-C. LIU, J. C. REED & W. R. CLARK. 1995. Bcl-2 blocks degranulation, but not Fas-based cell-mediated cytotoxicity. J. Immunol. **154:** 2023–2032.
22. LACRONIQUE, V., A. MIGNON, M. FABRE, B. VIOLLET, N. ROUQUET, T. MOLINA, A. PORTEU, A. HENRION, D. BOUSCARY, P. VARLET, V. JOULIN & A. KAHN. 1996. Bcl-2 protects from lethal hepatic apoptosis induced by an anti-Fas antibody in mice. Nature Med. **2:** 80–86.
23. RODRIGUEZ, I., K. MATSUURA, K. KHATIB, J. C. REED, S. NAGATA & P. VASSALLI. 1996. A bcl-2 transgene expressed in hepatocytes protects mice from fulminant liver destruction, but not from rapid death induced by anti-Fas antibody injection. J. Exp. Med. **183:** 1031–1036.
24. STRASSER, A., S. WHITTINGHAM, D. L. VAUX, M. L. BATH, J. M. ADAMS, S. CORY & A. W. HARRIS. 1991. Enforced bcl-2 expression in B-lymphoid cells prolongs antibody response and elicits autoimmune disease. Proc. Natl. Acad. Sci. U.S.A. **88:** 8661–8665.
25. MCDONNELL, T. J., N. DEANE, F. M. PLATT, G. NUNEZ, U. JAEGER, J. P. MCKEARN & S. J. KORSMEYER. 1989. Bcl-2-immunoglobulin transgenic mice demonstrate extended B cell survival and follicular lymphoproliferation. Cell **57:** 79–88.
26. KATSUMATA, M., R. M. SIEGEL, D. C. LOUIE, T. MIYASHITA, Y. TSUJIMOTO, P. C. NOWELL, M. I. GREENE & J. C. REED. 1992. Differential effects of bcl-2 on T and B cells in transgenic mice. Proc. Natl. Acad. Sci. U.S.A. **89:** 11376–11380.
27. YEH, T-M., S. J. KORSMEYER & J. M. TEALE. 1991. Skewed B cell V_H family repertoire in bcl-2-Ig transgenic mice. Int. Immunol. **3:** 1329–1333.
28. HARTLEY, S. B., M. P. COOKE, D. A. FULCHER, A. W. HARRIS, S. CORY, A. BASTEN & C. C. GOODNOW. 1993. Elimination of self-reactive B lymphocytes proceeds in two stages: arrested development and cell death. Cell **72:** 325–335.
29. NISITANI, S., T. TSUBATA, M. MURAKAMI, M. OKAMOTO & T. HONJO. 1993. The bcl-2 gene product inhibits clonal deletion of self-reactive B lymphocytes in the periphery, but not in the bone marrow. J. Exp. Med. **178:** 1247–1254.
30. ERIKSON, J., M. Z. RADIC, S. A. CAMPER, R. R. HARDY, C. CARMACK & M. WEIGERT. 1991. Expression of anti-DNA immunoglobulin transgenes in non-autoimmune mice. Nature **349:** 331–334.
31. HARDY, R. R., C. E. CARMACK, S. A. SHINTON, J. D. KEMP & K. HAYAKAWA. 1991. Resolution and characterization of pro-B and pre-B cell stages in normal mouse bone marrow. J. Exp. Med. **173:** 1213–1225.
32. REAP, E. A., N. J. FELIX, P. A. WOLTHUSEN, B. L. KOTZIN, P. L. COHEN & R. A. EISENBERG. 1995. Bcl-2 transgenic mice show profound enhancement of lymphadenopathy. J. Immunol. **155:** 5455–5462.
33. STRASSER, A., A. W. HARRIS, D. L. VAUX, E. WEBB, M. L. BATH, J. M. ADAMS & S. CORY. 1990. Abnormalities of the immune system induced by dysregulated bcl-2 expression in transgenic mice. Curr. Top. Microbiol. Immunol. **166:** 175–181.
34. TARLINTON, D., A. STRASSER, M. MCLEAN & A. BASTEN. 1995. D_H element reading frame selection is influenced by an Ig heavy chain transgene, but not by bcl-2. J. Immunol. **154:** 3341–3350.
35. STRASSER, A., A. W. HARRIS & S. CORY. 1991. Bcl-2 transgene inhibits T cell death and perturbs thymic self-censorship. Cell **67:** 889–899.

36. McDonnell, T. J., G. Nunez, F. M. Platt, D. Hockenberry, L. London, J. P. McKearn & S. J. Korsmeyer. 1990. Deregulated bcl-2-immunoglobulin transgene expands a resting, but responsive immunoglobulin M and D–expressing B cell population. Mol. Cell. Biol. **10:** 1901–1907.
37. Pauza, M. E., J. A. Rehmann & T. W. LeBien. 1993. Unusual patterns of immunoglobulin gene rearrangement and expression during human B cell ontogeny: human B cells can simultaneously express surface κ and λ light chains. J. Exp. Med. **178:** 139–149.
38. Roark, J. H., C. L. Kuntz, K-A. Nguyen, A. J. Caton & J. Erikson. 1995. Breakdown of B cell tolerance in a mouse model of SLE. J. Exp. Med. **181:** 1157–1167.
39. Tsao, B. P., K. Ohnishi, H. Cheroutre, B. Mitchell, M. Teitell, P. Mixter, M. Kronenberg & B. H. Hahn. 1992. Failed self-tolerance and autoimmunity in IgG anti-DNA transgenic mice. J. Immunol. **149:** 350–358.
40. Offen, D., L. Spatz, H. Escowitz, S. Factor & B. Diamond. 1992. Induction of tolerance to an IgG autoantibody. Proc. Natl. Acad. Sci. U.S.A. **89:** 8332–8336.
41. Imanishi-Kari, T., S. Bandyopadhay, P. Busto & C. A. Huang. 1993. Endogenous Ig production in μ transgenic mice. J. Immunol. **150:** 3311–3326.
42. Strasser, A., A. W. Harris, D. C. S. Huang, P. H. Krammer & S. Cory. 1995. Bcl-2 and Fas/APO-1 regulate distinct pathways to lymphocyte apoptosis. EMBO J. **14:** 6136–6147.
43. Tan, E. M. 1989. Antinuclear antibodies: diagnostic markers for autoimmune diseases and probes for cell biology. Adv. Immunol. **44:** 93–151.

Balancing Immunity, Autoimmunity, and Self-tolerance[a]

CHRISTOPHER C. GOODNOW

Howard Hughes Medical Institute
and
Department of Microbiology and Immunology
Stanford University School of Medicine
Stanford, California 94305

INTRODUCTION

Burnet's concept[1] of deleting self-reactive clones from the preimmune repertoire, leaving only nonself-reactive clones to fight infection, poses a central problem of balancing the opposing needs of self-tolerance and immunity. As pointed out by Nossal,[2] clonal deletion must logically have an affinity cutoff to avoid deleting most of the potential repertoire of B or T cells (FIGURE 1). The fact that self-reactive B and T cell clones can be found among circulating cells in the preimmune repertoire of healthy individuals and can be induced into autoaggression by particular immunization regimes has at various times been interpreted as either (a) the footprints of self-reactive clones that fall below the deletion cutoff or (b) evidence that self-tolerance is not acquired by clonal deletion at all.

Resolving how self-tolerance is actually acquired—and balanced against the need to fight infection—has depended on developing ways to track the fate of individual B or T lymphocyte clones within a diverse preimmune repertoire. Elucidation of the process for generating antibody and T cell receptor diversity in the 1980s finally provided two ways: (1) by following superantigen-reactive T cells bearing particular Vβ elements and (2) by following antigen-specific cells after elevating their frequency by fixing the diversity-generating machinery through introduction of prerearranged antibody H and L or TCR α and β transgenes. Examples of the B cell repertoires that result from fixing either H-chain diversity or both H- and L-chain diversity in antibody-transgenic mice are shown in FIGURE 2, panels D and B, respectively. This transgenic approach has turned out to have tremendous scope, particularly when combined with the ability to engineer by transgenesis new antigens that are expressed as part of the genetic self in different forms, concentrations, and tissue locations. Collectively, this ability to visualize repertoire selection *in vivo* has, first, confirmed the hypothesis that self-tolerance is acquired in part by clonal deletion. Second, these transgenic windows have provided views into a much more sophisticated process of clonal deletion and anergy than could have been imagined, presumably designed to

[a]This review has been adapted from a chapter by C. C. Goodnow in the CIBA Foundation Symposium, "The Molecular Basis of Cellular Defense Mechanisms", with permission from the CIBA Foundation.

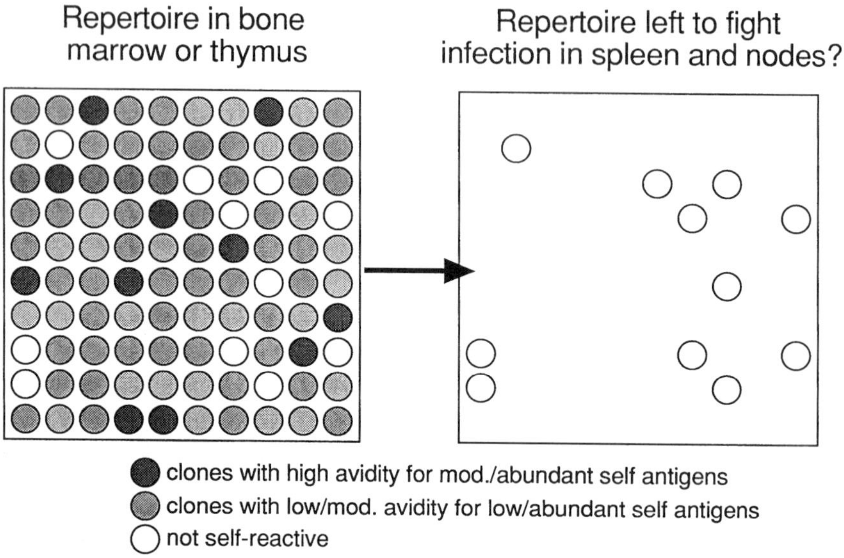

FIGURE 1. A schematic illustrating Burnet's model for acquisition of self-tolerance and the problem it poses for balancing tolerance and immunity.

balance self-tolerance by clonal deletion against the need to draw upon clonal diversity to fight infection. This review focuses on data from my laboratory relevant to the balance between immunity and tolerance; comprehensive reviews of the topic are published elsewhere.[3,4]

CLONAL DELETION THRESHOLDS

FIGURES 2D–2I show several examples of clonal deletion of self-reactive B cells, visualized in mice where H-chain diversity has been fixed by introducing a prerearranged H-chain transgene (Tg) encoding an antilysozyme antibody. In H-chain Tg mice where hen egg lysozyme (HEL) is genetically foreign (FIGURES 2D and 2H), subpopulations of B cells can be readily visualized in the spleen that bind lysozyme with distinct apparent affinities ranging from 10^{-9} M to less than 10^{-5} M, by pairing the transgenic H chain with different endogenous light chains.[5] By contrast, in H-chain Tg mice that have also inherited an HEL gene as part of the genetic self and thus express 1 nM soluble HEL in the bloodstream, the highest affinity self-reactive B cells are selectively deleted, whereas lower affinity cells are spared (FIGURE 2E).[6] Inheritance of a different HEL gene construct, with a different promoter and 10-fold higher circulating HEL, results in deletion of the highest affinity B cells and the lower affinity cells (FIGURE 2F).[6] The majority of HEL-binding B cells in these H-chain Tg mice nevertheless bind HEL with even lower affinity, so their receptors only saturate with monovalent HEL when 10–50 μM concentrations are used to stain and visualize them (FIGURE 2H). These very low affinity cells escape deletion by sHEL, but are

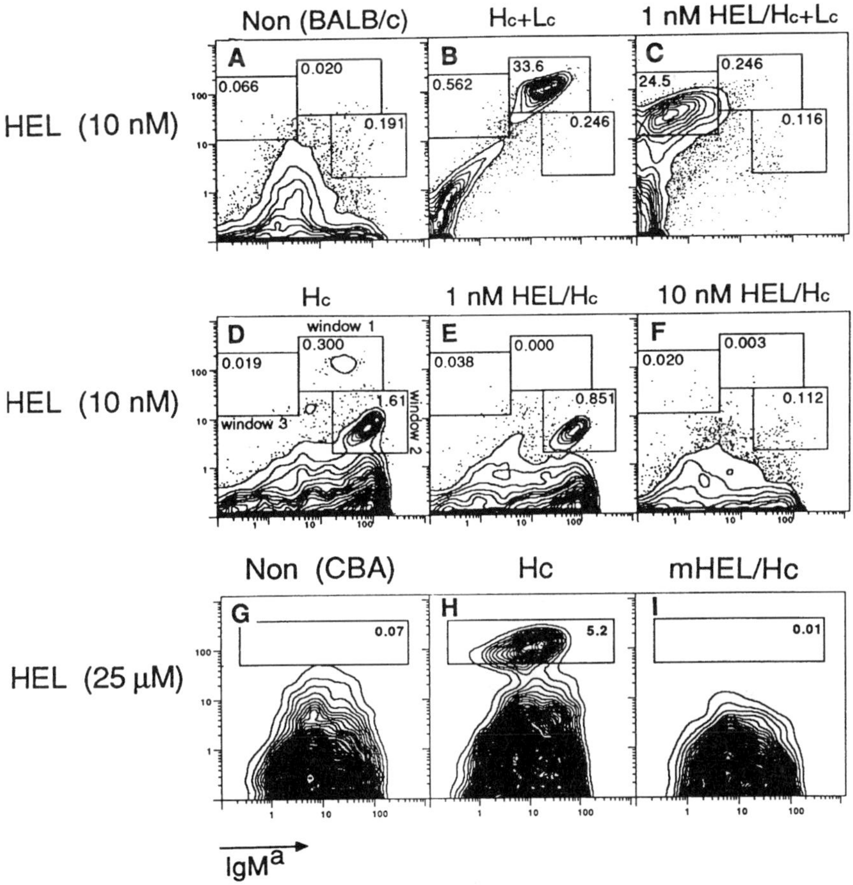

FIGURE 2. Visualization of self-reactive B cell clonal deletion and clonal anergy. Each panel shows spleen cells from different mice, stained by two-color immunofluorescence for cell surface IgM of the a-allotype (IgM^a) on the x-axis and for binding of HEL antigen on the y-axis. The concentration of HEL used to stain the cells is indicated. The upper row shows the rarity of high affinity HEL-binding B cells in the repertoire of normal mice (A), and the high frequency and homogeneity of HEL-binding B cells that result when both H- and L-chain diversity are fixed by H- and L-chain transgenes (B). In a littermate mouse that has also inherited a transgene producing soluble HEL self-antigen at 1 nM in serum as part of its genetic makeup (C), this homogeneous HEL-specific population is not deleted, but downregulates cell surface IgM as part of the desensitization process. The middle row shows the small subsets of high and medium affinity HEL-binding B cells present in an otherwise diverse repertoire when only the H-chain diversity is fixed by transgenesis (D). In a littermate mouse that has also inherited the gene producing 1 nM of serum HEL (E), the high affinity HEL-binding subset is deleted (window 1), but the medium affinity subset (window 2) is spared. The latter cells are nevertheless deleted when they develop in a mouse carrying an HEL gene with a different promoter that expresses 10-fold higher serum HEL (F). The bottom row (G–I) shows the entire pool of low, medium, and high affinity HEL-binding cells present in an H-chain transgenic mouse, revealed by staining with a very high concentration of HEL antigen (H). All of these B cells are deleted when they develop in a mouse carrying an HEL gene that has been modified to express HEL on the surface of neighboring cells in the bone marrow (mHEL) (I), where the array of self-antigen is recognized with high avidity. Data in panels A–F are reprinted from reference 6 with permission of MacMillan Magazines. Data in panels G–H are reprinted from reference 5 with permission of Oxford University Press.

eliminated in mice that inherit a third type of HEL transgene encoding the protein in a membrane-bound form (mHEL)[7] on the surface of cells exposed to the bloodstream (FIGURE 2I).[8] The membrane-bound lattice of self-antigen presumably cross-links HEL-binding surface immunoglobulins on B cells much more efficiently than the soluble form, so this increased avidity compensates for low intrinsic affinity.

Collectively, these results illustrate the fact that deletion of self-reactive clones is limited by thresholds determined by the amount of self-antigen and by the affinity and avidity with which a clone binds it. These thresholds have probably been set over evolutionary time by opposing forces that select for rapid antibody responses against infectious pathogens on the one hand and for minimal destruction of autologous tissues on the other. For example, stringent deletion of low affinity self-reactive B cells that recognize blood-cell surface antigens is almost certainly essential to survival because secretion even of low affinity, but high avidity, IgM antibodies to ABO carbohydrates would have devastating consequences in individuals whose erythrocytes and endothelium bore the corresponding antigens. By contrast, transient production of low or moderate avidity autoantibodies to oligovalent antigens dissolved in blood plasma, such as low affinity rheumatoid factors, appears tolerable in the short term due to the capacity of complement and the reticuloendothelial system to clear such immune complexes without serious immune pathology. Preserving such clones in the preimmune repertoire may be advantageous, by allowing them to be drawn upon immediately after infection if no other clone is available.

CLONAL ANERGY: ANTIGEN RECEPTOR DOWNREGULATION AND DESENSITIZATION

FIGURE 2 also shows an example of clonal anergy, an alternative strategy for acquiring self-tolerance in clones that bind to self at intermediate levels. In the example shown, the entire B cell repertoire has been fixed to have homogeneous HEL-reactivity by introducing prerearranged H- and L-chain transgenes (panel B). In a mouse that has inherited the sHEL gene as part of its genetic self, the HEL-reactive B cells are not deleted, but instead have decreased their surface IgM antigen receptor density by some 20-fold (panel C).[9] Interestingly, this is achieved not by decreasing IgM synthesis, but by blocking its egress from the endoplasmic reticulum.[10] The majority of HEL-binding receptors remaining on the self-reactive cells are of the IgD class. These are not blocked in their intracellular transport and are expressed on the surface in normal numbers;[9,10] however, they have a greatly reduced capacity to activate tyrosine phosphorylation of their intracellular ITAMs or of the pp72^{syk} tyrosine kinase, which together play essential roles in B cell antigen receptor signaling and activation.[11]

As a result of antigen receptor downregulation and desensitization, anergic self-reactive B cells cannot be triggered into mitosis through their antigen receptors by T-cell-independent routes of activation, and they require much more avid receptor cross-linking to induce CD86/B7.2 on their surface and to cooperate successfully with helper T cells.[9,11] Self-reactive B cells continually exposed to the moderate avidity soluble HEL self-antigen thus become functionally tolerant to that ligand much in the same way that cells become tolerant when chronically exposed to drugs or hormones, which is well known to involve receptor downregulation and desensitization.

Preserving clones in this desensitized state is an alternative strategy to balance tolerance and immunity because these cells can be called into clonal expansion and

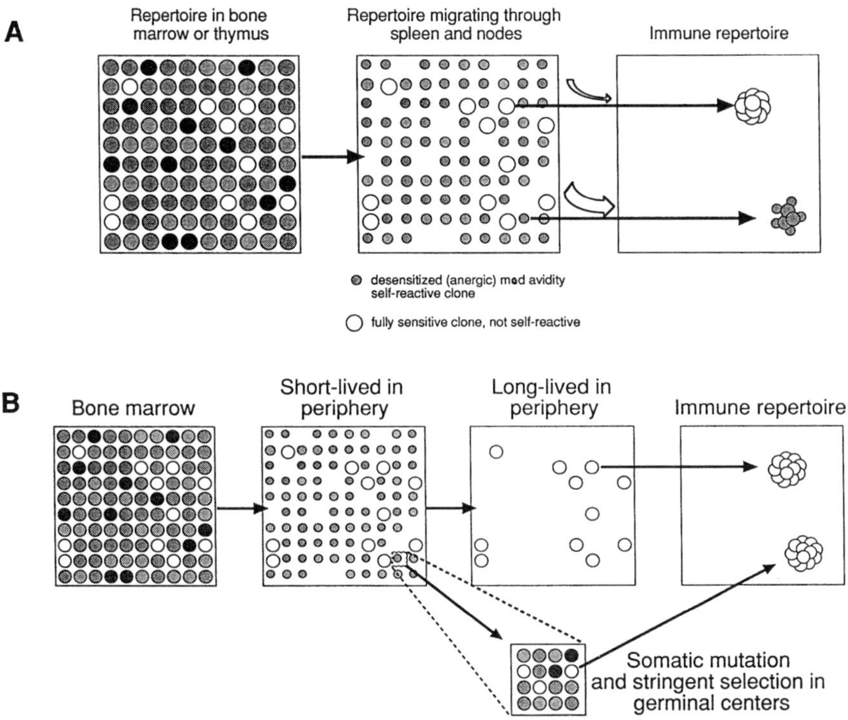

FIGURE 3. A schematic illustrating how B cell desensitization and peripheral deletion help to balance tolerance with autoimmunity. (A) High avidity self-reactive clones (dark gray) are deleted in the bone marrow so that they cannot participate in immune responses, whereas moderate avidity self-reactive clones (light gray) are exported to the spleen and lymph nodes in a desensitized self-tolerant state. The latter can be drawn nevertheless into a primary nonanamnestic antibody response, although they are absolutely dependent on cognate help from T cells and require a much stronger antigen receptor stimulus, and their net clonal expansion is markedly reduced. (B) Moderate avidity self-reactive clones are also filtered out in the periphery by competition for primary follicle niches, blocking their survival and recirculation so that the long-lived recirculating repertoire becomes dominated by clones with minimal self-reactivity. Moderate avidity self-reactive clones can also potentially be recruited into germinal centers in secondary follicles, where somatic hypermutation and stringent negative and positive selection can give rise to variants that have lost their self-reactivity.

antibody secretion if the need is great enough (FIGURE 3A). For that to happen, however, tolerant B cells must suddenly bind much more avidly to a foreign antigen such as membrane HEL and must immediately collaborate with nontolerant helper T cells.[11] Under those particular conditions, clonal expansion of desensitized self-reactive clones will nevertheless be rapidly overshadowed if any nonself-reactive clones are present with comparable avidity for the inciting foreign antigen because the receptors on the latter are not desensitized and, consequently, they proliferate approximately 10-fold more.[11] Transient production of low avidity autoantibodies at the outset of infection may thus be a small cost to pay for preserving repertoire diversity.

CLONAL DELETION TAKES PLACE AT SEVERAL DISTINCT CHECKPOINTS

Deletion of self-reactive B cells that bind with high avidity to self-antigens, as occurs in mice that inherit the mHEL form of antigen (FIGURE 2I), occurs in the bone marrow by developmental arrest and apoptosis, so as to render these clones completely unavailable for antibody responses.[8] By contrast, self-reactive cells that recognize the moderate avidity sHEL antigen in the H-chain Tg mice in FIGURES 2E and 2F are deleted in a different way and in a distinctly different site.[6] In this case, deletion of self-reactive B cells occurs after the cells have matured, become desensitized to sHEL, and emigrated from the bone marrow to the white pulp cords of the spleen or the paracortex of lymph nodes. After entering these peripheral lymphoid sites, the self-reactive B cells fail to continue their normal migration route into primary follicles and become stuck in the outer T cell zones, where they die prematurely by apoptosis within 1–3 days. Follicular exclusion depends on competition among B cells of different specificities, probably through a change in the relative tropism of the B cells towards an unknown set of migration cues that is brought about by continued antigen receptor signaling.[6,12] Interestingly, the antigen receptor signals that induce this change in migratory behavior involve intracellular signaling pathways that are not affected by receptor downregulation and desensitization.

Primary follicles in spleen and lymph node thus appear to function as filters in the preimmune repertoire, preferentially excluding moderate avidity self-antigen-binding B cells so that the accumulating long-lived repertoire becomes dominated by the least self-reactive clones available, even if these are initially produced at low frequency in the bone marrow (FIGURE 3B). Because the short-lived self-reactive cells that are excluded from recirculation are nevertheless transiently available to be drawn upon in the T zones, through reactivation by foreign antigens bound with high avidity (see above), deletion at this stage and site strikes a further balance between tolerance and immunity. Filtering B cells at the point of follicular entry appears to make a large impact on the repertoire of normal animals because a large fraction of B cells that are exported from the bone marrow are eliminated within 1–3 days in the same site and pattern once the recirculating pool has reached its mature size.[13] Moreover, the repertoire that is retained as long-lived recirculating cells in the adult is markedly skewed in V-region use, except when there are insufficient B cells to support such a competitive filtering process.[14,15]

When excluded self-reactive clones do become reactivated and drawn into clonal expansion by T cells in the T zone, a fraction of their progeny may enter the germinal centers of secondary follicles where further receptor diversification by somatic hypermutation occurs. Indeed, HEL-binding B cells that are activated by a cross-reactive foreign antigen can enter germinal centers of mice that express soluble HEL as genetic self, but are then eliminated very efficiently within these structures (K. Shokat & C. C. Goodnow, unpublished data). Deletion of self-reactive B cells occurs within germinal centers by a process of rapid cell death that can be mimicked by administering exogenous HEL antigen in soluble form.[16] Because the germinal center also positively selects emerging clones that bind more avidly to foreign antigens displayed by follicular dendritic cells, the germinal center output of mutated memory B cells and long-lived plasma cells is thus simultaneously enriched for antiforeign and stringently depleted of self-reactivity (FIGURE 3B). These clones come to dominate antibody responses, accounting for the exquisite fine specificity for foreign immunizing antigens and the lack of self-reactivity that are hallmarks of memory-type antibodies.

The effect of these filters in primary and secondary follicles is that self-reactive B cells are stringently deleted from the final immune repertoire of secreted antibodies and memory cells. Because these clones are deleted in a stepwise manner at multiple stages in the periphery rather than all at one step in the bone marrow, a more efficient balance is struck between tolerance and immunity because intermediate avidity self-reactive clones are still available: (A) to be drawn into primary nonanamnestic antibody responses in the T zones, where their immediate benefit in neutralizing microorganisms may outweigh any transient risk of immunopathology; and (B) to be drawn into germinal centers, where hypermutation and stringent selection can remove unwanted self-reactivity before contributing to the high-titer, long-lived anamnestic antibody response (FIGURE 3).

DECIDING B CELL FATE AT EACH CHECKPOINT

The fact that self-reactive B cells are deleted in the T zones and in germinal centers, perhaps more than in the bone marrow, focuses attention on the question of how clones passing through each checkpoint decide whether to adopt either a tolerant fate and die or an immune fate and proliferate.

Cues Deciding B Cell Fate in the Bone Marrow

In the bone marrow, B cells appear to use timing as a cue much as originally envisaged by Burnet[1] and Lederberg[17] (FIGURE 4A): if they are continually binding an antigen at this immature stage in their development, they are probably self-reactive. Indeed, immature B cells appear almost hardwired to respond to chronic antigen exposure by arresting their development, inhibiting their proliferative potential, and dying if antigenic stimulation is sustained.[2,8] The other chief factor determining B cell fate at this stage is the amount and avidity of the antigen bound. More antigen and greater cross-linking will result in a progressively increased magnitude of intracellular signaling to nuclear pathways such as ERK, NFκB, and JNK in B cells (J. Healy & C. C. Goodnow, unpublished data), and differences in the amount of these or other signals to the nucleus probably determine the extent to which B cells are terminated in the bone marrow.

The phosphorylation cascade from the antigen receptor to the nucleus is normally tuned so that only high avidity self-reactive B cells achieve a sufficient signal that they are arrested and deleted in the bone marrow, whereas clones with lower avidity have only a low rumble within them and are retained for export to the periphery. The importance of inheriting the right tuning set-point is illustrated by mouse mutations in two protein tyrosine phosphatases, SHP-1 (PTP1C) and CD45, that regulate the

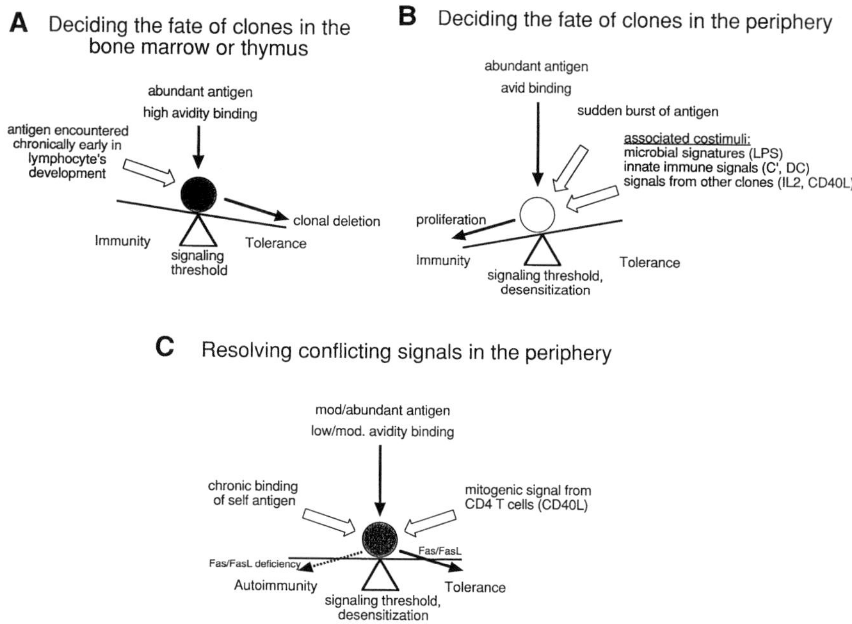

FIGURE 4. A schematic illustrating the interplay of cues that guide the decision between immunity and tolerance in immature and mature lymphocytes.

intracellular signaling response to antigen in B cells. HEL-specific B cells carrying a loss-of-function mutation in SHP-1, from the moth-eaten viable strain, mount an exaggerated intracellular calcium response to antigen demonstrating that SHP-1 normally tunes down this response.[18] Self-reactive cells with this signal-exaggerating mutation are developmentally arrested and deleted in the bone marrow if they develop in a mouse that has inherited the soluble HEL gene, encoding a moderate avidity autoantigen that only deletes at later checkpoints in the periphery under normal circumstances. Moreover, in the absence of any HEL ligand, the PTP1C-deficient B cells spontaneously downregulate their IgM receptors as they mature, suggesting that ligand-independent signaling by the antigen receptor complex occurs when SHP-1 is not present to oppose intrinsically active tyrosine kinases such as $pp72^{syk}$. Deletion of moderate avidity self-reactive B cells in the bone marrow as a result of exaggerated antigen receptor signaling is likely to explain the marked deficiency of mature recirculating B cells that occurs in moth-eaten viable mice.[18]

By contrast with SHP-1 deficiency, HEL-specific B cells lacking the CD45 tyrosine phosphatase have diminished intracellular calcium and ERK responses to antigen, confirming that the CD45 phosphatase tunes up signaling by antigen receptors.[19] Clonal selection of B cells with this signal-depressing mutation is also altered in the opposite direction. Thus, whereas CD45-deficient B cells are still deleted in the bone marrow if they develop in mice carrying the high avidity mHEL self-antigen, they are positively selected into the long-lived peripheral pool instead of being filtered out when they develop in mice carrying the moderate avidity sHEL autoantigen. In the absence of an exogenous HEL ligand, CD45-deficient HEL-specific B cells fail to persist after emigrating from the bone marrow, suggesting that a low level of tonic signaling by the antigen receptor may be necessary for mature B cells to stay alive and recirculate. When signaling is depressed by the CD45 mutation, the low tonic survival signal is only generated when soluble HEL autoantigen binds with moderate avidity. As a result, the recirculating repertoire is skewed in favor of moderate avidity self-reactive clones and away from the nonself-reactive cells that would normally be favored. The CD45-dependent signal that favors survival of mature B cells carrying the transgenic receptor may in principle have two origins: (1) it may result from basal ligand-independent tyrosine kinase activity associated with surface Ig; (2) it may result from weak engagement of the antigen receptors by some endogenous or exogenous antigen or ligand.

Cues Deciding B Cell Fate in the Periphery

Mature B cells use timing and costimuli as cues to determine whether to adopt an immune or tolerant fate (FIGURE 4B). Costimulatory cues—the body's red flags of infection—can come from (1) microbes themselves, such as LPS or double-stranded RNA; (2) the innate immune system, such as the complement fragment, C3d; or (3) other lymphocytes such as CD40L and IL4 from helper T cells. When these costimuli are coupled with an antigenic stimulus that appears as a sudden burst, this combination of timing and costimuli are both characteristic cues for infectious antigens and act in concert as cues to drive B cells into clonal expansion and antibody production (FIGURE 4B). By contrast, when antigen appears both in a constant monotonous way and in the absence of any costimulatory red flags, these are both characteristic presentations for self-antigens. In this case, mature B cells take these as cues to adopt tolerant fates either by desensitizing and downregulating their receptors[20] or by dying as a result of follicular exclusion.[12,16]

Moderate avidity self-tolerant B cells that chronically bind self-antigens—so that they desensitize their receptors and become trapped in the T zones—must nevertheless face conflicting cues frequently. The most common of these conflicting circumstances arises when a mature self-tolerant B cell, by virtue of its self-reactivity, has captured a foreign antigen through its association with a self-antigen. Examples include the capture by self-tolerant B cells of (a) virions whose envelopes are decorated with self-proteins and carbohydrates; (b) viral DNA binding proteins that are firmly attached to autologous chromatin; or (c) bacterial or viral antigens that are complexed with autologous IgG. In each case, B cells that bind the self-component of these complexes will present the foreign peptide moieties to nontolerant helper T cells in the T zones, eliciting CD40L expression on the T cells. At this stage, the B cell is faced with conflicting cues (FIGURE 4C). On the one hand, prior chronic antigen binding implies self-reactivity; on the other hand, though, reception of the mitogenic CD40L signal implies reactivity with infectious nonself. Desensitized self-reactive B cells that are trapped in the T zone in fact respond efficiently to CD40L,[11,21] potentially setting them on the course to clonal expansion.

The interacting pair of cell surface molecules, FasL and Fas (CD95), appear to function by resolving these conflicting cues to ensure that T cell help is not delivered inappropriately to self-tolerant B cells. This role of Fas and FasL is demonstrated by the outcome of *in vivo* interactions[22] between HEL-specific CD4 T cells and either nontolerant HEL-specific B cells that have grown up in animals where HEL was not part of the genetic self or tolerant (anergic) HEL-specific B cells that have grown up in the face of chronic receptor engagement by soluble HEL self-antigen.

When nontolerant B cells suddenly encounter HEL antigen just before interacting with T cells in an adoptive transfer, the B cells first become activated as judged by high expression of the T cell costimulatory molecule, CD86 (B7.2), and then are triggered into extensive clonal expansion and antibody production in a manner that is substantially dependent on CD40L.[12,18,22,23] Fas comes to be expressed at high levels on the initially naive B cells during their interactions with the T cells, but Fas does not trigger apoptosis in this context.[23] By contrast, HEL-tolerant B cells that have grown up chronically exposed to HEL do not become activated to express CD86 (B7.2) when they bind more HEL antigen, although they present HEL peptides efficiently.[11,12,24] Upon interaction with HEL-specific T cells, the self-tolerant B cells begin to activate in a CD40L-dependent manner and upregulate Fas, but FasL on the T cell then aborts the process by triggering their death. When the genes encoding Fas or FasL are defective in the B and T cell, respectively, CD40L-dependent activation of the self-tolerant B cells cannot be aborted and the cells proceed into cell cycle.[22,23]

Fas is thus expressed both on nontolerant B cells that have been acutely activated by antigen and T cells and on self-tolerant B cells that have been faced with the conflicting combination of prior chronic antigen exposure and the acute appearance of cognate T cell help. Fas only aborts clonal expansion of the self-tolerant cells, however, because their desensitized antigen receptors can no longer transmit signals that normally block Fas-induced death. The real-life importance of resolving this conflict is driven home by the severe autoantibody disorders that occur (rarely) in children with Fas deficiency[25,26] and by the massive accumulation of autoantibody-producing B cells in the T zones of mice with Fas deficiency.[27]

CLOSING COMMENTS

The glimpses into tolerance and how it is balanced with immunity, which I have summarized here, illustrate how the different tools now available for genetic analysis in mice can illuminate this complex physiological process. The use of transgenic animals allows repertoire diversity to be fixed in many different ways, enabling specific cells to be tracked in their native context. Transgenesis also enables new antigens to be added to the constellation encoded as genetic self and allows systematic changes in the way these antigens are presented to the immune system. The greatest opportunity for illuminating the balance between tolerance and immunity, however, comes from using these tools to pinpoint the effects of spontaneous and induced mutations in key molecules in the selection circuitry, illustrated by the SHP-1, CD45, FasL/Fas, and CD40L mutations discussed here. The key limitation to this approach currently lies in the very small number of strong, single-locus mutations known to affect tolerance and selection.

REFERENCES

1. BURNET, F. M. 1957. The Clonal Selection Theory of Acquired Immunity. Vanderbilt University Press. Nashville.
2. NOSSAL, G. J. V. 1983. Cellular mechanisms of immunologic tolerance. Annu. Rev. Immunol. **1:** 33–62.
3. GOODNOW, C. C., J. G. CYSTER, S. B. HARTLEY, S. E. BELL, M. P. COOKE, J. I. HEALY, S. AKKARAJU, J. C. RATHMELL, S. L. POGUE & K. M. SHOKAT. 1995. Self-tolerance checkpoints in B lymphocyte development. Adv. Immunol. **59:** 279–368.
4. GOODNOW, C. C. 1996. Balancing immunity and tolerance: deleting and tuning lymphocyte repertoires. Proc. Natl. Acad. Sci. U.S.A. **93:** 2264–2271.
5. HARTLEY, S. B. & C. C. GOODNOW. 1994. Censoring of self-reactive B cells with a range of receptor affinities in transgenic mice expressing heavy chains for a lysozyme-specific antibody. Int. Immunol. **6:** 1417–1425.
6. CYSTER, J. G., S. B. HARTLEY & C. C. GOODNOW. 1994. Competition for follicular niches excludes self-reactive cells from the recirculating B-cell repertoire. Nature **371:** 389–395.
7. HARTLEY, S. B., J. CROSBIE, R. BRINK, A. B. KANTOR, A. BASTEN & C. C. GOODNOW. 1991. Elimination from peripheral lymphoid tissues of self-reactive B lymphocytes recognizing membrane-bound antigens. Nature **353:** 765–768.
8. HARTLEY, S. B., M. P. COOKE, D. A. FULCHER, A. W. HARRIS, S. CORY, A. BASTEN & C. C. GOODNOW. 1993. Elimination of self-reactive B lymphocytes proceeds in two stages: arrested development and cell death. Cell **72:** 325–335.
9. GOODNOW, C. C., J. CROSBIE, S. ADELSTEIN, T. B. LAVOIE, S. J. SMITH-GILL, R. A. BRINK, H. PRITCHARD-BRISCOE, J. S. WOTHERSPOON, R. H. LOBLAY, K. RAPHAEL, R. J. TRENT & A. BASTEN. 1988. Altered immunoglobulin expression and functional silencing of self-reactive B lymphocytes in transgenic mice. Nature **334:** 676–682.
10. BELL, S. E. & C. C. GOODNOW. 1994. A selective defect in IgM antigen receptor synthesis and transport causes loss of cell surface IgM expression on tolerant B lymphocytes. EMBO J. **13:** 816–826.
11. COOKE, M. P., A. W. HEATH, K. M. SHOKAT, Y. ZENG, F. D. FINKELMAN, P. S. LINSLEY, M. HOWARD & C. C. GOODNOW. 1994. Immunoglobulin signal transduction guides the specificity of B cell–T cell interactions and is blocked in tolerant self-reactive B cells. J. Exp. Med. **179:** 425–438.

12. CYSTER, J. G. & C. C. GOODNOW. 1995. Antigen-induced exclusion from follicles and anergy are separate and complementary processes that influence peripheral B cell fate. Immunity **3:** 691–701.
13. CHAN, E. Y-T. & I. C. M. MACLENNAN. 1993. Only a small proportion of splenic B cells in adults are short-lived virgin cells. Eur. J. Immunol. **23:** 357–363.
14. MALYNN, B. A., G. D. YANCOPOULOS, J. E. BARTH, C. A. BONA & F. W. ALT. 1990. Biased expression of J_H-proximal V_H genes occurs in the newly generated repertoire of neonatal and adult mice. J. Exp. Med. **171:** 843–859.
15. GU, H., D. TARLINTON, W. MÜLLER, K. RAJEWSKY & I. FORSTER. 1991. Most peripheral B cells in mice are ligand-selected. J. Exp. Med. **173:** 1357–1371.
16. SHOKAT, K. M. & C. C. GOODNOW. 1995. Antigen-induced B cell death and elimination during germinal center immune responses. Nature **375:** 334–338.
17. LEDERBERG, J. 1959. Genes and antibodies. Science **129:** 1649–1653.
18. CYSTER, J. G. & C. C. GOODNOW. 1995. Protein tyrosine phosphatase 1C negatively regulates antigen receptor signaling in B lymphocytes and determines thresholds for negative selection. Immunity **2:** 13–24.
19. CYSTER, J. G., J. I. HEALY, K. KISHIHARA, T. W. MAK, M. L. THOMAS & C. C. GOODNOW. 1996. Regulation of B lymphocyte negative and positive selection by tyrosine phosphatase CD45. Nature **381:** 325–328.
20. GOODNOW, C. C., J. CROSBIE, H. JORGENSEN, R. A. BRINK & A. BASTEN. 1989. Induction of self-tolerance in mature peripheral B lymphocytes. Nature **342:** 385–391.
21. ERIS, J. M., A. BASTEN, R. A. BRINK, K. DOHERTY, M. R. KEHRY & P. D. HODGKIN. 1994. Anergic self-reactive B cells present self-antigen and respond normally to CD40-dependent T cell signals, but are defective in antigen-receptor-mediated functions. Proc. Natl. Acad. Sci. U.S.A. **91:** 4392–4396.
22. RATHMELL, J. C., M. P. COOKE, J. GREIN, W. HO, M. M. DAVIS & C. C. GOODNOW. 1995. Elimination of self-reactive B cells by CD4 T cells is disrupted by the lpr mutation in CD95 (Fas/Apo-1). Nature **376:** 181–184.
23. RATHMELL, J. C., S. TOWNSEND, J. C. XU, R. A. FLAVELL & C. C. GOODNOW. 1996. Expansion or elimination of B cells *in vivo*: dual roles for the CD40- and Fas (CD95)–ligands modulated by the B cell antigen receptor. Cell **87:** 319–329.
24. HO, W. Y., M. P. COOKE, C. C. GOODNOW & M. M. DAVIS. 1994. Resting and anergic B cells are defective in CD28-dependent costimulation of naive $CD4^+$ T cells. J. Exp. Med. **179:** 1539–1549.
25. RIEUX-LAUCAT, F., F. LEDEIST, C. HIVROZ, A. ROBERTS, K. DEBATIN, A. FISCHER & J. DEVILLARTAY. 1995. Mutations in Fas associated with human lymphoproliferative syndrome and autoimmunity. Science **268:** 1347–1349.
26. FISHER, G., F. ROSENBERG, S. STRAUS, J. DALE, L. MIDDLETON, A. LIN, W. STROBER, M. LENARDO & J. PUCK. 1995. Dominant interfering Fas gene mutations impair apoptosis in a human autoimmune lymphoproliferative syndrome. Cell **81:** 935–946.
27. JACOBSON, B. A., D. J. PANKA, K-A. NGUYEN, J. ERIKSON, A. ABBAS & A. MARSHAK-ROTHSTEIN. 1995. Anatomy of autoantibody production: dominant localization of antibody-producing cells to T cell zones in Fas-deficient mice. Immunity **3:** 509–519.

Fas-dependent and Fas-independent Mechanisms for Selection of the Mature Human B Cell Repertoire

THIERRY DEFRANCE,[a] GISÈLE BILLIAN,[a]
PETER H. KRAMMER,[b] AND CHANTAL LAGRESLE[a]

[a]*INSERM U 404*
"Immunité et Vaccination"
Institut Pasteur de Lyon
69365 Lyon Cedex 07, France

[b]*Tumor Immunology Program*
German Cancer Research Center
Heidelberg, Germany

INTRODUCTION

Immunization with a T cell–dependent antigen (Ag) induces the B cell clones bearing the appropriate antigenic specificity to initiate the formation of germinal centers (GC) where they differentiate into either precursors of plasma cells or memory B cells. Affinity maturation of the antibody (Ab) response is achieved within the GC by the mechanism of somatic mutations targeted to the Ig V genes. A process of positive selection based on the affinity for Ag binding allows for the recruitment of high affinity mutants into the memory B cell pool. Safeguard mechanisms are necessarily operating to preserve the specificity of the Ab response and to prevent the activation of self-reactive B cells during this Ag-driven maturation process. Indeed, self-tolerance may be endangered on two occasions during the formation of the B cell immune repertoire: first, because some autoreactive B cells can escape clonal deletion in the bone marrow; second, because the mechanism of somatic mutations of Ig V genes within the GC may generate B cell clones with antiself-reactivity. This latter possibility suggests the existence of a censoring mechanism capable of actively eliminating the self-reactive mutants in the GC.

In the present paper, we bring evidence that a process of negative selection, presenting similarities with the clonal deletion of immature self-reactive B cells in the bone marrow, is also operating within the GC. Our data suggest that the sole triggering of the Ag receptor can directly activate the cell death program in a GC B cell subset, in a Fas-independent fashion. By contrast, engagement of the B cell receptor (BCR) induces resistance against Fas-mediated killing in both naïve and memory B cells. These observations give rise to the idea that distinct intracellular signaling pathways may be coupled to the Ig receptor complex, depending on the B cell maturational stage. The role of Fas in preventing misdirected T cell help and in censoring of autoreactive B cells in the periphery is discussed.

DEVELOPMENTAL STAGES OF THE MATURE B CELL COMPARTMENT

It is now well established that human B cell subsets corresponding to distinct stages of the Ag-dependent maturation process can be identified and isolated on the basis of their differential expression of a set of surface markers.[1–3] Naïve B cells are defined by their high expression of IgD, IgM, and CD44 and by their lack of expression of GC-related markers such as CD38 and CD77. This population can be further subdivided into two cell types differing by their expression of CD23.[2,4] Until recently, the lack of expression of IgD and CD44 associated with the expression of CD38 was believed to be the hallmark of GC B cells. However, recent studies suggest that this initial definition of the GC compartment must be revised. First, CD44 has been reported to be expressed at low levels on a subset of centrocytes.[5,6] Second, we identified a novel subset of GC B cells that presents all the phenotypical and functional characteristics of the bona fide GC population, but also homogeneously expressed IgD.[7] Taken together, these findings are compatible with the notion that the GC comprises at least four fractions (FIGURE 1): the centroblasts ($IgD^-/CD38^+/CD44^-/CD77^+$), the centrocytes ($IgD^-/CD38^+/CD77^-$) divided into two subtypes by the expression or the absence of CD44, and an atypical IgD-bearing GC B cell population ($IgD^+/CD38^+/CD44^-/CD77^+$). Finally, it has now been convincingly demonstrated that memory B cells display a unique phenotype defined by the absence of IgD, CD38, and CD77 and by a high level of CD44 expression. This notion essentially stems from two sets of data: (a) the demonstration by Pascual and colleagues[2] that this particular population is characterized by the expression of heavily mutated V_H genes; (b) our observation that the capacity to generate a secondary *in vitro* Ab response to a recall Ag is restricted to these cells.[8]

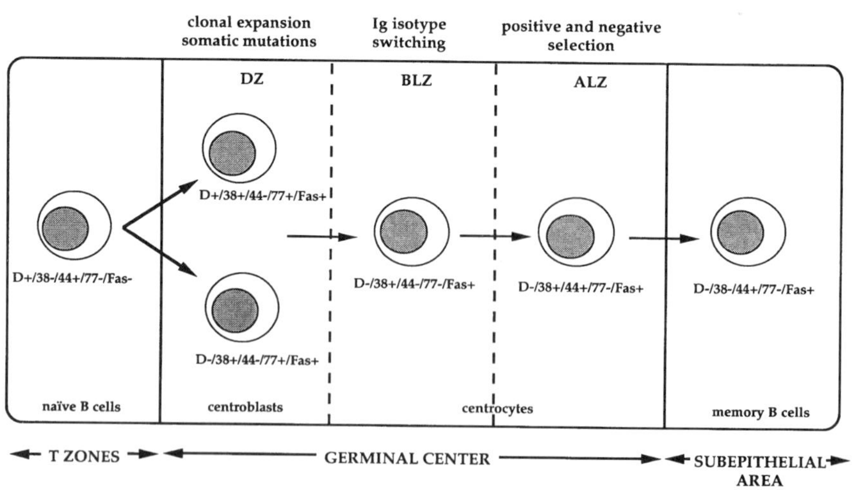

FIGURE 1. Putative scheme of B cell maturation during T-dependent responses (DZ: dark zone; BLZ: basal light zone; ALZ: apical light zone).

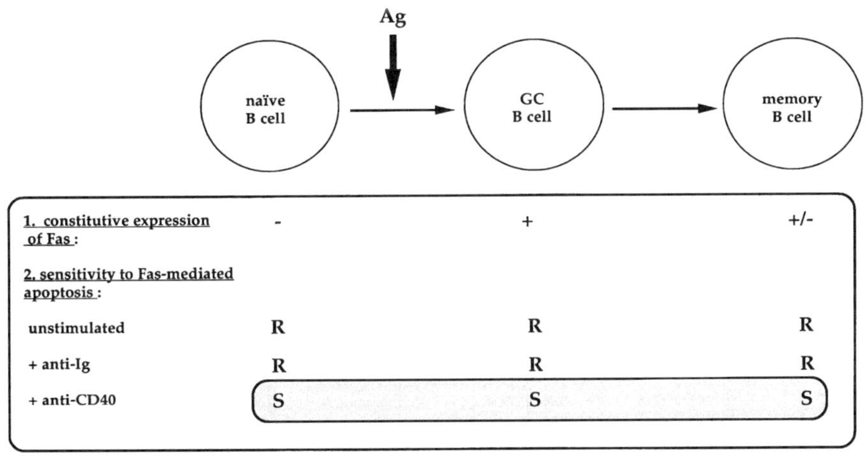

FIGURE 2. CD40 ligation induces the sensitivity of mature B cells to Fas-induced apoptosis (R: resistant; S: sensitive).

EXPRESSION AND FUNCTION OF FAS ON MATURE B CELL SUBSETS

The possibility to isolate different B cell compartments from human tonsils allowed us to study (a) the distribution of Fas on naïve, GC, and memory B cells in man and (b) the susceptibility of these human B cell subsets to the Fas-mediated death signal. Our results showed that Fas is constitutively expressed on both GC and memory B cells, but is absent on naïve B cells, thus implying that the induction of Fas on mature B cells coincides with the antigenic stimulation.[9,10] In spite of their high levels of constitutive expression of Fas, unstimulated GC and memory B cells are not susceptible to Fas-induced apoptosis *in vitro.* This finding suggests that Fas is not constitutively connected to the intracellular death-inducing pathway in mature human B cells. We observed that triggering of CD40, but not that of the BCR, confers on all B cell subsets (naïve B cells included) the susceptibility to Fas-mediated apoptosis. The acquisition of a Fas-sensitive phenotype is correlated with a strong upregulation of the membrane expression of Fas on all B cell subsets examined. These data are summarized in FIGURE 2.

CONCURRENT LIGATION OF CD40 AND THE BCR INDUCES FAS RESISTANCE IN HUMAN B CELLS

The data summarized above suggest the existence of a cross-talk between Fas and CD40 in B cells. As the ligands for both of these effector molecules are inducible on activated T cells, one can postulate that, in T-dependent responses, B cells can receive both differentiation and death signals from T helper cells. Thus, the Fas signaling pathway should be repressed during the effector phase of the response in order to avoid deletion of the Ag-activated B cell clones. We found that concurrent engagement of the BCR and CD40 protects both naïve and memory B cells, but not GC B cells, from Fas-mediated cell death.[10] Similar findings were also reported in the murine system.[11] These observations suggest that Fas could be instrumental in maintaining the specificity of the humoral response and in censoring self-reactive B

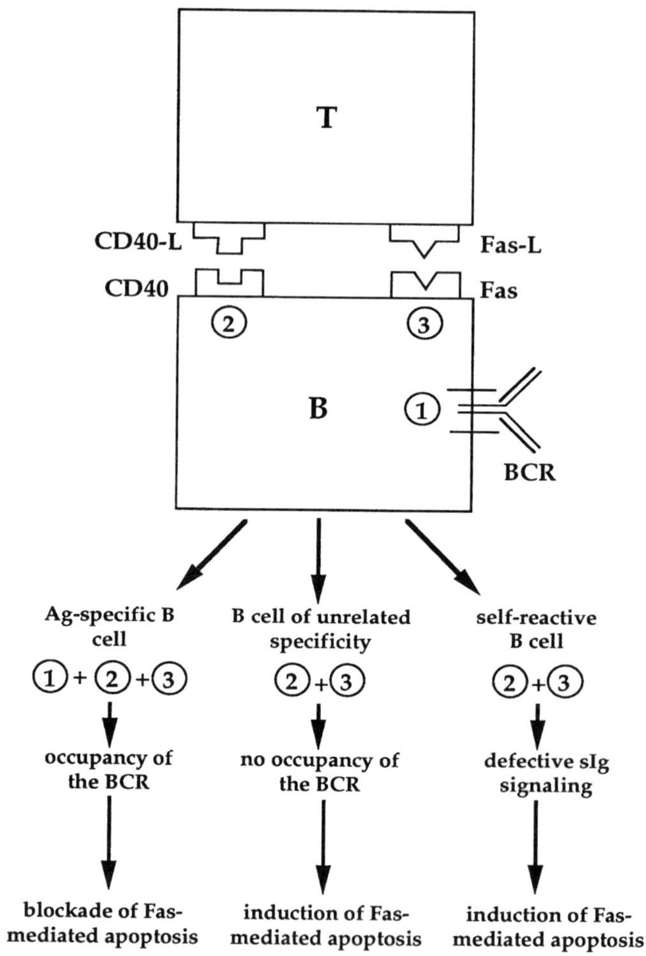

FIGURE 3. Hypothetical model for the immunoregulatory role of Fas on T-dependent B cell responses.

cells in the periphery. As shown in the hypothetical model depicted in FIGURE 3, B cells bearing the relevant antigenic specificity will be protected from Fas-induced killing due to the occupancy of the Ag receptor. By contrast, CD40-L-expressing T cells will induce the death of B cells lacking the appropriate antigenic specificity, through Fas-mediated cytotoxicity. CD40-mediated bystander stimulation of B cells may not be that uncommon *in vivo*, especially in the context of a primary response. Indeed, Ag presentation and subsequent activation of virgin T cells are achieved by dendritic cells (DCs) and not by B cells. Therefore, T lymphocytes expressing the CD40-L, consecutively to their priming by DCs, could potentially provide help to B cells, irrelevant of their antigenic specificity, as the CD40 signaling pathway is antigen-nonspecific and genetically unrestricted. Finally, the Fas/Fas-L system could also be involved in the demise of peripheral self-reactive B cells, as the impaired Ig signaling in tolerant self-reactive B cells[12] may preclude their protection from Fas-mediated killing.

EVIDENCE FOR A BCR-MEDIATED MECHANISM OF DELETION OF SELF-REACTIVE B CELLS WITHIN THE GC

Our observation that ligation of the BCR could not afford protection of GC B cells from Fas-induced apoptosis highlighted the unique nature of the sIg signaling at this particular maturational stage. This led us to investigate in more detail the outcome of the BCR triggering on the proliferative response of GC B cells. We reproducibly observed that the cross-linking of sIgs strongly antagonizes the CD40-mediated growth-response of GC B cells. Both entire anti-Ig Abs and $F(ab')_2$ fragments of anti-Ig Abs were equally effective in blocking the CD40-dependent proliferation of GC B cells, thus ruling out the involvement of $Fc\gamma$ receptors in this phenomenon. Subsequent experiments demonstrated that the inhibitory effect of anti-Ig Abs on GC B cell growth is mediated through the induction of apoptosis. Finally, the capacity of the BCR to transduce negative regulatory signals is confined to the GC B cell population because the ligation of sIgs failed to block the CD40-dependent proliferation of both naïve and memory B cells. The apoptotic signal delivered to GC B cells via ligation of sIgs is independent from the Fas/Fas-L system as a soluble Fas-Fc chimeric molecule failed to reverse the anti-Ig-mediated growth-inhibitory signal in GC B cell cultures. Two-step culture experiments revealed that a prior activation of GC B cells through CD40 is a prerequisite for inducing their sensitivity to the BCR-mediated apoptotic signal. Interestingly, CD40-activated GC B cells displayed marked phenotypical alterations when compared with freshly isolated GC B cells. In particular, the cell population emerging in CD40-stimulated GC B cell cultures was characterized by (a) the coexpression of CD38 and CD44, (b) an increased expression of sIgs, CD21, and CD45, and (c) a significant downregulation of the expression of CD77. Triple immunofluorescence stainings carried out on purified IgD^- B cells allowed the identification in fresh tonsil specimens of a minor subset of GC B cells presenting very similar phenotypical features (i.e., $CD38^+/CD44^{low}/CD21^{high}/CD77^{low}/sIg^{high}$). Our working hypothesis is that this particular GC B cell subset is representative of a population of centrocytes, possibly located in the apical light zone of the GC. This would imply that the *in vitro* CD40 stimulation induces the transition from the centroblastic to the centrocytic stage. We postulate that our *in vitro* findings relate to the mechanism of deletion of self-reactive B cells in GC previously reported by the groups of Goodnow and Nossal in murine models.[13,14]

DISCUSSION

Taken together, these observations address the issue of the nature of the molecular mechanisms that govern self/nonself-discrimination within the GC. We favor the hypothesis that the selection of the B cell repertoire within the GC is compatible with the two-signal model of Bretscher and Cohn.[15] According to this theory, the sole engagement of the BCR on centrocytes would induce their apoptosis, whereas the simultaneous triggering of the BCR and undefined costimulatory molecules would deliver a survival signal. This mechanism would allow for the elimination of self-reactive B cells that may arise in the GC as the consequence of somatic mutations (FIGURE 4). We have no direct evidence yet for the possible nature of the costimulatory signals required for positive selection in the GC. However, several key observations identify the CD19/CD21/TAPA-1 complex as a likely candidate (FIGURE 5). First, this complex has been demonstrated to be of critical importance for modulating the BCR-dependent B cell activation threshold.[16] Second, it was recently demonstrated that the humoral response to T-dependent Ag is dramatically perturbed in CR1/CR2/CR2 knockout mice.[17] Third, foreign Ags, which are trapped under the form of immune complexes on follicular dendritic cells, are expected to simultaneously engage the BCR and the CD19/CD21/TAPA-1 complex, whereas self-Ag should not. Finally, a recent report by Kozono and colleagues established that coligation of the complement receptors 1 and 2 with surface IgM prevents the B cell line WEHI 231 from entering apoptosis following sIg triggering.[18] Moreover, it is noteworthy that Ig signaling also triggers programmed cell death in group I Burkitt lymphoma cell lines, which are believed to represent the tumoral counterpart of GC B cells.[19,20] Taken together, our data are consistent with the hypothesis that germinal centers constitute the sites for both positive and negative selection of the mature B cell repertoire and

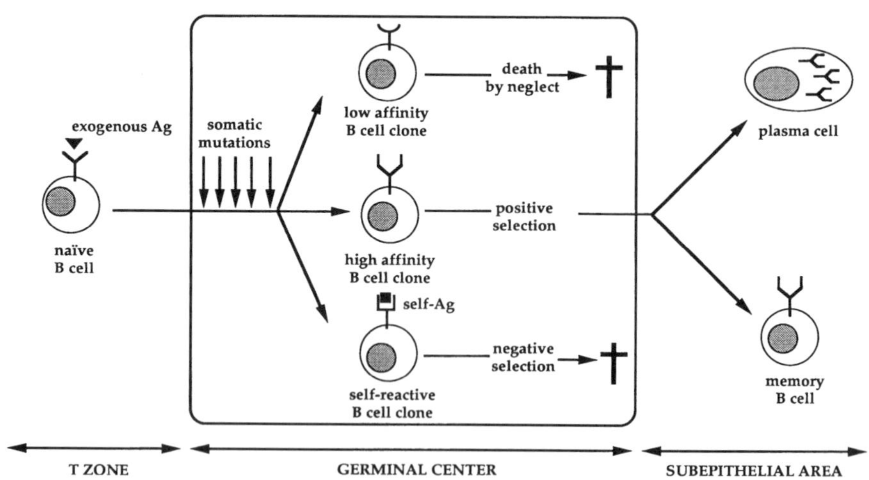

FIGURE 4. Germinal centers are the sites of both positive and negative selection of the mature B cell repertoire.

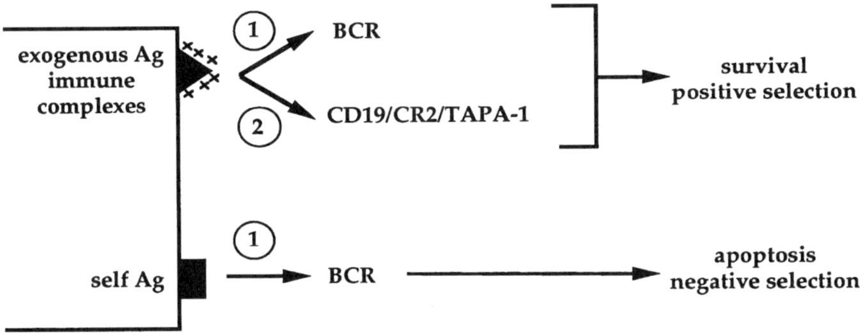

FIGURE 5. Hypothetical model illustrating the potential importance of the interplay between the BCR and the CD19/CR2/TAPA-1 complex for regulating the selection of the B cell repertoire within the germinal center.

suggest that elimination of self-reactive B cells in the periphery is a multistep process involving both Fas-dependent and Fas-independent mechanisms.

REFERENCES

1. Lagresle, C., C. Bella & T. Defrance. 1993. Phenotypical and functional heterogeneity of the IgD$^-$ B cell compartment: identification of two major tonsillar B cell subsets. Int. Immunol. **5:** 1259–1268.
2. Pascual, V., Y-J. Liu, A. Magalaski, O. De Bouteiller, J. Banchereau & J. D. Capra. 1994. Analysis of somatic mutations in five B cell subsets of human tonsil. J. Exp. Med. **180:** 329–339.
3. Liu, Y-J., C. Barthélémy, O. De Bouteiller, C. Arpin, I. Durand & J. Banchereau. 1995. Memory B cells from human tonsils colonize mucosal epithelium and directly present antigen to T cells by rapid up-regulation of B7-1 and B7-2. Immunity **2:** 239–248.
4. Liu, Y-J., F. Malisan, O. De Bouteiller, C. Guret, S. Lebecque, J. Banchereau, F. C. Mills, E. E. Max & H. Martinez-Valdez. 1996. Within germinal centers, isotype switching of immunoglobulin genes occurs after the onset of somatic mutations. Immunity **4:** 241–250.
5. Feuillard, J., D. Taylor, M. Casamayor-Palleja, G. D. Johnson & I. C. M. MacLennan. 1995. Isolation and characteristics of tonsil centroblasts with reference to Ig class switching. Int. Immunol. **7:** 121–130.
6. Kremmidiotis, G. & H. Zola. 1995. Changes in CD44 expression during B cell differentiation in the human tonsil. Cell. Immunol. **161:** 147–157.
7. Billian, G., C. Bella, P. Mondière & T. Defrance. 1996. Identification of a tonsil IgD$^+$ B cell subset with phenotypical and functional characteristics of germinal center B cells. Eur. J. Immunol. **26:** 1712–1719.
8. Silvy, A., C. Lagresle, C. Bella & T. Defrance. 1996. The differentiation of human memory B cells into specific antibody-secreting cells is CD40-independent. Eur. J. Immunol. **26:** 517–524.
9. Lagresle, C., C. Bella, P. T. Daniel, P. H. Krammer & T. Defrance. 1995. Regulation of germinal center B cell differentiation: role of the human APO-1/Fas (CD95) molecule. J. Immunol. **154:** 5746–5756.
10. Lagresle, C., P. Mondière, C. Bella, P. H. Krammer & T. Defrance. 1996. Concurrent engagement of CD40 and the antigen receptor protects naïve and memory human B cells from APO-1/Fas-mediated apoptosis. J. Exp. Med. **183:** 1–12.

11. ROTHSTEIN, T. L., J. K. M. WANG, D. J. PANKA, L. C. FOOTE, Z. WANG, B. STANGER, H. CUI, S. T. JU & A. MARSHAK-ROTHSTEIN. 1995. Protection against Fas-dependent Th-1-mediated apoptosis by antigen receptor engagement in B cells. Nature **374:** 163–165.
12. SHOKAT, K. M. & C. C. GOODNOW. 1995. Antigen-induced B-cell death and elimination during germinal-center immune responses. Nature **375:** 334–338.
13. COOKE, M. P., A. W. HEATH, K. M. SHOKAT, Y. ZENG, F. D. FINKELMAN, P. S. LINSLEY, M. HOWARD & C. C. GOODNOW. 1994. Immunoglobulin signal transduction guides the specificity of B cell–T cell interactions and is blocked in tolerant self-reactive B cells. J. Exp. Med. **179:** 425–438.
14. PULENDRAN, B., G. KANNOURAKIS, S. NOURI, K. G. C. SMITH & G. J. V. NOSSAL. 1995. Soluble antigen can cause enhanced apoptosis of germinal-center B cells. Nature **375:** 331–334.
15. BRETSCHER, P. & M. COHN. 1970. A theory of self-nonself discrimination: paralysis and induction involve the recognition of one and two determinants on an antigen, respectively. Science **163:** 1042–1049.
16. FEARON, D. T. & R. H. CARTER. 1995. The CD19/CR2/TAPA-1 complex of B lymphocytes: linking natural to acquired immunity. Annu. Rev. Immunol. **13:** 127–149.
17. AHEARN, J. M., M. B. FISCHER, D. CROIX, S. GOERG, M. MA, J. XIA, X. ZHOU, R. G. HOWARD, T. L. ROTHSTEIN & M. C. CARROLL. 1996. Disruption of the Cr2 locus results in a reduction in B-1a cells and in an impaired B cell response to T-dependent antigen. Immunity **4:** 251–262.
18. KOZONO, Y., R. C. DUKE, M. S. SCHLEICHER & V. M. HOLERS. 1995. Co-ligation of mouse complement receptors 1 and 2 with surface IgM rescues splenic B cells and WEHI-231 cells from anti-surface IgM-induced apoptosis. Eur. J. Immunol. **25:** 1013–1017.
19. GREGORY, C. D., T. TURSZ, C. F. EDWARDS, C. TETAUD, M. TALBOT, B. CAILLOU, A. B. RICKINSON & M. LIPINSKI. 1987. Identification of a subset of normal B cells with a Burkitt's lymphoma (BL)–like phenotype. J. Immunol. **139:** 313–318.
20. GREGORY, C. D., C. DIVE, S. HENDERSON, C. A. SMITH, G. T. WILLIAMS, J. GORDON & A. B. RICKINSON. 1991. Activation of Epstein-Barr virus protects human cells from death by apoptosis. Nature **349:** 612–614.

The Roles of B Cells in MRL/lpr Murine Lupus

OWEN CHAN,[a] MICHAEL P. MADAIO,[b] AND MARK J. SHLOMCHIK[a,c]

[a]*Section of Immunobiology*
Yale University School of Medicine
New Haven, Connecticut 06504

[b]*Renal Electrolyte Section*
University of Pennsylvania School of Medicine
Philadelphia, Pennsylvania 19104

[c]*Department of Laboratory Medicine*
Yale University School of Medicine
New Haven, Connecticut 06520

INTRODUCTION

Systemic autoimmune diseases are the result of complex interactions among T cells, B cells, and target tissues. Because of these interactions, it has been difficult to distinguish the contributions of various cell types to both the initiation of the autoimmune response and the resultant specific pathologic lesions. It has also been difficult to isolate the early events in what is undoubtedly a cascade of amplifying events, in part because of the interdependence of B and T cell activation.

To better address these issues, various genetic murine models of lupus, a prototypical human systemic autoimmune disease, have been developed.[1,2] Disease in these mice has been carefully described. Although no murine model exactly resembles human SLE, they have been very useful in identifying the mechanisms of pathogenesis and the roles of important cell types. For example, transfer of antibodies (Abs) and cells has allowed identification and characterization of pathogenic autoantibodies and cells.[3–5] Treatment of mice with anti-Thy1[6] or anti-CD4 Abs[7] has established important roles for $CD4^+$ T cells in auto-Ab production and disease. Although such studies have been informative, they are limited. In particular, it is not possible to reconstitute Ab-suppressed animals in order to prove the role of the cells in question and better define subsets of important cells. By crossing these murine lupus models with knockout mutations that affect T cells or B cells, a more precise elucidation may be possible of the role of T and B cell subsets and their interactions in autoimmune dysfunction. Because specific cells or molecules are eliminated in such mice without exogenous intervention, they can also serve as recipients in reconstitution experiments, which greatly extend the power of the analysis.

In this manuscript, we will summarize our own work using this approach on the role of B cells in nephritis and vasculitis and will present some new data on the role of B cells in spontaneous T cell activation.

NEPHRITIS AND VASCULITIS IN MRL/lpr × Jh KNOCKOUT F2 MICE

We previously showed, using F2 mice between Jh knockout (B-cell-deficient) homozygotes and MRL/lpr/lpr mice, that animals that were genotypically (Jh k/o)/(Jh k/o)/lpr/lpr and thereby lacked B cells also did not have pathologic evidence of autoimmune renal disease. Specifically, glomerulonephritis (GN), interstitial nephritis (IN), and vasculitis were all absent.[8]

The absence of GN was perhaps not surprising as previous work had suggested an important role for Ab in glomerular lesions. For example, recent work has shown that certain anti-DNA mAbs cause nephritis after injection into normal mice,[9–11] and certain rheumatoid factor (RF) cryoglobulins cause vasculitis and nephritis after injection.[12,13] There are probably several mechanisms by which Abs cause damage, including immune-complex deposition and direct binding to glomerular antigens (Ags).[11] There are, however, many instances in which auto-Ab production, such as anti-DNA, does not correlate with, or has been genetically separated from, GN. In some cases, high anti-DNA titers are present with little or no nephritis;[14,15] in others, low titers and little deposition accompany severe crescentic disease.[16,17] Thus, whether Ab alone is sufficient to cause full-blown glomerular disease remains to be determined. In particular, a direct role of B cells or T cells needs to be excluded, which will be the subject of future work.

The absence of IN and vasculitis was somewhat more surprising as most workers have cited the role of cellular components, particularly T cells and macrophages, in disease in these compartments.[18–20] Intense cellular inflammation often precedes Ig deposits along tubular basement membranes.[18] In addition, T cell lines have been isolated that cause IN upon injection.[21] However, lupus auto-Abs have not been reported to cause IN (see below). Models of experimentally induced IN have also been explored; in this case, pathogenetic mechanisms could be more clearly defined. Neilson and colleagues have pioneered this area using injection of tubular Ag in CFA. Their main findings are that T cells (both CD4 and CD8) are required and are pathogenic, although Ab is also made. These workers have also isolated T cell lines that cause disease when transferred under the kidney capsule.[20,22–24]

The relative roles of Ab and T cells in the pathogenesis of lupus vasculitis have been controversial.[11,19,25–27] A few pathogenic Abs that deposit in glomeruli also localize to vessels, although with the exception of some cryoglobulins[13] it is not clear that these glomerulonephritogenic Abs induce light microscopic changes in vessels. Berden *et al.*[25] found that Ig deposition correlated with inflammation in MRL/lpr mice. However, Moyer *et al.*[19] reported that perivascular lymphocytes and macrophages were present prior to vascular immune deposits; Ab deposition coincided with the later development of necrotizing vasculitis in older MRL/lpr mice. Jabs and Prendergast[26] and Tarkowski *et al.*[27] obtained similar results and in addition showed that CD4+ T cells predominated. These latter groups emphasized the cell-mediated nature of MRL/lpr vasculitis. Intriguingly, they did find B cells in the outer zone of the inflammatory infiltrate, providing a possible site for T-B collaboration and for T cells to become activated by autoreactive B cells. Cerny *et al.*[28] observed that anti-IgM treatment of C57BL6/lpr/lpr mice ameliorated nephritis, but did not affect vasculitis, suggesting that B cells/Ig are not required for the development of vasculitis. However, vasculitis was not detected in our B-less MRL/lpr mice, indicating that the vascular lesions were dependent on Ig deposition and/or the presence of B cells. At present, it is difficult to reconcile the differences observed between B-less mice and anti-IgM treatment. The presence of low levels of B cells, heterologous rabbit anti-serum, and presumably immune complexes in the anti-IgM-treated animals may have been sufficient to allow for the development of vasculitis. Again, this points out the limitations of the Ab-mediated cell suppression technique.

A POTENTIAL ROLE OF B CELLS AS ANTIGEN-PRESENTING CELLS (APCs) FOR AUTOREACTIVE T CELLS IN SPONTANEOUS AUTOIMMUNITY

In particular, because IN and vasculitis are putatively T cell–mediated, absence of these lesions in B-less mice raised the question of whether B cells are playing an additional role, aside from auto-Ab secretion, in pathogenesis. In principle, this question also applies to GN. The most likely role for B cells in autoimmune pathogenesis would be as APCs for T cell activation, although B cells are also known to secrete lymphokines. We therefore hypothesized that, in MRL/lpr mice, B cells are important APCs in promoting spontaneous T cell activation (FIGURE 1). Another feature of our initial data that supported this hypothesis was evidence that overall lymphoaccumulation (in terms of absolute cell numbers) in older lpr/lpr mice was inhibited, although the percentage of CD4−/CD8− (double negative: "DN") T cells was similar in B-less and B-sufficient lpr mice.[8] This suggested that B cells were in some way playing a role in the generation or maintenance of accumulating T cells.

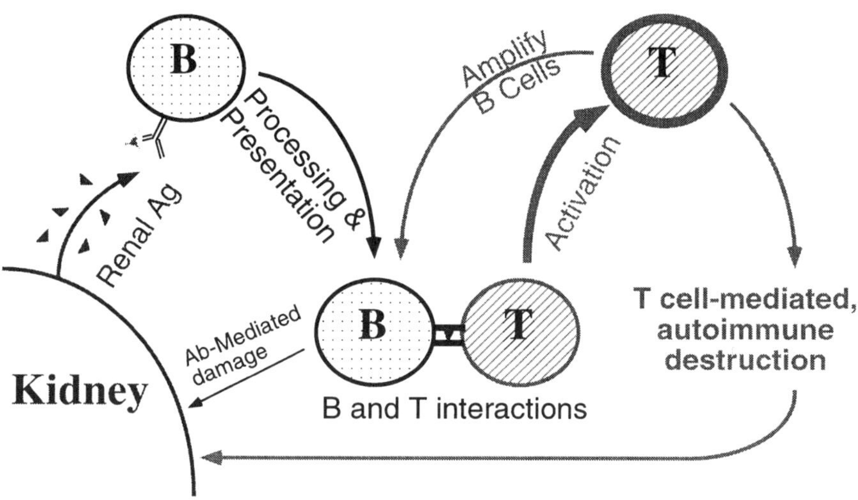

FIGURE 1. Potential roles of B cells in induction and amplification of autoimmunity.

The model presented in FIGURE 1 is an adaptation of a model proposed several years ago by Mamula and Janeway[29,30] as well as the Sercarz group[31,32] to explain phenomena observed in normal mice. For example, Mamula and colleagues developed a system in which B cells were thought to play an important role in induced autoimmunity in a normal mouse. Heterologous proteins that cross-reacted with self, such as human cytochrome c, were injected into normal mice. This induced a B and T cell response, of which only the B cell response was cross-reactive with mouse cytochrome c. When such mice were reimmunized with mouse cytochrome c, both a B and a T cell response ensued, with the T cell response now being specific for mouse cytochrome c. Mice immunized with mouse cytochrome c without prior immunization with human cytochrome c do not make such B and T cell responses.[29,30] The simplest model to explain these phenomena was that B cells primed initially with heterologous protein were later serving as APCs for peripheral T cells (either ignorant or anergic) that were specific for mouse cytochrome c. It is still unclear why these B cells could stimulate such autoreactive T cells, whereas such stimulation was undetectable in naive mice given the same mouse cytochrome c immunization. Among the possibilities to explain the T cell priming are the expansion of B cells, the efficiency of B cells as APCs, the induction of costimulatory molecules (which is more efficient in memory B cells), and some effect of the preexisting cross-reactive Ab to human cytochrome c. A similar phenomenon has been shown for immunization with small-nuclear ribonucleoprotein (snRNP)[33] and cryptic determinants of hen egg lysozyme.[34]

"Epitope spreading," in which a response to an initial autoepitope later expands to include other epitopes, is a variation on the cross-reactive priming theme that is particularly relevant to autoimmunity.[31] In the framework just outlined, B cells could be responsible for T cell epitope spreading by binding a whole particle, internalizing, and presenting multiple peptide epitopes in immunogenic form. T cells so stimulated could in turn help autoreactive B cells specific for various different epitopes of the auto-Ag, as long as those B cells could present the T cell epitope after internalizing and processing the particle.

Although this mechanism has obvious appeal in explaining progressive serologic autoimmunity in systemic autoimmune diseases, no direct evidence exists for it in spontaneous disease models. However, some features of human and murine lupus are suggestive. For example, the anti-Sm response in both MRL lupus-prone mice and humans occurs in only a fraction (25–50%) of individuals.[35,36] When it does occur, the response initially is often focused to one of the several proteins that comprise the Sm particle. Within a short period of time, though, immunoblotting can demonstrate that the response has spread to multiple other independent protein components of the particle—epitope spreading.[37] Presumably, this is dependent on B cell processing and presentation of the Sm particle.

LYMPHOACCUMULATION AND NEPHRITIS IN BACKCROSS MICE

The epitope idea as well as the unexpected finding that presumed T cell–mediated autoimmunity—IN and vasculitis—was absent in B-less MRL/lpr mice led us to investigate the effect of B cells on T cell activation in MRL/lpr mice. The long-term goal of these studies is to determine whether B cells are in fact important APCs for spontaneous activation of autoreactive T cells. Our initial experiments involved analysis of the T cell compartment of B-less MRL/lpr mice at a time when autoimmunity has begun in B-sufficient littermates. We analyzed lymph node (LN) and spleen for cell number and by FACS for DN T cells, presence of B cells, and markers of memory and activation phenotype on CD8 single-positive T cells. We also analyzed kidneys in these mice in order to confirm our previous results now that backcrossing had introduced >98% MRL genes into the mice being analyzed.

TABLE 1 summarizes the results of the analysis of glomerular, vascular, and interstitial renal disease in backcross-4 (BC4) and BC5 (to MRL) mice (and including similar data from a few additional F2 mice). We essentially confirmed our earlier findings in F2 mice that B-less lpr/lpr mice have minimal or background levels of disease in all compartments, whereas B-sufficient mice have flagrant disease. Thus, evidence obtained using genetically heterogeneous mice with 50% total MRL genes was confirmed in more genetically homogeneous mice with >97% MRL genes. TABLE 2 summarizes the results on total cell numbers and percentages of various T cell types in this latter cohort. Again, in the BC mice, we observed a diminution of lymphoaccumulation of DN T cells as well as CD4 and CD8 single-positive (SP) T cells. Indirectly, this suggests a role for B cells as APCs in the activation-dependent accumulation of such cells.

MEMORY AND ACTIVATION PHENOTYPES OF T CELLS IN B-LESS MRL/lpr MICE

Previous work by Giese and Davidson[38] established that both CD4 and CD8 positive T cells in older (>3-month) MRL/lpr mice were phenotypically either activated or memory-type cells. Evidence from anti-CD8-treated mice and CD8 and β2-microglobulin knockout mice suggests that the precursor for DN T cells is primarily a CD8+ T cell.[39–42] Therefore, we investigated the memory/activation of CD8+ T cells in B-less and B-sufficient mice. FIGURES 2 and 3 show data from a representative experiment. In both spleen and LN, the spontaneous accumulation of activation and memory phenotype CD8 T cells is clearly inhibited in the absence of B cells. Similar data have been obtained for CD4 T cells (not shown; Chan and Shlomchik, manuscript in preparation). In particular, the near-complete absence of naive phenotype cells in B-sufficient mice is not seen in B-deficient mice. This suggests that B cells may be responsible for efficiently inducing nearly all CD8 T cells to become activated. The mechanism behind the phenomenon remains to be determined, as does the Ag specificity of the activated T cells. As these cells were previously shown to be polyclonal and not particularly skewed in terms of Vβ family expression,[38,43,44] it seems unlikely that superantigens, as are known to be expressed on B cells, are responsible. It is also unclear why this phenomenon is Fas-dependent. In particular, is Fas-deficiency required in both the T and B cells? Because Fas-deficiency in the T cell per se seems to lead to its ultimate differentiation into a DN T cell,[45] it seems possible that Fas-deficiency may be required to allow the DN T cell to develop from a putative SP activated precursor, but may not be required in the T cell to

TABLE 1. Histologic Analysis of Kidneys from Mice of Various Genotypes[a]

Genotype	Generation[b]	Anatomic Site		
		Glomeruli	Interstitia	Vessels
B+ lpr/lpr	F1	1–2+, focal	2+, focal	2+, focal
	F1	2+	2–3+	4+, severe
	F1	3–4+, crescents	2+	3+, severe
	BC4	3+	3+	3+
	BC4	3+	3+	3+
	BC4	3+, focal and diffuse	2+	3+
B-less lpr/lpr	F1	0–1+	1+	0
	F1	0	0	0
	BC4	0–1+	1+	0
	BC4	0–1+	1+	0
	BC4	0	0	0
B-less CB.17		0	0	0
		0	0	0
		0	0	0

[a]Each line represents an individual mouse in the group. Mice—B+ l/l: MRL/lpr with B cells; B-less: homozygous Jh knockout; CB.17: a nonautoimmune mouse of BALB/c origin. All MRL/lpr-derived mice were 4 months old at sacrifice. CB.17 mice were 3 months old. Sections were prepared and read as described.[8] Disease was scored semiquantitatively according to the system in the following table:

Score	Glomerulonephritis	Interstitial Nephritis	Vessels
0–1+	focal, mild, or early proliferative	occasional, focal, or small pockets of MNC (10–15 cells)	occasional perivascular infiltrate
1–2+	moderate or definite proliferative; increased matrix	focal infiltrates (15–30 cells)	several foci of perivascular infiltrate; no necrosis
2–3+	diffuse and focal or diffuse proliferative	multifocal extensive infiltrates; with necrosis	multifocal perivascular; more extensive; +/− necrosis (3+)
3–4+	severe diffuse proliferative, with crescents/sclerosis	severe disease with extensive necrosis	multifocal or diffuse; extensive with necrosis

[b]F1 is an intercross of F1's with MRL/lpr mice (50% MRL genes); BC4 is an intercross with mice backcrossed four times to MRL/lpr (97% MRL genes). In the case of CB.17, similar backcrosses were done for three generations.

develop the activated or memory phenotype as an SP T cell in the first place. On the other hand, the SP activated T cell may be the target of most FasL-dependent regulation and the cells that we have observed may be accumulating as SP cells on their way to the DN fate.[46–50] In any case, these data link T cell activation of SP cells with the accumulation of DN T cells, further supporting the idea that DN T cells are postactivation products of SP T cell precursors.[49,50]

TABLE 2. Percentages and Total Numbers of Splenic Lymphocytes in B-less lpr/lpr Mice and Littermates[a]

Genotype	Cross	Age (Months)	Percentage of Total[b]				Total Cells (Millions)[c]				Total Cell Number (Millions)
			B Cell	CD8	CD4	DN	B Cell	CD8	CD4	DN	
B+ +/+	F1	6	27	12	16	2	23	10	13	2	84
	F1	6	12	13	11	4	9	10	9	3	77
		(mean ± SD)	20 ± 11	13 ± 0	13 ± 3	3 ± 1	16 ± 10	10 ± 0	11 ± 3	3 ± 1	81 ± 5
B-less +/+	F1	6	0	24	37	5	0	3	4	1	12
	F1	6	0	18	30	6	0	5	8	2	27
		(mean ± SD)	0 ± 0	21 ± 4	34 ± 5	6 ± 1	0 ± 0	4 ± 3	6 ± 3	1 ± 1	20 ± 11
B+ lpr/lpr	F1	6	18	3	18	34	74	12	76	139	410
	F1	6	11	2	15	38	12	2	16	39	105
	BC5	5	15	8	14	52	41	21	39	145	280
	BC4	5	6	2	5	22	14	5	11	50	225
	BC4	5	20	3	5	28	45	7	12	65	230
	BC4	5	9	3	6	26	19	6	13	53	200
	BC4	3	14	4	8	31	44	14	26	100	320
	BC4	3	5	2	7	30	19	8	25	112	375
	BC5	4.5	12	5	9	23	11	5	8	21	90
	BC5	4.5	9	8	10	30	11	10	12	36	122
	BC5	4.5	8	7	9	35	10	8	11	41	120
		(mean ± SD)	12 ± 5	4 ± 2	10 ± 4	32 ± 8	27 ± 21	9 ± 5	23 ± 20	73 ± 44	225 ± 111
B-less lpr/lpr	BC5	4.5	1	8	8	16	0	1	1	2	12
	BC4	5	1	3	3	9	2	3	4	12	130
	BC4	3	1	2	6	12	1	2	6	12	100
	BC4	3	1	2	7	14	1	2	7	14	100
		(mean ± SD)	1 ± 0	4 ± 3	6 ± 2	13 ± 3	1 ± 1	2 ± 1	4 ± 3	10 ± 6	86 ± 51

[a]Methods were as described.[8] Backcross nomenclature is as in TABLE 1. Each line represents a different mouse.
[b]Percentage of cells is of live (propidium iodide–excluding) cells as determined by FACS analysis.
[c]Total cell number is of nucleated splenocytes.

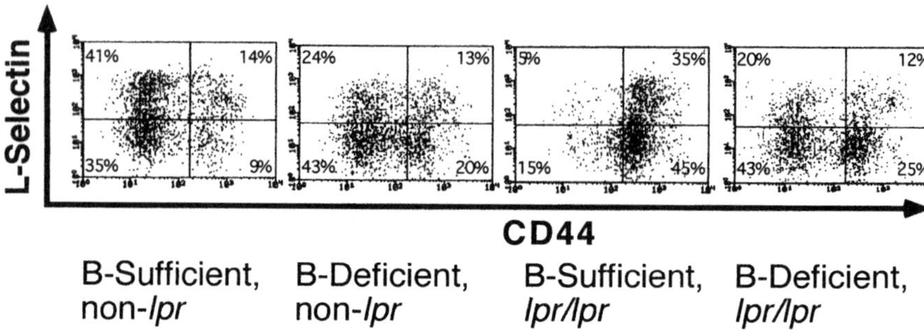

FIGURE 2. FACS analysis of CD8 T cell activation and memory phenotypes. Splenocytes from 5-month-old F1 intercross mice of the genotypes indicated under each plot were analyzed by three-color FACS. Dot plots show staining with anti-CD44 (Pgp-1, x-axis) and anti-L-selectin (MEL-14, y-axis) on cells gated for positive staining with anti-CD8. Numbers in the quadrants indicate the percentages of total CD8$^+$ cells. Representative animals of four different genotypes are shown. FIGURE 3 gives a summary of the same analysis on multiple animals.

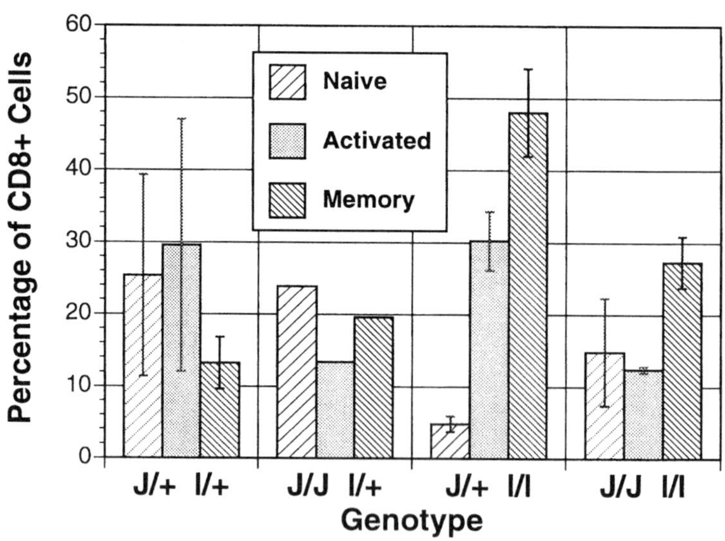

FIGURE 3. Summary of FACS analysis of CD8 T cell activation and memory phenotypes. FACS analysis performed as described in FIGURE 2 is summarized in the bar graph. Percentages of cells in the quadrants shown in FIGURE 2 are indicated on the y-axis. The x-axis gives the genotypes of four different groups—J/+ l/+: heterozygous for both Jh knockout and lpr (B-sufficient, non-lpr); J/J l/+: homozygous for the Jh knockout and heterozygous for lpr (B-less, non-lpr); J+ l/l: heterozygous for Jh knockout and homozygous for lpr (B-sufficient, lpr); J/J l/l: homozygous for both mutations (B-less, lpr). Error bars show 1 SD.

It seems likely, on the other hand, that Fas is required in the B cell.[4,51] It is reasonable to suppose, given the greater capacity of activated B cells that express costimulatory molecules[52–54] to activate T cells,[55,56] that the B cell APC for the spontaneous T cell activation is itself already activated. It is unknown whether Fas-deficiency in the B cell is required for the accumulation of activated B cells in MRL/lpr mice, but evidence that Fas-deficiency is required in the B cell for auto-Ab production[4,51] suggests that it is. In fact, the status of B cell activation in MRL/lpr mice requires further study. Presumably, reconstitution studies of B-less MRL/lpr mice could shed light on this question.

The Ag specificity and pathogenetic function of the spontaneously activated T cells in MRL/lpr mice are also unknown. Few groups have reported the isolation of autoreactive T cells with specificity for classical auto-Ags.[57–61] The hypothesis defined in FIGURE 1 suggests that autoreactive B cells are responsible for activating cognate T cells. By comparing T cell repertoires in B-less and B-sufficient mice, we may be able to establish this point and to better define the auto-Ag specificity of spontaneously activated T cells in this murine lupus model. As for pathogenesis, certainly both CD4 and CD8 SP cells have been identified in interstitial and vascular lesions (where CD4 cells predominate).[19,27] Little is known about the precise role of these cells in causing damage *in situ.* Presumably, cytotoxic CD8 T cells could cause direct cellular injury, as they are thought to do in GVHD (reviewed in reference 62). In this regard, it is interesting that B cells seem to be required to initiate GVHD in a murine minor Ag histoincompatibility model.[63] Cytokine secretion by both CD4 and CD8 T cells could also be important. Macrophages have been observed in both vasculitic and interstitial lesions, and cytokines that activate and recruit these are of likely importance.[26,64]

Thus, much remains to be defined about both the immune circuits that lead to T and B cell activation in systemic autoimmunity and the role of these cells in the pathogenesis of tissue damage. Autoimmune-prone mice deficient in T or B cells, in subsets of these cells, or deficient in particular costimulatory molecules involved in T-B collaboration should all be powerful tools for the experimental dissection of these processes. Future work will involve better characterization of these models as well as reconstitution of these deficient mice with specific subsets of missing lymphocytes or Abs.

ACKNOWLEDGMENTS

We thank Mark Mamula for a critical reading of the manuscript and Dennis Huszar for originally providing the Jh knockout mice.

REFERENCES

1. COHEN, P. L. & R. A. EISENBERG. 1991. Lpr and gld: single gene models of systemic autoimmunity and lymphoproliferative disease. Annu. Rev. Immunol. **9:** 243–269.
2. THEOFILOPOULOS, A. N. & F. J. DIXON. 1981. Etiopathogenesis of murine SLE. Immunol. Rev. **55:** 179–216.

3. Foster, M. H., B. Cizman & M. P. Madaio. 1993. Nephritogenic autoantibodies in systemic lupus erythematosus: immunochemical properties, mechanisms of immune deposition, and genetic origins. Lab. Invest. **69:** 494–507.
4. Sobel, E. S., T. Katagiri, K. Katagiri, S. C. Morris, P. L. Cohen & R. A. Eisenberg. 1991. An intrinsic B cell defect is required for the production of autoantibodies in the *lpr* model of murine systemic autoimmunity. J. Exp. Med. **173:** 1441–1449.
5. Sobel, E. S., P. L. Cohen & R. A. Eisenberg. 1993. Lpr T cells are necessary for autoantibody production in lpr mice. J. Immunol. **150:** 4160.
6. Wofsky, D., J. A. Ledbetter, P. L. Hendler & W. E. Seaman. 1985. Treatment of murine lupus with monoclonal anti–T cell antibody. J. Immunol. **134:** 852–857.
7. Santoro, T. J., J. P. Portanova & B. L. Kotzin. 1988. The contribution of L3T4+ T cells to lymphoproliferation and autoantibody production in MRL-lpr/lpr mice. J. Exp. Med. **167:** 1713–1718.
8. Shlomchik, M. J., M. P. Madaio, D. Ni, M. Trounstine & D. Huszar. 1994. The role of B cells in lpr/lpr-induced autoimmunity. J. Exp. Med. **180:** 1295–1306.
9. Dang, H. & R. J. Harbeck. 1984. The *in vivo* and *in vitro* glomerular deposition of isolated anti-double-stranded-DNA antibodies in NZB/W mice. Clin. Immunol. Immunopathol. **30:** 265–278.
10. Pankewycz, O. G., P. Migliorini & M. Madaio. 1987. Polyreactive autoantibodies are nephritogenic in murine lupus nephritis. J. Immunol. **139:** 3287–3294.
11. Vlahakos, D. V., M. H. Foster, S. Adams, M. Katz, A. A. Ucci, K. J. Barrett, S. K. Datta & M. P. Madaio. 1992. Anti-DNA antibodies form immune deposits at distinct glomerular and vascular sites. Kidney Int. **41:** 1690–1700.
12. Reininger, L., T. Berney, T. Shibata, F. Spertini, R. Merino & S. Izui. 1990. Cryoglobulinemia induced by a murine IgG3 rheumatoid factor: skin vasculitis and glomerulonephritis arise from distinct pathogenic mechanisms. Proc. Natl. Acad. Sci. U.S.A. **87:** 10038–10044.
13. Berney, T., T. Fulpius, T. Shibata, L. Reininger, J. Van Snick, H. Shan, M. Weigert, A. Marshak-Rothstein & S. Izui. 1992. Selective pathogenicity of murine rheumatoid factors of the cryoprecipitable IgG3 subclass. Int. Immunol. **4:** 93–99.
14. Eastcott, J. W., R. S. Schwartz & S. K. Datta. 1983. Genetic analysis of the inheritance of B cell hyperactivity in relation to the development of autoantibodies and glomerulonephritis in NZB × SWR crosses. J. Immunol. **131:** 2232–2239.
15. Davidson, W. F., J. B. Roths, K. L. Holmes, E. Rudikoff & H. C. Morse. 1984. Dissociation of severe lupus-like disease from polyclonal B cell activation and IL2 deficiency in C3H-*lpr/lpr* mice. J. Immunol. **133:** 1048–1056.
16. Nakajima, A., M. Azuma, S. Kodera, S. Nuriya, A. Terashi, M. Abe, S. Hirose, T. Shirai, H. Yagita & K. Okumura. 1995. Preferential dependence of autoantibody production in murine lupus on CD86 co-stimulatory molecule. Eur. J. Immunol. **25:** 3060–3069.
17. Kinjoh, K., M. Kyogoku & R. A. Good. 1993. Genetic selection for crescent formation yields mouse strain with rapidly progressive glomerulonephritis and small vessel vasculitis. Proc. Natl. Acad. Sci. U.S.A. **90:** 3413.
18. Halloran, P. F., J. Urmson, V. Ramassar, C. Laskin & P. Autenried. 1988. Increased class I and class II MHC products and mRNA in kidneys of MRL-lpr/lpr mice during autoimmune nephritis and inhibition by cyclosporine. J. Immunol. **141:** 2303–2312.
19. Moyer, C. F., J. D. Strandberg & C. L. Reinisch. 1987. Systemic mononuclear-cell vasculitis in MRL/Mp-lpr/lpr mice: a histologic and immunocytochemical analysis. Am. J. Pathol. **127:** 229–242.
20. Neilson, E. G. 1993. The nephritogenic T lymphocyte response in interstitial nephritis. Semin. Nephrol. **13:** 496–502.
21. Gallo, C. D., A. M. Jevnikar, D. C. Brennan, S. Florquin, S. A. Pacheco & V. R. Kelley. 1992. Autoreactive kidney-infiltrating T-cell clones in murine lupus nephritis. Kidney Int. **42:** 851.
22. Mann, R., B. Zakheim, M. Clayman, E. McCafferty, L. Michaud & E. G. Neilson. 1985. Murine interstitial nephritis. IV. Long-term cultured L3T4+ T cell lines transfer delayed expression of disease as I-A-restricted inducers of the effector T cell repertoire. J. Immunol. **135:** 286–293.

23. ZAKHEIM, B., E. MCCAFFERTY, S. M. PHILLIPS, M. CLAYMAN & E. G. NEILSON. 1984. Murine interstitial nephritis. II. The adoptive transfer of disease with immune T lymphocytes produces a phenotypically complex interstitial lesion. J. Immunol. **133:** 234–239.
24. HINES, W. H., T. P. HAVERTY, J. A. ELIAS, E. G. NEILSON & C. J. KELLY. 1989. T cell recognition of epithelial self. Autoimmunity **5:** 37–47.
25. BERDEN, J. H., L. HANG, P. J. MCCONAHEY & F. J. DIXON. 1983. Analysis of vascular lesions in murine SLE. I. Association with serologic abnormalities. J. Immunol. **130:** 1699–1705.
26. JABS, D. A. & R. A. PRENDERGAST. 1987. Reactive lymphocytes in lacrimal gland and vasculitic renal lesions of autoimmune MRL/lpr mice express L3T4. J. Exp. Med. **166:** 1198–1203.
27. TARKOWSKI, A., R. JONSSON, R. SANCHEZ, L. KLARESKOG & W. J. KOOPMAN. 1988. Features of renal vasculitis in autoimmune MRL lpr/lpr mice: phenotypes and functional properties of infiltrating cells. Clin. Exp. Immunol. **72:** 91–97.
28. CERNY, A., M. KIMOTO, A. W. HUGIN, R. MERINO & S. IZUI. 1989. Anti-IgM treatment of C57BL/6-lpr/lpr mice: depletion of B cells reduces lpr gene-induced lymphoproliferation and mononuclear cell vasculitis. Clin. Exp. Immunol. **77:** 124–129.
29. LIN, R-H., M. J. MAMULA, J. A. HARDIN & C. A. JANEWAY, JR. 1991. Induction of autoreactive B cells allows priming of autoreactive T cells. J. Exp. Med. **173:** 1433–1439.
30. MAMULA, M. J., R-H. LIN, C. A. JANEWAY, JR. & J. A. HARDIN. 1992. Breaking T cell tolerance with foreign and self co-immunogens: a study of autoimmune B and T cell epitopes of cytochrome c. J. Immunol. **149:** 789–795.
31. LEHMANN, P. V., E. E. SERCARZ, T. FORSTHUBER, C. M. DAYAN & G. GAMMON. 1993. Determinant spreading and the dynamics of the autoimmune T-cell repertoire. Immunol. Today **14:** 203–208.
32. LEHMANN, P. V., T. FORSTHUBER, A. MILLER & E. E. SERCARZ. 1992. Spreading of T-cell autoimmunity to cryptic determinants of an autoantigen. Nature **358:** 155–157.
33. MAMULA, M., S. FATENEJAD & J. CRAFT. 1994. B cells process and present lupus autoantigens that initiate autoimmune T cell responses. J. Immunol. **152:** 1453–1461.
34. MOUDGIL, K. D. & E. E. SERCARZ. 1993. Dominant determinants in hen egg white lysozyme correspond to the cryptic determinants within its self-homologue, mouse lysozyme: implications in shaping of the T cell repertoire and autoimmunity. J. Exp. Med. **178:** 2131–2138.
35. NOTMAN, D. D., N. KURATA & E. M. TAN. 1974. Profiles of antinuclear antibodies in systemic rheumatic diseases. Ann. Intern. Med. **83:** 464.
36. EISENBERG, R. A., E. M. TAN & F. J. DIXON. 1978. Presence of anti-Sm reactivity in autoimmune mouse strains. J. Exp. Med. **147:** 582.
37. FATENEJAD, S., W. BROOKS, A. SCHWARTZ & J. CRAFT. 1994. Pattern of anti–small nuclear ribonucleoprotein antibodies in MRL/Mp-lpr/lpr mice suggests that the intact U1 snRNP particle is their autoimmunogenic target. J. Immunol. **152:** 5523–5531.
38. GIESE, T. & W. F. DAVIDSON. 1992. Evidence for early onset, polyclonal activation of T cell subsets in mice homozygous for lpr. J. Immunol. **149:** 3097–3110.
39. KOH, D-R., A. HO, A. RAHEMTULLA, W-P. FUNG-LEUNG, H. GRIESSER & T-W. MAK. 1995. Murine lupus in MRL/*lpr* mice lacking CD4 or CD8 T cells. Eur. J. Immunol. **25:** 2558–2562.
40. MALDONADO, M. A., R. A. EISENBERG, E. ROPER, P. L. COHEN & B. L. KOTZIN. 1995. Greatly reduced lymphoproliferation in lpr mice lacking major histocompatibility complex class I. J. Exp. Med. **181:** 641–648.
41. MERINO, R., L. FOSSATI, M. IWAMOTO, S. TAKAHASHI, R. LEMOINE, N. IBNOUZEKRI, L. PUGLIATTI, J. MERINO & S. IZUI. 1995. Effect of long-term anti-CD4 or anti-CD8 treatment on the development of lpr CD4(−) CD8(−) double negative T cells and of the autoimmune syndrome in MRL-lpr. J. Autoimmun. **8:** 33–45.
42. OHTEKI, T., M. IWAMOTO, S. IZUI & H. R. MACDONALD. 1995. Reduced development of CD4(−)8(−)B220(+) T cells, but normal autoantibody production in lpr/lpr mice lacking major histocompatibility complex class I molecules. Eur. J. Immunol. **25:** 37–41.
43. HERRON, L. R., R. A. EISENBERG, E. ROPER, V. N. KAKKANAIAH, P. L. COHEN & B. L. KOTZIN. 1993. Selection of the T cell receptor repertoire in lpr mice. J. Immunol. **151:** 3450–3459.

44. SMYTH, L., M. HOWELL & I. N. CRISPE. 1992. Self-reactivity and the expression of memory markers vary independently in MRL-Mp+/+ and MRL-Mp-lpr/lpr mice. Dev. Immunol. **2:** 309–318.

45. WU, J., T. ZHOU, J. ZHANG, J. HE, W. C. GAUSE & J. D. MOUNTZ. 1994. Correction of accelerated autoimmune disease by early replacement of the mutated lpr gene with the normal Fas apoptosis gene in the T cells of transgenic MRL-lpr/lpr mice. Proc. Natl. Acad. Sci. U.S.A. **91:** 2344–2348.

46. VIGNAUX, F. & P. GOLSTEIN. 1994. Fas-based lymphocyte-mediated cytotoxicity against syngeneic activated lymphocytes: a regulatory pathway? Eur. J. Immunol. **24:** 923–927.

47. BOSSU, P., G. G. SINGER, P. ANDRES, R. ETTINGER, R. A. MARSHAK & A. K. ABBAS. 1993. Mature CD4+ T lymphocytes from MRL/lpr mice are resistant to receptor-mediated tolerance and apoptosis. J. Immunol. **151:** 7233–7239.

48. MIYAWAKI, T., T. UEHARA, R. NIBU, T. TSUJI, A. YACHIE, S. YONEHARA & N. TANIGUCHI. 1992. Differential expression of apoptosis-related Fas antigen on lymphocyte subpopulations in human peripheral blood. J. Immunol. **149:** 3753.

49. HUANG, L., K. SYE & I. N. CRISPE. 1994. Proliferation and apoptosis of B220+CD4−CD8− TCR$\alpha/\beta^{\text{intermediate}}$ T cells in the liver of normal adult mice: implication for lpr pathogenesis. Int. Immunol. **6:** 533–540.

50. HUANG, L. & I. N. CRISPE. 1993. Superantigen-driven peripheral deletion of T cells: apoptosis occurs in cells that have lost the α/β T cell receptor. J. Immunol. **151:** 1844–1851.

51. NEMAZEE, D., C. GUIET, K. BUERKI & A. MARSHAK-ROTHSTEIN. 1991. B lymphocytes from the autoimmune-prone mouse strain MRL/lpr manifest an intrinsic defect in tetraparental MRL/lpr DBA/2 chimeras. J. Immunol. **147:** 2536–2539.

52. DAMLE, N. K., P. S. LINSLEY & J. A. LEDBETTER. 1991. Direct helper T cell–induced B cell differentiation involves interaction between T cell antigen CD28 and B cell activation antigen B7. Eur. J. Immunol. **21:** 1277–1282.

53. LENSCHOW, D. J., A. I. SPERLING, M. P. COOKE, G. FREEMAN, L. RHEE, D. C. DECKER, G. GRAY, L. M. NADLER, C. C. GOODNOW & J. A. BLUESTONE. 1994. Differential up-regulation of the B7-1 and B7-2 costimulatory molecules after Ig receptor engagement by antigen. J. Immunol. **153:** 1990–1997.

54. KENNEDY, M. K., K. M. MOHLER, K. D. SHANEBECK, P. R. BAUM, K. S. PICHA, C. A. OTTEN-EVANS, C. A. JANEWAY & K. H. GRABSTEIN. 1994. Induction of B cell costimulatory function by recombinant murine CD40 ligand. Eur. J. Immunol. **24:** 116–123.

55. EYNON, E. E. & D. C. PARKER. 1992. Small B cells as antigen-presenting cells in the induction of tolerance to soluble protein antigens. J. Exp. Med. **175:**131.

56. LASSILA, O., O. VAINIO & P. MATZINGER. 1988. Can B cells turn on virgin T cells? Nature **334:** 253–255.

57. RAJAGOPALAN, S., T. ZORDAN, G. C. TSOKOS & S. K. DATTA. 1990. Pathogenic anti-DNA autoantibody-inducing T helper cell lines from patients with active lupus nephritis: isolation of $CD4^-8^-$ T helper cell lines that express the $\gamma\delta$ T-cell antigen receptor. Proc. Natl. Acad. Sci. U.S.A. **87:** 7020–7024.

58. SAINIS, K. & S. K. DATTA. 1988. $CD4^+$ T cell lines with selective patterns of autoreactivity as well as $CD4^-$ $CD8^-$ T helper cell lines augment the production of idiotypes shared by pathogenic anti-DNA autoantibodies in the NZB × SWR model of lupus nephritis. J. Immunol. **140:** 2215–2224.

59. MOHAN, C., S. ADAMS, V. STANIK & S. DATTA. 1993. Nucleosome: a major immunogen for pathogenic autoantibody-inducing T cells of lupus. J. Exp. Med. **177:** 1367–1381.

60. FERNANDEZ, B. R., M. KONSTADOULAKIS, K. BAUR, R. S. SCHWARTZ & M. P. MADAIO. 1991. Autoreactive T cells from MRL-lpr/lpr mice secrete multiple lymphokines and induce the production of IgG anti-DNA antibodies. J. Autoimmun. **4:** 563–576.

61. SHORES, E. W., R. A. EISENBERG & P. L. COHEN. 1988. T-B collaboration in the *in vitro* anti-Sm autoantibody response of MRL/Mp-lpr mice. J. Immunol. **140:** 2977–2982.

62. THEOBALD, M. 1995. Allorecognition and graft-versus-host disease. Bone Marrow Transplant. **15:** 489–498.

63. SCHULTZ, K. R., J. PAQUET, S. BADER & K. T. HAYGLASS. 1995. Requirement for B cells in T cell priming to minor histocompatibility antigens and development of graft-versus-host disease. Bone Marrow Transplant. **16:** 289–295.
64. KELLEY, V. R., R. D. BLOOM, M. A. YUI, C. MARTIN & D. PRICE. 1994. Pivotal role of colony stimulating factor-1 in lupus nephritis. Kidney Int. **45**(suppl.): S83–S85.

B Lymphocytes as Autoantigen-presenting Cells in the Amplification of Autoimmunity[a]

RITA ROTH, RENELLE J. GEE, AND MARK J. MAMULA[b]

Section of Rheumatology
Yale University School of Medicine
New Haven, Connecticut 06520

INTRODUCTION

The initiation of a T cell response to antigen requires at least two signals. One type of signal is conveyed through binding of the antigen-specific T cell receptor to a major histocompatibility complex (MHC) ligand displaying processed antigen on the surface of antigen-presenting cells (APCs). A second signal is delivered by antigen-nonspecific costimulatory molecules expressed on the same APC.[1,2] T cells not receiving costimulation, or the second signal, are rendered tolerant (or unresponsive) and are unable to produce certain cytokines.[1,3] The B7 family of costimulatory molecules including B7-1 and B7-2 provoke T cell responses by interacting with the counterreceptors CD28 and CTLA.[4–13] These two B7 molecules are expressed on activated B cells, activated monocytes/macrophages, and dendritic cells, but not on resting B cells. After B cell activation, B7-2 is expressed earlier and at higher levels than B7-1.[7,8,14–16] The interactive dynamics of these two costimulatory molecules are yet to be fully understood; however, some studies have suggested that B7-2-mediated costimulation is important in the initiation phase of a T cell response, whereas B7-1 may serve a role in maintaining and/or expanding the ongoing T cell response.[11,16–18] In addition, several recent studies have demonstrated that both B7 molecules deliver signals to regulate T cell cytokine production.[16,18–20] Finally, it has been indicated that B7-2-mediated costimulation may enhance a Th_2-type response, whereas B7-1 preferentially costimulates for a Th_1-type or cell-mediated response.

In the present study, we have investigated the conditions of costimulation that may be important in eliciting autoreactive T cell responses to a model self-protein, cytochrome *c* (cyt *c*), as well as to a target of lupus autoimmunity, the U1/Sm ribonucleoprotein (snRNP). To this end, previous reports have established that the normal lymphocyte repertoire contains autoreactive T cells that have escaped thymic T cell deletion and peripheral T cell anergy.[21–23] For example, T cell autoimmunity to cryptic self-peptides has been shown to arise in human disease and in animal models of multiple sclerosis and diabetes.[24–26] Although mice are unable to elicit B or T cell

[a]This work was supported by grants from the National Institutes of Health (Nos. AR41032 and AI36529) to M. J. Mamula.

[b]To whom all correspondence should be addressed.

responses to immunization with self–cyt *c* or self-snRNPs, tolerance can be broken by mechanisms of molecular mimicry or by cryptic self-peptides. In particular, B cells elicited by a foreign molecular mimic can bind and present immunogenic peptides of self–cyt *c*.[23,27,28] Here, we demonstrate that a cryptic self-peptide of mouse cyt *c*, residues 81–104, can elicit B cells that prime autoreactive T cells. A similar response can arise in T cell autoimmunity due to the snRNP autoantigen, where B cells (as APCs) are elicited with foreign molecular mimics. This mechanism relies on the presence of autoantigen-specific B cells bearing the cell surface costimulatory molecule B7-2. Thereafter, the T cell response diversifies to a variety of determinants on the self-antigen.

MATERIALS AND METHODS

Antigens

Commercially prepared rat heart cyt *c* (Sigma Chemical, St. Louis, Missouri) was used throughout this study. Rat cyt *c* has an amino acid sequence identical to mouse cyt *c* and is hereafter termed mouse cyt *c*. The polypeptide encompassing amino acids 81–104 of mouse cyt *c* was prepared as previously described.[23] Intact murine small ribonucleoproteins (snRNPs) were affinity-purified on an anti-7-methylguanosine column as previously reported.[29] The recombinant A protein of human snRNPs was also used in immunizations (a kind gift of Joe Craft).[30]

Mice and Immunizations

B cell donor B10.A mice [6–8 weeks of age (NIH, Bethesda, Maryland)] were immunized intraperitoneally (ip) with 100 μg of peptide fragment 81–104 of mouse cyt *c*, recombinant human snRNP A protein, or PBS, all emulsified 1:1 in CFA (Difco Laboratories, Detroit, Michigan). After 21 days, mice were boosted with 100 μg of the respective antigen or PBS emulsified 1:1 in IFA. At day 28, serum from B cell donor mice was assayed for the presence of antibodies to cyt *c*, human snRNP A protein, or murine snRNPs by conventional ELISA.

B cell–deficient mice (μ*MT*, 8–10 weeks old) originally generated in the laboratory of K. Rajewsky were the recipients of B cell adoptive transfers.[31] The μ*MT* mice were backcrossed (tenth generation) and maintained on the B10.A background in the animal-care facilities at Yale University. Mice made homozygous for the μ*MT* mutation lack B cells expressing B220, sIgM, or sIgD and have no detectable serum IgM (data not shown).

Antibodies and Flow Cytometry

Antibodies to B7-1 and B7-2 were kindly provided by D. Faherty and N. Nabavi of Hoffmann–La Roche (Nutley, New Jersey). The binding characteristics of rat anti-murine B7-1 (1G10, IgG_{2a}) and anti-B7-2 (2D10, IgG_{2b}) monoclonal antibodies (mAbs) have been described previously.[11,16,32,33] FITC-coupled anti-IgM (331.3) and FITC-anti-B220 (RA3-6B2) were a gift of M. J. Shlomchik (Yale University). The following mAbs were purchased from Pharmingen (San Diego, California): PE-anti-B220 mAb (RA3-6B2; rat IgG_{2a}); FITC-anti-mouse dendritic cell (4F7); purified rat IgG_{2a} (R35-95) and IgG_{2b} (R35-38), used as isotype controls; FITC-anti-CD54 (ICAM-1, 3E2, hamster IgG); PE-anti-HSA (M1/69, rat IgG_{2b}); and FITC-anti-CD62L (MEL-14, rat IgG_{2a}). Cell purifications were performed with culture supernatants of anti-Thy-1 (Y19), anti-CD4 (GK1.5), anti-CD8 (TIB 105 and TIB 210), and anti-Mac1 (TIB 128).

Cell surface staining with optimal concentrations of fluorochrome-conjugated mAbs was performed by conventional methods and samples were analyzed on a FACScan instrument (Becton Dickinson, Mountain View, California). In some experiments, cell sorting was performed with freshly isolated and stained B cells on a Becton Dickinson FACStar$^{plus®}$

Preparation of Cell Fractions

Immunizations, as described above, were performed in wild-type B10.A mice that served as B cell donors. Cell subsets were purified by complement-mediated lysis of erythrocyte-depleted spleen cells. Cells from donor mice and controls were incubated with a cocktail of anti-Thy-1 (Y19), anti-CD4 (GK1.5), anti-CD8 (TIB 105 and TIB 210), and anti-Mac1 (TIB 128) followed by complement lysis according to standard methodology.

Purification of B7-2^{pos}-B cells from B7-2^{neg}-B cells was performed by flow cytometry. In brief, purified B cells were incubated with biotinylated anti-B7-2 mAb, washed, and further incubated with streptavidin-coated magnetic beads (Biomag, Perspective Diagnostics, Cambridge, Massachusetts). Cells were then subjected to magnetic separation. The B7-2^{neg}-B cell fraction was further depleted of any remaining B7-2^{pos}-B cells by complement-mediated lysis in the presence of anti-B7-2 mAb. Cell populations were analyzed by flow cytometry for purity. Resulting B7-2^{neg}-B cell fractions stained negatively ($<1\%$) for FITC-anti-B7-2 mAb, whereas staining was $>96\%$ for B7-2^{pos}-B cell fractions, as determined by FACS® analysis. The overall yield of B7-2^{pos}-B cells was 7–10% of the purified B cell fraction. Purified B cell preparations were not contaminated with dendritic cells as analyzed by flow cytometry (data not shown).

Resting and LPS-activated B cells were analyzed for the expression of B7 molecules by flow cytometry according to the method of Chen and Nabavi.[32] Purified B cells (2×10^6/mL) were suspended in medium supplemented with 5% FCS and LPS (15 μg/mL) for 48 h prior to analysis.

Adoptive Cell Transfers and in Vivo *Antibody Treatment*

Purified subsets of splenic B cells (cell numbers are indicated in the figure legends below) of B10.A donor mice were suspended in 100 μL of PBS and injected subcutaneously in the left lower thigh of μ*MT* mice. Mice were then immunized with 100 μg of whole mouse cyt *c*/CFA, murine snRNPs/CFA, or PBS/CFA in the left footpad and into the base of the tail. In some experiments, animals were given daily ip injections of anti-B7-1 (100 μg), anti-B7-2 (100 μg), both antibodies (each 100 μg), or control rat Ig isotypes (100 μg in PBS) starting at the time of cell transfer. After 8 days, the draining left-side popliteal and inguinal LNs were aseptically collected, and single cell suspensions were analyzed for *in vitro* T cell proliferation and cytokine gene expression. In addition, LNCs were analyzed by flow cytometry for the presence of B cell populations relative to control μ*MT* recipient and normal B10.A mice. Each experimental condition was examined in a minimum of five mice.

Proliferation Assays

For *in vitro* proliferation assays, LNCs (5×10^5) were suspended in medium supplemented with 2.5% autologous, heat-inactivated mouse serum and were cultured with irradiated (2000 rad) splenic APCs (5×10^5), with or without antigen (final volume of 200 μL/well), in flat-bottomed 96-well microtiter plates (Costar, Cambridge, Massachusetts). After 3 days, cells were pulsed with 1 μCi of [^{3}H]thymidine/well for 18 h and harvested onto filters with a semiautomatic cell harvester (Skatron Instruments, Sterling, Virginia). Radioactivity was measured with a liquid scintillation counter (Betaplate, model 1205, LKB/Wallac, Gaithersburg, Maryland). The results presented in the figures below are means of duplicate wells. Standard deviations were less than 15%.

To analyze the ability of B7-2^{neg}-B cells to present antigen, T cell hybridomas (designated 11.1, E5, and 6.4.14) specific for mouse cyt *c* peptide 81–104 (10^5 cells) were cocultured with increasing numbers (10^4 to 10^6) of irradiated (1000 rad) B7-2^{neg}-B cells and cyt *c* peptide 81–104 (50 μg/mL). Culture supernatants were added to 5×10^3 CTLL cells, incubated overnight, and pulsed with [^{3}H]thymidine for 18 h. Cultures were harvested and radioactivity was measured as described above.

Antibody Analysis

Sera from B cell donor B10.A mice immunized with cyt *c* fragment 81–104 or immunized with recombinant A protein (of human snRNPs) were assayed by ELISA against native murine cyt *c* or native murine snRNPs, respectively. In brief, the antigens (10 μg/mL) were adsorbed overnight to microtiter plates in parallel assays. After incubation with 1% BSA in PBS, 1/100 dilutions of individual mouse serum were added, and plates were developed with goat anti-mouse IgG–alkaline phosphatase (Southern Biotechnology Associates, Birmingham, Alabama) and the substrate *p*-nitrophenylphosphate. Control sera were obtained from B10.A mice immunized with PBS/CFA.

RESULTS

Tolerance of Mice to Immunization with Self-protein

Maintenance of tolerance to self-protein is shown to occur in lymph node (LN) T cells from wild-type B10.A and syngeneic B cell–deficient (μ*MT*) mice immunized with self–cyt *c* (FIGURE 1A). LN T cells from these mice did not proliferate to *in vitro* restimulation with self–cyt *c* or to cyt *c* peptide 81–104. No significant T cell proliferation was noted with LNCs derived from cyt *c*–immunized μ*MT* mice reconstituted with B cells from syngeneic, wild-type B10.A mice (FIGURE 1A). In addition, no antibody responses in B10.A mice, μ*MT* mice, or B cell reconstituted μ*MT* mice were observed upon repeated immunizations with whole mouse cyt *c* (FIGURE 2 and data not shown). We have duplicated these observations with immunizations of intact murine snRNPs, the target of autoimmunity in murine (MRL strains) and human lupus. In a manner similar to immunizations with self–cyt *c*, our previous studies demonstrated that murine snRNPs elicit no B or T cell responses in wild-type B10.A or μ*MT* mice (data not shown).[29]

However, B cell–deficient mice will respond to immunization with peptide antigens (FIGURE 1B). We had previously found that the murine cyt *c* peptide 81–104 is unable to be processed and presented from the native whole cyt *c* protein by APCs.[23] Immunization with the 81–104 peptide elicits strong T cell responses in both wild-type B10.A and syngeneic μ*MT* mice. Clearly, T cells specific for this self-peptide have not been deleted or tolerized, most likely because these two functions of T cell tolerance are dependent on antigen processing functions. B cells, presumably as APCs, are not required to elicit anti-peptide T cell responses, although the magnitude of T cell responses in peptide-immunized μ*MT* mice is depressed by as much as 75% in comparison with responses in wild-type B10.A mice (FIGURE 1B). As previously reported, B cells may be more important in presenting peptides derived from protein antigen, whereas other APCs such as dendritic cells and macrophages may better present peptide antigens.[34] FIGURE 1B illustrates the crypticity of the cyt *c* 81–104 peptide. T cells elicited to this peptide are unable to respond to restimulation with native cyt *c*, demonstrating that APCs are unable to process and present this peptide from the native protein.

Cryptic Peptides Elicit Autoreactive B Cells

B10.A wild-type mice immunized with the cryptic peptide fragment 81–104 of cyt *c* produced autoantibodies specific for this peptide and whole mouse cyt *c*, as analyzed by ELISA (FIGURE 2). Soluble inhibition studies with native cyt *c* suggest that the anti-peptide antibodies bind native self (murine)–cyt *c*. The ability of anti-fragment 81–104 antibodies to bind whole mouse cyt *c* was not unexpected because its crystal structure indicates that this region is surface exposed on the whole protein.[35]

We next analyzed these autoreactive B cells for the expression of the costimulatory molecules B7-1 and B7-2 by flow cytometry. Freshly isolated, resting B cells from wild-type B10.A mice expressed little B7-2 on the cell surface (less than 3%,

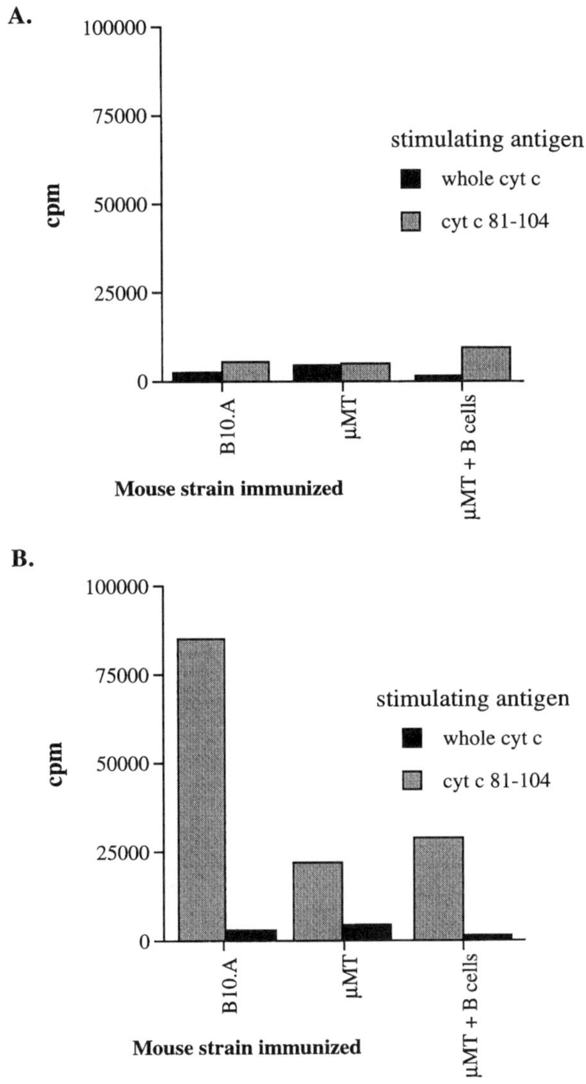

FIGURE 1. Mice are unresponsive to immunization with self–cyt *c* (A), but respond to self–cyt *c* peptide 81–104 (B). Wild-type B10.A mice, µ*MT* mice, and µ*MT* mice reconstituted with B cells (20×10^6) from normal, syngeneic B10.A mice were immunized with 100 µg of mouse cyt *c* (A) or cyt *c* peptide 81–104 (B) in CFA. Eight days later, standard proliferation assays were performed with draining LN cells and titrated amounts of mouse cyt *c* or cyt *c* peptide 81–104. Positive PPD (20 µg/mL) controls were 51,808 ± 1668 cpm.

data not shown). In contrast, 12–21% of resting B cells activated *in vitro* with lipopolysaccharide (LPS) stained positively for B7-1 (data not shown) and 50–58% for B7-2 (FIGURE 3B). Upon *in vivo* activation by immunization with the cyt *c* peptide 81–104 in CFA, B7-2 expression on B cells ranged from 3% to 7% (FIGURE 3A), whereas B7-1 expression was virtually undetectable on B7-1/B7-2 double-stained B cells (data not shown). However, sorting the purified B cell population into B7-2^{pos}-B cells revealed that 3–7% of the B7-2^{pos}-B cells also expressed B7-1 (FIGURE 3C). Approximately 17% of the B7-2^{pos} purified B cells were negative for B7-2, most likely due to the turnover (or short half-life) of surface B7-2. The sorted B7-2^{neg}-B cell fraction stained negatively for B7-1 (FIGURE 3D).

Finally, B7-2^{pos}- and B7-2^{neg}-B cell subsets expressed similar levels of MHC class II antigens, ICAM-1, heat-stable antigen, and L-selectin (CD62L) (data not shown).

Autoantigen-specific B7-2^{pos}-B Cells Break T Cell Tolerance to Self-proteins

In order to define the parameters crucial for T cell priming, we adoptively transferred subsets of B7-2^{pos}-B cells and B7-2^{neg}-B cells derived from donor mice immunized with cyt *c* peptide 81–104/CFA or PBS/CFA into μ*MT* mice (FIGURE 4A). The recipient mice were then immunized with whole cyt *c*. As measured by *in vitro* proliferative assays, B7-2^{pos}-B cells from cyt *c* fragment 81–104 immunized mice elicited a T cell proliferative response to mouse cyt *c* in the draining LNs of the recipient μ*MT* mice (FIGURE 4A). In the absence of immunization with cyt *c*, background levels of T cell proliferation were observed in mice (similar to mice immunized with PBS/CFA). Our previous studies and those described in FIGURE 1 demonstrated that murine cyt *c* 81–104 specific T cells do not respond to the native murine cyt *c* protein.[23] Therefore, the T cell response to whole cyt *c* represents novel,

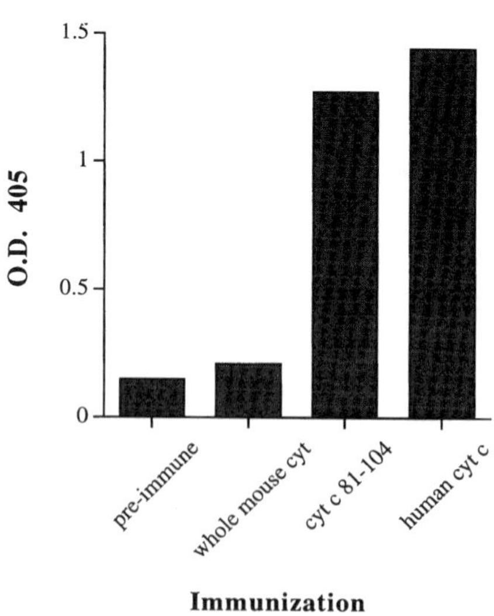

FIGURE 2. B cell responses in B10.A mice immunized with peptide fragment 81–104 of cyt *c*. Serum antibodies from B10.A mice immunized with whole mouse cyt *c*, fragment 81–104, or human cyt *c* were analyzed for their binding to mouse cyt *c* by ELISA. Whole murine cyt *c* was adsorbed to microtiter plates and incubated with 1/100 serum dilutions from B10.A mice immunized with the indicated antigens. Optical density (405 nm) was recorded after 30 minutes of substrate incubation.

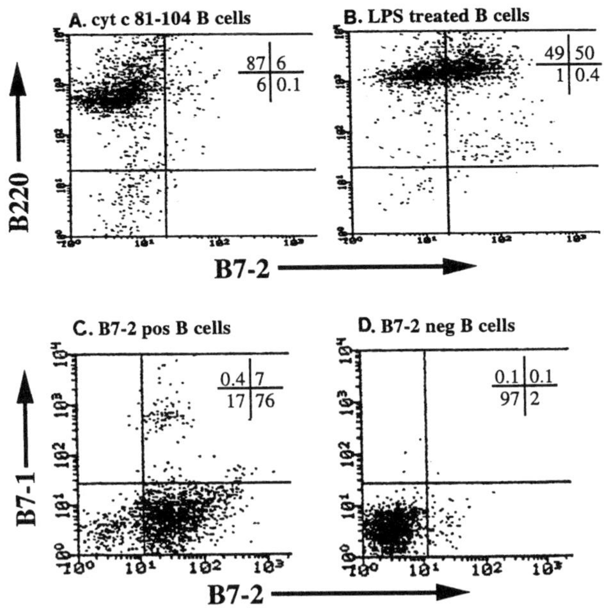

FIGURE 3. Flow cytometric analysis of B7 expression on B cells. Purified splenic B10.A B cells were double-stained with FITC-anti-B7-2 mAb and PE-anti-B220 or PE-anti-B7-1. FACS® analysis was performed with freshly isolated B cells from mice immunized with either cyt *c* fragment 81–104 in CFA (A) or LPS-treated B cells (B). B7-2-bearing B cells were purified as described in the text and were restained for the presence of B-7 molecules. B7-2^{pos}-B cells (C) and B7-2^{neg}-B cells (D) from peptide 81–104 immunized mice were double-stained with FITC-anti-B7-2 and PE-anti-B7-1 mAb and were analyzed by FACS®. The amount of cells in each quadrant is expressed as a percentage in the corresponding cross section. Log fluorescence intensities are shown on both axes of panels A–D.

noncryptic autoimmunity and not a transfer of 81–104 specific T cells from donor mice into recipient LNs.

In contrast to B7-2^{pos}-B cells, B7-2^{neg}-B cells were not able to elicit a T cell response to self–cyt *c* in recipient μ*MT* mice (FIGURE 4A). Also, LN cells of control μ*MT* mice reconstituted with nonspecific B7-2^{pos}-B cells or B7-2^{neg}-B cells derived from PBS/CFA-immunized donor mice failed to respond to mouse cyt *c* (data not shown).

The failure of B7-2^{neg}-B cells of peptide-immunized donor mice to activate naive T cells could be ascribed to their inability to present antigen because of the absence of costimulatory molecules. To address this point, we cocultured increasing numbers of B7-2^{neg}-B cells from cyt *c* fragment 81–104 immunized mice with T cell hybridomas specific for the cyt *c* peptide 81–104. Our results revealed that B7-2^{neg}-B cells were indeed potent APCs in presenting the peptide 81–104 to the T cell hybridomas. In addition, LPS treatment of B7-2^{neg}-B cell populations elicited cyt *c* binding antibodies, demonstrating the presence of cyt *c*–specific B cells in the B7-2^{neg} population (data not shown).

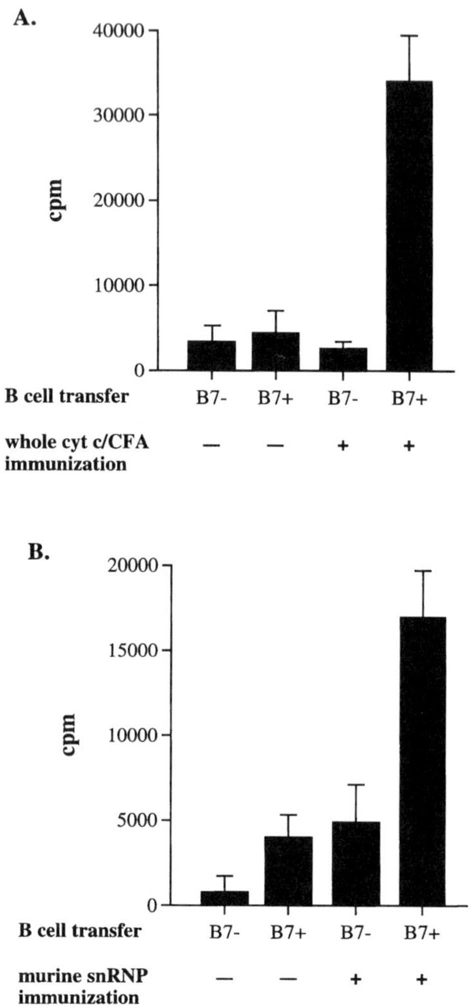

FIGURE 4. B7-2^{pos}-B cells from mice immunized with a cryptic self-peptide or a foreign molecular mimic elicit autoreactive T cell responses. T cell proliferative responses to mouse cyt *c* (A) or mouse snRNPs (B) were analyzed in μ*MT* mice reconstituted with B7+/− B cells from antigen-primed donor mice (cyt *c* 81–104 peptide in panel A or recombinant human snRNP A protein in panel B). B cells from wild-type B10.A immunized mice were separated into B7-2^{pos}- and B7-2^{neg}-B cell fractions. Purified B cell subsets (10^5 cells) were injected subcutaneously into μ*MT* mice that were subsequently immunized with or without mouse cyt *c* or mouse snRNPs in CFA (as indicated). Eight days later, mice were sacrificed, and *in vitro* proliferation of single cell suspensions prepared from draining popliteal and inguinal LNs was measured with titrated amounts of mouse cyt *c* or murine snRNPs.

We next examined the ability of B cells specific for the lupus autoantigen, snRNPs, to activate autoreactive T cells. In this system, donor mice were immunized with a molecular mimic, recombinant human A protein of human snRNPs. Our previous studies demonstrated that mice immunized with the human A protein generate antibodies capable of binding the murine A protein.[29] Akin to our studies with cytochrome *c*, mice are completely unresponsive to immunization with self-snRNPs. However, we previously found that coimmunization of mice with self-snRNPs along with the human A protein elicited T cell responses specific for the murine snRNP complex.[29] We hypothesized that B cells elicited to the foreign, cross-reactive A protein were able to present self-snRNPs in an immunogenic manner. FIGURE 4B confirms this hypothesis and again suggests that the B cells must be capable of binding the autoantigen and must possess B7-2 costimulatory molecules in order to elicit an autoreactive T cell response.

Anti-B7 Antibody Prevents in Vivo *T Cell Priming to Self-protein*

To examine the contribution of the B7 costimulatory molecules in T cell priming to the cyt *c* autoantigen, experimental μ*MT* mice (as described above) received daily injections (ip) with 100 μg of anti-B7-1, anti-B7-2, or both antibodies. After 8 days of treatment, the *in vitro* proliferative response to cyt *c* was inhibited by over 80% by both LN cells isolated from anti-B7-1- and anti-B7-2-treated mice (FIGURE 5). Simultaneous administration of anti-B7-1 and anti-B7-2 antibodies completely abolished the T cell response. In contrast, the isotype-matched rat IgG (IgG_{2a} and/or IgG_{2b}) control antibodies did not significantly suppress the T cell responses.

We were also interested in understanding the role of B7 molecules in spontaneous models of lupus autoimmunity. We chose the MRL lpr/lpr and MRL +/+ mouse strains, which spontaneously develop anti-snRNP and/or anti-double-stranded DNA autoantibodies along with autoimmune pathology such as glomerulonephritis and vasculitis.[36,37] This study consisted of four different treatment groups—those receiving anti-B7-1, anti-B7-2, and anti-B7-1/B7-2 together, and a control group receiving isotype-matched antibody. MRL lpr/lpr and MRL +/+ mice (30 mice in each group) were treated for 8 weeks (three times per week) beginning at 4 weeks of age. The mice were bled biweekly and an analysis of autoantibodies was performed by immunofluorescence, ELISA for anti-DNA and anti-snRNP, immunoblotting for anti-snRNP, and immunoprecipitations. This extensive series of studies revealed that the treatment group did not statistically differ from untreated controls for any of the autoantibody responses examined (data not shown). Specificities and titers of autoantibody subsets

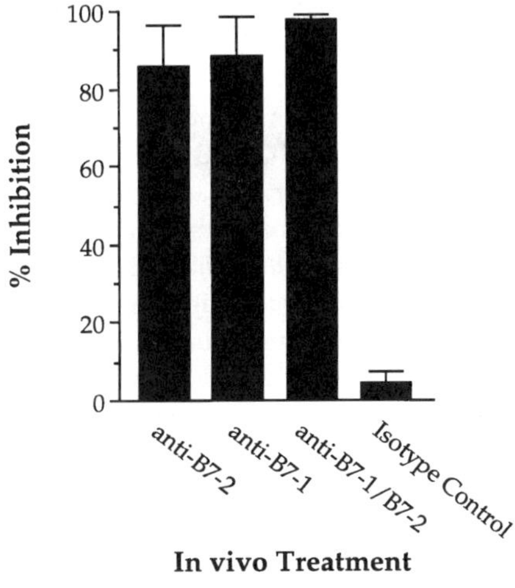

FIGURE 5. Cell proliferation after *in vivo* treatment of recipient mice with anti-B7 mAbs. Recipient μ*MT* mice reconstituted with B7-2^pos^-B cells (10^5) and immunized with whole mouse cyt *c* were daily injected ip with 100 μg of anti-B7-1, anti-B7-2, both antibodies, or isotype controls (IgG_{2a}, IgG_{2b}, or both). As in FIGURE 4, standard LN proliferation assays were performed after 8 days and results are expressed as % inhibition. Data represent the means of 5–7 mice and SD.

(anti-DNA and anti-snRNP) did not change between anti-B7 groups and sham control groups in comparison with untreated MRL mice. Because the antibody treatment protocol was used under physiologically relevant conditions (such as those used for *in vivo* inhibition studies), it is possible that lupus autoimmunity, as spontaneously developing in the MRL mouse, may circumvent or perhaps not be dependent on the B7 costimulatory pathway. The observations are in contrast to a recent study where anti-DNA antibody responses and corresponding autoimmune histopathology are less severe in murine models treated with CTLA4Ig, a treatment that interferes with the B7/CD28 pathway.[38]

DISCUSSION

The present study demonstrates that autoreactive T cells are readily elicited in B cell–deficient mice upon the adoptive transfer of autoantigen-specific B7-2^{pos}-B cells. The successful T cell priming by this B cell subset relied upon both their specificity to self-protein and the expression of the B7-2 costimulatory molecule.

Autoantigen-specific B Cells Activate Autoreactive T Cells

Autoantigen-specific B cells were elicited in wild-type mice by immunization with the cryptic self-peptide 81–104 of mouse cyt *c* or with the recombinant human A ribonucleoprotein (snRNP), a molecular mimic of the target of lupus autoimmunity in human and murine models of SLE. The induction of the B cells was likely to occur with the help of T cells initially primed by nonspecific APCs such as dendritic cells (FIGURE 6).[39] Here, we support this postulate in that immunization of μ*MT* mice with the peptide 81–104 of cyt *c* elicited strong peptide-specific LN T cell responses in the absence of B cell APCs. In contrast, LN T cells of μ*MT* mice immunized with the whole mouse cyt *c* remained unresponsive, suggesting that resident nonspecific APCs were not able to present the mouse cyt *c* protein in an immunogenic manner. A recent study indicates that B cells, as APCs, may be critical in processing and presenting protein antigen, whereas other APCs (macrophages and dendritic cells) may be more efficient at presenting peptide antigen.[34]

Nonspecific B7-2^{pos}-B cells also failed to elicit autoreactive T cells, emphasizing the requirement for autoantigen-specific B cell APCs in this autoimmune response. Peptide-specific B cells bind and process the native cyt *c* antigen via the surface exposure of region 81–104 on the native cyt *c* autoantigen.[35] These B cells process and present immunogenic self-peptides distinct from those presented by nonspecific APCs such as macrophages and dendritic cells. The latter APC population likely presents peptides to which T cells have become deleted or tolerized, whereas antigen-specific B cells present unique (or cryptic) self-determinants easily recognized by the T cell repertoire.

It is well established that B cells bind antigen via specific cell surface receptors in order to efficiently function as APCs. As demonstrated by Rock *et al.* and Lanzavecchia, B cells present antigen up to 10,000-fold more efficiently by receptor-mediated

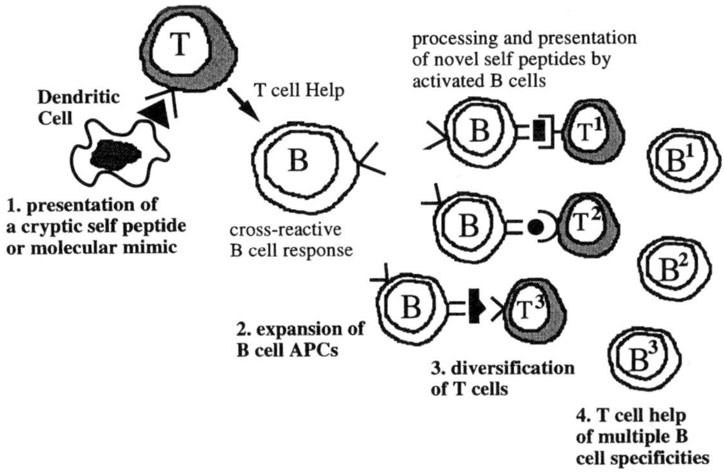

FIGURE 6. Mechanism of inducing B cells as autoantigen-presenting cells in the activation of autoimmune T cells.

uptake as compared to nonspecific uptake of antigen.[40–42] Based on our own B cell trafficking studies (not reported here), we find that approximately 300 resident B7-2^{pos}-B cells are sufficient to elicit detectable T cell autoimmunity. Although we have not yet determined the role of recirculating B cell APCs that may enter the LNs at later time points, it appears that B7-2^{pos}-B cells may be important APCs under physiologic conditions where low antigen concentrations prevail, such as in autoimmunity to intracellular autoantigens in systemic lupus erythematosus (SLE).

In contrast to B7-2^{pos}-B cells, adoptively transferred B7-2^{neg}-B cells, which made up the large majority (90%) of the unseparated B cell population, did not activate naive T cells in cyt *c*–immunized μ*MT* mice. However, the B7-2^{neg}-B cells did present antigen to previously primed T cells. We also do not know whether the B7-2^{neg}-B cells induce unresponsiveness (tolerance or anergy) in T cells as found to occur with small resting B cells.[43–45]

In contrast to our results, it has been suggested that B cells (either activated or resting) do not prime naive CD4 T cells, but instead serve as a mechanism to tolerize naive T cells.[43–46] These studies contend that dendritic cells and/or macrophages are responsible for T cell priming, whereas B cells stimulate only previously primed T cells. However, the present and previous *in vivo* studies attribute to B cells a critical role in breaking T cell tolerance to self-protein. In support of our studies, Ho *et al.* have demonstrated that only B cells activated by the engagement of the B cell receptor with antigen, which induced upregulation of B7-related surface molecules, lead to complete T cell activation.[47] The fact that naive T cells are particularly dependent on costimulation and are activated only by dendritic cells and preactivated B cells, but not by resting B cells and macrophages, has previously been established with transgenic naive T cells by Croft *et al.*[48,49] In addition, Cassell and Schwartz have shown that peptide-activated B cells activate naive T cells by involving B7-related costimulatory molecules.[50] They conclude that B cells are less potent APCs as compared with dendritic cells because they express lower levels of B7-related molecules and lack costimulatory ligands expressed on dendritic cells. Together, these studies emphasize the importance of the activation state of a B cell at the time of encountering a T cell in that quantitative and qualitative aspects of costimulation determine the ability and efficiency to activate naive T cells. As noted by Metlay *et al.*, the lower potency of activated B cells as compared to nonspecific APCs could ascribe B cells as featured APCs to activate a subset of T cells.[51]

Costimulation through B7-2 Is a Prerequisite for Priming of Autoreactive T Cells

Our results showing that recipient mice treated with anti-B7-2 mAb were unresponsive to immunization with cyt *c* strongly support the role of B7-2 as a major costimulatory molecule in the initiation of an immune response. Moreover, the first signaling for the activation of naive T cells may have occurred through the interaction of the B7-2 molecule with the T cell counterreceptor CD28. This suggestion is based on the findings that CD28 is constitutively expressed on naive T cells, whereas CTLA4, another ligand for B7-2, is expressed only on activated T cells.[12,52,53] We also made this conclusion by ignoring a possible immediate upregulation of B7-1 after the adoptive transfer of the B7-2^{pos}-B cell subset into recipient mice. Upregulation of B7-1 has been shown to occur through stimuli such as cross-linking of MHC class II molecules or surface Ig cross-linking by antigen.[33,54] Because treatment with anti-B7-2 mAb resulted in complete inhibition of the T cell response, signaling through (already expressed and/or possibly upregulated) B7-1 alone could not initiate the activation of naive T cells.

Recent studies have also demonstrated the important contribution of the B7 molecules in directing the outcome of the T cell effector function.[18,19] B7-1 has been reported to drive Th_1-type T cell responses, whereas B7-2 directs a Th_2-like response. In our experiments, cytokine gene expression of LNCs from mice reconstituted with B7-2^{pos}-B cells and immunized with cyt *c* encoded for a Th_0-like response and/or both a Th_1- and Th_2-like response (data not shown). In the absence of costimulation through B7-1, these autoreactive B cells primed T cells to express lower IFN-γ, perhaps a Th_2-enhanced response.

Our results provide strong evidence for a multistep mechanism involved to break T cell tolerance to self-protein *in vivo*. The initial step in the mechanism involves the processing and presentation of cryptic self-peptides (or peptides of molecular mimics) by dendritic cells. The dendritic cells present these peptides in the priming of naive T cells, which in turn provide help to evolving B cell responses. These B cell responses may be limited in their specificity, but are capable of binding native self-proteins, if present. These B cells, as APCs, are able to bind, process, and present self-antigen and bear conventional costimulatory molecules such as B7-1 and B7-2. These B cells process antigen in a manner distinct from other APCs via the protection of particular determinants bound to surface immunoglobulin. A subsequent second tier of T cell priming arises due to a diverse set of novel self-determinants. Several recent studies emphasize the ability of antigen-specific B cells to direct or modulate the expression of individual peptides from processed proteins.[55,56] Finally, the diverse array of T cells are capable of driving B cell responses, again with diverse specificity. These diverse responses to foreign antigen would clearly provide a selective advantage in clearing pathogenic challenges. However, this same mechanism, when directed at self-antigens, may provide a basis for autoimmune-mediated pathology.[57,58]

SUMMARY

The exact role of B cells in antigen presentation to naive T cells *in vivo* is presently not known. Here, we demonstrate the ability of a B cell subset consisting of B7-2^{pos}-B cells to prime autoreactive T cells in B cell–deficient mice. In contrast, B cell–deficient mice are unable to mount a similar initiation and expansion of the autoimmune response. The expression of the B7-2 costimulatory molecule as well as the specificity to a self-antigen, either murine cytochrome *c* or murine ribonucleoproteins (the target of autoimmunity in SLE), enabled B cells as antigen-presenting cells to induce naive lymph node T cells to proliferate and to express IFN-γ, IL-4, IL-5, and IL-10 cytokine mRNAs. In contrast, neither adoptively transferred B7-2^{neg}-B cells nor nonspecific B7-2^{pos}-B cells were able to activate naive T cells. In addition, anti-B7-2 treatment prevented the *in vivo* expression of the IL-4, IL-5, and IFN-γ cytokine mRNA responses. Our results suggest a major role of autoantigen-specific B7-2^{pos}-B cells in breaking T cell tolerance to self-antigen.

ACKNOWLEDGMENTS

We are grateful to C. Janeway and R. Flavell for their critical review of this manuscript and to D. Faherty and N. Nabavi of Hoffmann–La Roche (Nutley, New Jersey) and M. J. Shlomchik of Yale University for the generous supply of monoclonal antibodies. We also thank the expert technical assistance of T. Taylor in flow cytometry studies.

REFERENCES

1. SCHWARTZ, R. H. 1988. Acquisition of immunologic tolerance. Cell **57:** 1073–1081.
2. BRETSCHER, P. 1992. The two-signal model of lymphocyte activation twenty-one years later. Immunol. Today **13:** 74–76.
3. HARDING, F. A., J. G. MCARTHUR, J. A. GROSS, D. H. RAULET & J. P. ALLISON. 1992. CD28-mediated signalling co-stimulates murine T cells and prevents induction of anergy in T-cell clones. Nature **356:** 607–609.
4. FREEMAN, G. J., G. S. GRAY, C. D. GIMMI, D. B. LOMBARD, L-J. ZHOU, M. WHITE, J. D. FINGEROTH, J. G. GRIBBEN & L. M. NADLER. 1991. Structure, expression, and T cell costimulatory activity of the murine homologue of the human B lymphocyte activation antigen B7. J. Exp. Med. **174:** 625–631.

5. FREEMAN, G. J., F. BORRIELLO, R. J. HODES, H. REISER, J. G. GRIBBEN, J. W. NG, J. KIM, J. GOLDBERG, K. HATHCOCK, G. LASZLO, L. A. LOMBARD, S. WANG, G. S. GRAY, L. M. NADLER & A. H. SHARPE. 1993. Murine B7-2, an alternative CTLA4 counter-receptor that costimulates T cell proliferation and interleukin-2 production. J. Exp. Med. **178:** 2185–2192.
6. LENSCHOW, D. J., G. H-T. SU, L. A. ZUCKERMAN, N. NABAVI, C. J. JELLIS, G. S. GRAY, J. MILLER & J. A. BLUESTONE. 1993. Expression and functional significance of an additional ligand for CTLA4. Proc. Natl. Acad. Sci. U.S.A. **90:** 11054–11058.
7. HATHCOCK, K. S., G. LASZLO, H. B. DICKLER, J. BRADSHAW, P. LINSLEY & R. J. HODES. 1993. Identification of an alternative CTLA-4 ligand costimulatory for T cell activation. Nature **362:** 905–907.
8. AZUMA, M., D. ITO, H. YAGITA, K. OKUMURA, J. H. PHILLIPS, L. L. LANIER & C. SOMOZA. 1993. B70 antigen is a second ligand for CTLA-4 and CD28. Nature **366:** 76–79.
9. FREEMAN, G. J., F. BORRIELLO, R. J. HODES, H. REISER, K. S. HATHCOCK, G. LASZLO, A. J. MCKNIGHT, J. KIM, L. DU, D. B. LOMBARD, G. S. GRAY, L. M. NADLER & A. H. SHARPE. 1993. Uncovering of functional alternative CTLA-4 counter-receptor in B7-deficient mice. Science **262:** 907–909.
10. FREEMAN, G. J., J. G. GRIBBEN, V. A. BOUSSIOTIS, J. W. NG, V. A. RESTIVO, L. A. LOMBARD, G. S. GRAY & L. M. NADLER. 1993. Cloning of B7-2: a CTLA-4 counter-receptor that costimulates human T cell proliferation. Science **262:** 909–911.
11. CHEN, C., D. A. FAHERTY, A. GAULT, S. E. CONNAUGHTON, G. D. POWERS, D. I. GODFREY & N. NABAVI. 1994. Monoclonal antibody 2D10 recognizes a novel T cell costimulatory molecule on activated murine B lymphocytes. J. Immunol. **152:** 2105–2114.
12. LINSLEY, P. S., W. BRADY, L. GROSMAIRE, A. ARUFFO, N. K. DAMLE & J. A. LEDBETTER. 1991. Binding of the B cell activation antigen B7 to CD28 costimulates T cell proliferation and interleukin-2 mRNA accumulation. J. Exp. Med. **173:** 721–730.
13. LINSLEY, P. S., W. BRADY, M. URNES, L. S. GROSMAIRE, N. K. DAMLE & J. A. LEDBETTER. 1991. CTLA-4 is a second receptor for the B cell activation antigen B7. J. Exp. Med. **174:** 561–570.
14. HATHCOCK, K. S., G. LASZLO, C. PUCILLO, P. LINSLEY & R. J. HODES. 1994. Comparative analysis of B7-1 and B7-2 costimulatory ligands: expression and function. J. Exp. Med. **180:** 631–640.
15. LENSCHOW, D. J., A. I. SPERLING, M. P. COOKE, G. FREEMAN, L. RHEE, D. C. DECKER, G. GRAY, L. M. NADLER, C. C. GOODNOW & J. A. BLUESTONE. 1994. Differential upregulation of the B7-1 and B7-2 costimulatory molecules after Ig receptor engagement by antigen. J. Immunol. **153:** 1990–1997.
16. CHEN, C., A. GAULT, L. SHEN & N. NABAVI. 1994. Molecular cloning and expression of early T cell costimulatory molecule-1 and its characterization as B7-2 molecule. J. Immunol. **152:** 4929–4936.
17. DAMLE, N. K., K. KLUSSMAN, G. LEYTZE, A. ARUFFO, P. S. LINSLEY & J. A. LEDBETTER. 1993. Costimulation with integrin ligands, intercellular adhesion molecule-1 or vascular cell adhesion molecule-1, augments activation-induced death of antigen-specific $CD4^+$ T lymphocytes. J. Immunol. **151:** 2368–2379.
18. FREEMAN, G. J., V. A. BOUSSIOTIS, A. ANUMANTHAN, G. M. BERNSTEIN, X-Y. KE, P. D. RENNERT, G. S. GRAY, J. G. GRIBBEN & L. M. NADLER. 1995. B7-1 and B7-2 do not deliver identical costimulatory signals, since B7-2 but not B7-1 preferentially costimulates the initial production of IL-4. Immunity **2:** 523–532.
19. KUCHROO, V. K., M. P. DAS, J. A. BROWN, A. M. RANGER, S. S. ZAMVIL, R. A. SOBEL, H. L. WEINER, N. NABAVI & L. H. GLIMCHER. 1995. B7-1 and B7-2 costimulatory molecules activate differentially the Th1/Th2 developmental pathways: application to autoimmune disease therapy. Cell **80:** 707–718.
20. THOMPSON, C. B. 1995. Distinct roles for the costimulatory ligands B7-1 and B7-2 in T helper cell differentiation? Cell **81:** 979–982.
21. SCHILD, H., O. ROTZSCHKE, H. KALBACHER & H. G. RAMMENSEE. 1990. Limit of T cell tolerance to self proteins by peptide presentation. Science **247:** 1587–1589.
22. GAMMON, G., E. E. SERCARZ & G. BENICHOU. 1991. The dominant self and the cryptic self: shaping the autoreactive T-cell repertoire. Immunol. Today **12:** 193–195.

23. MAMULA, M. J. 1993. The inability to process a self-peptide allows autoreactive T cells to escape tolerance. J. Exp. Med. **177:** 567–571.
24. LEHMANN, P. V., T. FORSTHUBER, A. MILLER & E. E. SERCARZ. 1992. Spreading of T cell autoimmunity to cryptic determinants of an autoantigen. Nature **358:** 155–157.
25. SERCARZ, E. E., P. V. LEHMANN, A. AMETANI, G. BENICHOU, A. MILLER & K. MOUDGIL. 1993. Dominance and crypticity of T cell antigenic determinants. Annu. Rev. Immunol. **11:** 729–766.
26. MARKOVIC-PLESE, S., H. FUKAURA, J. ZHANG, A. AL-SABBAGH, S. SOUTHWOOD, A. SETTE, V. K. KUCHROO & D. A. HAFLER. 1995. T cell recognition of immunodominant and cryptic proteolipid protein epitopes in humans. J. Immunol. **155:** 982–992.
27. LIN, R-H., M. J. MAMULA, J. A. HARDIN & C. A. JANEWAY, JR. 1991. Induction of autoreactive B cells allows priming of autoreactive T cells. J. Exp. Med. **173:** 1433–1439.
28. MAMULA, M. J., R-H. LIN, C. A. JANEWAY, JR. & J. A. HARDIN. 1992. Breaking T cell tolerance with foreign and self co-immunogens: a study of autoimmune B and T cell epitopes of cytochrome *c*. J. Immunol. **149:** 789–795.
29. MAMULA, M. J., S. FATENEJAD & J. CRAFT. 1994. B cells process and present lupus autoantigens that initiate autoimmune T cell responses. J. Immunol. **152:** 1453–1461.
30. LUTZ-FREYERMUTH, C., C. C. QUERY & J. KEENE. 1990. Quantitative determination that one of the two potential RNA-binding domains of the A protein component of the U1 small nuclear ribonucleoprotein complex binds with high affinity to stem-loop II of U1 RNA. Proc. Natl. Acad. Sci. U.S.A. **87:** 693–697.
31. KITAMURA, D., J. ROES, R. KUHN & K. RAJEWSKY. 1991. A B cell–deficient mouse by targeted disruption of the membrane exon of the immunoglobulin μ chain gene. Nature **350:** 423–426.
32. CHEN, C. & N. NABAVI. 1994. *In vitro* induction of T cell anergy by blocking B7 and early T cell costimulatory molecule ETC-1/B7-2. Immunity **1:** 147–154.
33. NABAVI, N., G. J. FREEMAN, A. GAULT, D. GODFREY, L. M. NADLER & L. H. GLIMCHER. 1992. Signalling through the MHC class II cytoplasmic domain is required for antigen presentation and induces B7 expression. Nature **360:** 266–268.
34. CONSTANT, S., D. SANT'ANGELO, T. PASQUALINI, T. TAYLOR, D. LEVIN, R. FLAVELL & K. BOTTOMLY. 1995. Peptide and protein antigens require distinct antigen-presenting cell subsets for the priming of $CD4^+$ T cells. J. Immunol. **154:** 4915–4923.
35. TAKANO, T. & R. E. DICKERSON. 1981. Conformational change of cytochrome *c*. I. Ferrocytochrome *c* structure refined at 1.5-angstrom resolution. J. Mol. Biol. **153:** 79–94.
36. ANDREWS, B. S., R. A. EISENBERG, A. N. THEOFILOPOULOS, S. IZUI, C. B. WILSON, P. J. MCCONAHEY, E. D. MURPHY, J. B. ROTHS & F. J. DIXON. 1978. Spontaneous murine lupus-like syndromes: clinical and immunopathological manifestations in several strains. J. Exp. Med. **148:** 1198–1215.
37. EISENBERG, R. A., E. M. TAN & F. J. DIXON. 1978. Presence of anti-Sm reactivity in autoimmune mouse strains. J. Exp. Med. **147:** 582–587.
38. FINK, B. K., P. S. LINSLEY & D. WOFSY. 1994. Treatment of murine lupus with CTLA4Ig. Science **265:** 1225–1227.
39. MAMULA, M. J. & C. A. JANEWAY, JR. 1993. Do B cells drive the diversification of immune responses? Immunol. Today **14:** 151–152.
40. ROCK, K. L., B. BENACERRAF & A. K. ABBAS. 1984. Antigen presentation by hapten-specific B lymphocytes. I. Role of surface immunoglobulin receptors. J. Exp. Med. **160:** 1102–1113.
41. LANZAVECCHIA, A. 1985. Antigen-specific interactions between T and B cells. Nature **314:** 537–539.
42. LANZAVECCHIA, A. 1990. Receptor-mediated antigen uptake and its effect on antigen presentation to class II–restricted T lymphocytes. Annu. Rev. Immunol. **8:** 773–793.
43. EYNON, E. E. & D. C. PARKER. 1992. Small B cells as antigen-presenting cells in the induction of tolerance to soluble protein antigens. J. Exp. Med. **175:** 131–138.
44. FUCHS, E. J. & P. MATZINGER. 1992. B cells turn off virgin, but not memory T cells. Science **258:** 1156–1159.
45. GILBERT, K. M. & W. O. WEIGLE. 1994. Tolerogenicity of resting and activated B cells. J. Exp. Med. **179:** 249–258.

46. RONCHESE, F. & B. HAUSMANN. 1993. B lymphocytes *in vivo* fail to prime naive T cells, but can stimulate antigen-experienced T lymphocytes. J. Exp. Med. **177:** 679–690.
47. HO, W. Y., M. P. COOKE, C. C. GOODNOW & M. M. DAVIS. 1994. Resting and anergic B cells are defective in CD28-dependent costimulation of naive $CD4^+$ T cells. J. Exp. Med. **179:** 1539–1549.
48. CROFT, M., D. D. DUNCAN & S. L. SWAIN. 1992. Response of naive antigen-specific $CD4^+$ T cells *in vitro*: characteristics and antigen-presenting cell requirements. J. Exp. Med. **176:** 1431–1437.
49. CROFT, M., L. M. BRADLEY & S. L. SWAIN. 1994. Naive versus memory CD4 T cell response to antigen: memory cells are less dependent on accessory cell costimulation and can respond to many antigen-presenting cell types including resting B cells. J. Immunol. **152:** 2675–2685.
50. CASSELL, D. J. & R. H. SCHWARTZ. 1994. A quantitative analysis of antigen-presenting cell function: activated B cells stimulate naive CD4 T cells, but are inferior to dendritic cells in providing costimulation. J. Exp. Med. **180:** 1829–1840.
51. METLAY, J. P., E. PURE & R. M. STEINMAN. 1989. Control of the immune response at the level of antigen-presenting cells: a comparison of the function of dendritic cells and B lymphocytes. Adv. Immunol. **47:** 45–116.
52. LINSLEY, P. S., P. M. WALLACE, J. JOHNSON, M. G. GIBSON, J. L. GREENE, J. A. LEDBETTER, C. SINGH & M. A. TEPPER. 1992. Immunosuppression *in vivo* by a soluble form of the CTLA-4 T cell activation molecule. Science **257:** 792–795.
53. LINSLEY, P. S., J. L. GREENE, P. TAN, J. BRADSHAW, J. A. LEDBETTER, C. ANASETTI & N. K. DAMLE. 1992. Coexpression and functional cooperation of CTLA-4 and CD28 on activated T lymphocytes. J. Exp. Med. **176:** 1595–1604.
54. FREEMAN, G. J., A. S. FREEDMAN, J. M. SEGIL, G. LEE, J. F. WHITMAN & L. M. NADLER. 1989. B7, a new member of the Ig superfamily with unique expression on activated and neoplastic B cells. J. Immunol. **143:** 2714–2722.
55. DAVIDSON, H. W. & C. WATTS. 1989. Epitope directed processing of specific antigen by B lymphocytes. J. Cell Biol. **109:** 85–92.
56. WATTS, C. & A. LANZAVECCHIA. 1993. Suppressive effect of antibody on processing of T cell epitopes. J. Exp. Med. **178:** 1459–1463.
57. MAMULA, M. J. 1995. Lupus autoimmunity: from peptides to particles. Immunol. Rev. **144:** 301–314.
58. MAMULA, M. J. & J. CRAFT. 1994. Expression of self antigenic determinants: implications for tolerance and autoimmunity. Curr. Opin. Immunol. **6:** 882–886.

In Vivo Consequences of B Cell Superantigen Immunization

GREGG J. SILVERMAN, JAYAKAR V. NAYAK, RAYMOND WAGENKNECHT, AND KLAUS WARNATZ

Sam and Rose Stein Institute for Research on Aging
and
Theodore Gildred Cancer Center
Department of Medicine
University of California, San Diego
La Jolla, California 92093

During the development of the B cell repertoire, the greatest diversity of immune cells with binding specificities for potential pathogens is retained, whereas clones with potentially harmful autoreactivity are deleted. We have hypothesized that there are exogenous (and perhaps endogenous) proteins that can influence large-scale shifts in B cell clonal representation due to unconventional variable (V) region–mediated binding interactions analogous to those of T cell superantigens.[1,2] This hypothesis was originally instigated by observations of the *in vitro* binding properties of staphylococcal protein A (SpA). We found that this 45-kDa bacterial membrane protein has sites for specific Fab-binding interactions that are restricted to the products of the human V_H3 gene family[1,3,4] (reviewed in reference 5). This binding capacity is also displayed by B cell receptors (BCR) from the structurally related V_HIII clan genes in other mammalian species, which in the mouse include the V_H families J606 and S107 (T15)[6] and likely other related families. SpA binding capacity correlates with conserved V_HIII clan–specific sequences. Analyses using synthetic peptides have supported our initial speculation that these binding interactions involve the V_H framework 3 subdomain, which is distinct from the conventional antigen binding pocket.[7] To date, antibodies with SpA binding activity have been characterized, which derive from 16 of the ~20 potentially functional human V_H3 gene segments. Phage-display library studies have suggested that there is a hierarchy among human V_H genes for relative SpA binding capacity, and antibodies encoded by the V_H26c/V3-23 gene can encode for antibodies with the best SpA binding affinity.[4,8] Importantly, the V_H26c/V3-23 gene contains one of the most highly conserved V_H FR1/FR3 surfaces in the human immune system.[9] The V_H26c/V3-23 gene is also closest to the consensus sequence of germline human V_H3 gene segments.[10] Moreover, this gene is the most highly expressed V_H gene in the human primary immune repertoire.[11] Differential H-L chain pairing studies demonstrated that specific L chain usage does not define SpA binding activity, and alternate L chain usage resulted in, at most, a 4-fold change on relative affinity.[4] Fab-mediated SpA binding capacity is also little affected by the composition of the V_HCDR3 created by V-D-J rearrangement; however, the relative size of the CDR3 may indirectly affect relative affinity.[2,4,5] These unconventional BCR binding interactions confer SpA with the ability to interact with a 100–1000-fold greater proportion of the antigen receptors of B cells than generally bind a common protein antigen.[12] Collectively, these data document the *in vitro* properties of a B cell superantigen.

The structure of SpA is well suited for the cross-linking of membrane-bound BCR. It is composed of five extracellular domains in tandem, E, D, A, B, C, and an additional transmembrane domain, X.[13–16] Each of these extramembrane domains consists of 58–61 amino acids that are about 80% homologous at a protein level.[15] Whereas a single domain of SpA can express a site for V_H3 Fab binding interactions, a single molecule of multidomain native SpA is capable of simultaneously binding two or more V_HIII-encoded BCR.[8] SpA binding affinities up to 5×10^{-7} M for V_H3 Fab and avidities of 5×10^{-9} M for intact V_H3 IgM have been documented by surface plasmon resonance determinations,[8] which are equivalent to many conventional induced primary antibody responses.

Although much is now known about the BCR binding properties of SpA, the immune response to *in vivo* challenge has not been previously investigated. In the design of these studies, we reasoned that the impact of experimental exposure to a B cell superantigen may be greatest during the early development of the immune system, before an equilibrium in the mature lymphocyte repertoire is established. We therefore utilized a protocol previously employed to investigate the neonatal response to immunization of BALB/c mice with a bacterial T cell superantigen.[17] Pregnant BALB/cbyJ mice were obtained (Jackson Labs) and, for the first two weeks of life, neonatal mice received intraperitoneal immunizations with a chemically modified form of SpA, termed modified SpA (MS), that retains V_HIII binding specificity, but is devoid of Fc binding activity.[12] Control animals were immunized with the conventional protein immunogens, bovine serum albumin, or phycoerythrin (PE) (Molecular Probes, Eugene, Oregon), which had been previously used in flow cytometric studies of postimmunization antigen-specific B cells.[18,19] The effect on the composition of the B cell repertoire was assessed in multiparameter flow cytometric studies, and the antibody response was evaluated by ELISA.

All determinations were made in comparison to age-matched animals that had received equivalent immunizations with a control protein antigen or buffer alone. MS binding was not detected among Thy-1^+ cells (T cells) or $B220^-$ mononuclear cells in blood and spleen as all MS binding was associated with $B220^+$ surface (s)IgM^+ cells (B lymphocytes). As demonstrated in FIGURE 1, in naive adult mice or mice that received control immunizations, about 4–8% of sIgM-positive B cells in blood or spleen bound to PE-labeled MS. Similarly, among $B220^+$ cells, 4–8% bound labeled MS. Binding of PE-labeled MS was completely inhibited by unlabeled MS or native SpA. Inhibition of MS binding following preincubation of the labeled MS with a monoclonal human V_H3 IgG indicated that these binding interactions involved the V_H3 Fab binding site of SpA.

Following neonatal treatment with MS, the relative level of MS binding was decreased for 3–7 days and the same basal level of MS binding was exhibited for 2–4 weeks thereafter. Challenge by subcutaneous injection with small doses (50–100 μg) of MS precipitated in alum failed to induce a detectable antibody response in neonatally treated animals during the first 5 weeks of life, which is consistent with

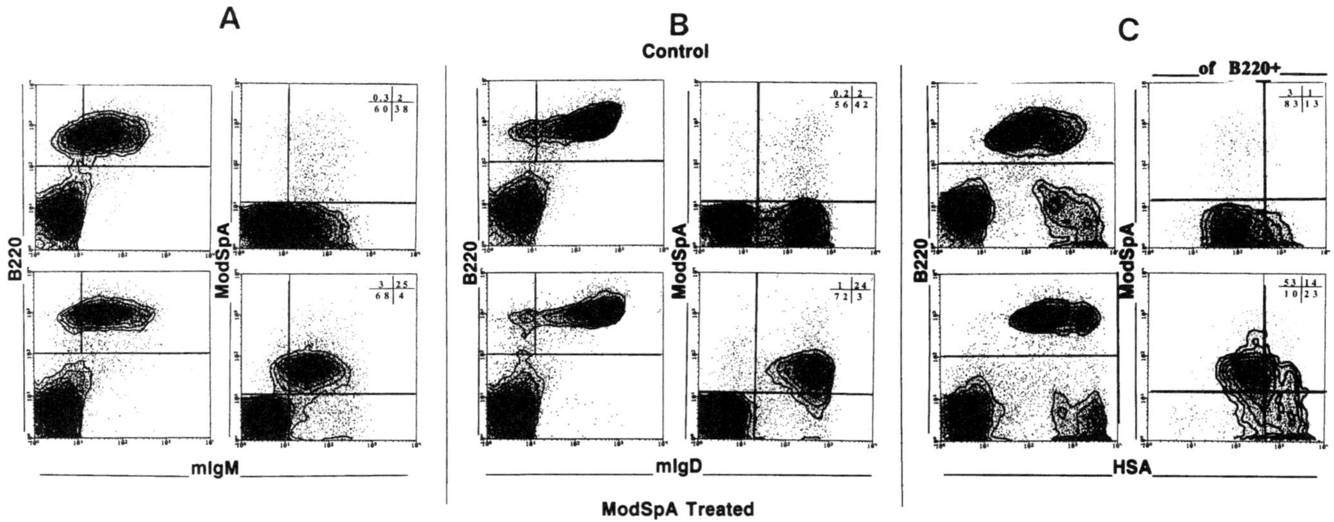

FIGURE 1. The effect on the peripheral B cells of neonatal immunization with a B cell superantigen. Neonatal BALB/c mice were treated with either a control protein antigen, phycoerythrin (top), or chemically modified SpA (MS) (bottom). The peripheral blood mononuclear cells of 15-week-old adult mice were examined, at 3 months following the last immunization. Each pair of panels represents the findings from three-color flow cytometry studies of lymphocyte-gated (FSC versus SSC) cells from a representative MS-treated mouse (bottom) and a phycoerythrin (PE)–treated mouse (top). Panels A (left): in the control mouse, about 5% of $sIgM^+$ (clone 11/41) cells bind labeled MS; in the MS-treated mouse, about 86% of $sIgM^+$ cells bind labeled MS. Panels B (middle): in the control mouse, about 4.5% of $sIgD^+$ (clone AMS 9.1) cells bind labeled MS; in the MS-treated mouse, about 89% of $sIgD^+$ cells bind labeled MS. Panels C (right): roughly the same distribution of heat-stable antigen (HSA; clone M1/69) is seen on $B220^+$ (clone RA3-6B2) cells from the control and MS-treated mice. At far right, the panels depict the gating on $B220^+$ cells: in the control mouse, about 4% of $B220^+$ cells bind labeled MS; in the MS-treated mouse, ~67% of $B220^+$ cells bind labeled MS. Significantly, in the MS-treated mouse, the representation of B cells that bind MS appears to be increased in both the HSA^{hi} and HSA^{low} populations. This suggests that the shift toward increased representation of MS-specific B cells is also present among lymphocytes that have been newly generated in the bone marrow (i.e., HSA^{hi}).[25] In animals with peripheral expansions of MS-binding B cells, less than 1% of $B220^-$ cells were MS-reactive in analyses without the lymphocyte gates, and these cells were predominantly $Mac1^+$ (not shown). In naive animals, this percentage was much lower.

previous descriptions of a period of neonatal tolerance.[20–22] Following this period of tolerance, every animal that was neonatally treated with MS experienced large increases in the proportion of peripheral B lymphocytes that bound MS and, in most animals, 70–90% of B cells bound MS. In these posttreatment animals, B cells with MS binding capacity displayed the same surface phenotype present in control mice, regarding expression of B220, the ratio of B cells that express κ and λ, surface IgM, surface IgD, and heat-stable antigen (HSA) (FIGURE 1). In addition, although the proportion of B cells with MS binding capacity was increased, there was no change in the number of B220-positive B cells in the blood or in the distribution of Thy-1 (T cells) to B cells. Therefore, neonatal treatment results in a 10–20-fold increase in the relative representation of B cells specific for the MS protein antigen, but not in an overall expansion of B cells in the periphery. In comparison, even after hyperimmunization with a conventional protein antigen (such as PE), the frequency of antigen-specific B cells detected by flow cytometric analyses does not exceed 1–2% of the peripheral B cell pool.[18]

In certain animals, peripheral blood was sequentially sampled over time, up to 1 year after the last MS exposure. Unexpectedly, these studies demonstrated that there was no decrement in binding levels over time. Notably, the relative proportion of B cells with MS binding capacity was maintained in each animal. This suggested the following: once a set point for the composition of the peripheral B cell pool was attained, it was retained by some internal immunoregulatory mechanism(s). When the levels of MS binding by splenic and blood mononuclear cells were compared, in every case there was concordance (binding by B cells was within 10%) between the relative levels in these two subcompartments. This indicated that B cells in these anatomic sites were in equilibrium.

The levels of MS-specific IgG antibodies in MS-treated animals were significantly elevated (2.5–20×) compared to control animals. However, there was no correlation between the frequency of peripheral B cells with MS binding capacity, the absolute level of MS-specific IgG antibodies, or the MS-specific IgG/total IgG ratio. Importantly, control animals neonatally treated with PE also developed increased levels of IgG antibodies to PE with the same time course as detected in the MS-treated animals. When the levels of B cells specific for MS were assessed in these animals using the PE-labeled MS, the levels of MS-binding B cells were indistinguishable from those of age-matched untreated animals. These studies suggest that cytophilic (passively absorbed serum) antibodies do not affect these determinations of cellular MS binding capacity. However, additional studies will further evaluate for these types of artifacts.

These initial observations appear to provide evidence that a protein antigen, such as SpA, which has unconventional V_H3 family–restricted BCR binding properties, can influence the *in vivo* composition of the B cell repertoire by inducing cellular population shifts that are orders of magnitude greater than occur in responses to conventional protein antigens. These studies therefore suggest that SpA can act as a superantigen for B lymphocytes.

Studies in progress seek to better define the stage(s) of maturation at which B cells can be selected by this prototypic B cell superantigen. The finding that neonatal immunization may result in the vast majority of peripheral B cells displaying this binding specificity suggests that this exposure results in alterations in clonal selection in the bone marrow and in the peripheral selection of the long-lived recirculating pool. Each day, an estimated 1.5×10^7 B cells are newly generated in adult bone marrow, the primary site of B cell generation, but only a small proportion of the newly generated B cells gain entry into the pool of mature peripheral B cells.[23,24] The mechanisms responsible for selection of the repertoire are currently undefined, but the superantigen-challenge model introduced here may offer a means to investigate the development of the primary repertoire in the central compartment.

REFERENCES

1. SILVERMAN, G. J. 1992. Human antibody responses to bacterial antigens: studies of a model conventional antigen and a proposed model B cell superantigen. Int. Rev. Immunol. **9:** 57–78.
2. SILVERMAN, G. J., P. ROBEN, J-P. BOUVET & M. SASANO. 1995. Superantigen properties of a human sialoprotein involved in gut-associated immunity. J. Clin. Invest. **96:** 417–426.
3. SASSO, E. H., G. J. SILVERMAN & M. MANNIK. 1989. Human IgM molecules that bind staphylococcal protein A contain V_HIII H chains. J. Immunol. **142:** 2778–2783.
4. SASANO, M., D. R. BURTON & G. J. SILVERMAN. 1993. Molecular selection of human antibodies with an unconventional bacterial B cell superantigen. J. Immunol. **151:** 5822–5839.
5. SILVERMAN, G. J. 1996. B-cell superantigens and the somatic diversification of immune repertoires: molecular and cellular implications. *In* Human B-Cell Superantigens. M. Zouali, Ed. Landes Co. Austin, Texas.
6. SEPPALA, I., M. KAARTINEN, S. IBRAHIM & O. MAKELA. 1990. Mouse Ig coded by V_H families S107 or J606 binds to protein A. J. Immunol. **145:** 2989–2993.
7. HAKODA, M., N. KAMATANI, S. KURUMANDA, S. KASHIWAZAKI & G. J. SILVERMAN. 1995. Involvement of framework region 3 of V_H3 IgM in the binding of the B cell superantigen, staphylococcal protein A. Arthritis Rheum. **38:** S190.
8. ROBEN, P., A. SALEM & G. J. SILVERMAN. 1995. V_H3 antibodies bind domain D of staphylococcal protein A. J. Immunol. **154:** 6437–6446.
9. SCHROEDER, H. W., JR., J. L. HILLSON & R. M. PERLMUTTER. 1990. Structure and evolution of mammalian V_H families. Int. Immunol. **2:** 41–50.
10. SCHROEDER, H. W., JR., F. MORTARI, S. SHIOKAWA, P. M. KIRKHAM, R. A. ELGAVISH & F. E. BERTRAND III. 1995. Developmental regulation of the human antibody repertoire. Ann. N.Y. Acad. Sci. **764:** 242–260.
11. STEWART, A. K., C. HUANG, B. D. STOLLAR & R. S. SCHWARTZ. 1993. High-frequency representation of a single V_H gene in the expressed human. J. Exp. Med. **177:** 1227.
12. SILVERMAN, G. J., M. SASANO & S. B. WORMSLEY. 1993. Age-associated changes in binding of human B lymphocytes to a V_H3-restricted unconventional bacterial antigen. J. Immunol. **151:** 5840–5855.
13. SJODAHL, J. 1977. Structural studies on the four repetitive Fc-binding regions in protein A from *Staphylococcus aureus.* Eur. J. Biochem. **78:** 471–479.
14. LOFDAHL, S., B. GUSS, M. UHLEN, L. PHILIPSON & M. LINDBERG. 1983. Gene for staphylococcal protein A. Proc. Natl. Acad. Sci. U.S.A. **80:** 697–701.
15. UHLEN, M., B. GUSS, B. NILSSON, S. GATENBECK, L. PHILIPSON & M. LINDBERG. 1984. Complete sequence of the staphylococcal gene encoding protein A: a gene evolved through multiple duplications. J. Biol. Chem. **259:** 1695–1702.
16. MOKS, T., L. ABRAHMSEN, B. NILSSON, U. HELLMAN, J. SJOQUIST & M. UHLEN. 1986. Staphylococcal protein A consists of five IgG-binding domains. Eur. J. Biochem. **156:** 637–643.
17. WHITE, J., A. HERMAN, A. M. PULLEN, R. KUBO, J. W. KAPPLER & P. MARRACK. 1989. The V beta–specific superantigen staphylococcal enterotoxin B: stimulation of mature T cells and clonal deletion in neonatal mice. Cell **56:** 27–35.

18. HAYAKAWA, K., R. ISHII, K. YAMASAKI, T. KISHIMOTO & R. R. HARDY. 1987. Isolation of high-affinity memory B cells: phycoerythrin as a probe for antigen-binding cells. Proc. Natl. Acad. Sci. U.S.A. **84:** 1379–1383.
19. SCHITTEK, B. & K. RAJEWSKY. 1990. Maintenance of B-cell memory by long-lived cells generated from proliferating precursors. Nature **346:** 749–751.
20. TERRES, G. & W. L. HUGHES. 1959. Acquired immune tolerance in mice to crystalline bovine serum albumin. J. Immunol. **83:** 459–467.
21. THORBECKE, G. J., G. W. SISKIND & N. J. GOLDBERGER. 1961. The induction in mice of sensitization and immunological unresponsiveness by neonatal injection of bovine gamma-globulin. J. Immunol. **87:** 147–152.
22. SISKIND, G. W., P. Y. PATERSON & L. THOMAS. 1963. Induction of unresponsiveness and immunity in newborn and adult mice with pneumococcal polysaccharide. J. Immunol. **90:** 929–934.
23. OPSTELTEN, D. & D. G. OSMOND. 1983. Pre-B cells in mouse bone marrow: immunofluorescence stathmokinetic studies of the proliferation of cytoplasmic μ-chain-bearing cells in normal mice. J. Immunol. **131:** 2635–2640.
24. DEENEN, G. J., I. VAN BALEN & D. OPSTELTEN. 1990. In rat B lymphocyte genesis, sixty percent is lost from the bone marrow at the transition of non-dividing pre-B to sIgM+ B lymphocyte. Eur. J. Immunol. **20:** 557.
25. ALLMAN, D. M., S. E. FERGUSON, V. M. LENTZ & M. P. CANCRO. 1993. Peripheral B cell maturation. II. Heat-stable antigen (hi) splenic B cells are an immune developmental intermediate in the production of long-lived marrow-derived B cells. J. Immunol. **151:** 4431–4444.

Immunoglobulin J Chain

An Early Differentiation Marker of Human B Cells

JIRI MESTECKY,[a,b] ITARU MORO,[c] ZINA MOLDOVEANU,[a]
TOMIHISA TAKAHASHI,[a,c] TAKASHI IWASE,[c]
HIROMI KUBAGAWA,[d] AND MAX D. COOPER[a,b,c,e]

[a]*Department of Microbiology*
[b]*Department of Medicine*
[c]*Department of Pediatrics*
University of Alabama at Birmingham
Birmingham, Alabama 35294

[d]*Department of Pathology*
Nihon University
Tokyo, Japan

[e]*Howard Hughes Medical Institute*
Birmingham, Alabama 35294

INTRODUCTION

Joining (J) chain is a glycosylated polypeptide that displays a single Ig domain-like structure and is linked by disulfide bridges to the penultimate Cys residues of the α and μ chains of polymeric IgA and IgM, respectively.[1,2] Immunohistochemical and biosynthetic studies indicated that, in normal cells, J chain is present in the cytoplasm, but not on the plasma membrane of polymeric IgA- or IgM-producing cells. In normal mucosal tissues and sites of inflammation, the presence of J chain is not restricted to cells producing IgA or IgM; IgG- as well as IgD-containing cells are also J chain–positive, although the free J chain is not secreted by such cells.[1,2]

J CHAIN EXPRESSION IN HUMAN MYELOMA CELLS

In contrast to the cells from normal bone marrow, IgA-, IgG-, IgD-, or only L chain (either κ or λ)–containing plasma cells from patients with multiple myeloma frequently display intense staining with anti–J chain reagents.[3] Furthermore, bone marrow aspirates from four patients with suspected plasma cell dyscrasia indicated the presence of cells staining intensely for J chain, but frequently negative for either H or L chains.[4] The J chain–positive cells displayed morphological features of lymphoblasts and plasma cells, and comprised 5.6–28.5% of the nucleated cells. Trace amounts of free J chain were detectable in serum and/or urine from two such patients. These results indicate that J chain can be expressed in the bone marrow plasma cells of myeloma patients in the absence of Ig H and L chains and thus can represent a novel phenotype.

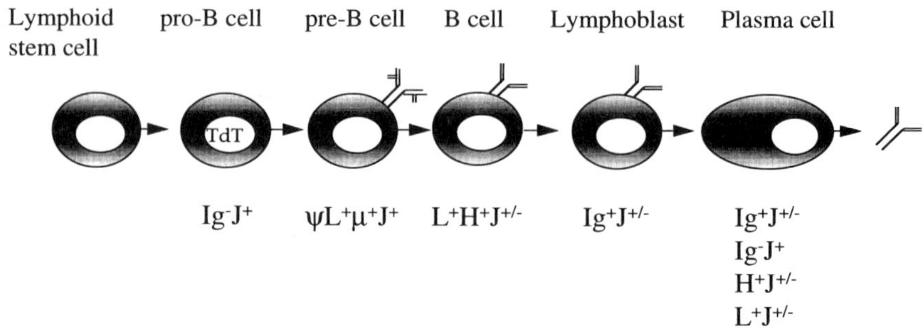

FIGURE 1. Expression patterns of the J chain in human lymphoid cells. For altered J chain expression patterns in pathological conditions, see TABLE 1 and the text.

J CHAIN EXPRESSION IN HUMAN LEUKEMIC CELLS AND ESTABLISHED CELL LINES

Because the earlier studies of Ig-secreting lymphoblastoid cell lines indicated that such cells frequently contain intracellular J chain irrespective of the Ig isotype,[5] we attempted to relate the expression of J chain to the stage of human B cell differentiation (see FIGURE 1 and TABLE 1). Bone marrow, peripheral blood cells, and leukemic cells representative of early stages of differentiation along the B cell pathway (null,

TABLE 1. Expression of Human J Chain in Normal or Pathological Lymphoid Cells[a]

	Pro-B Cells	Pre-B Cells	B Cells	Lymphoblasts	Plasma Cells
Embryonic or fetal liver	+ (6 weeks)	+ (7–8 weeks)	+		
Lymph nodes			+/−	+/−	+/−
Spleen			+/−	+/−	+/−
Mucosal tissues				+/−	+/−
Pokeweed mitogen-stimulated peripheral blood lymphocytes				+/−	+/−
Epstein-Barr virus–transformed cells and cell lines	+	+	+	+/−	+/−
Bone marrow					
normal					−
multiple myeloma				+/−	+/−
Acute lymphocytic leukemia (peripheral blood or bone marrow	+/−	+/−	+/−		

[a]Determined by polymerase chain reaction, immunofluorescence, immunoelectron microscopy, Western blotting, immunoprecipitation, radioimmunoassay, and/or enzyme-linked immunoassay.

pre-B, and B cells) were examined by immunohistochemical and immunochemical techniques for the presence of intracellular and secreted J and μ chains.[6] Cells positive for intracellular J chain, but negative for μ chain, constituted 20–90% of the total, and low levels of J chain were detectable in supernatants of lysed cells. Two leukemic cell lines of pre-B cell phenotype expressed intracytoplasmic J chain. These results suggested that J chain expression is an early event in B cell differentiation and may precede μ chain synthesis. This conclusion was strengthened by immunological and genetic studies of EBV-transformed human fetal bone marrow depleted of B cells.[7] Although such transformed precursors were Ig-negative and maintained their Ig genes in the germline configuration or had undergone DJ or abortive VDJ rearrangement, they displayed prominent expression of J chain, several B and plasma cell maturation markers, and plasma cell morphology.

Finally, using polymerase chain reaction with primers specific for human J and μ chains, we have detected J chain, but not μ chain, mRNA in fetal liver at the sixth gestational week. The μ chain mRNA became detectable 1–2 weeks later.[8] Therefore, the J chain appears to be the first Ig-related polypeptide expressed during differentiation of cells along the B cell axis; however, its expression is upregulated as a function of B cell differentiation.[2]

CONCLUSIONS

Correlative studies of J chain expression in human lymphoid cells at various stages of differentiation along the B cell pathway indicate that this polypeptide is produced from the earliest stages to terminally differentiated plasma cells. In such cells, the J chain expression is regulated independently of the production of either H or L chains. Because J chain is also expressed in many invertebrate species[9] that do not produce Ig, and its DNA sequence displays a high degree of structural homology to its vertebrate counterparts, we conclude that J chain is a highly conserved gene product that arose before the evolution of Ig molecules.

REFERENCES

1. MESTECKY, J. & J. R. MCGHEE. 1987. Adv. Immunol. **40:** 153–245.
2. KOSHLAND, M. E. 1974. Annu. Rev. Immunol. **3:** 425–453.
3. MESTECKY, J., J-L. PREUD'HOMME, S. S. CRAGO, E. MIHAESCO, J. T. PRCHAL & A. J. OKOS. 1980. Clin. Exp. Immunol. **39:** 371–385.
4. MESTECKY, J., Z. MOLDOVEANU, B. A. JULIAN & J. T. PRCHAL. 1990. Am. J. Med. **88:** 411–416.
5. KUTTEH, W. H., Z. MOLDOVEANU, S. J. PRINCE, R. KULHAVY, F. ALONSO & J. MESTECKY. 1983. Mol. Immunol. **9:** 967–976.
6. HAJDU, I., Z. MOLDOVEANU, M. D. COOPER & J. MESTECKY. 1983. J. Exp. Med. **158:** 1993–2006.
7. KUBAGAWA, H., P. D. BURROWS, C. E. GROSS, J. MESTECKY & M. D. COOPER. 1988. Proc. Natl. Acad. Sci. U.S.A. **85:** 875–879.
8. IWASE, T., I. SAITO, T. TAKAHASHI, L. CHU, T. USAMI, J. MESTECKY & I. MORO. 1993. Cell Struct. Funct. **18:** 297–302.
9. TAKAHASHI, T., T. IWASE, N. TAKENOUCHI, M. SAITO, K. KOBAYASHI, Z. MOLDOVEANU, J. MESTECKY & I. MORO. 1996. Proc. Natl. Acad. Sci. U.S.A. **93:** 1886–1891.

Inducible Fas-Resistance Mediated by IL-4 in Activated B Cells[a]

LINDA C. FOOTE, ANN MARSHAK-ROTHSTEIN, AND THOMAS L. ROTHSTEIN[b]

Departments of Microbiology and Medicine
Boston University Medical Center
Boston, Massachusetts 02118

Activated $CD4^+$ Th1 cells express Fas ligand and induce cytotoxicity in target cells through a Fas-dependent, apoptotic mechanism. B cells can be targets for this form of cell death; however, the sensitivity of B cell targets to Fas-mediated apoptosis is regulated by specific receptor signals. In particular, CD40 cross-linking induces susceptibility to Fas-induced cell death, whereas antigen receptor engagement blocks Fas killing in otherwise susceptible targets.[1] We examined additional receptors that might influence Fas-mediated apoptosis by determining the capacity of several lymphokines to downregulate Fas signaling for cell death. B cells were stimulated for 2 days with a cross-linked CD40/CD8α fusion protein, in the presence or absence of lymphokine, and were then tested as targets for cytotoxicity mediated by AE7 effector cells in 4-hour, lectin-dependent, ^{51}Cr release assays. IL-4 substantially reduced Fas-dependent, Th1 cell–mediated cytotoxicity (Th1-CMC). CD40L-stimulated B cells treated with IL-4 expressed surface Fas at a level comparable to that of B cells exposed to CD40L alone, ruling out the simple mechanism of a change in Fas expression. Furthermore, dual (CD40L plus IL-4) treated B cells were resistant to lysis produced by recombinant FasL (kindly provided by David Lynch, Immunex, Seattle, Washington), ruling out a mechanism based on inducible expression of a putative viability receptor that might interact with another T cell ligand. Thus, it seems most likely that IL-4-mediated Fas-resistance results from a loss or suppression of the Fas-triggered intracellular signals that lead to cell death.

In several respects, IL-4-induced resistance to Th1-CMC differed from that produced by anti-Ig. First, IL-4 was a little less effective than anti-Ig, typically producing about half the level of Fas-resistance as measured by the effector:target cell ratio needed to produce equivalent levels of killing in resistant and sensitive B cell targets (about 10-fold for IL-4 and greater than 20-fold for anti-Ig). Second, the time course for IL-4-induced Fas-resistance was more protracted than that for anti-Ig; although both produced maximal Fas-resistance when present during the last 24 hours of 2-day cultures, the effect of IL-4 was minimal at 6 hours (prior to the end of the 2-day cultures), whereas the anti-Ig effect was well developed at this time. Third, IL-4-induced Fas-resistance was unaffected by PKC depletion, whereas anti-Ig-induced Fas-resistance was PKC-dependent. These findings suggested that IL-4 and

[a]This work was supported by Public Health Service Grant No. AI29690.
[b]To whom all correspondence should be addressed.

anti-Ig may trigger separate pathways that oppose Fas, and this is supported by the observation that suboptimal doses of these reagents acted in synergy to produce marked resistance to Fas-mediated apoptosis.

It has been reported that anergic, autoreactive B cells are ultimately deleted via a Fas-dependent pathway[2] and that, in Fas-deficient mice, autoantibody-producing B cells are found in T cell–rich regions of the inner PALS.[3] Our findings, in combination with these reports, suggest that inducible Fas-resistance may contribute to autoantibody formation. To evaluate this possibility, sera from IL-4-overexpressing transgenic mice[4] (kindly provided by Abul Abbas, Harvard Medical School, Boston, Massachusetts) were tested for autoantibody expression using fixed HEp-2 cells. Two such sera expressed clearly evident cytoplasmic immunofluorescence, which was not observed with sera from normal animals. Thus, IL-4 may act to protect autoreactive B cells from the Fas deletional pathway, providing the opportunity for further development and differentiation.

We propose, then, under certain circumstances of extreme immunological stress, that the anergic B cell pool may be protected against Fas-mediated apoptosis and thereby join the immunocompetent B cell population. This could act to enhance immunity against microorganisms whose antigenic determinants cross-react with self and may reflect the relative balance of Th1 cells, which express FasL, and Th2 cells, which lack FasL, but express IL-4. The net result of these processes would be a predisposition to the production of autoreactive antibodies.

REFERENCES

1. ROTHSTEIN, T. L., J. K. M. WANG, D. J. PANKA, L. C. FOOTE, Z. WANG, B. STANGER, H. CUI, S-T. JU & A. MARSHAK-ROTHSTEIN. 1995. Nature **374:** 163–166.
2. RATHMELL, J. C., M. P. COOKE, W. Y. HO, J. GREIN, S. E. TOWNSEND, M. M. DAVIS & C. C. GOODNOW. 1995. Nature **376:** 181–184.
3. JACOBSON, B. A., D. J. PANKA, K-A. NGUYEN, J. ERIKSON, A. K. ABBAS & A. MARSHAK-ROTHSTEIN. 1995. Immunity **3:** 509–519.
4. TEPPER, R. I., D. A. LEVINSON, B. Z. STANGER, J. CAMPOS-TORRES, A. K. ABBAS & P. LEDER. 1990. Cell **62:** 457–467.

Markedly Diminished Radiation-induced Lymphocyte Apoptosis in *lpr* Mice Suggests a Role for Fas in Eliminating Damaged Cells

ELIZABETH A. REAP, KEVIN ROOF, KENRICK MAYNOR, AND PHILIP L. COHEN[a]

Departments of Medicine and Microbiology/Immunology
University of North Carolina School of Medicine
Chapel Hill, North Carolina 27599-7280

Cross-linking of cell surface Fas (CD95) mediates rapid apoptosis.[1] The insight that the autoimmune and lymphoproliferative disorder of *lpr* and *gld* mice is due to mutations in Fas and Fas ligand (FasL), respectively, has heightened interest in the biological significance of the Fas receptor.[2] Through induction of cell death, Fas controls the extent of T cell receptor–mediated T cell responses in the periphery and mediates a major part of cytotoxic T cell killing.[3] Fas-FasL interactions may also limit the clonal expansion of B lymphocytes.[4]

In this study, we undertook to examine whether Fas was involved in the apoptosis induced by ionizing radiation. Apoptosis after exposure to gamma radiation occurs rapidly and is mediated by both nuclear and membrane events.[5] Because *lpr* mice are deficient in surface Fas, their sensitivity to cell death induced by gamma radiation was studied to determine the participation of Fas in this phenomenon. The relative resistance of *lpr* lymphocytes to radiation-induced apoptosis, together with the increased expression of Fas on irradiated normal spleen cells, suggests that part of the apoptosis induced by radiation and other forms of cell injury may be mediated by Fas-FasL interactions.

METHODS

Mice

Five- to eight-month-old C57BL/6 (B6) and C57BL/6-*lpr/lpr* (B6/*lpr*) mice were from our breeding colony.

Radiation

Mice received 150 R of gamma radiation from a ^{137}Cs source and were sacrificed within 1 hour.

[a]To whom all correspondence should be addressed.

Quantitation of Apoptosis

Apoptosis was measured by flow cytometry as previously reported.[6] Single spleen cell suspensions were washed; resuspended in RPMI 1640 media supplemented with 10% fetal calf serum, glutamine, pyruvate, penicillin-streptomycin, and nonessential amino acids; and cultured overnight in 24-well plates. Cell surface markers were identified by direct immunofluorescence using FITC-conjugated anti-Thy 1.2, anti-CD4, and anti-IgM. After surface staining, cells were fixed in ethanol and nuclei were stained with propidium iodide. Cells were analyzed using a Becton-Dickinson FACScan with Cytomation software.

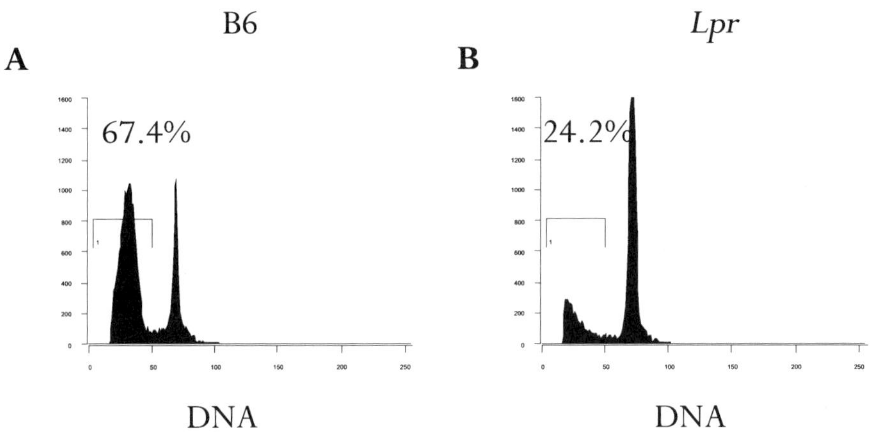

FIGURE 1. Spleen cells from B6 (A) or B6/*lpr* mice (B) were cultured overnight after irradiation. After permeabilization, cellular DNA was stained with propidium iodide and the DNA content of individual cells was assessed by flow cytometry. Numbers above bracketed areas indicate the percent of cells with subdiploid DNA content, representing cells undergoing apoptosis. These data are from a representative experiment.

RESULTS AND DISCUSSION

Although B6/*lpr* cells underwent considerable cell death following irradiation, apoptosis was substantially less than observed for control B6 spleen cells (FIGURE 1). Both T and B cells from B6/*lpr* showed decreased radiation sensitivity (not shown) and this was not limited to the abnormal CD4−CD8− T cells because B6/*lpr* CD4+ cells were markedly less radiation-sensitive than control CD4+ cells (FIGURE 2). Heat-shock treatment (incubation for 30 minutes at 43 °C in a shaking water bath) induced much less apoptosis in B6/*lpr* as compared to B6.

One possible explanation for our results is that Fas expression on normal cells is enhanced after radiation or heat shock and plays a role in the apoptosis of injured cells. As assessed by immunofluorescent staining with the Jo2 monoclonal anti-Fas antibody, Fas expression is indeed enhanced in irradiated B6 cells, even in unirradiated cells cultured overnight.

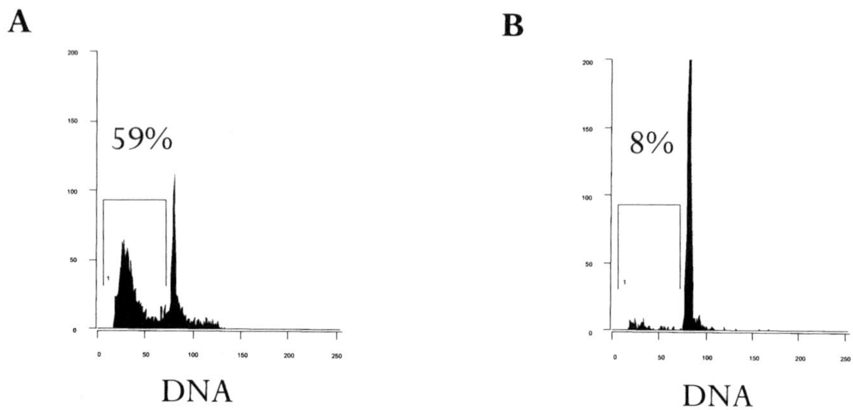

FIGURE 2. Irradiated spleen cells were cultured as in FIGURE 1 (A & B) and were stained using FITC anti-CD4 and then (for DNA content) using propidium iodide. Data shown represent the DNA content of CD4-positive cells and are from a representative experiment.

These studies suggest to us a possible novel function for Fas and FasL in the elimination by apoptosis of injured cells. We propose that the immune system may perform a kind of immunological surveillance using FasL-bearing cells to eliminate Fas-expressing cells. Some of these may have acquired Fas in response to injury, as a consequence of senescence, or as a normal event in an evolving immune response. Their elimination by apoptosis may be an important means of disposing of potentially inflammatory cell debris.

REFERENCES

1. DHEIN, J., P. T. DANIEL, B. C. TRAUTH, A. OEHM, P. MOLLER & P. H. KRAMMER. 1992. Induction of apoptosis by monoclonal antibody anti-APO-1 class switch variants is dependent on cross-linking of APO-1 cell surface antigens. J. Immunol. **149:** 3166–3173.
2. WATANABE-FUKUNAGA, R., C. I. BRANNAN, N. G. COPELAND, N. A. JENKINS & S. NAGATA. 1992. Lymphoproliferation disorder in mice explained by defects in Fas antigen that mediates apoptosis. Nature **356:** 314–317.
3. SINGER, G. G., A. C. CARRERA, A. MARSHAK-ROTHSTEIN, C. MARTINEZ & A. K. ABBAS. 1994. Apoptosis, Fas, and systemic autoimmunity: the MRL-lpr/lpr model. Curr. Opin. Immunol. **6:** 913–920.
4. GARRONE, P., E. M. NEIDHARDT, E. GARCIA, L. GALIBERT, C. VAN KOOTEN & J. BANCHEREAU. 1995. Fas ligation induces apoptosis of CD40-activated human B lymphocytes. J. Exp. Med. **182:** 1265–1273.
5. HAIMOVITZ-FRIEDMAN, A., C. C. KAN, D. EHLEITER, R. S. PERSAUD, M. MCLOUGHLIN, Z. FUKS & R. N. KOLESNICK. 1994. Ionizing radiation acts on cellular membranes to generate ceramide and initiate apoptosis. J. Exp. Med. **180:** 525–535.
6. REAP, E. A., D. LESLIE, M. ABRAHAMS, R. A. EISENBERG & P. L. COHEN. 1995. Apoptosis abnormalities of splenic lymphocytes in autoimmune lpr and gld mice. J. Immunol. **154:** 936–943.

Ig-specific T Cells Regulate the Fate of the B Cells during the Immune Response in a TCR Transgenic Mouse Model

F. GRANUCCI,[a] M. RESCIGNO,[a] P. CORBELLA,[a]
R. LONGHI,[b] AND P. RICCIARDI-CASTAGNOLI[a]

[a]*Cellular and Molecular Pharmacology Center*
Consiglio Nazionale delle Ricerche
20129 Milan, Italy

[b]*Hormone Chemistry Center*
Consiglio Nazionale delle Ricerche
20131 Milan, Italy

Tolerance is the property by which the immune system is unresponsive to self-constituent. It is achieved by either clonal deletion or functional silencing (anergy). The tolerance-inducing capacity of three major groups of self-antigens—thymic-presented, tissue-sequestered, and circulating proteins—has been studied. In the thymus, T cells recognizing a self-protein epitope are deleted during the T cell differentiation process. In the periphery, anergy or clonal deletion of T cells specific for tissue-sequestered self-antigens has also been shown.

As far as circulating proteins are concerned, both thymic deletion and peripheral anergy have been described, with the exception of the immunoglobulins (Igs). In fact, anti-idiotype specific T cells were not deleted in the thymus unless the idiotype was expressed within the thymus as a transgene or by injecting a nonphysiological amount of the immunoglobulin.[1] Thus, circulating Igs do not seem to be able to induce thymic deletion and the peripheral function of anti-Ig T cells remains to be investigated.

RESULTS AND DISCUSSION

To study the fate of anti-Ig T cells, a mouse transgenic for the IgG2a^b-specific T cell receptor (TCR) was produced. The original T cell clone (B5) is a CD4$^+$, Th1, I-A^d restricted clone.[2] We selected B5 because it has been shown to suppress the Igh-1b allotype *in vivo*.[2] The epitope recognized by the B5 TCR was mapped in the CH3 domain of IgG2a^b. The transgenic mice were generated on two different genetic backgrounds: Igh-1a/a (Tg$^+$b$^-$, not expressing the self-antigen) and Igh-1a/b (Tg$^+$b$^+$, expressing the self-antigen). Surprisingly, transgenic T cells were not deleted in the thymus and did not become tolerant in the periphery as they could be activated to proliferate *in vitro* in response to the specific peptide.[3] To test the *in vivo* activity of transgenic T cells, self-antigen serum levels were measured. IgG2a^b serum levels (FIGURE 1A) were undetectable with ELISA (sensitivity: 3 ng/mL), whereas IgG2a^a levels were comparable with those of nontransgenic mice (FIGURE 1B); furthermore,

$\gamma 2a^b$-secreting cells were consistently undetectable as estimated by the ELISPOT assay. In order to challenge the immune system and increase $IgG2a^b$ serum levels, transgenic mice were immunized with *S. typhimurium* on days 0 and 7. Three weeks after immunization, a peak level of 10 μg/mL of $\gamma 2a^b$ protein was reached, which was almost 60 times lower than that reached in the control mice (FIGURE 1C). As the other isotypes and the $IgG2a^a$ were unaffected (data not shown), IgE serum levels were 5 times higher than in the nontransgenic animals. Four weeks after immunization, a decrease in $IgG2a^b$ was associated with an increase in IgE levels (FIGURE 1D). Interestingly, the increased IgE's in the transgenic F1 (Igh-1a/b) were all of the b allotype, indicating that they derive from $IgG2a^b$-positive cells (FIGURE 1E). We can

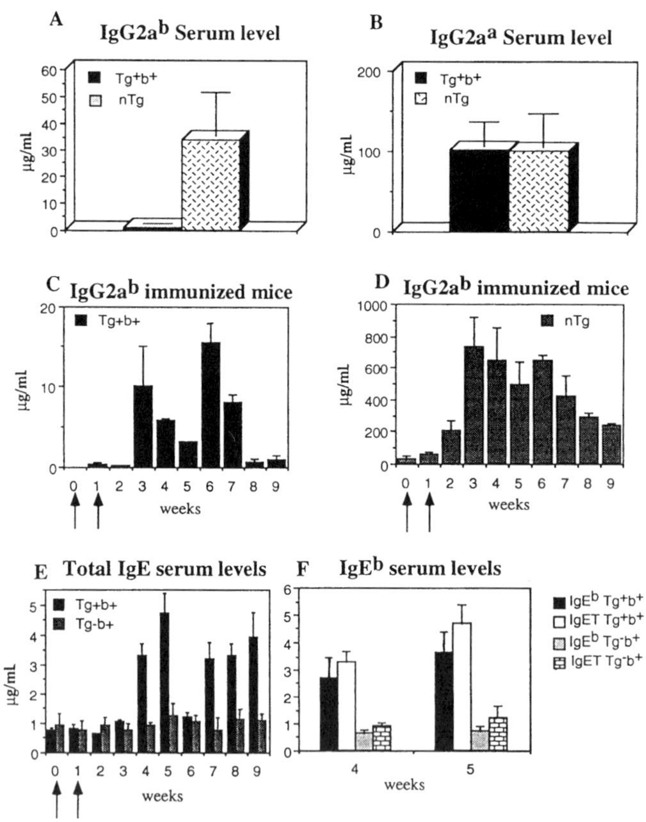

FIGURE 1. Serum levels of (A) $IgG2a^b$ and (B) $IgG2a^a$ in Tg^+b^+ mice and in controls. $IgG2a^b$ and $IgG2a^a$ serum levels in 4- to 6-week-old mice were measured using solid-phase ELISA. Transgenic mice were immunized on day 0 and day 7 with *S. typhimurium* (arrows) and the immune response was followed from 0 to 9 weeks. (C) Transgenic and (D) nontransgenic mice $IgG2a^b$ total serum levels during the immune response. (E) IgE total serum levels and (F) IgE^b in comparison with total IgE serum levels in transgenic mice and in controls at 4 and 5 weeks after the immunization.

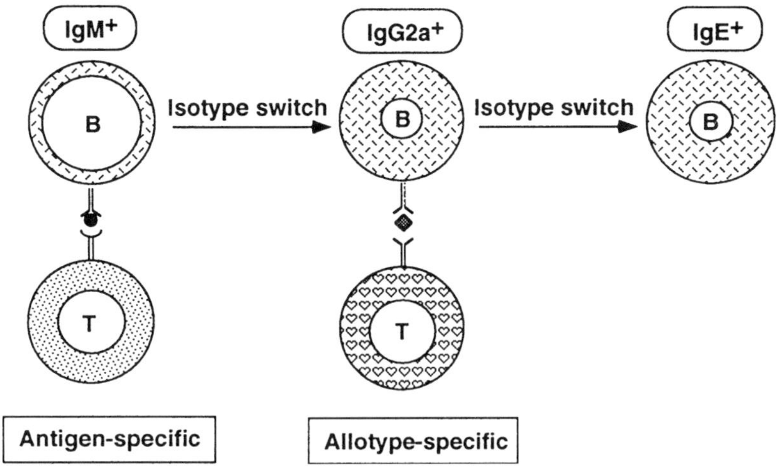

FIGURE 2. Proposed model of B cell fate during the immune response. Antigen-specific T cells interact with IgM-positive B cells that induce their maturation and class switch. After this process, the IgM-positive B cells become IgG2a^b-expressing cells that can present epitopes of $\gamma 2a^b$ and interact with allotype-specific transgenic T cells. A further class switch of the B cell is then induced by this interaction.

thus assume that the mechanism by which the B cells are silenced is the induction of a further switch to IgE mediated by transgenic T cells.

The B cells follow a singular fate: after antigen encounter, IgM-positive cells interact with antigen-specific T cells, which induce their maturation and class switch (FIGURE 2); when IgM-expressing B cells become IgG2a^b-positive, they can present epitopes of the $\gamma 2a^b$ immunoglobulin and can interact with the antiallotype transgenic T cells. The result of this *in vivo* interaction induces a further switch to IgE, as shown by the b-allotype IgE production. Given that transgenic T cells are not deleted in the thymus and are functional in the periphery, all of these findings indicate that Ig-specific T cells could exist in normal individuals and may represent a late-acting form of T cells involved in the regulation of the immune response.

REFERENCES

1. BOGEN, B., Z. DEMBIC & S. WEISS. 1993. Clonal deletion of specific thymocytes by an immunoglobulin idiotype. EMBO J. **12:** 357–363.
2. BARTNES, K. & K. HANNESTAD. 1991. Igh-1b-specific CD4$^+$CD8$^-$ T cell clones of the Th1 subset selectively suppress the Igh-1b allotype *in vivo*. Eur. J. Immunol. **21:** 2365–2371.
3. GRANUCCI, F., M. RESCIGNO, G. MARCONI, M. FOTI & P. RICCIARDI-CASTAGNOLI. 1996. Ig-specific T cell receptor–transgenic T cells are not deleted in the thymus and are functional *in vivo*. J. Exp. Med. **183:** 203–213.

Expression of the Tyrosine Kinase Lyn during B Cell Receptor Engagement and Apoptosis

SYLVIE HUCK[a] AND MONCEF ZOUALI[a]

Département d'Immunologie
Institut Pasteur
75015 Paris, France

Maintenance of B cell tolerance to self operates through several mechanisms, including clonal deletion, clonal anergy, clonal ignorance, competitive elimination for follicular entry, and receptor editing.[1] In systemic autoimmunity, however, antiself high-affinity antibodies are overexpressed and the corresponding B cells exhibit an intrinsic abnormality.[2] Such an alteration raises the question of the emergence and the clonal survival, as well as the death of antiself high-affinity B cells in diseased subjects, with evidence for both accelerated and reduced apoptosis (reviewed in reference 3). In an attempt to uncover the mechanisms of the production of aggressive autoantibodies in the disease of systemic lupus erythematosus (SLE), we began exploring the influence of structural components of the B cell receptor (BcR) on survival of autoreactive human B cells.

In an initial set of experiments, we used two murine cell lines (CTLL, a cytotoxic T cell line; and WEHI-231, an IgM$^+$ pre-B cell line) to investigate a potential relationship between apoptosis and Lyn, a tyrosine kinase that plays a central role in signal transduction of B cells.[4] Apoptosis was induced in CTLL cells by IL-2 deprivation for 12 hours and WEHI-231 cells were treated with two concentrations of anti-IgM antibodies (0.5 and 1 μg/mL) for 24 hours. Because the protein tyrosine kinase Lyn plays a crucial role in transducing signals that control B cell proliferation and differentiation, we examined its expression in our system by Western blotting using an anti-Lyn monoclonal antibody (Santa Cruz Biotechnology, Santa Cruz, California). We found that the two forms of the Lyn gene products, $p56^{lyn}$ and $p53^{lyn}$, are expressed in WEHI-231 cells, but not in CTLL cells. However, we noted the presence of an additional band of approximately 52-kDa molecular weight in anti-IgM-treated apoptotic WEHI-231 cells (FIGURE 1).

In recent studies, it was shown that deletion of the protein tyrosine kinase Lyn in mice results in an autoimmune syndrome reminiscent of SLE.[5,6] We therefore began exploring the role of this kinase in B cell tolerance and apoptosis. Here, we made the observation that expression of an additional Lyn-related protein is specifically induced during apoptosis. Further probing of the B cell receptor and its accessory molecules will be important to determine the relationship between the activation stage, the autoreactivity, and the clonal fate of various B cell subpopulations from SLE subjects.

[a]Investigators of the Institut National de la Recherche et de la Santé Médicale (INSERM).

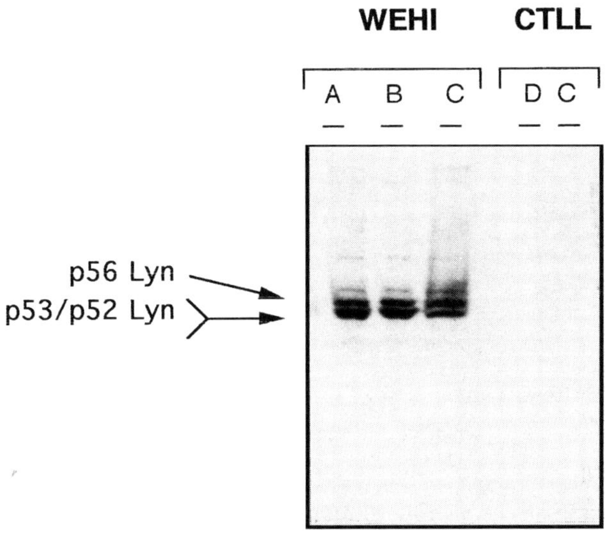

FIGURE 1. Lyn expression in control cells and in apoptotic cells. The p56/p53 Lyn proteins, which come from two alternatively spliced mRNAs, are involved in signal transduction through the BcR. As expected, Lyn is not expressed in CTLL cells. p56 is rapidly downregulated when the BcR is activated, but the level becomes equivalent to the nonapoptotic control after 24 hours. p53 expression seems to increase in apoptotic cells after 24-hour treatment, and an additional lower band (p52) is observed. Terms: (A) cells treated with 1 μg/mL of anti-IgM for 24 hours; (B) cells treated with 0.5 μg/mL of anti-IgM for 24 hours; (C) untreated control cells; (D) cells deprived of IL-2 for 12 hours.

REFERENCES

1. Goodnow, C. C., J. G. Cyster, S. B. Hartley, S. E. Bell, M. P. Cooke, J. I. Healy, S. Akkaraju, J. C. Rathmell, S. L. Pogue & K. P. Shokat. 1995. Self-tolerance checkpoints in B lymphocyte development. Adv. Immunol. **59:** 279–368.
2. Bensimon, C., P. Chastagner & M. Zouali. 1994. Human lupus anti-DNA autoantibodies undergo essentially primary V_{kappa} gene rearrangements. EMBO J. **13:** 2951–2962.
3. Huck, S. & M. Zouali. 1996. DNA methylation: a potential pathway to abnormal autoreactive lupus B cells. Clin. Immunol. Immunopathol. **80:** 1–8.
4. Bolen, J. B., R. B. Rowley, C. Spana & A. Y. Tsygankov. 1992. The Src family of tyrosine protein kinases in hemopoietic signal transduction. FASEB J. **6:** 3403–3409.
5. Hibbs, M. L., D. M. Tarlinton, J. Armes, D. Grail, G. Hodgson, R. Maglitto, S. A. Stacker & A. R. Dunn. 1995. Multiple defects in the immune system of Lyn-deficient mice, culminating in autoimmune disease. Cell **83:** 301–311.
6. Nishizumi, H., I. Taniuchi, Y. Yamanashi, D. Kitamura, D. Ilic, S. Mori, T. Watanabe & T. Yamamoto. 1995. Impaired proliferation of peripheral B cells and indication of autoimmune disease in Lyn-deficient mice. Immunity **3:** 549–560.

Lupus Humoral Autoimmunity after Short Peptide Immunization[a]

JUDITH A. JAMES, R. HAL SCOFIELD,
AND JOHN B. HARLEY

Arthritis and Immunology Program
Oklahoma Medical Research Foundation
and
Department of Medicine
University of Oklahoma Health Sciences Center
and
Department of Veterans Affairs Medical Center
Oklahoma City, Oklahoma 73104

Anti-Sm is a common and specific autoantibody found in systemic lupus erythematosus. The peptide, PPPGMRPP, is found in Sm B/B′ and is an early target of the autoimmune response in some anti-Sm precipitin–positive patient sera.[1] Rabbits and some strains of inbred mice develop anti-Sm autoantibodies with B cell epitope spreading of the autoimmune response after immunization with this peptide on an MAP™ backbone of branching lysines.[2] In addition to generating antibodies that bind PPPGMRPP and other spliceosomal peptides (as well as the Sm and nRNP proteins), these animals variably develop positive antinuclear antibodies (ANA), anti-double-stranded DNA antibodies (dsDNA), proteinuria, elevated creatinine, seizures, alopecia, and thrombocytopenia. Rabbits immunized with control protocols develop none of these features of lupus nor of autoimmunity.[2]

This common antigenic target of Sm B/B′, PPPGMRPP, is very similar to a region of the Epstein-Barr nuclear antigen-1 (EBNA-1) protein, PPPGRRP. We have previously reported that lupus patients, but not normals nor patients with other autoimmune diseases, have antibodies that bind this region of EBNA-1.[1] In addition, both the major autoantigenic target of Sm D in lupus and EBNA-1 have repeated glycine-arginine sequences.[3,4] These glycine-arginine repeats of the EBNA-1 protein specifically bind human lupus sera.[4,5]

Two rabbits have been immunized, using a protocol previously published,[2] with the PPPGRRP-MAP™ peptide of EBNA-1. Both rabbits mount an immune response to the peptide of immunization (FIGURE 1, panel A). In addition, early in the immunization protocol these rabbits both develop antibodies that cross-react with the PPPGMRPP-MAP™ peptide of Sm B/B′ (FIGURE 1, panel B). Neither of these animals have antibodies that bind any of three different Ro/SSA-MAP™ peptides.

[a]This work was supported by the National Institutes of Health (Grant Nos. AR42474, AI24717, AR42460, AR31584, and GM14841), the United States Department of Veterans Affairs, the Oklahoma Lupus Foundation, the Presbyterian Health Foundation, the Warren Foundation, and the Noble Foundation.

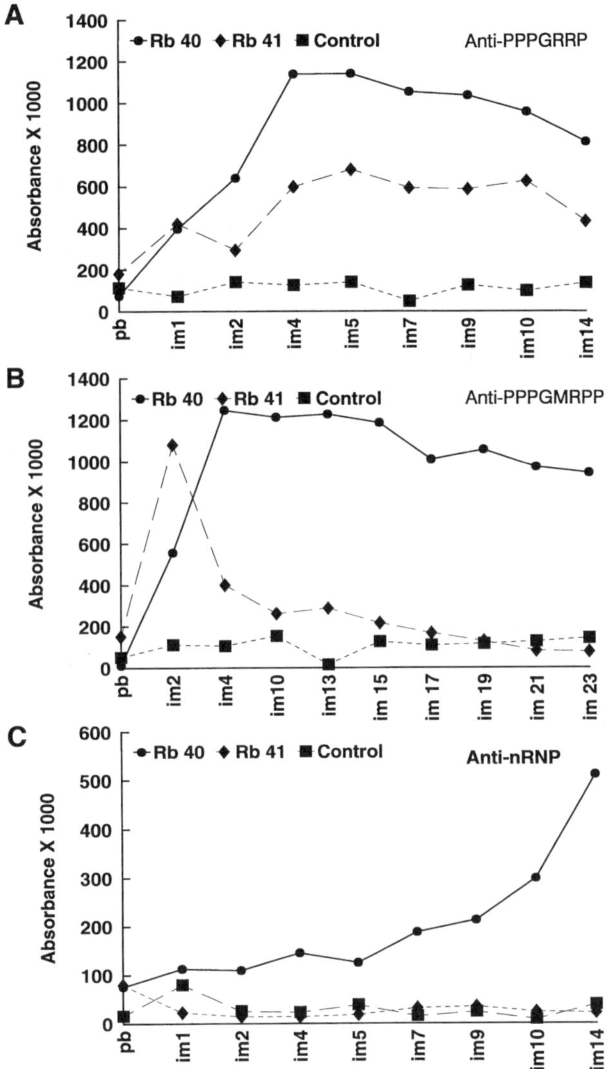

FIGURE 1. Binding of PPPGRRP-MAP™-immunized rabbit sera and a Freund's control serum to the PPPGRRP-MAP™, PPPGMRPP-MAP™, and nRNP antigens. Panel A presents the binding of these PPPGRRP-MAP™-immunized rabbits to the PPPGRRP-MAP™ peptide of immunization by standard ELISA. Various immunized bleeds are presented in chronological order along the x-axis. Panel B displays the binding of these same rabbit sera to the PPPGMRPP-MAP™ peptide of Sm B/B′. Panel C shows the binding of these sera to the whole nRNP antigen. (Note that pb indicates the preimmune sera, and the im 1 through 14 sera were collected at 2 to 52 weeks after initial immunization.)

However, one of these rabbits quickly loses antibody binding to the PPPGMRPP-MAP™ peptide. The rabbit with persistently high titers of anti-PPPGMRPP antibodies also develops antibodies against the Sm and nRNP whole antigens (FIGURE 1, panel C).

The rabbit that mounts an immune response against the whole nRNP protein behaves in a way very similar to those rabbits previously immunized with PPPGMRPP-MAP™.[2] This rabbit develops a positive nuclear speckled ANA (titer of 1:360). In addition, this rabbit develops anti-dsDNA antibodies to 1:90 (*Crithidia lucillea* assay). This rabbit also makes a humoral immune response to various regions of the Sm B/B′ and Sm D proteins as shown in FIGURE 2. Many of the same regions bound by this

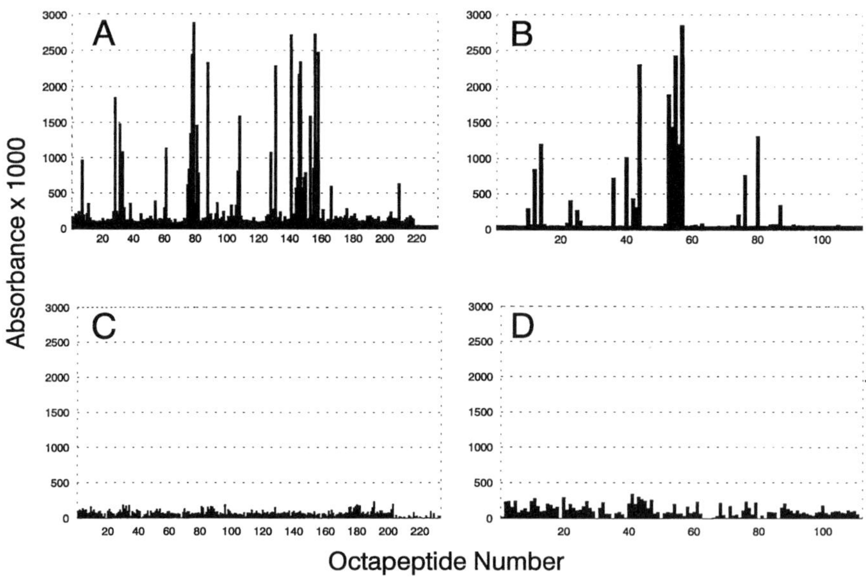

FIGURE 2. Serum binding of a rabbit immunized with the PPPGRRP-MAP™ sequence of EBNA-1 to the overlapping octapeptides of Sm B/B′ and Sm D. Panel A presents the binding of Rabbit 40 serum collected 86 days after initial immunization with the overlapping octapeptides of Sm B/B′. Panel B presents the reactivity of this same rabbit serum with the overlapping octapeptides of Sm D. Panel C shows the binding of Rabbit 41 serum collected 86 days after initial immunization with the overlapping octapeptides of Sm B/B′; this serum binding to Sm D peptides is presented in panel D.

peptide-immunized rabbit are also bound by SLE patient sera, as well as by animals immunized with PPPGMRPP-MAP™. (Curiously, this animal has not developed antibodies that bind the glycine-arginine repeat of Sm D.) These data suggest that this rabbit immunized with a segment of EBNA-1 breaks tolerance to his own spliceosomal proteins.

The second rabbit succeeded in suppressing or avoiding an autoimmune anti-Sm response. Serum from this animal was ANA-negative; there was no anti-dsDNA, no antibody that convincingly bound any of the other octapeptides from Sm B/B′ nor D, and no anti-Sm B/B′ nor Sm D binding in Western blot.

Both rabbits generated an antibody response against PPPGRRP and also initially against PPPGMRPP. In one animal, these antibodies appear to be cross-reactive with Sm, leading to the capacity to present this autoantigen (via class II) and then to develop lupus autoimmunity. The other animal, however, developed only peptide-specific antibodies and its immune response never became directed against the whole Sm protein. These observations are consistent with the paradigm previously offered for the critical events in human lupus from an antigenically cross-reactive intact structure to presentation to autoimmunity.[2]

REFERENCES

1. JAMES, J. A. & J. B. HARLEY. 1992. Linear epitope mapping of an Sm B/B′ polypeptide. J. Immunol. **148:** 2074–2079.
2. JAMES, J. A., T. GROSS, R. H. SCOFIELD & J. B. HARLEY. 1995. Immunoglobulin epitope spreading and autoimmune disease after peptide immunization: Sm B/B′–derived PPPGMRPP and PPPGIRGP induce spliceosome autoimmunity. J. Exp. Med. **181:** 453–461.
3. ROKEACH, L. A., J. A. HASELBY & S. O. HOCH. 1988. Molecular cloning of a cDNA encoding the human Sm-D autoantigen. Proc. Natl. Acad. Sci. U.S.A. **85:** 4832–4836.
4. JAMES, J. A., M. J. MAMULA & J. B. HARLEY. 1994. Sequential autoantigenic determinants of the small nuclear ribonucleoprotein Sm D shared by human lupus autoantibodies and MRL lpr/lpr antibodies. Clin. Exp. Immunol. **98:** 419–426.
5. BARAKAT, S., J. P. BRIAND, J. C. WEBER, M. H. V. REGENMORTEL & S. MULLER. 1990. Recognition of synthetic peptides of Sm-D autoantigen by lupus sera. Clin. Exp. Immunol. **81:** 256–262.

The Regulation of Murine Lupus[a]

STANFORD L. PENG[b,c,d] AND JOE CRAFT[b]

[b]*Section of Rheumatology*
Yale University School of Medicine
New Haven, Connecticut 06510

[c]*Department of Biology*
Yale University
New Haven, Connecticut 06510

INTRODUCTION

Systemic lupus erythematosus (SLE) remains a paradigm of systemic autoimmunity. Murine models for SLE include several inbred strains, all of which develop anti-double-stranded (ds) DNA autoantibodies and glomerulonephritis.[1] The congenic MRL/Mp-+/+ (MRL/+) and MRL/Mp-*lpr/lpr* strains in particular develop a broad, multiorgan autoimmune response extraordinarily reminiscent of SLE, including the development of anti-dsDNA autoantibodies and the SLE-specific anti-Sm,[2] anti-ribosome P,[3] and anti-Su[4] specificities. These mice develop glomerulonephritis,[5] vasculitis,[6] arthritis,[7] and cerebritis[8] due to the development of pathogenic autoantibody-containing immune complexes, as well as subsequent autoimmune end-organ infiltration.[9] Numerous investigations into the pathogenesis of SLE have focused upon these mice as models for systemic autoimmunity. This review discusses the current understanding of murine lupus, emphasizing recent work in MRL mice that provides evidence for an intricate regulatory network in systemic autoimmunity.

A BRIEF NATURAL HISTORY OF LUPUS-PRONE B CELLS

Central and essential components of murine lupus remain autoreactive B cells,[10] which are overrepresented and substantially activated in lupus-prone mice.[11] Although some genetic studies have found that end-organ disease may occasionally develop in the absence of B cell hyperactivity,[12,13] the brisk onset of murine lupus most closely correlates with the presence of polyclonal activation.[11] This phenomenon likely reflects a generalized immune dysregulation, as suggested by several studies demon-

[a]This report is based partially upon a dissertation submitted to fulfill in part the requirements for the degree of Doctor of Philosophy in Yale University. The work was supported in part by grants from the NIH (Nos. AR40072 and AR42475), the Arthritis and Lupus Foundations, and their Connecticut chapters, as well as by donations to Yale Rheumatology in the memories of Irene Feltman, Albert L. Harlow, and Chantal Marquis (to J. Craft).

[d]S. L. Peng was supported by the Medical Scientist Training Program at Yale University School of Medicine.

strating that lupus-prone mice possess intrinsic B cell defects,[14–17] which may result in defective tolerance induction[18,19] and/or aberrant selection of abnormal B cell clones.[20] Such alterations in B cell homeostasis probably allow select autoreactive clones, stimulated by self-antigens or antigens cross-reactive with self,[21] to proliferate and activate, resulting in polyclonal (or multiclonal, as termed by Klinman and Steinberg) B cell activation.[22]

Despite the broad autoreactivity implicit in such a model, an important feature of the lupus autoantibody response remains the extraordinary affinity and pathogenicity of some autoantibodies. Many autoantibodies display evidence of somatic mutation and affinity maturation[23–25] in conjunction with pathogenicity,[26,27] although germline-encoded and/or polyreactive antibodies have also been found to induce tissue injury.[28] In addition, typical autoimmune responses in lupus-prone mice increase in intensity and affinity over time,[29–31] together suggesting that significant features of autoimmune B cell responses involve selection by antigen as well as T cells that provide autoantigen-specific help.[32–34] Consequently, lupus autoimmunity must involve both intrinsic and extrinsic B cell regulatory effects.

THE ROLE OF αβ T CELLS IN MURINE LUPUS

αβ T cells remain the most popularly regarded effector cells in the extrinsic propagation of B cell autoimmunity.[35] They have been considered essential for the development of lupus by inducing isotype switching and affinity maturation,[36–40] although direct demonstrations of such phenomena have not been described. Still, the importance of αβ T cells in disease has been supported by studies involving helper autoreactive αβ T cell lines, which are capable of inducing lupus pathology *in vivo.*[41,42] Other manipulations of the lupus immune system provide further evidence: neonatal thymectomy,[43] anti-Thy-1 antibody treatment,[44] anti-CD4 antibody treatment,[45,46] MHC class II deficiency,[47] and CD4 deficiency[48] all significantly diminish autoantibody titers and renal disease.

These studies provide a simple, concise model for lupus, in which pathogenic autoantibody production by B cells requires autoreactive $CD4^+$ αβ T cell help. Such a view, however, does not account for the ontogeny of such T cells, which continues to elude many investigations. Some of these autoreactive αβ T cells may have resulted from defective central and/or peripheral tolerance,[49,50] but the majority of lupus-prone mice possess normal thymic and peripheral tolerance.[51–53] The *lpr* mutation, which is considered to confer lupus to several "normal" mouse strains, consists of a functional defect in the Fas apoptosis antigen[54] and results in defective peripheral tolerance of B cells[55] and T cells;[56,57] however, this effect only accelerates, rather than initiates, primary disease processes unique to the respective backgrounds against which the mutation is crossed.[58] Thus, MRL mice, which themselves develop lupus, progress to intense, accelerated disease in the presence of *lpr*; on the other hand, C3H/*lpr* and C57BL/6/*lpr* mice develop virtually negligible end-organ lesions. Consequently, the promotion of lupus by αβ T cells likely reflects more complex regulatory alterations beyond the simple activation of autoreactive T cells. Rather, systemic autoimmunity likely involves dysregulation within other populations of lymphoid cells as well.

To address the potential importance of αβ T cell–independent mechanisms in murine lupus, recent studies have examined the development of disease in lupus-prone MRL mice congenitally deficient in αβ T cells.[59] Here, a germline TCR α −/− mutation was used to dissociate clearly αβ T cell–dependent from αβ T cell–independent mechanisms. TCR α −/− lupus-prone mice developed a significant, although partially penetrant, lupus phenotype, producing antinuclear antibodies as well as anti-dsDNA and anti-snRNP autoantibodies at frequencies similar to TCR α +/+ counterparts. Some animals developed hypergammaglobulinemia of the IgG1, IgG2a, and IgE isotypes, and accumulated substantial amounts of immune complexes in their kidneys, as detected by direct immunofluorescence of native IgG. These findings were quite surprising, in light of the widely held tenets regarding the necessity of αβ T cells.

Indeed, αβ T cell–independent lupus constituted a relatively subdued, albeit respectable, disease phenotype. Despite the incompletely penetrant class-switched hypergammaglobulinemia, αβ T cell–deficient mice as a whole failed to develop significantly elevated titers of all class-switched immunoglobulins compared to TCR α +/+ mice. Also, despite substantial autoantibody levels, the qualities of TCR α −/− autoantibodies were clearly distinct: antinuclear antibodies, as detected by the fluorescent antinuclear antibody test, were of lower intensities than TCR α +/+ antibodies; and their anti-dsDNA and anti-snRNP antibodies, as detected by ELISA, were of low specificity and/or affinity, as determined by the *Crithidia luciliae* immunofluorescent test and ^{35}S-immunoprecipitation assay, respectively. Furthermore, TCR α −/− mice failed to develop significantly elevated titers of kappa rheumatoid factor, unlike their T cell–sufficient littermates, and their renal disease was delayed: whereas TCR α +/+ *lpr* mice developed substantial glomerular, interstitial, and perivascular infiltrates by 12 weeks of age, TCR α −/− kidneys remained mostly unaffected, as judged by light microscopy, despite the presence of substantial immune complexes at 24 weeks of age.

These findings thus provide a cautious demonstration of αβ T cell–dependent mechanisms in the enhancement of murine lupus. The less-impressive qualities of TCR α −/− immunoglobulins, autoantibodies, and renal disease suggest that αβ T cells induce class-switching to pathogenic immunoglobulin isotypes and induce antigen-specific selection, and possibly affinity maturation, of B cell autoimmunity. At the same time, however, the development of substantial anti-dsDNA and anti-snRNP autoantibodies in TCR α −/− mice demonstrates the potential importance of αβ T cell–independent mechanisms. Indeed, older TCR α −/− mice develop significant light-microscopic kidney disease, along with increased mortality and compromised renal function, irrespective of Fas phenotype, thus constituting an incontrovertible lupus phenotype that may reflect not only the absence of regulatory αβ T cells in TCR α −/− MRL/+ mice, but the absence of helper αβ T cells in TCR α −/− MRL/*lpr* mice.[60] The regulation of murine lupus therefore does not end with helper αβ T cells and B cells.

THE ROLE OF γδ T CELLS IN MURINE LUPUS

Relatively little work has addressed the roles of non-αβ T cells in systemic autoimmune responses, despite a substantial number of intriguing immunological studies. Although their function remains on the whole unassigned,[61] recent studies have pointed toward a role for γδ T cells in the regulation of immune responses,[62] particularly at epithelial surfaces.[63–65] γδ T cells have been shown to provide both helper and regulatory functions in several nonautoimmune systems,[63,64,66–68] as well as some organ-specific autoimmune syndromes, such as experimentally induced arthritis[69–71] and uveitis.[72] Still, γδ T cells remain largely unexplored in systemic autoimmunity, although one study in humans with SLE has described the isolation of γδ T cells that help autoantibody production.[73]

Recent work has addressed the roles of γδ T cells in systemic autoimmunity by examining lupus-prone mice deficient in αβ T cells, γδ T cells, or both.[74] Here, the germline TCR β −/− and TCR δ −/− mutations were used to eliminate T cell subsets selectively. In this system, γδ T cells performed a predominantly regulatory function because TCR δ −/− mice displayed significantly more intense hypergammaglobulinemia and autoantibody titers. TCR δ −/− *lpr* animals developed increased peripheral cell counts of $CD4^-CD8^-B220^+$ αβ T cells, which reflect autoreactive cells unable to complete activation-induced cell death.[75–77] Mortality and renal disease were also augmented in TCR δ −/− mice, which contained more severe glomerular, interstitial, and perivascular lesions. γδ T cells thus regulate both αβ T cell and B cell autoreactivity.

γδ T cells were also found capable of performing a significant helper function in systemic autoimmunity, by comparison of TCR β −/− and TCR β −/− TCR δ −/− mice. TCR β −/− mice recapitulated the partially penetrant autoimmune syndrome of TCR α −/− mice (arguing against a significant role for the minor population of TCR $\alpha^-\beta^+$ cells sometimes implicated as functional in the latter mice[78,79]). TCR β −/− TCR δ −/− mice, on the other hand, failed to develop significant titers of class-switched immunoglobulins or autoantibodies, nor did they develop immune-complex renal disease. γδ T cells were responsible for the production of IL-2 and IL-4, as well as a significant portion of IFN-γ in TCR β −/− animals. γδ T cells thus are capable of providing significant T cell–dependent help; coupled with data from TCR α −/− mice, these findings suggest that γδ T cells may effect systemic humoral autoimmunity with end-organ consequences, although their ramifications lack the severity of αβ T cell–dependent help.

OTHER LYMPHOID CELLS IN MURINE LUPUS

Very little information is available regarding the possible contributions of non-T, non-B cells to murine lupus. Many molecular abnormalities in macrophages from lupus-prone mice have been described, but most have not provided clear insight into their role in disease pathogenesis.[1] One recent study, however, has found that Th1

$CD4^+$ $\alpha\beta$ T cells delete activated macrophages via Fas,[80] and another study has demonstrated that macrophages may present autoantigens to and activate T cells.[81] Other studies have raised interest in the possible roles of natural killer (NK) cells, which likely regulate autoimmune responses,[82] but are diminished in activity in lupus-prone mice.[83–85] As such, it is interesting to note that some TCR β −/− TCR δ −/− lupus-prone mice develop peculiar, but severe, renal lesions consisting of glomerular hypercellularity as well as perivascular and interstitial mononuclear infiltrates, despite the absence of renal immune deposits and B cell activation (unpublished data); thus, this suggests that one or more of such non-T, non-B cell lymphoid cells may further contribute to murine lupus by cellular autoimmune pathology. The physiological roles of both macrophages and NK cells, however, remain largely to be determined.

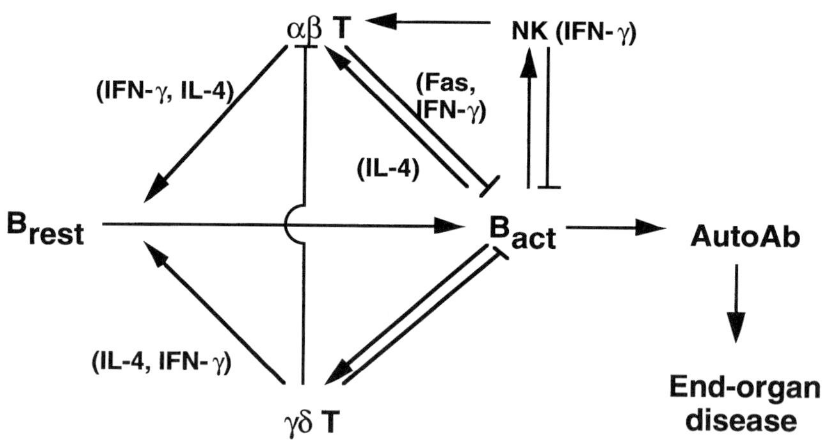

FIGURE 1. A simplified model for murine lupus including regulatory interactions among T cells, B cells, and NK cells. See text for details.

A WORKING MODEL FOR THE REGULATION OF MURINE LUPUS

Together, these recent findings suggest a complex, circular regulatory network in systemic autoimmunity (FIGURE 1). The pathway most central to the development of lupus involves the activation of autoreactive B cells, resulting in autoantibody production and immune-complex-mediated end-organ disease. It remains unclear what specific forces drive lupus B cell activation, but both $\alpha\beta$ and $\gamma\delta$ T cells are capable of promoting B cell autoimmunity, with the former providing the more-significant source of T cell help. Another possibility includes intrinsic B cell hyperactivity, a trait common to all lupus-prone strains,[11] but the virtual absence of hypergammaglobulinemia and autoantibodies in TCR β −/− TCR δ −/− lupus-prone mice would suggest that polyclonal B cell activation, although perhaps a prerequisite for murine lupus, cannot progress to pathogenic disease in the absence of

T cell help. As other possible B cell activators, NK cells have been demonstrated to promote immunoglobulin synthesis by B cells;[86,87] however, the TCR β −/− TCR δ −/− phenotype also argues against a significant role for NK cells in the promotion of B cell autoantibody production. Rather, NK cells likely play a predominantly regulatory role in the suppression of B cell autoimmunity,[82–85] perhaps via IFN-γ, which inhibits,[88–90] or via Fas ligand (FasL), which deletes[91,92] activated B cells. T cells, both αβ and γδ, thus provide the significant majority of the extrinsic factors that drive autoreactive B cells.

At the same time, both αβ and γδ T cells also likely play regulatory roles. Indeed, the primary role for γδ T cells appears to involve the downregulation of systemic autoimmunity, as illustrated by TCR δ −/− lupus-prone mice. These cells likely regulate αβ T cells because γδ T cell–deficient lupus-prone mice contain greater numbers of conventional αβ T cells, but normal or reduced numbers of B cells (unpublished data), and γδ T cells have been demonstrated to exert cytotoxic activity against antigen-specific targets.[93] Alternatively, γδ T cells may perform a modulatory function, as illustrated by the phenotypes of TCR α −/− and TCR β −/− mice, which develop a predominantly IgG1 and IgE hypergammaglobulinemia suggestive of a γδ T cell–dependent, IL-4-predominant environment.[59,67] As such, the IgG1 isotype, which predominates the autoantibodies of TCR α −/− and TCR β −/− mice, is notable for its poor complement fixation ability,[94] and IL-4 is notable for its Th2-modulating capability.[95] Because murine lupus is characterized by an IFN-γ-predominant, Th1-like environment,[22] γδ T cells may modulate autoimmunity toward a protective phenotype, involving somewhat protective Th2-like IgG1 autoantibodies that guard against the pathogenicity of complement-fixing IgG2a, IgG2b, and IgG3 antibodies. Modulation in T cell–dependent autoimmunity also likely exists in the αβ T cell compartment, where activated B cells promote IL-4 production and Th2 modulation.[96] In addition, Th1 αβ T cells likely regulate activated autoreactive B cells via FasL and IFN-γ.[89,92] These studies collectively imply an extraordinarily complex network in the regulation of autoimmunity.

This working model provides a conglomerated view that synthesizes current knowledge. In MRL/+ animals, B cell hyperactivity eventually activates helper T cells, leading to T cell–dependent autoantibody production and disease. Here, αβ T cells exert a significant regulatory role via FasL, and thus TCR α −/− Fas+ mice develop increased autoantibody titers and hypergammaglobulinemia, in association with disease-related mortality.[60] In MRL/*lpr* animals, FasL-dependent regulation of B cells is not possible, so αβ T cells perform a primarily helper function, and TCR α −/− *lpr* mice develop reduced disease, although they still continue to produce autoantibodies and develop end-organ disease due to γδ T cell–dependent help. The primary role for γδ T cells, however, remains the downregulation of autoimmunity, as illustrated by TCR δ −/− mice irrespective of Fas genotype.[74] Finally, NK cells exert primarily a regulatory influence[82–85] because TCR β −/− TCR δ −/− mice fail to develop significant levels of class-switched immunoglobulins or autoantibodies. Thus, lupus autoimmunity involves complex regulatory interactions still incompletely understood, but it is now clear that these interactions do not simply involve conventional αβ T cell help to autoreactive B cells.

REFERENCES

1. THEOFILOPOULOS, A. N. & F. J. DIXON. 1985. Murine models of systemic lupus erythematosus. Adv. Immunol. **37**(269): 269–390.
2. EISENBERG, R. A., E. M. TAN & F. J. DIXON. 1978. Presence of anti-Sm reactivity in autoimmune mouse strains. J. Exp. Med. **147**(2): 582–587.
3. BONFA, E., A. MARSHAK-ROTHSTEIN, H. WEISSBACH, N. BROT & K. ELKON. 1988. Frequency and epitope recognition of anti-ribosome P antibodies from humans with systemic lupus erythematosus and MRL/lpr mice are similar. J. Immunol. **140**(10): 3434–3437.
4. TREADWELL, E. L., P. COHEN, D. WILLIAMS, K. O'BRIEN, A. VOLKMAN & R. EISENBERG. 1993. MRL mice produce anti-Su autoantibody, a specificity associated with systemic lupus erythematosus. J. Immunol. **150**(2): 695–699.
5. HEWICKER, M. & G. TRAUTWEIN. 1986. Glomerular lesions in MRL mice: a light and immunofluorescence microscopic study. Zentralbl. Veterinaermed. Reihe B **33**(10): 727–739.
6. HEWICKER, M. & G. TRAUTWEIN. 1987. Sequential study of vasculitis in MRL mice. Lab. Anim. **21**(4): 335–341.
7. HEWICKER, M., L. H. GARCES, E. KROMSCHRÖDER & G. TRAUTWEIN. 1988. Beitrag zur Pathogenese der spontanen chronischen Polyarthritis der MRL-Mäuse. Z. Rheumatol. **47**(4): 219–226.
8. ALEXANDER, E. L., E. D. MURPHY, J. B. ROTHS & G. E. ALEXANDER. 1983. Congenic autoimmune murine models of central nervous system disease in connective tissue disorders. Ann. Neurol. **14**(2): 242–248.
9. HEWICKER, M., E. KROMSCHRÖDER & G. TRAUTWEIN. 1990. Detection of circulating immune complexes in MRL mice with different forms of glomerulonephritis. Z. Verstierkd. **33**(4): 149–156.
10. SHLOMCHIK, M. J., M. P. MADAIO, D. NI, M. TROUNSTEIN & D. HUSZAR. 1994. The role of B cells in lpr/lpr-induced autoimmunity. J. Exp. Med. **180**(4): 1295–1306.
11. KLINMAN, D. M. & A. D. STEINBERG. 1987. Systemic autoimmune disease arises from polyclonal B cell activation. J. Exp. Med. **165**(6): 1755–1760.
12. DATTA, S. K., F. L. OWEN, J. E. WOMACK & R. J. RIBLET. 1982. Analysis of recombinant inbred lines derived from "autoimmune" (NZB) and "high leukemia" (C58) strains: independent multigenic systems control B cell hyperactivity, retrovirus expression, and autoimmunity. J. Immunol. **129**(4): 1539–1544.
13. EASTCOTT, J. W., R. S. SCHWARTZ & S. K. DATTA. 1983. Genetic analysis of the inheritance of B cell hyperactivity in relation to the development of autoantibodies and glomerulonephritis in NZB × SWR crosses. J. Immunol. **131**(5): 2232–2239.
14. KATAGIRI, T., P. L. COHEN & R. A. EISENBERG. 1988. The *lpr* gene causes an intrinsic T cell abnormality that is required for hyperproliferation. J. Exp. Med. **167**(3): 741–751.
15. NEMAZEE, D., C. GUIET, K. BUERKI & A. MARSHAK-ROTHSTEIN. 1991. B lymphocytes from the autoimmune-prone mouse strain MLR/lpr manifest an intrinsic defect in tetraparental MRL/lpr in equilibrium DBA/2 chimeras. J. Immunol. **147**(8): 2536–2539.
16. PERKINS, D. L., R. M. GLASER, C. A. MAHON, J. MICHAELSON & A. MARSHAK-ROTHSTEIN. 1990. Evidence for an intrinsic B cell defect in lpr/lpr mice apparent in neonatal chimeras. J. Immunol. **145**(2): 549–555.
17. SOBEL, E. S., T. KATAGIRI, K. KATAGIRI, S. C. MORRIS, P. L. COHEN & R. A. EISENBERG. 1991. An intrinsic B cell defect is required for the production of autoantibodies in the lpr model of murine systemic autoimmunity. J. Exp. Med. **173**(6): 1441–1449.
18. ROARK, J. H., C. L. KUNTZ, K-A. NGUYEN, L. MANDIK, M. CATTERMOLE & J. ERIKSON. 1995. B cell selection and allelic exclusion of an anti-DNA Ig transgene in MRL-lpr/lpr mice. J. Immunol. **154**(9): 4444–4455.
19. ROARK, J. H., C. L. KUNTZ, K-A. NGUYEN, A. J. CATON & J. ERIKSON. 1995. Breakdown of B cell tolerance in a mouse model of systemic lupus erythematosus. J. Exp. Med. **181**(3): 1157–1167.
20. JACOBSON, B. A., D. J. PANKA, K-A. NGUYEN, J. ERIKSON, A. K. ABBAS & A. MARSHAK-ROTHSTEIN. 1995. Anatomy of autoantibody production: dominant localization of antibody-producing cells to T cell zones in Fas-deficient mice. Immunity **3**(4): 509–519.

21. HARDIN, J. A. 1986. The lupus autoantigens and the pathogenesis of SLE. Arthritis Rheum. **29**(4): 457–460.
22. KLINMAN, D. M. & A. D. STEINBERG. 1995. Inquiry into murine and human lupus. Immunol. Rev. **144:** 157–193.
23. BLOOM, D. D., J. L. DAVIGNON, M. W. RETTER, M. J. SHLOMCHIK, D. S. PISETSKY, P. L. COHEN, R. A. EISENBERG & S. H. CLARKE. 1993. V region gene analysis of anti-Sm hybridomas from MRL/Mp-lpr/lpr mice. J. Immunol. **150**(4): 1591–1610.
24. SHLOMCHIK, M. J., A. H. AUCOIN, D. S. PISETSKY & M. G. WEIGERT. 1987. Structure and function of anti-DNA autoantibodies derived from a single autoimmune mouse. Proc. Natl. Acad. Sci. U.S.A. **84**(24): 9150–9154.
25. SHLOMCHIK, M. J., A. MARSHAK-ROTHSTEIN, C. B. WOLFOWICZ, T. L. ROTHSTEIN & M. G. WEIGERT. 1987. The role of clonal selection and somatic mutation in autoimmunity. Nature **328**(6133): 805–811.
26. DANG, H. & R. J. HARBECK. 1984. The *in vivo* and *in vitro* glomerular deposition of isolated anti-double-stranded-DNA antibodies in NZB/W mice. Clin. Immunol. Immunopathol. **30**(2): 265–278.
27. VLAHAKOS, D. V., M. H. FOSTER, S. ADAMS, M. KATZ, A. A. UCCI, K. J. BARRETT, S. K. DATTA & M. P. MADAIO. 1992. Anti-DNA antibodies form immune deposits at distinct glomerular and vascular sites. Kidney Int. **41**(6): 1690–1700.
28. PANKEWYCZ, O. G., P. MIGLIORINI & M. P. MADAIO. 1987. Polyreactive autoantibodies are nephritogenic in murine lupus nephritis. J. Immunol. **139**(10): 3287–3294.
29. BURLINGAME, R. W., R. L. RUBIN, R. S. BALDERAS & A. N. THEOFILOPOULOS. 1993. Genesis and evolution of antichromatin autoantibodies in murine lupus implicates T-dependent immunization with self antigen. J. Clin. Invest. **91**(4): 1687–1696.
30. AMOURA, Z., H. CHABRE, S. KOUTOUZOV, C. LOTTON, A. CABRESPINES, J. F. BACH & L. JACOB. 1994. Nucleosome-restricted antibodies are detected before anti-dsDNA and/or antihistone antibodies in serum of MRL-Mp lpr/lpr and +/+ mice, and are present in kidney eluates of lupus mice with proteinuria. Arthritis Rheum. **37**(11): 1684–1688.
31. FATENEJAD, S., W. BROOKS, A. SCHWARTZ & J. CRAFT. 1994. Pattern of anti-small nuclear ribonucleoprotein antibodies in MRL/Mp-lpr/lpr mice suggests that the intact U1 snRNP particle is their autoimmunogenic target. J. Immunol. **152**(11): 5523–5531.
32. SHORES, E. W., R. A. EISENBERG & P. L. COHEN. 1986. Role of the Sm antigen in the generation of anti-Sm autoantibodies in the SLE-prone MRL mouse. J. Immunol. **136**(10): 3662–3667.
33. MOHAN, C., S. ADAMS, V. STANIK & S. K. DATTA. 1993. Nucleosome: a major immunogen for pathogenic autoantibody-inducing T cells of lupus. J. Exp. Med. **177**(5): 1367–1381.
34. SHAN, H., M. J. SHLOMCHIK, A. MARSHAK-ROTHSTEIN, D. S. PISETSKY, S. LITWIN & M. G. WEIGERT. 1994. The mechanism of autoantibody production in an autoimmune MRL/*lpr* mouse. J. Immunol. **153**(11): 5104–5120.
35. MOHAN, C. & S. K. DATTA. 1995. Lupus: key pathogenic mechanisms and contributing factors. Clin. Immunol. Immunopathol. **77**(3): 209–220.
36. ANDO, D. G., E. E. SERCARZ & B. H. HAHN. 1987. Mechanisms of T and B cell collaboration in the *in vitro* production of anti-DNA antibodies in the NZB/NZW F1 murine SLE model. J. Immunol. **138**(10): 3185–3190.
37. DATTA, S. K., H. PATEL & D. BERRY. 1987. Induction of a cationic shift in IgG anti-DNA autoantibodies: role of T helper cells with classical and novel phenotypes in three murine models of lupus nephritis. J. Exp. Med. **165**(5): 1252–1268.
38. NAIKI, M., B. L. CHIANG, D. CAWLEY, A. ANSARI, S. J. ROZZO, B. L. KOTZIN, A. ZLOTNIK & M. E. GERSHWIN. 1992. Generation and characterization of cloned T helper cell lines for anti-DNA responses in NZB.H-2bm12 mice. J. Immunol. **149**(12): 4109–4115.
39. SOBEL, E. S., V. N. KAKKANAIAH, M. KAKKANAIAH, R. L. CHEEK, P. L. COHEN & R. A. EISENBERG. 1994. T-B collaboration for autoantibody production in lpr mice is cognate and MHC-restricted. J. Immunol. **152**(12): 6011–6016.
40. MOHAN, C., Y. SHI, J. D. LAMAN & S. K. DATTA. 1995. Interaction between CD40 and its ligand gp39 in the development of murine lupus nephritis. J. Immunol. **154**(3): 1470–1480.

41. Adams, S., P. Leblanc & S. K. Datta. 1991. Junctional region sequences of T-cell receptor beta-chain genes expressed by pathogenic anti-DNA autoantibody-inducing helper T cells from lupus mice: possible selection by cationic autoantigens. Proc. Natl. Acad. Sci. U.S.A. **88**(24): 11271–11275.
42. Mao, C., G. E. Osman, S. Adams & S. K. Datta. 1994. T cell receptor alpha-chain repertoire of pathogenic autoantibody-inducing T cells in lupus mice. J. Immunol. **152**(3): 1462–1470.
43. Steinberg, A. D., J. B. Roths, E. D. Murphy, R. T. Steinberg & E. S. Raveche. 1980. Effects of thymectomy or androgen administration upon the autoimmune disease of MRL/Mp-lpr/lpr mice. J. Immunol. **125**(2): 871–873.
44. Seaman, W. E., D. Wofsy, J. S. Greenspan & J. A. Ledbetter. 1983. Treatment of autoimmune MRL/lpr mice with monoclonal antibody to Thy-1.2: a single injection has sustained effects on lymphoproliferation and renal disease. J. Immunol. **130**(4): 1713–1718.
45. Wofsy, D. & W. E. Seaman. 1987. Reversal of advanced murine lupus in NZB/NZW F1 mice by treatment with monoclonal antibody to L3T4. J. Immunol. **138**(10): 3247–3253.
46. Santoro, T. J., J. P. Portanova & B. L. Kotzin. 1988. The contribution of L3T4+ T cells to lymphoproliferation and autoantibody production in MRL-lpr/lpr mice. J. Exp. Med. **167**(5): 1713–1718.
47. Jevnikar, A. M., M. J. Grusby & L. H. Glimcher. 1994. Prevention of nephritis in major histocompatibility complex class II–deficient MRL-*lpr* mice. J. Exp. Med. **179**(4): 1137–1143.
48. Koh, D-R., A. Ho, A. Rahemutulla, W-P. Fung-Leung, H. Griesser & T-W. Mak. 1995. Murine lupus in MRL/*lpr* mice lacking CD4 or CD8 T cells. Eur. J. Immunol. **25:** 2558–2562.
49. Adams, S., T. Zordan, K. Sainis & S. Datta. 1990. T cell receptor V_β genes expressed by IgG anti-DNA autoantibody-inducing T cells in lupus nephritis: forbidden receptors and double-negative T cells. Eur. J. Immunol. **20**(7): 1435–1443.
50. Singh, R. R., V. Kumar, F. B. Ebling, S. Southwood, A. Sette, E. E. Sercarz & B. H. Hahn. 1995. T cell determinants from autoantibodies to DNA can upregulate autoimmunity in murine systemic lupus erythematosus. J. Exp. Med. **181**(6): 2017–2027.
51. Kotzin, B. L., J. W. Kappler, P. C. Marrack & L. R. Herron. 1989. T cell tolerance to self antigens in New Zealand hybrid mice with lupus-like disease. J. Immunol. **143**(1): 89–94.
52. Singer, P. A., R. S. Balderas, R. J. McEvilly, M. Bobardt & A. N. Theofilopoulos. 1989. Tolerance-related V_β clonal deletions in normal CD4−8−, TCR-αβ+, and abnormal lpr and gld cell populations. J. Exp. Med. **170**(6): 1869–1877.
53. Herron, L. R., R. A. Eisenberg, E. Roper, V. N. Kakkanaiah, P. L. Cohen & B. L. Kotzin. 1993. Selection of the T cell receptor repertoire in lpr mice. J. Immunol. **151**(7): 3450–3459.
54. Watanabe-Fukunaga, R., C. I. Brannan, N. G. Copeland, N. A. Jenkins & S. Nagata. 1992. Lymphoproliferation disorder in mice explained by defects in Fas antigen that mediates apoptosis. Nature **356**(6367): 314–317.
55. Rathmell, J. C. & C. C. Goodnow. 1994. Effects of the lpr mutation on elimination and inactivation of self-reactive B cells. J. Immunol. **153**(6): 2831–2842.
56. Singer, G. G. & A. K. Abbas. 1994. The Fas antigen is involved in peripheral, but not thymic deletion of T lymphocytes in T cell receptor transgenic mice. Immunity **1**(5): 365–371.
57. Van Parijs, L., A. Ibraghimov & A. K. Abbas. 1996. The roles of costimulation and Fas in T cell apoptosis and peripheral tolerance. Immunity **4**(3): 321–328.
58. Izui, S., V. E. Kelley, K. Masuda, H. Yoshida, J. B. Roths & E. D. Murphy. 1984. Induction of various autoantibodies by mutant gene *lpr* in several strains of mice. J. Immunol. **133**(1): 227–233.
59. Peng, S. L., M. P. Madaio, D. P. M. Hughes, I. N. Crispe, M. J. Owen, L. Wen, A. C. Hayday & J. Craft. 1996. Murine lupus in the absence of αβ T cells. J. Immunol. **156**(10): 4041–4049.
60. Peng, S. L., J. Cappadona, J. F. Madison, M. P. Madaio, M. J. Owen, A. C. Hayday & J. Craft. 1996. Pathogenesis of autoimmunity in αβ T cell–deficient lupus-prone mice. Submitted.
61. Janeway, C. A., Jr., B. Jones & A. Hayday. 1988. Specificity and function of T cells bearing γδ receptors. Immunol. Today **9**(3): 73–76.

62. FERRICK, D. A., M. D. SCHRENZEL, T. MULVANIA, B. HSIEH, W. G. FERLIN & H. LEPPER. 1995. Differential production of interferon-γ and interleukin-4 in response to Th1- and Th2-stimulating pathogens by γδ T cells *in vivo*. Nature **373**(6511): 255–257.

63. FUJIHASHI, K., T. TAGUCHI, W. K. AICHER, J. R. MCGHEE, J. A. BLUESTONE, J. H. ELDRIDGE & H. KIYONO. 1992. Immunoregulatory functions for murine intraepithelial lymphocytes: γ/δ T cell receptor–positive (TCR^+) T cells abrogate oral tolerance, while α/β TCR^+ T cells provide B cell help. J. Exp. Med. **175**(3): 695–707.

64. MCMENAMIN, C., C. PIMM, M. MCKERSEY & P. G. HOLT. 1994. Regulation of IgE responses to inhaled antigen in mice by antigen-specific γδ T cells. Science **265**(5180): 1869–1871.

65. SUZUKI, T., K. HIROMATSU, Y. ANDO, T. OKAMOTO, Y. TOMODA & Y. YOSHIKAI. 1995. Regulatory role of γδ T cells in uterine intraepithelial lymphocytes in maternal antifetal immune response. J. Immunol. **154**(9): 4476–4484.

66. VAN VLASSELAER, P., H. GASCAN, R. DE WAAL MALEFYT & J. E. DE VRIES. 1992. IL-2 and a contact-mediated signal provided by $TCR\alpha\beta^+$ or $TCR\gamma\delta^+$ $CD4^+$ T cells induce polyclonal Ig production by committed human B cells: enhancement by IL-5; specific inhibition of IgA synthesis by IL-4. J. Immunol. **148**(6): 1674–1684.

67. WEN, L., S. J. ROBERTS, J. L. VINEY, F. S. WONG, C. MALLICK, R. C. FINDLY, Q. PENG, J. E. CRAFT, M. J. OWEN & A. C. HAYDAY. 1994. Immunoglobulin synthesis and generalized autoimmunity in mice congenitally deficient in αβ(+) T cells. Nature **369**(6482): 654–658.

68. HORNER, A. A., H. JABARA, N. RAMESH & R. S. GEHA. 1995. γ/δ T lymphocytes express CD40 ligand and induce isotype switching in B lymphocytes. J. Exp. Med. **181**(3): 1239–1244.

69. PETERMAN, G. M., C. SPENCER, A. I. SPERLING & J. A. BLUESTONE. 1993. Role of γδ T cells in murine collagen-induced arthritis. J. Immunol. **151**(11): 6546–6558.

70. MAEDA, T., I. SAIKAWA, T. HOTOKEBUCHI, Y. SUGIOKA, M. ETO, Y. MURAKAMI & K. NOMOTO. 1994. Exacerbation of established collagen-induced arthritis in mice treated with an anti–T cell receptor antibody. Arthritis Rheum. **37**(3): 406–413.

71. PELEGRÍ, C., P. KÜHNLEIN, E. BUCHNER, C. B. SCHMIDT, A. FRANCH, M. CASTELL, T. HÜNIG, F. EMMRICH & R. W. KINNE. 1996. Depletion of γ/δ T cells does not prevent or ameliorate, but rather aggravates, rat adjuvant arthritis. Arthritis Rheum. **39**(2): 204–215.

72. THURAU, S. R., P. KÜHNLEIN, T. HÜNIG & G. WILDNER. 1995. The role of gamma-delta T cells in induction and suppression of autoimmune uveitis (abstract). Immunobiology **194:** 157.

73. RAJAGOPALAN, S., T. ZORDAN, G. C. TSOKOS & S. K. DATTA. 1990. Pathogenic anti-DNA autoantibody-inducing T helper cell lines from patients with active lupus nephritis: isolation of $CD4^-8^-$ T helper cell lines that express the γδ T-cell antigen receptor. Proc. Natl. Acad. Sci. U.S.A. **87**(18): 7020–7024.

74. PENG, S. L., M. P. MADAIO, A. C. HAYDAY & J. CRAFT. 1996. Propagation and regulation of systemic autoimmunity by γδ T cells. J. Immunol. **157:** in press.

75. BUDD, R. C. & P. F. MIXTER. 1995. The origin of $CD4^-CD8^-TCR\alpha\beta^+$ thymocytes: a model based on T-cell receptor avidity. Immunol. Today **16**(9): 428–431.

76. BRAUN, M. Y., B. LOWIN, L. FRENCH, H. ACHA-ORBEA & J. TSCHOPP. 1996. Cytotoxic T cells deficient in both functional Fas ligand and perforin show residual cytolytic activity, yet lose their capacity to induce lethal acute graft-versus-host disease. J. Exp. Med. **183**(2): 657–661.

77. RENNO, T., M. HAHNE, J. TSCHOPP & H. R. MACDONALD. 1996. Peripheral T cells undergoing superantigen-induced apoptosis *in vivo* express B220 and upregulate Fas and Fas ligand. J. Exp. Med. **183**(2): 431–437.

78. MIZOGUCHI, A., E. MIZOGUCHI, C. CHIBA, G. M. SPIEKERMANN, S. TONEGAWA, C. NAGLER-ANDERSON & A. K. BHAN. 1996. Cytokine imbalance and autoantibody production in T cell receptor-α mutant mice with inflammatory bowel disease. J. Exp. Med. **183**(3): 847–856.

79. EICHELBERGER, M., A. MCMICKLE, M. BLACKMAN, P. MOMBAERTS, S. TONEGAWA & P. C. DOHERTY. 1995. Functional analysis of the TCR $\alpha^-\beta^+$ cells that accumulate in the pneumonic lung of influenza virus–infected TCR-$\alpha^{-/-}$ mice. J. Immunol. **154**(4): 1569–1576.

80. ASHANY, D., X. SONG, E. LACY, J. NIKOLIC-ZUGIC, S. M. FRIEDMAN & K. B. ELKON. 1995. Th1 CD4+ lymphocytes delete activated macrophages through the Fas/APO-1 antigen pathway. Proc. Natl. Acad. Sci. U.S.A. **92**(24): 11225–11229.

81. MICHAËLSSON, E., M. HOLMDAHL, A. ENGSTRÖM, H. BURKHARDT, A. SCHEYNIUS & R. HOLMDAHL. 1995. Macrophages, but not dendritic cells, present collagen to T cells. Eur. J. Immunol. **25**(8): 2234–2241.

82. TAKEDA, K. & G. DENNERT. 1993. The development of autoimmunity in C57BL/6 lpr mice correlates with the disappearance of natural killer type 1–positive cells: evidence for their suppressive action on bone marrow stem cell proliferation, B cell immunoglobulin secretion, and autoimmune symptoms. J. Exp. Med. **177**(1): 155–164.

83. KATZ, P., A. M. ZAYTOUN, J. H. LEE, JR., R. S. PANUSH & S. LONGLEY. 1982. Abnormal natural killer cell activity in systemic lupus erythematosus: an intrinsic defect in the lytic event. J. Immunol. **129**(5): 1966–1971.

84. STRANNEGÄRD, Ö., S. HERMODSSON & G. WESTBERG. 1982. Interferon and natural killer cells in systemic lupus erythematosus. Clin. Exp. Immunol. **50**(2): 246–252.

85. SIBBITT, W. L., JR., P. M. MATHEWS & A. D. BANKHURST. 1983. Natural killer cell in systemic lupus erythematosus: defects in effector lytic activity and response to interferon and interferon inducers. J. Clin. Invest. **71**(5): 1230–1239.

86. SNAPPER, C. M., H. YAMAGUCHI, M. A. MOORMAN, R. SNEED, D. SMOOT & J. J. MOND. 1993. Natural killer cells induce activated murine B cells to secrete Ig. J. Immunol. **151**(10): 5251–5260.

87. GRAY, J. D. & D. A. HORWITZ. 1995. Activated human NK cells can stimulate resting B cells to secrete immunoglobulin. J. Immunol. **154**(11): 5656–5664.

88. MICHAEL, A., J. J. HACKETT, M. BENNETT, V. KUMAR & D. YUAN. 1989. Regulation of B lymphocytes by natural killer cells: role of IFN-γ. J. Immunol. **142**(4): 1095–1101.

89. ABED, N. S., J. H. CHACE & J. S. COWDERY. 1994. T cell–independent and T cell–dependent B cell activation increases IFN-γR expression and renders B cells sensitive to IFN-γ-mediated inhibition. J. Immunol. **153:** 3369–3377.

90. WILDER, J. A., C. Y. KOH & D. YUAN. 1996. The role of NK cells during *in vivo* antigen-specific antibody responses. J. Immunol. **156**(1): 146–152.

91. ARASE, H., N. ARASE & T. SAITO. 1995. Fas-mediated cytotoxicity by freshly isolated natural killer cells. J. Exp. Med. **181**(3): 1235–1238.

92. RATHMELL, J. C., M. P. COOKE, W. Y. HO, J. GREIN, S. E. TOWNSEND, M. M. DAVIS & C. C. GOODNOW. 1995. CD95 (Fas)–dependent elimination of self-reactive B cells upon interaction with $CD4^+$ T cells. Nature **376**(6536): 181–184.

93. DAVIS, M. M. & Y. CHIEN. 1995. Issues concerning the nature of antigen recognition by αβ and γδ T-cell receptors. Immunol. Today **16**(7): 316–318.

94. MILETIC, V. D. & M. M. FRANK. 1995. Complement-immunoglobulin interactions. Curr. Opin. Immunol. **7:** 41–47.

95. MOSMANN, T. R. & S. SAD. 1996. The expanding universe of T-cell subsets: Th1, Th2, and more. Immunol. Today **17**(3): 138–146.

96. STOCKINGER, B., T. ZAL & D. GRAY. 1996. B cells solicit their own help from T cells. J. Exp. Med. **183**(3): 891–899.

Initiation of Autoimmunity to Self-proteins Complexed with Viral Antigens[a]

WESTLEY H. REEVES, XINGWEN DONG, JINGSONG WANG, AND KIMBERLY HAMILTON

Departments of Medicine and Microbiology/Immunology
Thurston Arthritis Research Center
and
UNC Lineberger Comprehensive Cancer Center
University of North Carolina
Chapel Hill, North Carolina 27599-7280

AUTOANTIBODY PRODUCTION CHARACTERIZES SYSTEMIC LUPUS ERYTHEMATOSUS (SLE)

SLE is a systemic autoimmune disease characterized serologically by the production of antinuclear antibodies.[1] The antigens recognized by these autoantibodies are primarily components of multicomponent particles, such as small nuclear ribonucleoproteins, nucleosomes, RNA polymerases, and ribosomes. Specific autoantibodies in SLE are thought to be produced mainly by conventional B cells requiring T cell help,[2] although the production of low-affinity, polyreactive autoantibodies by the B1 subset also has been reported.[3] The mechanisms of autoantibody production in SLE remain incompletely understood, but abnormalities in maintaining immune tolerance or unresponsiveness may play a central role. The predominance of autoantibodies along with their T cell dependence suggests that autoreactive T as well as B cells may contribute to the disease. Several mechanisms are responsible for immunological unresponsiveness to self-antigens. Autoreactive cells may be deleted (clonal elimination) or rendered anergic (clonal anergy). Alternatively, they may ignore self-antigens.

B AND T CELL TOLERANCE

Autoreactive B cells are subject to both elimination and functional silencing (anergy) at several stages in their development.[4,5] For this reason, it may be more accurate to regard B cell tolerance as a series of checkpoints along the differentiation pathway rather than simply deletion versus anergy.[5] Because autoreactive B cells are continuously generated by hypermutation in secondary lymphoid organs after formation of the preimmune repertoire, these also must be eliminated or silenced. In part,

[a]This work was supported by Grant Nos. P50-AR42573 and R01-AR40391 from the United States Public Health Service and by grants from the Arthritis Foundation.

this occurs because the binding of a hapten to B cell surface immunoglobulin in the absence of a second signal delivered by T cells causes anergy or deletion.[6,7] This is likely to explain the observation that regions of amino acid sequence difference between an immunizing antigen and the host organism's corresponding protein are antigenic, whereas shared determinants generally are not[8,9] (FIGURE 1B). In this view, the provision of T cell help is a critical determinant of whether an autoreactive B cell is

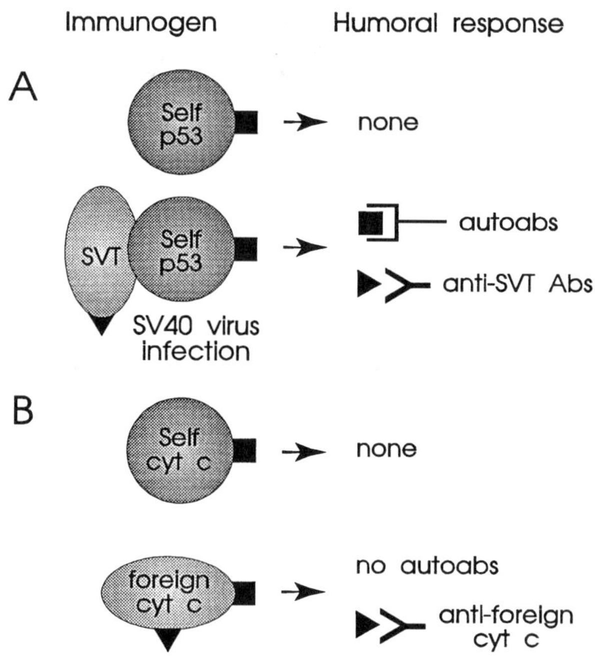

FIGURE 1. B cell tolerance in two models. (A) Although rodent B cells are normally tolerant to p53, autoantibodies to epitopes of self-p53 (square) are produced along with anti-SVT antibodies when mice or hamsters are infected with SV40. It has been proposed that these autoantibodies are the result of a hapten-carrier-like mechanism, in which self-p53 is the hapten and SVT acts as a carrier. (B) Immunization with foreign cytochrome c (cyt c) may be analogous to the situation in panel A. Rabbits are tolerant of their own cytochrome c. When immunized with foreign cytochrome c, they produce antibodies specific for epitopes of the foreign antigen that are not shared with self (triangle). Antibodies to epitopes of self–cytochrome c (square) are not produced, even though linked to an immunogenic carrier (foreign cytochrome c).

activated or tolerized.[7] Other factors, such as antigen valency, concentration, or affinity, also may play an important role.[10] Triggering of B cell tolerance requires a certain threshold of antigen concentration and receptor affinity.[11] B cells appear to ignore self-antigens present at concentrations below this threshold and therefore are neither tolerized nor activated. Such B cells potentially can be activated if exposed to higher levels of the antigen along with antigen-specific T cell help.

Deletion, anergy, and ignorance also contribute to T cell unresponsiveness to self. In animal lupus models, there is little evidence for a global abnormality in thymic deletion of autoreactive T cells,[12] making it more likely that autoimmunity results from the escape of autoreactive cells from a state of anergy or indifference. As is true of B cells, T cell antigen receptor occupancy is insufficient for activation, and clonal expansion requires a second costimulatory signal delivered by antigen-presenting cells (APCs).[13] In the absence of a second signal, T cell receptor occupancy can result in anergy or death. Naive T cells appear to require that the costimulatory signal be provided by professional APCs (dendritic cells), whereas memory T cells can receive this signal from B cells.[14] Viewed this way, the activation of naive T cells may depend on the relative likelihood that an antigen is presented by professional APCs (e.g., dendritic cells) versus nonprofessional APCs (e.g., B cells). T cells that recognize a self-antigen may be more likely to see it on the surface of a nonprofessional APC, whereas T cells recognizing a foreign antigen may be more likely to see it on a dendritic cell.[7,15]

Ignorance is an additional mechanism of T cell unresponsiveness. Some self-proteins are encountered by the immune system at levels too low to trigger either T cell activation or tolerance. This may reflect either their low abundance or sequestration in "immunologically privileged sites."[16] Like B cells exposed to levels of antigen below the triggering threshold, T cells recognizing such antigens are neither activated nor deleted or rendered anergic, and they remain in a state of immunological ignorance.[17]

The presence of ignorant autoreactive T cells has important implications for the pathogenesis of autoimmunity. The expressed T cell repertoire is controlled, in part, by MHC-linked genes through a determinant selection mechanism in which immunodominant peptides bind to MHC molecules that can present the peptide, but not to MHC molecules that do not present the peptide.[18,19] As a consequence, T cell responses to an exogenous antigen are focused onto a limited number of major T cell inducing determinants rather than being broadly directed against all portions of the antigen.[18] Similarly, tolerance is focused onto a limited number of dominant epitopes,[20] and T cells responsive to self-peptides that are presented at low levels (due to inefficient processing or poor binding to MHC molecules) remain ignorant. Hindering structures on naturally processed fragments that differentially affect presentation by different MHC molecules can have important effects on T cell repertoire selection.[18] These include structural constraints imposed by the tertiary structure of a protein and intermolecular contacts between subunits of an oligomeric antigen.[21,22] For example, recognition of the human chorionic gonadotropin (hCG) α/β dimer by α-specific T cell hybridomas is dramatically reduced compared to free hCG α or heat-dissociated dimers, suggesting that the quaternary structure of hCG affects presentation of antigenic determinants of the monomers by interfering with degradation into peptides capable of binding MHC molecules. The effects of hindering structures can be overcome by artificially processing a self-antigen with cyanogen bromide, resulting in the activation of autoreactive T cells specific for "cryptic" epitopes of self.[23] We have obtained evidence that protein-protein interactions between a self-protein (p53) and a foreign antigen (SV40 large T antigen, SVT) may enhance the processing of cryptic p53 peptides, leading to the activation of autoreactive "ignorant" T cells.[24] This results in the production of autoantibodies against the nuclear protein, p53. Unlike artificial processing with cyanogen bromide, complexes of p53 and SVT are generated naturally in the context of SV40 virus infection.

AUTOIMMUNITY TO p53 IN RODENTS WITH SV40-INDUCED TUMORS

Our work on p53 was prompted by the observations of two groups that autoantibodies to the p53 tumor suppressor protein are present in sera from hamsters or mice bearing SV40-induced tumors or infected with SV40 (TABLE 1).[25,26] In addition to anti-SVT antibodies, these sera contained antibodies recognizing a 53-kDa cellular protein that formed a complex with SVT in SV40-transformed cells. The p53 protein was found later to be tumor suppressor protein.[27] Binding of SVT inactivates the tumor suppressor function of p53[28] and, at the same time, markedly increases its half-life.[29,30] Thus, 3T3 cells have 20- to 50-fold lower levels of p53 than SV40-transformed or SV40-infected 3T3 cells. The central portion of p53 (amino acids 94–293) mediates its interaction with SVT (FIGURE 2).[27,31,32] Tumor-promoting mutations are focused within five conserved regions of p53, four of which are located within the SVT binding domain.[27] Other viral antigens, including the adenovirus E1B 55K protein[33] and the human papillomavirus (HPV) E6 protein,[34] also interact with p53 (FIGURE 2). However, unlike SVT, the HPV E6 protein increases the rate of p53 degradation and it is virtually undetectable in HPV-infected cells.[34]

The presence of anti-p53 antibodies in sera from tumor-bearing mice originally was thought to be a consequence of a "hapten-carrier" mechanism, in which p53 was analogous to a hapten and SVT to the carrier (FIGURE 1A).[25,26] Similarly, although transgenic mice expressing the membrane-associated glycoprotein of vesicular stomatitis virus (VSV-G) are tolerant to this "self"-antigen, autoantibodies are induced when the mice are infected with wild-type VSV.[35] Thus, it has been suggested that T cells specific for other components of the VSV virion may provide help to VSV-G-specific B cells, resulting in autoantibody production.

There are difficulties with that model, however. Immunization of experimental animals with the homologue of a self-antigen results in the production of antibodies specific for antigenic determinants unique to the immunizing antigen (FIGURE 1B).[8,9] Thus, a rabbit immunized with foreign cytochrome c develops primarily antibodies recognizing epitopes that differ between rabbit cytochrome c and the immunogen.[9]

TABLE 1. Induction of Autoantibodies to p53 Tumor Suppressor Protein by SV40 Virus in Rodents

Species	How Immunized	Reference
mouse	transfer of SV40-transformed SVT2 cells	25, 26
hamster	transfer of SV40-transformed SVT5 C12 cells	25
hamster	injected with 10^8 PFU of SV40 strain 776	26

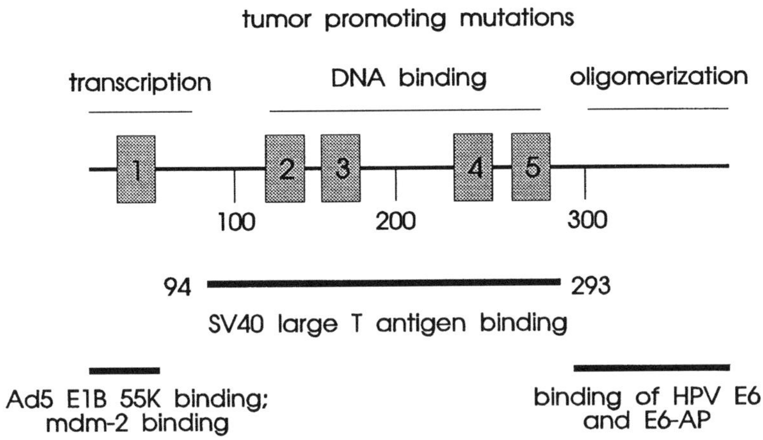

FIGURE 2. Interactions of p53 with viral antigens. Diagram of the primary structure of p53 (top) indicating functional domains mediating transcriptional activation, DNA binding, and oligomerization. Shaded boxes indicate the locations of five highly conserved regions in which mutations associated with human tumors are clustered. Regions of the protein involved in interactions with viral-transforming proteins are shown below, including the central domain implicated in binding of SVT (amino acids 94–293), as well as C-terminal and N-terminal domains that bind adenovirus E1B 55K protein and the human papillomavirus E6/E6-associated protein, respectively.

Autoantibodies are not produced. The same general principle underlies the ability to generate antisera specific for allogeneic MHC molecules.[7] Viewed this way, it is unclear why autoantibodies to p53 should be generated in mice immunized with p53/SVT complexes because B cell tolerance mechanisms might be expected to inactivate the p53-responsive B cells. One possibility was that SV40-transformed tumor cells were providing a costimulatory signal that interfered with B cell tolerance. A second possibility was that the autoantibodies actually recognized somatically mutated p53,[36] although this has not been confirmed in other systems.[37] Finally, it was possible that SVT binding altered the conformation of mouse p53 so that it was seen by both B and T cells as foreign. We have investigated these possibilities by immunizing BALB/c mice with recombinant mouse p53 bound to SVT.

INDUCTION OF ANTI-p53 AUTOANTIBODIES BY RECOMBINANT p53/SVT COMPLEXES EXPRESSED IN A BACULOVIRUS SYSTEM

To exclude the possibility that the tumor cells were providing a second signal required for the production of anti-p53 autoantibodies, mouse p53, SVT, and p53/SVT complexes were expressed in Sf-9 insect cells using the recombinant baculoviruses vEV55p53 and vEV55SVT.[38] The antigens were affinity-purified on protein A–Sepharose CL-4B beads coated with murine monoclonal antibodies specific for either p53 (PAb 122) or SVT (PAb 101) as illustrated in FIGURE 3. In our standard immunization

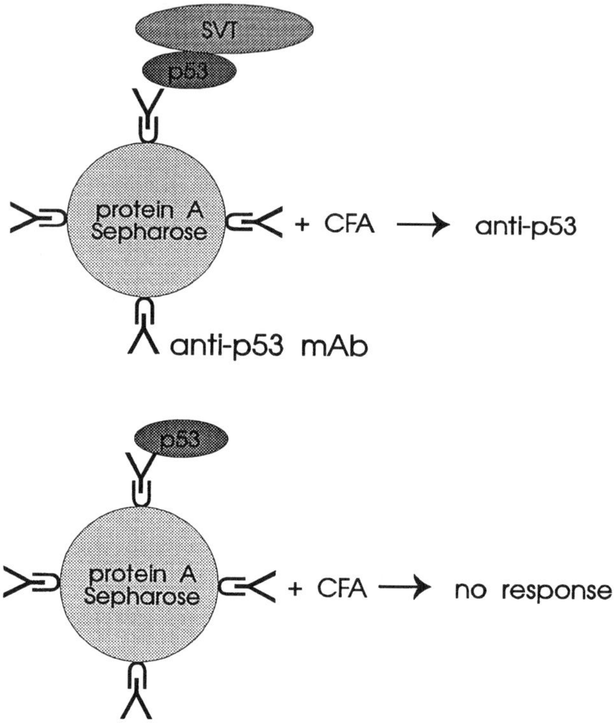

FIGURE 3. Diagram of p53 and SVT immunogens. Murine p53 and SVT were expressed in Sf-9 insect cells using recombinant baculoviruses vEV55p53 and vEV55SVT, respectively, and were purified onto monoclonal antibody–coated protein A–Sepharose CL-4B beads as illustrated. The diagram shows the use of PAb 122 (anti-p53) to affinity-purify recombinant mouse p53, or p53/SVT complexes, which can be assembled either *in vivo* in doubly infected Sf-9 cells or *in vitro* on p53-coated beads incubated with extract from Sf-9 cells infected with vEV55SVT. Similarly, SVT or p53/SVT complexes can be affinity-purified onto beads coated with PAb 101 (anti-SVT). Beads carrying p53, SVT, or p53/SVT antigens are washed extensively with PBS, emulsified in complete (or incomplete) Freund's adjuvant, and injected. Mice are immunized with beads carrying 1 μg of p53 in the form of either free p53 (bottom) or p53/SVT complexes (top).

protocol, BALB/c mice are injected with 1 μg of mouse p53, either by itself or in the form of p53/SVT complexes, on protein A–Sepharose beads. The first dose of antigen is emulsified in complete Freund's adjuvant, followed by two subsequent immunizations with the same antigen in incomplete adjuvant.[24]

Complexes of p53 and SVT affinity-purified on PAb 122 (anti-p53) and complexes purified on PAb 101 (anti-SVT) were both immunogenic (FIGURE 4). BALB/c mice immunized three times with p53/SVT complexes that were affinity-purified on PAb 101–protein A–Sepharose beads developed anti-p53 antibodies that efficiently immunoprecipitated mouse p53 from extracts of Sf-9 cells infected with vEV55p53 (FIGURE 4, top panel, right) as well as anti-SVT antibodies (bottom panel, right). Autoantibodies to p53 were not produced by mice immunized with SVT alone, although these mice produced high levels of anti-SVT antibodies (FIGURE 4, right). Similarly, mice immunized with p53/SVT complexes that were affinity-purified on PAb 122 beads developed autoantibodies to p53 as well as anti-SVT antibodies (FIGURE 4, left). In contrast, mice immunized with p53 alone developed neither anti-p53 nor anti-SVT antibodies (FIGURE 4, left).[24] These data indicate that immunization of mice with

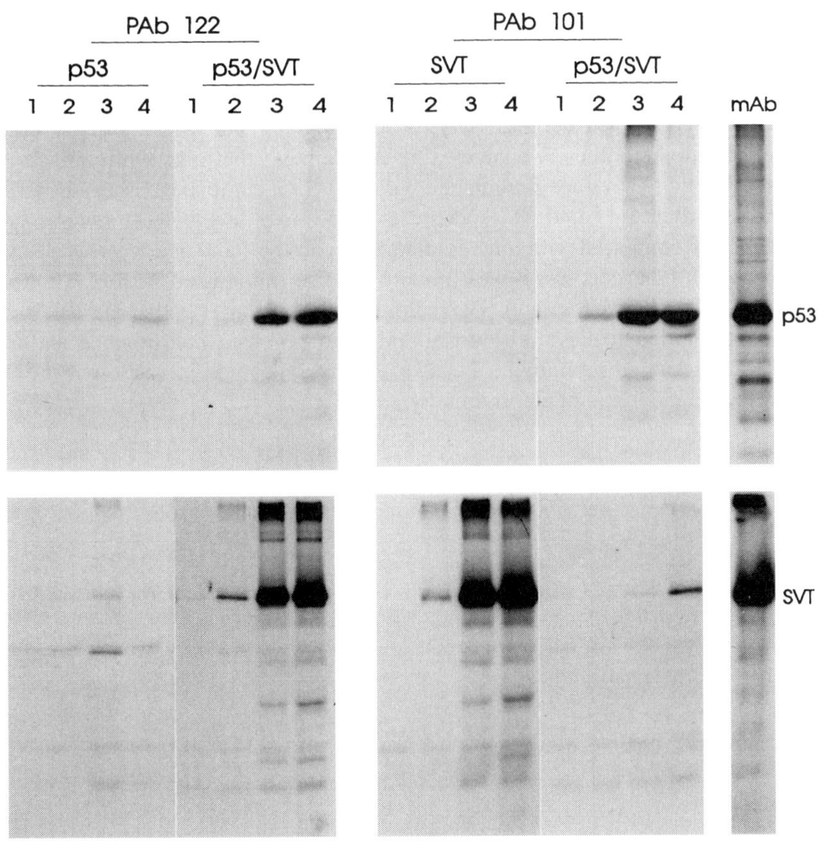

FIGURE 4. Immunoprecipitation of p53 and SVT using sera from mice immunized with p53/SVT, p53, or SVT. (Left) Serial sera from representative BALB/c mice immunized three times at 2-week intervals with 1 μg of p53 alone or with 1 μg of p53 bound to SVT and attached to PAb 122–coated protein A–Sepharose beads were tested for immunoprecipitation of radiolabeled extracts from Sf-9 cells infected with vEV55p53 (top panel) or vEV55SVT (bottom panel).[24] Lane 1, preimmune serum; lanes 2–4, sera obtained 2 weeks after immunizations at days 0, 14, and 28, respectively. (Right) Serial sera from mice immunized three times with 1 μg of SVT alone or with 1 μg of SVT bound to p53 and attached to PAb 101–coated protein A–Sepharose beads were tested for immunoprecipitation of radiolabeled extracts from Sf-9 cells infected with vEV55p53 (top panel) or vEV55SVT (bottom panel).[24] Lane 1, preimmune serum; lanes 2–4, sera obtained 2 weeks after immunizations at days 0, 14, and 28, respectively.

mouse p53 complexes with SVT can induce humoral autoimmunity to p53, suggesting that *in vivo* infection with SV40 is not required for the induction of autoimmunity. Also, the induction of autoimmunity by recombinant wild-type mouse p53 suggests that somatic mutation of the self-antigen was not a major factor. Finally, the data suggest that the anti-p53 antibodies were not a population of anti-SVT antibodies that recognized a cross-reactive epitope of p53, an interpretation that also is supported by Western blot analysis using affinity-purified anti-p53 and anti-SVT antibodies.[24]

ROLE OF ADJUVANT AND PHYSICAL ASSOCIATION BETWEEN p53 AND SVT

Adjuvant appears to be unnecessary for inducing autoantibodies to p53, although the level of autoantibodies is enhanced by immunizing the mice with antigen plus adjuvant (FIGURE 5). In mice immunized with p53/SVT complexes on beads without adjuvant, the total IgG and the specific anti-p53 IgG levels were both reduced proportionately compared with mice immunized with the same antigen plus adjuvant (not shown). In other studies, it was found that mice immunized with p53 (affinity-purified on PAb 122 beads) and SVT (affinity-purified on PAb 101 beads) in two separate sites failed to develop autoantibodies to p53, but did produce anti-SVT antibodies (X. Dong, submitted). Thus, a direct association of p53 with SVT is required for the induction of autoimmunity.

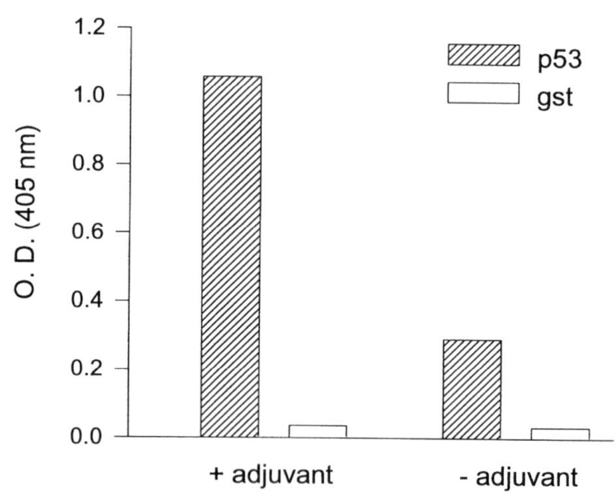

FIGURE 5. Adjuvant is not necessary for induction of autoantibodies to p53. Mice were immunized three times with p53/SVT complexes that were affinity-purified on PAb 122–coated protein A–Sepharose beads. One group received affinity-purified antigen plus complete Freund's adjuvant (first immunization) or incomplete adjuvant (second and third immunizations). The other group received the same antigen in PBS. Anti-p53 antibodies were measured by ELISA using a gst-p53 fusion protein as antigen. Hatched bars: reactivity of serum (1:500 dilution) with gst-p53-coated wells; open bars: reactivity with gst-coated wells.

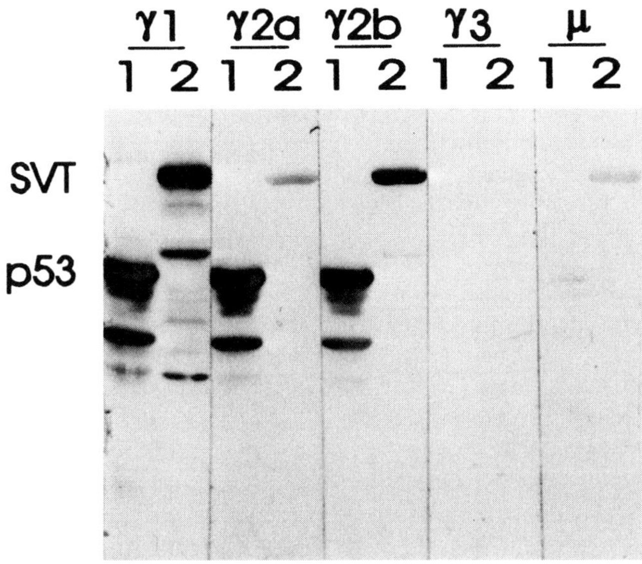

FIGURE 6. Isotypes of anti-p53 and anti-SVT antibodies. Immunoblot analysis of serum (1:500 dilution) from representative BALB/c mice immunized three times with p53/SVT complexes (1 μg of p53 bound to SVT on PAb 101–coated beads). Lane 1: reactivity with mouse p53 (from vEV55p53-infected Sf-9 cells); lane 2: reactivity with SVT (from vEV55SVT-infected Sf-9 cells). Blots were probed with isotype-specific goat anti-mouse immunoglobulin antibodies at a 1:1000 dilution. Positions of SVT and p53 are indicated on the left.

HUMORAL RESPONSE TO SELF-p53

Titers of the anti-p53 autoantibodies induced by immunizing with p53/SVT complexes were as high as 1:25,000. Both IgG and IgM autoantibodies were present. Immunoblot analysis using mouse p53 and SVT from extracts of Sf-9 cells infected with vEV55p53 or vEV55SVT, respectively, is shown in FIGURE 6. In all mice tested, the predominant isotype of anti-p53 as well as anti-SVT antibodies was IgG1. In most mice, lower levels of IgG2a and IgG2b anti-p53 and/or anti-SVT antibodies were also detected. Because IgG1, IgG2a, and IgG2b are generally considered to be "T cell–dependent" subclasses, these data suggested that either SVT- or p53-responsive T cells were involved in autoantibody production.

ROLE OF AUTOREACTIVE T CELLS IN AUTOANTIBODY PRODUCTION

To further evaluate whether T cells specific for SVT were providing help to B cells producing autoantibodies to p53, BALB/c mice that were primed previously with p53/SVT complexes were immunized with p53 alone. Unexpectedly, the titer of anti-p53 autoantibodies increased, whereas the level of anti-SVT antibodies remained nearly constant,[24] suggesting that autoreactive T cells responsive to murine p53 were generated by immunizing mice with p53/SVT complexes. More recently, we have found that spleen and lymph node T cells isolated from mice immunized once with p53/SVT complexes exhibited a proliferative response to mouse p53 *in vitro* (X. Dong *et al.*, submitted). Priming BALB/c mice with SVT did not enhance anti-p53 autoantibody production when the mice were challenged subsequently with p53/SVT complexes, despite the fact that these mice displayed a strong *in vitro* proliferative response to SVT. T cell proliferation *in vitro* to mouse p53 was directed primarily against the carboxyl-terminal two-thirds of the protein and was inhibited strongly by anti-CD4 antibodies as well as anti-I-A and anti-I-E antibodies. In contrast, anti-CD8 antibodies had no effect on *in vitro* T cell proliferation. Moreover, autoantibodies to p53 were not generated in C57BL/6 CD4 (−/−) mice immunized with p53/SVT complexes, but could be induced in control C57BL/6 mice (X. Dong *et al.*, submitted). These data suggest that autoreactive, p53-responsive, helper T cells participate in the production of autoantibodies to p53.

A MODEL FOR THE ACTIVATION OF AUTOREACTIVE T AND B CELLS IN MICE IMMUNIZED WITH p53/SVT COMPLEXES

The experiments described above suggest that the "hapten-carrier" model proposed initially is unlikely to explain the production of autoantibodies to p53 in mice immunized with complexes or recombinant mouse p53 and SVT. Once tolerance is broken with p53/SVT complexes, autoantibody production can be boosted with mouse p53 alone. In addition, autoreactive T cells responsive to mouse p53 *in vitro* are activated. Finally, priming with SVT had little effect on the subsequent autoantibody response to p53 upon challenging with p53/SVT complexes. Taken together, the data strongly suggest that the activation of SVT-responsive T cells is not critical for inducing autoimmunity to p53. The same is likely to be true of autoantibody production to p53 in mice or hamsters with SV40-induced tumors (TABLE 1).

To understand the induction of autoimmunity to p53, it will be necessary to explain the activation of autoreactive B as well as T cells. Our data are consistent with the following working model for the activation of p53-responsive T cells in mice immunized with p53/SVT complexes. The binding of SVT to p53 causes significant alterations in the p53 protein's conformation, reflected in altered recognition by monoclonal antibodies[39] and a greatly reduced susceptibility to intracellular degradation.[29,30] The binding of SVT is likely to serve as a hindering structure that alters the pattern of processing of p53 after the complex is taken up by APCs. Altering the quaternary and/or tertiary structure of p53 as a consequence of its interaction with SVT may change the pattern of antigen processing in a manner analogous to that seen in studies of the hCG α/β dimer.[22] This could enhance the presentation of minor T cell epitopes by professional antigen-presenting cells (FIGURE 7). In the absence of SVT binding, these minor peptides may be generated at levels below the threshold required for T cell activation or tolerization. Ignorant T cells specific for such minor epitopes could be activated if the threshold level is reached due to formation of p53/SVT complexes. Unlike the artificial processing necessary to activate T cells specific for cryptic epitopes of lysozyme,[23] this is an example of "naturally" altered antigen processing of a self-protein during a viral infection. A population of activated CD4+ p53-responsive T cells may then activate autoreactive B cells producing anti-p53 autoantibodies.

Because tolerance also occurs in the B cell compartment, the question is raised whether p53-reactive B cells escape from a state of anergy or are in an ignorant state from which they can be activated if provided with appropriate T cell signals. As

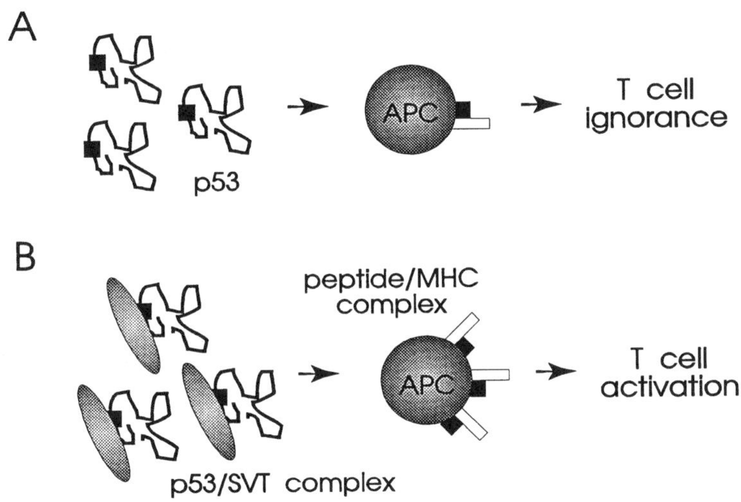

FIGURE 7. A model for the activation of autoreactive T cells by p53/SVT complexes. (A) A minor epitope of self-p53 (black square) is presented inefficiently by APCs. This may reflect degradation by endosomal proteases or other mechanisms. The level of peptide associated on the surface of the APC with class II MHC (open rectangle) does not reach the threshold necessary to induce either T cell activation or tolerance. Consequently, T cells ignore it. (B) Binding of SVT to self-p53 enhances the processing of the minor T cell epitope (black square) by APCs. The level of peptide associated with class II MHC on the surface of the APC reaches the threshold needed to cause T cell activation. Because T cells responsive to the peptide-MHC complex have not previously been tolerized (due to previous failure to reach the threshold level), they now can be activated.

discussed above, an effective antigen threshold (a function of concentration, valency, and affinity for surface Ig receptors) may be required to inactivate autoreactive B cells.[5] B cells carrying surface Ig receptors specific for an epitope unique to a minor conformational state of self-p53 may not be inactivated (FIGURE 8). The conformation of a protein is flexible, and localized areas of its surface can undergo reversible fluctuations in shape,[8] generating potential B cell epitopes. Depending on the equilibrium between different conformational states, B cells carrying surface Ig receptors for these potential epitopes may or may not be tolerized.

We suggest that the binding of SVT may freeze p53 in a minor conformational state, as indicated by reactivity with monoclonal antibody PAb 246.[39] B cells specific for these minor epitopes could be activated if appropriate T cell help is provided. There is considerable evidence that the binding of an antibody can also trap antigen in a minor conformational state.[8] The activation of B cells could have further conse-

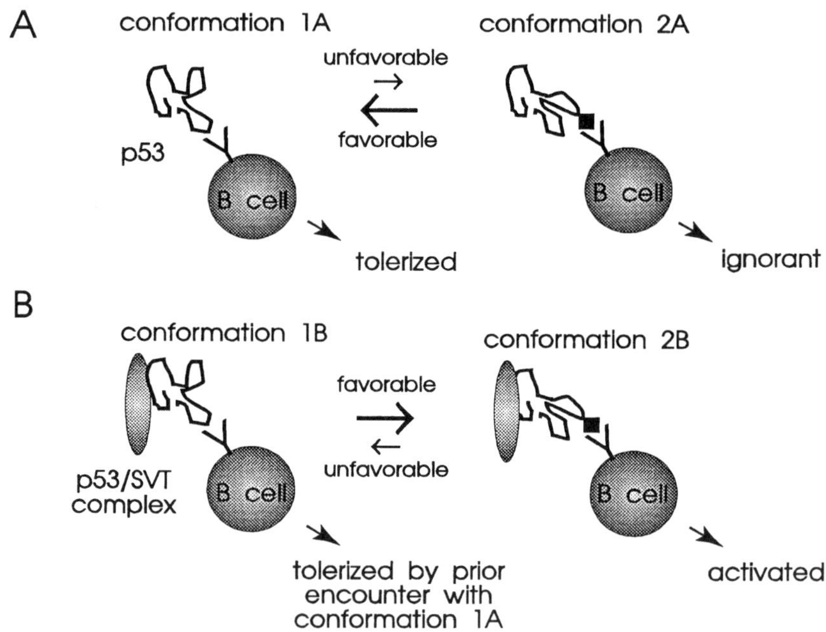

FIGURE 8. A model for the activation of autoreactive B cells by p53/SVT complexes. (A) Two conformational states of self-p53 are depicted, one energetically favorable and the other unfavorable. B cells with high-affinity surface Ig receptors capable of recognizing the abundant conformation 1 are tolerized, whereas those capable of recognizing conformation 2 remain ignorant due to its low abundance. (B) Binding of SVT to p53 alters the equilibrium between conformations 1 and 2 by stabilizing conformation 2. B cells with high-affinity surface Ig receptors capable of recognizing conformation 1 remain tolerized because they have encountered form 1A previously at a level that induces unresponsiveness or deletion. In contrast, B cells capable of recognizing conformation 2 have not been tolerized because of the low abundance of form 2A. They can be activated by p53-responsive T cells after exposure to the higher levels of form 2A, which is stabilized by the binding of SVT. Autoantibodies specific for this conformational state can be detected because, although they recognize only a small fraction of the total p53 (conformation 2A), they stabilize that state, driving the equilibrium to the right.

quences for the development of autoimmunity. By focusing antigen on their surface Ig receptors, activated B cells can present antigen up to 10,000-fold more efficiently than macrophages,[40] greatly enhancing the presentation of minor T cell epitopes. Thus, although p53/SVT complexes may be required to reach the threshold necessary for a primary T cell response, the ability to boost autoantibody production using mouse p53 alone[24] might be explained by the more-efficient generation of this minor T cell epitope by activated autoreactive B cells. In other words, the dose of self-p53 needed to boost secondary T cell responses to a minor epitope may be considerably lower than that needed to trigger the primary response, as suggested previously.[41]

This model could explain other poorly understood features of autoantibodies in systemic autoimmune diseases. It has been noted previously that the specificities of autoantibodies in SLE are highly restricted[42] and that autoantibodies in SLE tend to recognize functional or active sites.[43] In addition, autoantibodies developing spontaneously in lupus exhibit different specificities than polyclonal antisera raised against the same protein in rabbits.[43] Finally, the common existence of autoantibodies that stabilize the conformation of self-antigens, including the Ku-DNA-PK_{cs} complex[44] and the U1 snRNP (M. Satoh *et al.*, submitted), has been described. Stabilizing autoantibodies recognizing a minor conformational state of a self-antigen could trap the protein in that state,[8] driving the equilibrium toward that conformation (FIGURE 8). Thus, certain autoantibodies may play a role in perpetuating autoimmunity by increasing the effective concentration of minor forms of a self-antigen.

Autoantibodies that stabilize a minor conformation of a self-antigen also may be involved in the recruitment of additional autoreactive T cell populations. Induction of new autoantibodies to the snRNP/Sm antigens by immunizing MRL mice with anti-Sm-D monoclonal antibodies could be an example of this phenomenon.[45,46] Autoantibody induction does not appear to be due to an idiotype–anti-idiotype mechanism, nor does it appear to operate by enhancing Fc-mediated uptake of antigen-antibody complexes.[46] The binding of anti-Sm-D antibodies to snRNPs could trigger autoantibody production in a manner analogous to the binding of SVT to p53.

IMPLICATIONS FOR THE VIRAL INDUCTION OF AUTOIMMUNITY

There is considerable evidence that viral infections can induce autoimmunity.[47–49] In reovirus infection, autoimmunity appears to target only those tissues in which the virus actually multiplies,[49] suggesting that close proximity of the virus and specific autoantigens is a critical factor.

There are several models for the role of viral infection in triggering autoimmunity. Immunological cross-reactivity of a viral antigen with a self-antigen can lead to the production of a population of antiviral antibodies cross-reacting with autoantigens.[50] There is also evidence that virally induced ectopic production of certain cytokines or MHC antigens can trigger autoimmunity.[51] The induction of antigen-specific autoimmunity as a consequence of the binding of a viral antigen to a self-protein represents a novel pathway for the viral induction of autoimmunity. In this model, autoimmunity may be triggered as a "hit-and-run" event because transient exposure to the self-nonself complex induces a long-lived immune response directed against the self component that appears to be maintained independently of continued exposure to the foreign antigen. Although it is not yet clear whether this mechanism is responsible for the restricted specificities of autoantibodies in lupus, further investigation of the importance of this pathway in systemic autoimmune disease seems warranted.

ACKNOWLEDGMENTS

We thank L. K. Miller (University of Georgia) for providing the baculovirus vectors, vEV55p53 and vEV55SVT, and D. Benjamin (University of Virginia) for helpful discussions.

REFERENCES

1. TAN, E. M. 1989. Antinuclear antibodies: diagnostic markers for autoimmune diseases and probes for cell biology. Adv. Immunol. **44:** 93–151.
2. SOBEL, E. S., V. N. KAKKANAIAH, M. KAKKANAIAH, R. L. CHEEK, P. L. COHEN & R. A. EISENBERG. 1994. T-B collaboration for autoantibody production in lpr mice is cognate and MHC-restricted. J. Immunol. **152:** 6011–6016.
3. CASALI, P., S. E. BURASTERO, J. E. BALOW & A. L. NOTKINS. 1989. High-affinity antibodies to ssDNA are produced by CD-5 cells in systemic lupus erythematosus patients. J. Immunol. **143:** 3476–3483.
4. NOSSAL, G. J. 1994. Negative selection of lymphocytes. Cell **76:** 229–239.
5. GOODNOW, C. C., J. G. CYSTER, S. B. HARTLEY, S. E. BELL, M. P. COOKE, J. I. HEALY, S. AKKARAJU, J. C. RATHMELL, S. L. POGUE & K. P. SHOKAT. 1995. Self-tolerance checkpoints in B lymphocyte development. Adv. Immunol. **59:** 279–368.
6. LINTON, P. J., A. RUDIE & N. R. KLINMAN. 1991. Tolerance susceptibility of newly generated memory B cells. J. Immunol. **146:** 4099–4104.
7. MATZINGER, P. 1994. Tolerance, danger, and the extended family. Annu. Rev. Immunol. **12:** 991–1045.
8. CRUMPTON, M. J. 1974. Protein antigens: the molecular bases of antigenicity and immunogenicity. *In* The Antigens. Volume 2. M. Sela, Ed.: 1–72. Academic Press. New York.
9. JEMMERSON, R. & E. MARGOLIASH. 1979. Topographic antigenic determinants on cytochrome c: immunoadsorbent separation of the rabbit antibody populations directed against horse cytochrome c. J. Biol. Chem. **254:** 12706–12716.
10. DINTZIS, R. J., M. OKAJIMA, M. H. MIDDLETON, G. GREENE & H. M. DINTZIS. 1989. The immunogenicity of soluble haptenated polymers is determined by molecular mass and hapten valence. J. Immunol. **143:** 1239–1244.
11. DRESSER, D. W. & N. A. MITCHISON. 1968. The mechanism of immunological paralysis. Adv. Immunol. **8:** 129–181.
12. KOTZIN, B. L., S. K. BABCOCK & L. R. HERRON. 1988. Deletion of potentially self-reactive T cell receptor specificities in L3T4$^-$, Lyt-2$^-$ T cells of *lpr* mice. J. Exp. Med. **168:** 2221–2229.
13. LINSLEY, P. S., W. BRADY, L. GROSMAIRE, A. ARUFFO, N. K. DAMLE & J. A. LEDBETTER. 1991. Binding of the B cell activation antigen B7 to CD28 costimulates T cell proliferation and interleukin-2 mRNA accumulation. J. Exp. Med. **173:** 721–730.
14. FUCHS, E. J. & P. MATZINGER. 1992. B cells turn off virgin, but not memory T cells. Science **258:** 1156–1159.
15. JANEWAY, C. A., JR. & K. BOTTOMLY. 1994. Signals and signs for lymphocyte responses. Cell **76:** 275–285.
16. ANDO, K., L. G. GUIDOTTI, A. CERNY, T. ISHIKAWA & F. V. CHISARI. 1994. CTL access to tissue antigen is restricted *in vivo*. J. Immunol. **153:** 482–488.
17. MURAKAMI, M., T. TSUBATA, M. OKAMOTO, A. SHIMIZU, S. KUMAGAI, H. IMURA & T. HONJO. 1992. Antigen-induced apoptotic death of Ly-1 B cells responsible for autoimmune disease in transgenic mice. Nature **357:** 77–80.
18. BRETT, S. J., K. B. CEASE & J. A. BERZOFSKY. 1988. Influences of antigen processing on the expression of the T cell repertoire: evidence for MHC-specific hindering structures on the products of processing. J. Exp. Med. **168:** 357–373.
19. BUUS, S., A. SETTE, S. M. COLON, C. MILES & H. M. GREY. 1987. The relation between major histocompatibility complex (MHC) restriction and the capacity of Ia to bind immunogenic peptides. Science **235:** 1353–1358.

20. CIBOTTI, R., J. M. KANELLOPOULOS, J. P. CABANIOLS, O. HALLE-PANENKO, K. KOSMATOPOULOS, E. SERCARZ & P. KOURILSKY. 1992. Tolerance to a self protein involves its immunodominant, but does not involve its subdominant determinants. Proc. Natl. Acad. Sci. U.S.A. **89:** 416–420.
21. ATASSI, M. Z., M. YOSHIOKA & G. S. BIXLER. 1989. T cells specific for alpha-beta interface regions of hemoglobin recognize the isolated subunit, but not the tetramer, and indicate presentation without processing. Proc. Natl. Acad. Sci. U.S.A. **86:** 6729–6733.
22. ROUAS, N., S. CHRISTOPHE, F. HOUSSEAU, D. BELLET, J. G. GUILLET & J. M. BIDART. 1993. Influence of protein-quaternary structure on antigen processing. J. Immunol. **150:** 782–792.
23. OKI, A. & E. SERCARZ. 1985. T cell tolerance studied at the level of antigenic determinants. I. Latent reactivity to lysozyme peptides that lack suppressogenic epitopes can be revealed in lysozyme-tolerant mice. J. Exp. Med. **161:** 897–911.
24. DONG, X., K. J. HAMILTON, M. SATOH, J. WANG & W. H. REEVES. 1994. Initiation of autoimmunity to the p53 tumor suppressor protein by complexes of p53 and SV40 large T antigen. J. Exp. Med. **179:** 1243–1252.
25. LANE, D. P. & L. V. CRAWFORD. 1979. T antigen bound to a host protein in SV40-transformed cells. Nature **278:** 261–263.
26. LINZER, D. I. H. & A. J. LEVINE. 1979. Characterization of a 54K dalton cellular SV40 tumor antigen present in SV40-transformed cells and uninfected embryonal carcinoma cells. Cell **17:** 43–52.
27. PRIVES, C. & J. J. MANFREDI. 1993. The p53 tumor suppressor protein: meeting review. Genes Dev. **7:** 529–534.
28. BARGONETTI, J., I. REYNISDOTTIR, P. N. FRIEDMAN & C. PRIVES. 1992. Site-specific binding of wild-type p53 to cellular DNA is inhibited by SV40 T antigen and mutant p53. Genes Dev. **6:** 1886–1898.
29. OREN, M., W. MALTZMAN & A. J. LEVINE. 1981. Post-translational regulation of the 54K cellular tumor antigen in normal and transformed cells. Mol. Cell. Biol. **1:** 101–110.
30. REICH, N. C., M. OREN & A. J. LEVINE. 1983. Two distinct mechanisms regulate the levels of a cellular tumor antigen, p53. Mol. Cell. Biol. **3:** 2143–2150.
31. RUPPERT, J. M. & B. STILLMAN. 1993. Analysis of a protein-binding domain of p53. Mol. Cell. Biol. **13:** 3811–3820.
32. JENKINS, J. R., P. CHUMAKOV, C. ADDISON, H. W. STURZBECHER & A. WADE-EVANS. 1988. Two distinct regions of the murine p53 primary amino acid sequence are implicated in stable complex formation with simian virus 40 T antigen. J. Virol. **62:** 3903–3906.
33. LOWE, S. W. & H. E. RULEY. 1993. Stabilization of the p53 tumor suppressor is induced by adenovirus 5 E1A and accompanies apoptosis. Genes Dev. **7:** 535–545.
34. CROOK, T., J. A. TIDY & K. H. VOUSDEN. 1991. Degradation of p53 can be targeted by HPV E6 sequences distinct from those required for p53 binding and trans-activation. Cell **67:** 547–556.
35. ZINKERNAGEL, R. M., S. COOPER, J. CHAMBERS, R. A. LAZZARINI, H. HENGARTNER & H. ARNHEITER. 1990. Virus-induced autoantibody response to a transgenic viral antigen. Nature **345:** 68–71.
36. WINTER, S. F., J. D. MINNA, B. E. JOHNSON, T. TAKAHASHI, A. F. GAZDAR & D. P. CARBONE. 1992. Development of antibodies against p53 in lung cancer patients appears to be dependent on the type of p53 mutation. Cancer Res. **52:** 4168–4174.
37. SCHLICHTHOLZ, B., Y. LEGROS, D. GILLET, C. GAILLARD, M. MARTY, D. LANE, F. CALVO & T. SOUSSI. 1992. The immune response to p53 in breast cancer patients is directed against immunodominant epitopes unrelated to the mutational hot spot. Cancer Res. **52:** 6380–6384.
38. O'REILLY, D. R. & L. K. MILLER. 1988. Expression and complex formation of simian virus 40 large T antigen and mouse p53 in insect cells. J. Virol. **62:** 3109–3119.
39. YEWDELL, J. W., J. V. GANNON & D. P. LANE. 1986. Monoclonal antibody analysis of p53 expression in normal and transformed cells. J. Virol. **59:** 444–452.
40. LANZAVECCHIA, A. 1985. Antigen-specific interaction between T and B cells. Nature **314:** 537–539.
41. CEROTTINI, J. C. & H. R. MACDONALD. 1989. The cellular basis of T-cell memory. Annu. Rev. Immunol. **7:** 77–89.

42. Elkon, K., E. Bonfa, R. Llovet, W. Danho, H. Weissbach & N. Brot. 1988. Properties of the ribosomal P2 protein autoantigen are similar to those of foreign protein antigens. Proc. Natl. Acad. Sci. U.S.A. **85:** 5186–5189.
43. Chan, E. K. & E. M. Tan. 1987. Human autoantibody-reactive epitopes of SS-B/La are highly conserved in comparison with epitopes recognized by murine monoclonal antibodies. J. Exp. Med. **166:** 1627–1640.
44. Satoh, M., A. K. Ajmani, L. P. Stojanov, J. J. Langdon, T. Ogasawara, J. Wang, M. A. Dooley, H. Richards, J. B. Winfield, T. H. Carter *et al.* 1996. Autoantibodies that stabilize the molecular interaction of the Ku and p350 subunits of DNA-dependent protein kinase. Clin. Exp. Immunol. **105:** 460–467.
45. Stocks, M. R., D. G. Williams & R. N. Maini. 1987. Differential induction of lupus-associated antinuclear antibodies in MRL mice by monoclonal anti-Sm antibodies. Clin. Exp. Immunol. **67:** 492–499.
46. Eisenberg, R. A., D. S. Pisetsky, S. Y. Craven, J. P. Grudier, M. A. O'Donnell & P. L. Cohen. 1990. Regulation of the anti-Sm autoantibody response in systemic lupus erythematosus mice by monoclonal anti-Sm antibodies. J. Clin. Invest. **85:** 86–92.
47. Kaplan, M. E. & E. M. Tan. 1968. Antinuclear antibodies in infectious mononucleosis. Lancet **1:** 561–563.
48. Wolfgram, L. J., K. W. Beisel & N. R. Rose. 1985. Heart-specific autoantibodies following murine coxsackievirus B3 myocarditis. J. Exp. Med. **161:** 1112–1121.
49. Onodera, T., A. Toniolo, U. R. Ray, A. B. Jenson, R. A. Knazek & A. L. Notkins. 1981. Virus-induced diabetes mellitus. XX. Polyendocrinopathy and autoimmunity. J. Exp. Med. **153:** 1457–1473.
50. Oldstone, M. B. A. 1987. Molecular mimicry and autoimmune disease. Cell **50:** 819–820.
51. Gianani, R. & N. Sarvetnick. 1996. Viruses, cytokines, antigens, and autoimmunity. Proc. Natl. Acad. Sci. U.S.A. **93:** 2257–2259.

Nucleosome-driven Autoimmune Response in Lupus

Pathogenic T Helper Cell Epitopes and Costimulatory Signals

SYAMAL K. DATTA AND ARUNAN KALIYAPERUMAL

Departments of Medicine (Arthritis Division) and Microbiology/Immunology
Northwestern University Medical School
Chicago, Illinois 60611

INTRODUCTION

Autoantibodies that bind DNA play a major role in the development of lupus nephritis, yet B cells of normal subjects produce natural anti-DNA autoantibodies.[1] Moreover, DNA is only a target antigen and not the primary immunogen because deliberate immunization with DNA does not lead to SLE.[2] To address these complexities and paradoxes of lupus and to identify the primary immunogen(s) that drives the autoimmune response in this disease, we cloned and analyzed the structures and specificities of the receptors expressed by the select population of T and B cells that are responsible for the pathogenesis of lupus nephritis.

SIGNAL 1

Immunogen for the Pathogenic Autoantibody-inducing T Helper Cells of Lupus

Murine Lupus—Lessons from the NZB × SWR Model

The New Zealand Black (NZB) mice are autoimmune, but they rarely develop glomerulonephritis. However, when NZB mice are crossed with the NZW or the SWR strain, the F_1 progeny, called BWF_1 and SNF_1, respectively, will develop severe lupus nephritis that resembles human lupus very closely.[3–8] Moreover, analogous to human SLE, the BWF_1 or SNF_1 mice develop the disease without superimposition of any of the genes that secondarily accelerate lupus in the MRL-*lpr* or BXSB models, thus permitting a dissection of the *primary* factors in the development of SLE.[9,10] However, the NZW mice (parents of BWF_1) are not normal; they themselves are autoimmune and lupus-prone, and they produce high levels of retroviruses, just like the NZB strain.[11,12] The SWR mice, on the other hand, are nonautoimmune and virus-free.[4–8] Hence, the normal SWR mice have served as valuable genetic tools for dissecting the roles of various NZB traits in the etiology of autoimmune disease. Retroviruses were considered to be the etiologic agents of lupus for several decades and considerable resources were spent pursuing the "lupus virus."[13–21] Genetic studies with NZB × SWR crosses revealed the NZB genes responsible for the high level of expression of retroviruses and gp70, but those genes could be segregated from the development of SLE.[4–7] We showed that the retroviruses in NZB were endogenous, thus being another target autoantigen, but not the cause of autoimmunity. Our results were later replicated.[22–24] We and others showed that endogenous retroviruses could be induced by immunologic stimulation and that these retroviruses probably evolved by incorporating host genetic sequences.[25–27] Therefore, it is not surprising that endogenous A-type retroviruses are activated in Sjögren's syndrome or that the *gag* core protein that binds to and stabilizes the retroviral RNA genome shares homology and serological cross-reactivity with host ribonucleoproteins.[28,29] Expression of MCF-like retroviral genes, which was proclaimed to be another causal factor,[30] can also be dissociated from lupus, as those endogenous viral genes are expressed by normal nonautoimmune mice as well.[30,31] Thus, the genetic test with the NZB × SWR crosses changed the emphasis and direction of lupus research, from the pursuit of a viral etiology to elucidating basic defects in the immune system.[8,31–34] Remarkably, when the NZB mice are crossed with other normal strains, such as C57BL/6 or AKR, lupus is suppressed in their F_1 progeny.[3] Therefore, the NZB × SWR cross has also been useful in identifying the genetic factors contributed by a "normal" nonautoimmune strain in the development of autoimmune disease.

Pathogenic Autoantibody-producing B Cells

The above studies led us to ask why the SNF_1 progeny, but not the NZB parents, uniformly develop lupus nephritis. We found that the SNF_1 mice produce a select population of pathogenic anti-DNA autoantibodies that are qualitatively different from the nonpathogenic or "natural" anti-DNA antibodies produced by the NZB parents. The pathogenic autoantibodies of SNF_1 belong to the complement-fixing IgG class; they are also predominantly cationic in charge. Moreover, their antigen-combining sites are closely related, sharing a recurrent idiotype and similar antigenic fine-specificity patterns.[35–38] These autoantibodies are representative of the antibodies found in renal lesions of lupus and are capable of causing immune-deposit glomerulonephritis when administered *in vivo.*[37,39] Sequence analysis showed that the pathogenic autoantibodies consist of clonally related sets of autoantibodies sharing highly homologous V_H regions with numerous basic residues generated by somatic mutation.[35,40] However, a cationic net charge by itself[41] is not sufficient for the antigenic specificity of the autoantibodies. Many highly cationic antibodies are not specific for DNA.[42,43] Moreover, monoclonal anti-DNA autoantibodies with a neutral net charge can be pathogenic, but their V regions always contain cationic residues.[44–47] Even before sequencing studies of hybridoma-selected anti-DNA autoantibodies were done,[40,46–49] clonally restricted, cationic anti-DNA autoantibodies were found to be produced by unselected lupus B cells during active disease, both *in vivo* as detected in lupus sera, as well as *ex vivo* in short-term cultures.[42,43] Immune complexes containing the cationic anti-DNA autoantibodies probably initiate lupus nephritis by binding to negatively charged proteoglycans in glomerular basement membrane.[42,43,50,51] Recent studies suggest that this glomerular binding is probably mediated via histones in nucleosomes with which these autoantibodies react strongly.[52–55]

Pathogenic Autoantibody-inducing T Helper Cells

The V_H gene that encodes a major family of pathogenic anti-DNA autoantibodies is inherited by the SNF_1 mice from the normal SWR parent.[56,57] However, in the SNF_1 progeny only, the select population of B cells that produce the pathogenic anti-DNA autoantibodies are expanded by special subsets of T helper (Th) cells.[42] Although their antigenic specificities were not known, we could clone the Th cells by selecting for their special *functional* property, as they selectively induced the production of pathogenic antinuclear antibodies when cocultured with syngeneic B cells.[58,59] Only ~12% of 268 "autoreactive" clones derived from T cells that are activated *in vivo* in mice with lupus nephritis have this unique functional ability.[59,60] Therefore, these are special *autoimmune* Th cells, distinct from the "autoreactive" T cells that accompany immunization with exogenous antigens.[61] We thus focused on these particular Th cells that we had characterized functionally to be of pathogenic relevance in lupus.

Nucleosomes—Immunogens for the Pathogenic Th Cells of Lupus

In SNF_1 or other lupus mice, the Th cells with the strongest pathogenic autoantibody-inducing ability are $CD4^+$ and representative clones rapidly induce the development of lupus nephritis when injected *in vivo*.[59,60] The T cell receptor (TCR) genes expressed by these pathogenic Th cells of SLE are heterogeneous.[60,62] Strikingly, though, their V-D-J or V-J junctional region (CDR3 loops) sequences invariably contain one or more negatively charged residues generated by *N*-nucleotide additions.[60,62] These results indicated for the first time that the pathogenic Th cells are probably specific for some reciprocally charged, autoantigenic peptide(s).[60,62] Cationic proteins, such as histones, complexed with DNA could be taken up and processed by the anti-DNA B cells of lupus, or those B cells could process and present their own cationic, anti-DNA antibody-derived idiopeptides. This scheme proposed by us in 1990[60,63] also took into account the preferential and cognate interaction between these Th cells and the cationic anti-DNA-producing B cells. Interactions of reciprocally charged residues in TCR-CDR3 loops with their corresponding antigenic peptides were confirmed in other systems.[64]

Indeed, we found that about half of the pathogenic autoantibody-inducing Th clones from SNF_1 lupus mice are specific for nucleosomal antigen(s) presented by $I\text{-}A^d$ or $I\text{-}A^q$ molecules.[54] Furthermore, we detected nucleosome-primed T cells in lupus-prone mice, but not in normal strains, months before serologic manifestations of autoimmunity, thus predicting the development of lupus nephritis well in advance.[54] Also, immunization of preautoimmune lupus mice (but not normal animals) with pure mononucleosomes markedly accelerated the development of severe lupus nephritis.[54] Crude preparations of nucleosomes can stimulate B cells of normal as well as lupus mice as a polyclonal mitogen.[65] However, the pathogenic autoantibodies in lupus have the features of an antigen-driven response.[46,47,66] Moreover, the mere presence of nucleosomes in the serum could not explain the mechanism of autoimmunization as nucleosomes are released normally into circulation every day as a result of apoptosis of cells, and in substantial amounts in patients undergoing chronic hemodialysis, without the development of lupus.[67–69] Therefore, our identification of the nucleosome as a major *lupus-specific* immunogen for the pathogenic anti-DNA autoantibody-inducing Th cells is a major step towards understanding the etiologic mechanism of the disease.[54] These observations have brought a resurgence of interest in the serologic phenomena of nucleoprotein-binding versus DNA-binding autoantibodies in lupus. Indeed, pathogenic autoantibodies found initially in lupus sera are primarily directed against nucleosomal antigens.[52–55,70–74]

Identifying the Critical Th Cell Epitopes in Nucleosomes

Identification of the Th cell autoepitopes will help in understanding how the pathogenic Th cells of lupus emerge and will eventually lead to the development of peptide-based tolerogenic therapy. Mononucleosomes consist of dsDNA wrapped around a core octamer of histones: two of each histone H2A, H2B, H3, and H4.[75] Mononucleosome presentation could be blocked by inhibitors of endosomal proteases, leupeptin and pepstatin A, suggesting that the histone components of the nucleosomes harbor the relevant epitopes for the pathogenic Th cells of lupus.[54] However, the majority of the nucleosome-specific, pathogenic Th clones of lupus do not respond to histones free of DNA.[54] The histone peptide epitopes that are critical for the pathogenic Th cells could be protected during antigen processing, by contacting with DNA in the nucleosome, or these Th clones could be recognizing processed nucleotides (from the DNA) complexed with peptides from the histones, as in the case of T cells recognizing haptenated peptides or nucleotides.[76–78] Furthermore, nucleosomes as a whole could be taken up more efficiently by anti-DNA antibody receptors on the pathogenic B cells[54,79,80] or by special nucleosome receptors found on all types of APCs.[81,82] Therefore, in order to identify the critical autoepitopes, we are undertaking two approaches: (a) synthesize overlapping peptides spanning all four core histones and then test the pathogenic Th cells of lupus for response to the synthetic peptides and (b) elute MHC class II–bound, naturally processed peptides from appropriate APC lines pulsed with nucleosomes. The eluted peptides are being fractionated by HPLC and the fractions that stimulate the pathogenic Th cells are being analyzed by mass spectrometry and sequenced. Our initial studies show that the disease-relevant, Th cell autoepitopes are buried in the core histones in the nucleosome.[83]

Diversification of Pathogenic Help

Remarkably, each of the nucleosome-specific Th clones from SNF_1 lupus mice can augment the production of multiple IgG autoantibodies when cocultured with syngeneic splenic B cells. Moreover, the levels of IgG antinucleosomal autoantibodies induced by the pathogenic Th clones are several orders of magnitude higher than autoantibodies to dsDNA, ssDNA, or histones.[54] These results indicated that a single lupus Th clone can help a dsDNA-specific, ssDNA-specific, histone-specific, or nucleosome-specific B cell because each of these B cells, by binding to its respective

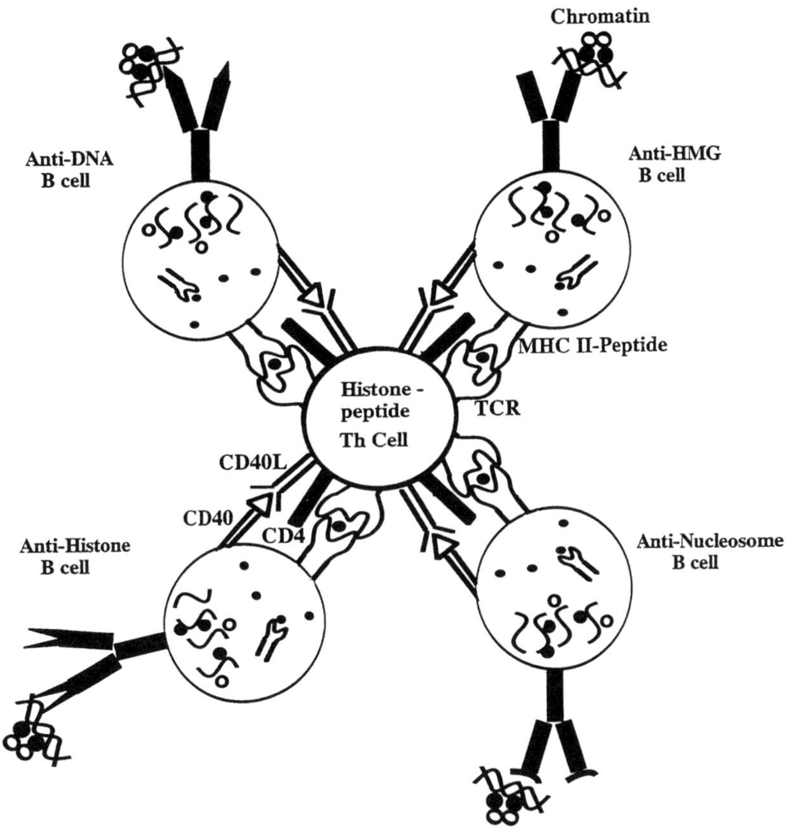

FIGURE 1. Intermolecular help diversifies pathogenic autoantibody production. In this example, a single Th cell that is specific for a nucleosomal histone peptide can help B cells specific for DNA, or others specific for nucleosomes, histones, or the nonhistone chromosomal protein HMG.[54,84] Each of these types of B cells will bind to its respective epitope in chromatin, will take up and process the whole chromatin particle, and will then present the relevant peptide epitope in the core histone to this particular Th clone. The peptide epitope for the Th clone is in the region of the histone that contacts with DNA in the nucleosome, thus being protected during antigen processing.[83] This type of help involving different molecular epitopes in the complex chromatin particle is also relevant in the case of the other pathogenic autoantibody-inducing Th cells of lupus that are specific for HMG or other nucleosomal core histone peptides.[54,83,84]

epitope on the whole chromatin, can take it up and process and then present the relevant peptide epitope in the chromatin to the Th clone (FIGURE 1). This type of intermolecular help, involving different molecular epitopes in the complex nucleosomes, is also seen in human lupus[84] and in autoimmune responses to RNP particles in SLE.[85,86]

Susceptible B Cells—Intrinsic Defects

The pathogenic Th cells of lupus mice induce the production of cationic anti-DNA autoantibodies only by SNF_1 B cells, but not by the parental NZB or SWR B cells, indicating that these autoimmune Th cells interact with a select population of susceptible B cells in a cognate manner.[42,58] However, a central tolerance defect in deleting autoimmune B cells[87] may not be the primary problem in *spontaneous* SLE because peripheral B cells of normal mice can also produce pathogenic autoantibodies with allogeneic T cell help or by other means.[46,88,89] Nevertheless, an intrinsic hyperactivity of B cells, due to Fas defect in lpr mice, due to expression of unknown stimulatory molecules in BXSB mice,[90–92] or due to hyperexpression of costimulatory molecules, such as CD40-L, in human lupus,[93] could rescue the autoimmune B cells from apoptosis and could make them more efficient in presenting nucleosomal autoantigens (see below).

Human Lupus—Similar Mechanisms of Pathogenic Autoimmune Response

SLE in humans is of course genetically more complex and heterogeneous.[94,95] However, we and others found that lupus nephritis in humans is also associated with the production of cationic IgG anti-DNA autoantibodies,[37,42,43,50,51,96,97] with evidence of class switching, clonal expansion,[42,43] and somatic mutations that generate cationic residues in their autoantibody V regions.[46,98] The production of these pathogenic autoantibodies is driven by special Th cells that are found in patients with active lupus nephritis, but not in normal subjects or patients in remission.[43] We could also clone these autoimmune Th cells of human lupus by selecting for their special functional property.[43,63] Among 396 T cell lines that were established by limiting dilution cultures of spontaneously activated T cells from five patients with lupus nephritis, only 59 ($\sim$15%) had the ability to selectively augment the production of pathogenic anti-DNA autoantibodies when cultured with autologous B cells.[63] Even though certain double-negative ($CD4^-/CD8^-$) Th cells, as well as certain $CD8^+$ Th cells, are important components of this autoantibody-inducing T cell population, their contribution is probably secondary in SLE.[43,63,99,100] The $CD4^+$ Th cells are the prime movers in the pathogenic autoimmune response because they are most prevalent among the autoimmune Th clones[49,59] and they also are the strongest helpers, increasing pathogenic anti-DNA autoantibody production up to 250-fold when cocultured with autologous B cells.[63]

We found that the TCR-CDR3 loops of the autoimmune Th clones of human lupus display recurrent motifs of charged residues,[84] similar to our results in murine SLE.[60,62] Remarkably, in four of the five patients analyzed, the frequency of Va8 gene usage was markedly and selectively increased among their pathogenic autoantibody-inducing Th clones.[84] Interestingly, human T cell lines specific for another charged autoantigen, myelin basic protein, also use Va8 genes predominantly.[101] Finally, several sets of independently derived Th clones from each lupus patient shared identical TCR a, TCR b, or both TCRs.[84] This feature could again be due to selection of these Th cells by certain autoantigens.

The finding of charged residues in the TCRs of pathogenic autoantibody-inducing Th clones[84] led us to test their response to candidate autoantigens bearing charged residues.[102] These autoantigens are recurrently found to be the targets of autoantibodies in lupus and are associated with anti-DNA autoantibody production. We also took into account the observation that the lupus Th clones preferentially provide cognate help to the select population of B cells that produce pathogenic anti-DNA autoantibodies.[43,63] Therefore, those autoimmune B cells probably in turn present some autoantigen to these Th cells to perpetuate the pathogenic autoimmune response in human lupus,[43,63] similar to the situation in murine SLE.[58,60,85,103–105]

Immunogens for the Pathogenic Th Cells of Human Lupus—Nucleosomes Again

We found that the pathogenic autoantibody-inducing Th clones of human lupus respond to highly charged nucleosomal proteins, that is, histones or the nonhistone chromosomal protein HMG.[84] The anti-DNA B cells that these Th cells specifically help probably take up DNA-bound HMG or histones and present to the Th cells. Thus, the Th cell and B cell epitopes are on different molecules within the same chromatin particle, allowing for cognate interaction between the two types of cells—intermolecular help.[54,106,107] Interestingly, as in the case of murine lupus, the majority of the human lupus Th clones responded to HMG or histones only when presented as a complex with DNA.

Immunization of mice with various DNA-binding proteins of exogenous or endogenous origin along with adjuvant leads to the production of anti-DNA autoantibodies, particularly in lupus-prone genetic backgrounds.[86,108–110] However, our studies identified which of the naturally occurring autoantigens were recognized by the *spontaneously arising* Th cells of lupus that drive the production of pathogenic anti-DNA autoantibodies. Our studies also indicate that the autoimmune response in lupus is not as heterogeneous and polyclonal as it appears from the diversity of autoantibodies in this disease.[94] There is an underlying connection between the different autoimmune B cells as each of them could share help from the same Th cell specific for an endogenous chromosomal protein epitope[54,84,111] (FIGURE 1). This interaction between the autoimmune T and B cells of human lupus is cognate, being HLA-DR-restricted in the panel of Th clones that we tested. A similar cognate interaction occurs in murine SLE.[42,54,58,112–115] Thus, we have identified the nature of the primary immunogen(s) that will bring the pathogenic T and B cells together to trigger the autoimmune response in lupus. As in the case of murine lupus, we are now trying to identify the critical T cell epitopes in the complex autoantigens in order to define "Signal 1" in the cognate interaction between the pathogenic T and B cells of human lupus.

SIGNAL 2

Role of CD40-mediated Costimulatory Signal in Pathogenic Autoantibody Production

Murine Lupus

The studies described so far clearly indicate that production of pathogenic autoantibodies in lupus is driven by an antigen-specific cognate interaction. However, other studies[116,117] have suggested that the polyclonal B cell hyperactivity that is manifest in lupus from early life[31,118,119] or some other intrinsic B cell abnormality is the primary defect in SLE, sufficient by itself to cause lupus nephritis without T cell help.

During cognate, contact-dependent help for antibody production, a ligand for CD40, called CD40-L, is transiently expressed on activated, $CD4^+$ Th cells and it binds to CD40 on the antigen-specific B cells, transducing a second signal that is essential for B cell growth and differentiation[120–126] (also see articles elsewhere in this volume). The CD40-transduced signal also prevents apoptosis of germinal center B cells that have encountered antigen.[127–135] The CD40-L (gp39) until recently was thought to be transiently expressed, mainly by $CD4^+$ T cells, upon activation.[120,124,136–140]

To establish the importance of a contact-dependent, cognate interaction between the pathogenic Th and B cells of lupus, we first tested the effect of an antibody to CD40-L in blocking the pathogenic autoimmune response in SNF_1 lupus mice.[141] We found that the interaction between CD40-L on autoimmune Th cells and CD40 on B cells is important in the spontaneous autoimmune response and blocking this interaction at a particular window of time in the natural history of lupus mice produces unexpected long-term benefits.[141] The antibody to CD40-L could block the autoantibody-inducing ability of the Th clones, as well as freshly isolated lupus Th cells, as tested by coculturing them with syngeneic B cells. Interestingly, unmanipulated SNF_1 lupus mice had markedly increased numbers of CD40-L^+ T cells in their spleens as early as 1 month of age. By contrast, in normal mice, this type of increase in CD40-L^+ cells is seen only after deliberate immunization.[122,142,143] Coincidentally, T cells responsive to nucleosomal antigens are also detectable in these lupus-prone SNF_1 mice as early as 1 month of age,[54] whereas pathogenic autoantibodies are serologically detectable in these mice later, namely, 3 to 5 months of age.[8,37] Remarkably, upon anti-CD3 activation, a significantly higher proportion of T cells from lupus mice expressed CD40-L, suggesting an inherent difference from T cells of normal mice.

A brief anti-CD40-L antibody treatment had a profound long-term effect on the development of *spontaneous* lupus nephritis in SNF_1 mice. Because the lupus mice begin to express elevated levels of IgG autoantibodies in their serum between 3 to 5 months and begin to develop nephritis around 6 months of age,[8,9,37,54] we decided to inject the anti-CD40-L antibody at 3 months of age when the population of pathogenic autoantibody-producing B cells are probably just beginning to expand. Surprisingly, development of lupus nephritis was delayed in the treated mice many months (observed up to 9 months posttherapy) after the anti-CD40-L antibody had been cleared from their system. The serum levels of pathogenic autoantibodies were also markedly decreased in the anti-CD40-L-treated group. In experimental autoimmune diseases deliberately induced by injection of autoantigens, anti-CD40-L antibody also blocks autoantibody responses.[122,144,145]

What caused the sustained beneficial effect in the SNF_1 lupus mice? We first examined the T cells in the anti-CD40-L-treated mice. Because CD40, the receptor for CD40-L, is also expressed by non-B cells, such as dendritic cells, macrophages, and thymic epithelial cells,[121] anti-CD40-L could have blocked the development and maturation of pathogenic T cells. Furthermore, the interaction between T and B cells is bidirectional, that is, the CD40-L → CD40 interaction also leads to enhanced B7 family → CD28 interaction, thus leading to expansion of not only the B cells, but the Th cells.[121,146–148] However, the pathogenic autoantibody-inducing Th cells were left intact or were replenished quickly in the anti-CD40-L-treated mice, indicating that these Th cells could utilize alternative accessory signals for their expansion. In contrast, the pathogenic B cells in the anti-CD40-L-treated mice were profoundly affected, even many months after the disappearance of the anti-CD40-L antibody from their system—B cells from the treated mice were unable to produce pathogenic autoantibodies even with appropriate T cell help.[141] In the natural history of lupus, once autoimmune memory B cells are generated, they may further amplify the autoimmune response by efficiently presenting nucleosomal and other autoantigens to the pathogenic Th cells.[10,54,149] The brief anti-CD40-L therapy may also check this amplification process. Further studies will determine if the pathogenic B cells are deleted or are rendered anergic by the brief anti-CD40-L therapy. Moreover, the anti-CD40-L therapy in lupus mice,[141] although brief, could render autoimmune B cells tolerogenic by diminishing their costimulatory ability and APC function.[121,146,150,151]

Anti-CD40-L-treated lupus mice[141] or normal mice[143,144] did not develop any generalized immunodeficiency or hyper-IgM syndrome that is found in patients with genetic defects of CD40-L expression (reviewed in reference 152). This preferential effect could occur because the CD40-L molecule is only transiently expressed on activated T cells and, in lupus, most of the T cells that are activated are the pathogenic Th cells that drive B cells to make the nephritogenic autoantibodies. Moreover, the B cells capable of producing pathogenic autoantibodies were eventually replenished because the briefly treated mice eventually developed lupus nephritis of delayed onset. Thus, the long-term beneficial effect of anti-CD40-L therapy was most probably mediated by checking the expansion of autoimmune memory B cells that are committed to produce the pathogenic autoantibodies.

Human Lupus

In humans with active lupus, we found a greater than 20-fold increase in CD40-L-expressing $CD4^+$ T cells without any exogenous stimulation.[93] However, the expression of CD40-L by lupus T cells by mitogenic stimulation could still be downregulated by CD40 molecules on autologous B cells.[93] Therefore, this negative feedback mechanism found in normal T cells[153–155] is still intact in lupus. Active lupus patients also had an equally marked increase in CD8$^+$ T cells expressing CD40-L.[93] This observation could explain the unusual helper activity of CD8 T cells in SLE.[43,100]

Most surprisingly, patients with active disease also had a marked increase in B cells that spontaneously expressed high levels of CD40-L.[93] Normal human B cells have to be stimulated with calcium ionophore, phorbol ester, and IL-2 to express low levels of CD40-L.[156] In contrast, the spontaneous expression of CD40-L by lupus B cells was as high as that found in activated T cells.[93] Thus, in addition to being costimulated by CD40-L$^+$ T cells, the lupus B cells could amplify and perpetuate the autoimmune response further by interacting with CD40 on other autoimmune B cells, as well as on follicular dendritic cells in the germinal center.[156,157] The unexpectedly long-term benefit of a brief anti-CD40-L therapy in murine lupus[141] indicates that CD40-L–CD40 interactions in a variety of immunocytes are involved in pathogenic autoantibody production in SLE. Indeed, the nephritogenic autoantibodies of lupus are Th1-dependent[83] and the development of Th1 cells is determined by CD40-L–CD40 interactions between T cells and macrophages or dendritic cells.[158]

On the other hand, lupus patients in *remission* had low levels of CD40-L$^+$ T and B cells, in the range of normal subjects.[93] However, upon stimulation with *suboptimal* doses of mitogens, the upregulation of CD40-L expression in these T and B cells was markedly greater than normal. These results indicate that an intrinsic defect in CD40-L regulation or a lowering of the threshold for CD40-L expression exists in lupus, in addition to autoantigen-driven activation.[93] Abnormalities in other signal transduction pathways have also been detected in lupus T cells.[159,160]

A monoclonal antibody to human CD40-L significantly blocked the *in vitro* production of pathogenic antinuclear autoantibodies by lymphocytes from lupus patients with active and established disease. Therefore, the pathogenic B cells of lupus can be downregulated and they are not totally autonomous due to some intrinsic defect. The autoimmune B cells in human and murine lupus (except MRL-lpr) may be as susceptible to apoptosis as normal antigen-driven B cells unless they are rescued by the CD40-mediated second signal.[128–131,161]

These studies show that anti-CD40-L therapy will be effective in lupus, a *spontaneous* autoimmune disease. The disease mechanisms in the SNF_1 lupus mice are almost identical to human SLE.[42,43,54,58,63,84] Therefore, the long-term benefit of a brief anti-CD40-L therapy in these mice is relevant to developing similar treatment in human SLE. Indeed, anti-CD40-L therapy was beneficial even at a time when early autoimmune abnormalities were manifest in the lupus mice. This suggests that anti-CD40-L therapy might be beneficial in newly diagnosed lupus patients or in patients in the early stages of disease flare-up. Conversely, blocking the B cell → T cell interaction by CTLA4Ig that interferes with CTLA4/CD28 signaling by the B7 family of molecules also has a beneficial effect on murine lupus.[162] The mechanism of the therapeutic effect of CTLA4Ig has yet to be studied, but it is probably mediated through its indirect effect on the CD40-L → CD40 signaling pathway.[121,146–148]

FUTURE DIRECTIONS

Specific immunotherapy for human SLE can be eventually designed based on these studies. Once the pathogenic Th cell epitopes in the nucleosomes are identified, autoantigen-mediated signal 1 to the Th cells could be blocked,[163,164] in combination with anti-CD40-L therapy to block CD40-mediated signal 2 to the pathogenic autoantibody-producing B cells. Thus, instead of blocking signals 1 and 2 for either the autoimmune T cell or the autoimmune B cell,[165] both of these major players in the pathogenic unit could be blocked by combination therapy.

It is not clear how autoimmunization against nucleosomes occurs in lupus. These autoantigens are released normally as a product of apoptosis,[67,166] without the development of lupus.[68] Obviously, fundamental defects in the immune system play an initiating role, and environmental factors then contribute to the autoimmune response.[46,108,110,111,167,168] Perhaps, abnormal autoantigen processing and presentation lead to the early expansion of nucleosome-specific T cells in lupus. Intrinsic B and T cell defects, such as hyperexpression of CD40-L, could contribute to this process and sustain it. However, why is the autoimmune response skewed toward apoptotic antigens in lupus? How are nucleosome-specific T cells positively selected in the thymus? Do nucleosome-specific B and T cells have a special survival advantage and, if so, what are the mechanisms? These are some of the pressing questions in lupus research that we and others will attempt to answer in the near-future.

REFERENCES

1. Stewart, A., C. Huang, A. Long, B. Stollar & R. Schwartz. 1992. Immunol. Rev. **128:** 101–122.
2. Madaio, M. P., S. Hodder, R. S. Schwartz & B. D. Stollar. 1984. J. Immunol. **132:** 872–876.
3. Howie, J. B. & B. J. Helyer. 1968. Adv. Immunol. **9:** 215–268.
4. Datta, S. K. & R. S. Schwartz. 1976. Nature **263:** 412–415.
5. Datta, S. K. & R. S. Schwartz. 1977. Virology **83:** 449–452.
6. Datta, S. K., N. Manny, C. Andrzejewski, J. Andre-Schwartz & R. S. Schwartz. 1978. J. Exp. Med. **147:** 854–871.
7. Datta, S. K., P. J. McConahey, N. Manny, A. N. Theofilopoulos, F. J. Dixon & R. S. Schwartz. 1978. J. Exp. Med. **147:** 872–881.
8. Eastcott, J. W., R. S. Schwartz & S. K. Datta. 1983. J. Immunol. **131:** 2232–2239.
9. Datta, S. K. 1989. Clin. Immunol. Immunopathol. **51:** 141–156.
10. Sercarz, E. E. & S. K. Datta. 1994. Curr. Opin. Immunol. **6:** 875–881.
11. Kelly, V. E. & A. Winkelstein. 1980. Clin. Immunol. Immunopathol. **16:** 142–150.
12. Yoshiki, T., R. C. Mellors, M. Strand & J. T. August. 1974. J. Exp. Med. **140:** 1011–1027.
13. Schwartz, R. S. 1975. N. Engl. J. Med. **293:** 132–138.
14. Lewis, R. M., W. Tannenberg, C. Smith & R. S. Schwartz. 1974. Nature **252:** 78–79.
15. Talal, N. 1970. Arthritis Rheum. **13:** 887–894.
16. Lambert, P. H. & F. J. Dixon. 1970. Clin. Exp. Immunol. **6:** 829–839.
17. Levy, J. A. 1975. J. Rheumatol. **2:** 135–148.
18. Panem, S., N. G. Ordonez, W. H. Kerstein, A. I. Katz & B. H. Spargo. 1976. N. Engl. J. Med. **295:** 470–475.

19. MELLORS, R. C. & J. W. MELLORS. 1976. Proc. Natl. Acad. Sci. U.S.A. **73:** 233–237.
20. MARKENSON, J. A. & P. E. PHILLIPS. 1978. Arthritis Rheum. **21:** 266–270.
21. STRAND, M. & J. T. AUGUST. 1974. J. Virol. **14:** 1584–1596.
22. DAVIDSON, W. F. 1982. J. Immunol. **129:** 751–758.
23. ANDREW, J., L. M. HANG, A. N. THEOFILOPOULOS & F. J. DIXON. 1986. J. Exp. Med. **163:** 458–462.
24. KIMURA, M., T. ANDOH & K. KAI. 1980. Arthritis Rheum. **23:** 111–113.
25. DATTA, S. K. & R. S. SCHWARTZ. 1976. Eur. J. Cancer **12:** 977–988.
26. LEVY, J. A., S. K. DATTA & R. S. SCHWARTZ. 1977. Clin. Immunol. Immunopathol. **7:** 262–268.
27. BISHOP, J. M. 1983. Annu. Rev. Biochem. **52:** 301–354.
28. GARRY, R. F., C. D. FERMIN, D. J. HART, S. S. ALEXANDER, L. A. DONEHOWER & H. LUO-ZHANG. 1990. Science **250:** 1127–1129.
29. QUERRY, C. C. & J. D. KEENE. 1987. Cell **51:** 211–220.
30. KRIEG, A. M. & A. D. STEINBERG. 1990. J. Clin. Invest. **86:** 809–816.
31. DATTA, S. K., F. L. OWEN, J. E. WOMACK & R. J. RIBLET. 1982. J. Immunol. **129:** 1539–1544.
32. PISETSKY, D. S., G. A. MCCARTY & D. V. PETERS. 1980. J. Exp. Med. **152:** 1302–1310.
33. COHEN, P. L. & R. A. EISENBERG. 1982. J. Exp. Med. **156:** 173–180.
34. CHIANG, B-L., E. BEARER, A. ANSARI, K. DORSHKIND & M. E. GERSHWIN. 1990. J. Immunol. **145:** 94–101.
35. GAVALCHIN, J., J. NICKLAS, J. W. EASTCOTT, M. P. MADAIO, B. D. STOLLAR, R. S. SCHWARTZ & S. K. DATTA. 1985. J. Immunol. **134:** 885–894.
36. GAVALCHIN, J., R. A. SEDER & S. K. DATTA. 1987. J. Immunol. **138:** 128–137.
37. GAVALCHIN, J. & S. K. DATTA. 1987. J. Immunol. **138:** 138–148.
38. DATTA, S. K. & J. GAVALCHIN. 1986. Ann. N.Y. Acad. Sci. **475:** 47–58.
39. VLAHAKOS, D. V., M. H. FOSTER, S. ADAMS, M. KATZ, A. A. UCCI, K. J. BARRETT, S. K. DATTA & M. P. MADAIO. 1992. Kidney Int. **41:** 1690–1700.
40. O'KEEFE, T. L., S. BANDYOPADHYAY, S. K. DATTA & T. IMANISHI-KARI. 1990. J. Immunol. **144:** 4275–4283.
41. SELA, M., E. MOZES, G. M. SHEARER & Y. KARNIELY. 1970. Proc. Natl. Acad. Sci. U.S.A. **67:** 1288–1293.
42. DATTA, S. K., H. PATEL & D. BERRY. 1987. J. Exp. Med. **165:** 1252–1268.
43. SHIVAKUMAR, S., G. C. TSOKOS & S. K. DATTA. 1989. J. Immunol. **143:** 103–112.
44. TSAO, B. P., F. M. EBLING, C. ROMAN, N. PANOSIAN-SAHAKIAN, K. CALAME & B. H. HAHN. 1990. J. Clin. Invest. **85:** 530–540.
45. KIEBER-EMMONS, T., M. H. FOSTER, W. V. WILLIAMS & M. P. MADAIO. 1994. Immunol. Res. **13:** 172–185.
46. DIAMOND, B., J. B. KATZ, E. PAUL, C. ARANOW, D. LUSTGARTEN & M. D. SCHARFF. 1992. Annu. Rev. Immunol. **10:** 731–757.
47. RADIC, M. Z. & M. WEIGERT. 1994. Annu. Rev. Immunol. **12:** 487–520.
48. TILLMAN, D. M., N-T. JOU, R. J. HILL & T. N. MARION. 1992. J. Exp. Med. **176:** 761–779.
49. SHLOMCHIK, M. J., M. MASCELLI, H. SHAN, M. Z. RADIC, D. PISETSKY, A. MARSHAK-ROTHSTEIN & M. WEIGERT. 1990. J. Exp. Med. **171:** 265–292.
50. EBLING, F. & B. H. HAHN. 1980. Arthritis Rheum. **23:** 392–403.
51. GAUTHIER, V. J. & M. MANNIK. 1990. J. Immunol. **145:** 3348–3352.
52. SCHMIEDKE, T. M. J., F. W. STOCKL, R. WEBER, Y. SUGISAKI, S. R. BATSFORD & A. VOGT. 1989. J. Exp. Med. **169:** 1879–1894.
53. KRAMERS, C., M. N. HYLKEMA, M. C. J. VAN BRUGGEN, R. VAN DE LAGEMAAT, H. B. P. M. DIJKMAN, K. J. M. ASSMANN, R. J. T. SMEENK & J. H. M. BERDEN. 1994. J. Clin. Invest. **94:** 568–577.
54. MOHAN, C., S. ADAMS, V. STANIK & S. K. DATTA. 1993. J. Exp. Med. **177:** 1367–1381.
55. OHNISHI, K., F. M. EBLING, B. MITCHELL, R. R. SINGH, B. H. HAHN & B. P. TSAO. 1994. Int. Immunol. **6:** 817–827.

56. GHATAK, S., K. SAINIS, F. L. OWEN & S. K. DATTA. 1987. Proc. Natl. Acad. Sci. U.S.A. **84:** 6850–6853.
57. O'KEEFE, T. L., S. K. DATTA & T. IMANISHI-KARI. 1992. Eur. J. Immunol. **22:** 619–624.
58. SAINIS, K. & S. K. DATTA. 1988. J. Immunol. **140:** 2215–2224.
59. ADAMS, S., T. ZORDAN, K. SAINIS & S. K. DATTA. 1990. Eur. J. Immunol. **20:** 1435–1443.
60. ADAMS, S., P. LEBLANC & S. K. DATTA. 1991. Proc. Natl. Acad. Sci. U.S.A. **88:** 11271–11275.
61. ZAUDERER, M. & K. NATARAJAN. 1990. Immunol. Rev. **116:** 160.
62. MAO, C., G. E. OSMAN, S. ADAMS & S. K. DATTA. 1994. J. Immunol. **152:** 1462–1470.
63. RAJAGOPALAN, S., T. ZORDAN, G. C. TSOKOS & S. K. DATTA. 1990. Proc. Natl. Acad. Sci. U.S.A. **87:** 7020–7024.
64. JORGENSEN, J. L., U. ESSER, P. A. REAY, B. FAZEKAS DE ST. GROTH & M. M. DAVIS. 1992. Nature **355:** 224–230.
65. ATKINSON, M. J., D. A. BELL & S. K. SINGHAL. 1985. J. Immunol. **135:** 2524–2533.
66. DATTA, S. K., S. RAJAGOPALAN, T. L. O'KEEFE, S. GHATAK & T. IMANISHI-KARI. 1992. Pathogenic anti-DNA autoantibodies and pathogenic autoantibody-inducing T cells. *In* Molecular Immunobiology of Self-reactivity. C. A. Bona & A. Kaushik, Eds.: 133–153. Dekker. New York.
67. RUMORE, P. & C. STEINMAN. 1990. J. Clin. Invest. **86:** 69–74.
68. FOURNIE, G. J., J. LULE, J-M. DUEYMES, F. LAVAL, I. DELOBLE, I. VERNIER & J. P. POURAT. 1989. Am. J. Nephrol. **9:** 384–391.
69. ATANASSOV, C., J. P. BRIAND, D. BONNIER, M. H. V. VAN REGENMORTEL & S. MULLER. 1991. Clin. Exp. Immunol. **86:** 124–133.
70. ROTHFIELD, N. F. & B. D. STOLLAR. 1967. J. Clin. Invest. **46:** 1785–1794.
71. BURLINGAME, R. W., R. L. RUBIN, R. S. BALDERAS & A. N. THEOFILOPOULOS. 1993. J. Clin. Invest. **91:** 1687–1696.
72. BURLINGAME, R. W., M. L. BOEY, G. STARKEBAUM & R. L. RUBIN. 1994. J. Clin. Invest. **94:** 184–192.
73. CHABRE, H., Z. AMOURA, J-C. PIETTE, P. GODEAU, J-F. BACH & S. KOUTOUZOV. 1995. Arthritis Rheum. **38:** 1485–1491.
74. BERNSTEIN, K. A., R. DIVALERIO & J. B. LEFKOWITH. 1995. J. Immunol. **154:** 2424–2433.
75. USACHENKO, S. I., S. G. BAVYKIN, I. M. GAVIN & E. M. BRADBURY. 1994. Proc. Natl. Acad. Sci. U.S.A. **91:** 6845–6849.
76. KASIBHATLA, S., E. A. NALEFSKI & A. RAO. 1993. J. Immunol. **151:** 3140–3151.
77. GANJU, R. K., S. T. SMILEY, J. BAJORATH, J. NOVOTNY & E. L. REINHERZ. 1992. Proc. Natl. Acad. Sci. U.S.A. **89:** 11552–11556.
78. CONSTANT, P., F. DAVODEAU, M-A. PEYRAT, Y. POQUET, G. PUZO, M. BONNEVILLE & J-J. FOURNIE. 1994. Science **264:** 267–270.
79. CARSON, D. A. 1991. J. Immunol. **146:** 1–3.
80. TAN, E. M. 1989. Adv. Immunol. **44:** 93–151.
81. FREED, A. C., S. H. HEFENEIDER, C. VEDDER, K. KHAW, A. C. BAKKE, S. L. MCCOY & R. M. BENNETT. 1994. Arthritis Rheum. **37:** supplement R5 (abstract).
82. KOUTOUZOV, S., A. CABRESPINES, Z. AMOURA, H. CHABRE, C. LOTTON & J-F. BACH. 1996. Eur. J. Immunol. **26:** 472–486.
83. KALIYAPERUMAL, A., C. MOHAN, W. WU & S. K. DATTA. 1996. J. Exp. Med. **183:** 2459–2469.
84. DESAI-MEHTA, A., C. MAO, S. RAJAGOPALAN, T. ROBINSON & S. K. DATTA. 1995. J. Clin. Invest. **95:** 531–541.
85. MAMULA, M. J., S. FATENEJAD & J. CRAFT. 1994. J. Immunol. **152:** 1453–1461.
86. JAMES, J. A., T. GROSS, R. H. SCOFIELD & J. B. HARLEY. 1995. J. Exp. Med. **181:** 453–461.
87. NEMAZEE, D. & K. BURKI. 1989. Nature **337:** 562–566.
88. GLEICHMANN, E., E. H. VAN ELVEN & J. P. W. VAN DER VEEN. 1982. Eur. J. Immunol. **12:** 152–159.
89. MOENS, U., O-M. SETERNES, A. W. HEY, Y. SILSAND, T. TRAAVIK, B. JOHANSEN & O. P. REKVIG. 1995. Proc. Natl. Acad. Sci. U.S.A. **92:** 12393–12397.

90. COHEN, P. L. & R. A. EISENBERG. 1991. Annu. Rev. Immunol. **9:** 243–269.
91. PERKINS, D. L., R. M. GLASER, C. A. MAHON, J. MICHAELSON & A. MARSHAK-ROTHSTEIN. 1990. J. Immunol. **145:** 549–555.
92. IZUI, S., R. MERINO, L. FOSSATI & M. IWAMOTO. 1994. Int. Rev. Immunol. **11:** 211–230.
93. DESAI-MEHTA, A., L. LU, R. RAMSEY-GOLDMAN & S. K. DATTA. 1996. J. Clin. Invest. **97:** 2063–2073.
94. HARLEY, J. B., A. L. SESTAK, L. G. WILLIS, S. M. FU, J. A. HANSEN & M. REICHLIN. 1989. Arthritis Rheum. **32:** 826–836.
95. BOUMPAS, D. T., H. A. AUSTIN, B. J. FESSLER, J. E. BALOW, J. H. KLIPPEL & M. D. LOCKSHIN. 1995. Ann. Intern. Med. **122:** 940–950.
96. SUENAGA, R. & N. I. ABDOU. 1993. Clin. Exp. Immunol. **94:** 418–422.
97. SUZUKI, N., T. HARADA, Y. MIZUSHIMA & T. SAKANE. 1993. J. Immunol. **151:** 1128–1136.
98. WINKLER, T. H., H. FEHR & J. R. KALDEN. 1992. Eur. J. Immunol. **22:** 1719–1728.
99. RAJAGOPALAN, S., C. MAO & S. K. DATTA. 1992. Clin. Immunol. Immunopathol. **62:** 344–350.
100. LINKER-ISRAELI, M., F. P. QUISIMORO & D. A. HORWITZ. 1990. Arthritis Rheum. **33:** 1216–1225.
101. UTZ, U., J. A. BROOKS, H. F. MCFARLAND, R. MARTIN & W. E. BIDDISON. 1994. Proc. Natl. Acad. Sci. U.S.A. **91:** 5567–5571.
102. BRENDEL, V., J. DOHLMAN, B. E. BLAISDELL & S. KARLIN. 1991. Proc. Natl. Acad. Sci. U.S.A. **88:** 1536–1540.
103. LANZAVECCHIA, A. 1985. Nature **314:** 537–539.
104. MALYNN, B. A. & H. H. WORTIS. 1984. J. Immunol. **132:** 2253–2258.
105. ROCK, K. L., B. BENACERRAF & A. K. ABBAS. 1984. J. Exp. Med. **160:** 1102–1113.
106. LAKE, P. & N. A. MITCHISON. 1976. Cold Spring Harbor Symp. Quant. Biol. **41:** 589–595.
107. LEHMAN, P., T. FORSTHUBER, A. MILLER & E. SERCARZ. 1992. Nature **358:** 155–157.
108. DESAI, D. D., M. R. KRISHNAN, J. T. SWINDLE & T. N. MARION. 1993. J. Immunol. **151:** 1614–1626.
109. KANAI, Y., O. TAKEDA, Y. KANAI, K. MIURA & Y. KUROSAWA. 1994. Immunol. Lett. **39:** 83–89.
110. FREDRIKSEN, K., A. OSEI, A. SUNDSFJORD, T. TRAAVIK & O. P. REKVIG. 1994. Eur. J. Immunol. **24:** 66–70.
111. PUCCETTI, A., M. P. MADAIO, G. BELLESE & P. MIGLIORINI. 1995. J. Exp. Med. **181:** 1797–1804.
112. ANDO, D. G., E. E. SERCARZ & B. H. HAHN. 1987. J. Immunol. **138:** 3185–3190.
113. SOBEL, E. S., V. N. KAKKANAIAH, M. KAKKANAIAH, R. L. CHEEK, P. L. COHEN & R. A. EISENBERG. 1994. J. Immunol. **152:** 6011–6016.
114. NAIKI, M., B-L. CHIANG, D. CAWLEY, A. ANSARI, S. J. ROZZO, B. L. KOTZIN, A. ZLOTNIK & M. E. GERSHWIN. 1992. J. Immunol. **149:** 4109–4115.
115. PORTANOVA, J. P., R. E. ARNDT & B. L. KOTZIN. 1988. J. Immunol. **140:** 755–760.
116. KLINMAN, D. M. & A. D. STEINBERG. 1987. J. Exp. Med. **165:** 1755–1760.
117. REININGER, L., T. RADASZKIEWICZ, M. KOSCO, F. MELCHERS & A. G. ROLNIK. 1992. J. Exp. Med. **176:** 1343–1353.
118. DATTA, S. K. & R. S. SCHWARTZ. 1978. Genetic, viral, and immunologic aspects of autoimmune disease in NZB mice. *In* Genetic Control of Autoimmune Disease. N. R. Rose, P. E. Bigazzi & N. L. Warner, Eds.: 192–206. Elsevier/North-Holland. Amsterdam/New York.
119. MERINO, R., M. IWAMOTO, L. FOSSATI & S. IZUI. 1993. J. Immunol. **151:** 6509–6516.
120. NOELLE, R. J., J. A. LEDBETTER & A. ARUFFO. 1992. Immunol. Today **13:** 431–433.
121. CLARK, E. A. & J. A. LEDBETTER. 1994. Nature **367:** 425–428.
122. ROY, M., T. WALDSCHMIDT, A. ARUFFO, J. A. LEDBETTER & R. J. NOELLE. 1993. J. Immunol. **151:** 2497–2510.
123. BANCHEREAU, J., F. BAZAN, D. BLANCHARD, F. BRIERE, J. P. GALIZI, C. VAN KOOTEN, Y. J. LIU, F. ROUSSET & S. SAELAND. 1994. Annu. Rev. Immunol. **12:** 881–922.

124. LEDERMAN, S., M. J. YELLIN, G. INGHIRAMI, J. J. LEE, D. M. KNOWLES & L. CHESS. 1992. J. Immunol. **149:** 3817–3826.
125. SPRIGGS, M. K., R. J. ARMITAGE, L. STROCKBINE, K. N. CLIFFORD, B. M. MACDUFF, T. A. SATO, C. R. MALISZEWSKI & W. C. FANSLOW. 1992. J. Exp. Med. **176:** 1543–1550.
126. STAMENKOVIC, I., E. A. CLARK & B. SEED. 1989. EMBO J. **8:** 1403–1410.
127. LEDERMAN, S., M. J. YELLIN, A. M. CLEARY, A. PERNIS, G. INGHIRAMI, L. E. COHN, L. R. COVEY, J. L. LEE, P. ROTHMAN & L. CHESS. 1994. J. Immunol. **152:** 2163–2171.
128. LIU, Y-J., D. E. JOSHUA, G. T. WILLIAMS, C. A. SMITH, J. GORDON & I. C. M. MACLENNAN. 1989. Nature **342:** 929–931.
129. TSUBATA, T., J. WU & T. HONJO. 1993. Nature **364:** 645–648.
130. ROTHSTEIN, T. L., J. K. M. WANG, D. J. PANKA, L. C. FOOTE, Z. WANG, B. STANGER, H. CUI, S-T. JU & A. MARSHAK-ROTHSTEIN. 1995. Nature **374:** 163–165.
131. PARRY, S. L., J. HASBOLD, M. HOLMAN & G. G. B. KLAUS. 1994. J. Immunol. **152:** 2821–2829.
132. REN, C. L., T. MORIO, S. M. FU & R. S. GEHA. 1994. J. Exp. Med. **179:** 673–680.
133. FARIS, M., F. GASKIN, J. T. PARSONS & S. M. FU. 1994. J. Exp. Med. **179:** 1923–1931.
134. WORTIS, H. H., M. TEUTSCH, M. HIGER, J. ZHENG & D. C. PARKER. 1995. Proc. Natl. Acad. Sci. U.S.A. **92:** 3348–3352.
135. SCHATTNER, E. J., K. B. ELKON, D-H. YOO, J. TUMANG, P. H. KRAMMER, M. K. CROW & S. M. FRIEDMAN. 1995. J. Exp. Med. **182:** 1557–1565.
136. LANE, P. J. L., A. TRAUNECKER, S. HUBELE, S. INUI, A. LANZAVECCHIA & D. GRAY. 1992. Eur. J. Immunol. **22:** 2573–2578.
137. ARMITAGE, R. J., W. C. FANSLOW, L. STROCKBINE, T. A. SATO, K. N. CLIFFORD, B. M. MACDUFF, S. D. ANDERSON, T. GIMPLE, C. R. DAVIS-SMITH, C. R. MALISZEWSKI, E. A. CLARK, C. A. SMITH, K. H. GRABSTEIN, D. COSMAN & M. K. SPRIGGS. 1992. Nature **357:** 80–82.
138. GRAF, D., U. KORTHAUER, H. W. MAGES, G. SENGER & R. A. KROCZEK. 1992. Eur. J. Immunol. **22:** 3191–3194.
139. NOELLE, R. J., M. ROY, D. M. SHEPHERD, I. STAMENCOVIC, J. A. LEDBETTER & A. ARUFFO. 1992. Proc. Natl. Acad. Sci. U.S.A. **89:** 6550–6554.
140. GAUCHAT, J-F., J. P. AUBRY, G. MAZZEI, P. LIFE, T. JOMOTTE, G. ELSON & J-Y. BONNEFOY. 1993. FEBS Lett. **315:** 259–266.
141. MOHAN, C., Y. SHI, J. D. LAMAN & S. K. DATTA. 1995. J. Immunol. **154:** 1470–1480.
142. VAN DEN EERTWEGH, A. J. M., R. J. NOELLE, M. ROY, D. M. SHEPHERD, A. ARUFFO, J. A. LEDBETTER, W. J. A. BOERSMA & E. CLASSEN. 1993. J. Exp. Med. **178:** 1555.
143. FOY, T. M., D. M. SHEPHERD, F. H. DURIE, A. ARUFFO, J. A. LEDBETTER & R. J. NOELLE. 1993. J. Exp. Med. **178:** 1567–1575.
144. DURIE, F. H., R. A. FAVA, T. M. FOY, A. ARUFFO, J. A. LEDBETTER & R. J. NOELLE. 1993. Science **261:** 1328–1330.
145. GRIGGS, N. D., S. S. AGERSBORG, R. J. NOELLE, J. A. LEDBETTER, P. S. LINSLEY & K. S. K. TUNG. 1996. J. Exp. Med. **183:** 801–810.
146. RANHEIM, E. A. & T. J. KIPPS. 1993. J. Exp. Med. **177:** 925–935.
147. KLAUS, S. J., L. M. PINCHUK, H. D. OCHS, C-L. LAW, W. C. FANSLOW, R. J. ARMITAGE & E. A. CLARK. 1994. J. Immunol. **152:** 5643–5652.
148. DE BOER, M., A. KASRAN, J. KWEKKEBOOM, H. WALTER, P. VANDENBERGHE & J. L. CEUPPENS. 1993. Eur. J. Immunol. **23:** 3120–3125.
149. SINGH, R. R., V. KUMAR, F. M. EBLING, S. SOUTHWOOD, A. SETTE, E. E. SERCARZ & B. H. HAHN. 1995. J. Exp. Med. **181:** 2017–2027.
150. BUHLMANN, J. E., T. M. FOY, A. ARUFFO, K. M. CRASSI, J. A. LEDBETTER, W. R. GREEN, J. C. XU, L. D. SHULTZ, D. ROOPESIAN, R. A. FLAVELL, L. FAST, R. J. NOELLE & F. H. DURIE. 1995. Immunity **2:** 645–653.
151. KENNEDY, M. K., K. M. MOHLER, K. D. SHANEBECK, P. R. BAUM, K. S. PICHA, C. A. OTTENE-EVANS, C. A. JANEWAY & K. H. GRABSTEIN. 1994. Eur. J. Immunol. **24:** 116–123.
152. HILL, A. & H. CHAPEL. 1993. Nature **361:** 494.

153. CASTLE, B. E., K. KISHIMOTO, C. STEARNS, M. L. BROWN & M. R. KEHRY. 1993. J. Immunol. **151:** 1777–1788.
154. YELLIN, M. J., K. SIPPEL, G. INGHIRAMI, L. R. COVEY, J. J. LEE, J. SINNING, E. A. CLARK, L. CHESS & S. LEDERMAN. 1994. J. Immunol. **152:** 598–608.
155. VAN KOOTEN, C. V., C. GAILLARD, J-P. GALLIZI, P. HERMANN, F. FOSSIEZ, J. BANCHEREAU & D. BLANCHARD. 1994. Eur. J. Immunol. **24:** 787–792.
156. GRAMMER, A. C., M. C. BERGMAN, Y. MIURA, K. FUJITA, L. S. DAVIS & P. E. LIPSKY. 1995. J. Immunol. **154:** 4996–5010.
157. FACCHETTI, F., C. APPIANI, L. SALVI, J. LEVY & L. D. NOTARANGELO. 1995. J. Immunol. **154:** 6624–6633.
158. STUBER, E., W. STROBER & M. NEURATH. 1996. J. Exp. Med. **183:** 693–698.
159. VASSILOPOULOS, D., B. KOVACS & G. C. TSOKOS. 1995. J. Immunol. **155:** 2269–2281.
160. KAMMER, G. M., I. KHAN & C. MALEMUD. 1994. J. Clin. Invest. **94:** 422–430.
161. WANG, Z., J. G. KARRAS, R. G. HOWARD & T. L. ROTHSTEIN. 1995. J. Immunol. **155:** 3722–3725.
162. FINCK, B. K., P. S. LINSLEY & D. WOFSY. 1994. Science **265:** 1225–1227.
163. DEMAGISTRIS, M. T., J. ALEXANDER, M. COGGESHALL, A. ALTMAN, F. C. A. GAETA, H. M. GREY & A. SETTE. 1992. Cell **68:** 625–634.
164. SLOAN-LANCASTER, J., B. D. EVAVOLD & P. M. ALLEN. 1994. J. Exp. Med. **180:** 1195–1205.
165. BRESTCHER, P. A. & M. COHN. 1970. Science **169:** 1042–1049.
166. CASCIOLA-ROSEN, L. A., G. ANHALT & A. ROSEN. 1994. J. Exp. Med. **179:** 1317–1330.
167. GILKESON, G. S., A. M. M. PIPPEN & D. S. PISETSKY. 1995. J. Clin. Invest. **95:** 1398–1402.
168. DONG, X., K. J. HAMILTON, M. SATOH, J. WANG & W. H. REEVES. 1994. J. Exp. Med. **179:** 1243–1252.

Phenotypic and Functional Characterization of Human Tonsillar Subepithelial (SE) B Cells[a]

MARIELLA DONO,[b] SIMONA ZUPO,[b]
VITO L. BURGIO,[c] ADRIANO AUGLIERA,[b]
CARLO TACCHETTI,[d] ANNA FAVRE,[d] CARLO E. GROSSI,[d,e]
NICHOLAS CHIORAZZI,[f] AND MANLIO FERRARINI[b]

[b]*Servizio di Immunologia Clinica*
Istituto Nazionale per la Ricerca sul Cancro
IST
16132 Genova, Italy

[c]*Istituto di 1[a] Clinica Medica Generale e Terapia Medica*
Università "La Sapienza"
00100 Roma, Italy

[d]*Istituto di Anatomia Umana Normale*
Università di Genova
16132 Genova, Italy

[e]*Servizio di Patologia Clinica*
Istituto Nazionale per la Ricerca sul Cancro
IST
16132 Genova, Italy

[f]*Department of Medicine*
North Shore University Hospital
New York University School of Medicine
Manhasset, New York 11030

INTRODUCTION

In the past, mature B cells were considered to be a homogeneous population of cells, the function of which consisted in the production of antibodies of increasing affinity upon appropriate antigenic stimulation. The current views, however, attribute a more complex role to B cells. B cells can release cytokines, which are responsible for various functions such as the induction of the inflammatory response, the promotion of hematopoiesis, and the initiation of an acute phase reaction.[1] Moreover, B cells can adsorb, process, and present antigens to T cells. In addition, they express surface molecules that, upon interaction with complementary structures of T cells, participate in the mutual process of activation of both T and B cells.[2]

[a]This work was supported in part by grants from AIRC, ISS Progetto AIDS, CNR (P. F. Ingegneria Genetica and ACRO), Fondazione Andrea Cesalpino, and NIH (No. AI 10811).

Recent data indicate that mature B cells are heterogeneous and that they display different phenotype, morphology, and functional features depending upon the anatomical site where they home in the peripheral lymphoid tissues.[3–6]

In peripheral lymphoid organs, B cells are found predominantly in the lymphoid follicles, where they accumulate both in the germinal centers (GC) and in the follicular mantles (FM).[7] Studies with panels of anti-B cell mAb have disclosed that GC and FM B cells have a different phenotype and can thus be separated when B cells are prepared in suspension.[8–10] Functionally, GC B cells are characterized by a special propensity for apoptosis which, however, can be prevented if certain signals are delivered to the cells by other cells and/or by cytokines.[8,9] Spontaneous apoptosis and rescue mediated by different signals, including antigenic stimulation, may constitute the basic mechanisms of B cell selection in the GC.[5,7] This results in the survival of only those cells that are capable of producing antibodies of relatively high affinity for the stimulating antigen. So far, much less is known about the FM B cells and their relationships with GC B cells, although data have been collected that indicate that they primarily comprise virgin B cells and produce IgM antibodies (upon stimulation with polyclonal B cell activators).[10–12]

The use of B cell–specific mAb has led to the identification of another subset of B cells that are phenotypically distinct from those located in the lymphoid follicles. The prototypic cells of these extrafollicular B cells[13,14] are the B cells of the splenic marginal zone (MZ).[15,16] The MZ is defined as the outermost area of the splenic white pulp and has been traditionally thought to comprise resident (nonrecirculating) B cells endowed with the capacity to respond to polysaccharide (T-independent type 2 or TI-2) antigens.[14–21] Cells with a phenotype similar to that of the splenic MZ B cells have been found in defined areas of other peripheral lymphoid organs. It is generally assumed that, in man, the B cells of the subepithelial (SE) areas of the tonsils, of the subcapsular sinus of lymph nodes, of the thymic medulla, and of the dome region of Peyer's patches are the equivalent of the splenic MZ B cells.[13,22–25] The functional data on these human B cell subset populations are scarce, particularly because of the difficulties related to their separation and purification. Most of the available data come from studies on the splenic MZ of mice and rats, both *in vivo* and *in vitro.*[17–19,26] However, some observations, particularly at the clinical level, suggest functional similarities of these cells with the human splenic MZ B cells.[27,28]

In recent years, in an attempt to gain further insight into the human extrafollicular B cells, our laboratories have undertaken studies aimed at characterizing and purifying tonsillar subepithelial B cells *in vitro*. This review will briefly summarize the results of such studies and will compare the features of SE B cells with those of FM and GC B cells.

IN SITU DEFINITION OF THE PHENOTYPIC, ULTRASTRUCTURAL, AND CYTOCHEMICAL FEATURES OF TONSILLAR SE B CELLS

These studies have led to the definition of certain features of SE B cells that can help in distinguishing them from both GC and FM B cells. *In situ* staining with mAbs demonstrated that the cells located underneath the epithelial cryptae and also within the epithelial lining of the tonsils are represented primarily by B cells. In these areas, there are a few macrophages (some of which are clearly activated) and T cells. SE B cells can be identified through the expression of pan-B cell markers (CD20 or CD19), although characteristically they express low levels or no CD21, CD22, and CD24. CD10 and CD77, which are abundantly expressed by GC B cells, are virtually absent in SE B cells, whereas CD38 (another typical GC B cell marker) is present only on a minority of SE B cells that appear to be activated. There is, however, a substantial proportion of CD38+ plasma cells and of activated macrophages in the SE area. The typical marker of FM B cells, CD23, is absent in the SE B cells. Likewise, CD39 mAbs, although staining strongly FM B cells, fail to stain SE B cells, except for a few activated B cells. CD44, which is abundant on FM B cells, is dishomogeneously expressed by SE B cells and at a lower level. This marker is typically absent in GC B cells. Ki67, a marker of cycling cells, is expressed by GC B cells, but is virtually absent in the FM and SE areas. The predominant surface isotype of SE B cells is IgM, whereas IgD is much less expressed (FIGURE 1), and IgA and IgG are found on a minority of cells. This is at variance with that determined for GC B cells, which bear mainly surface IgG, and for FM B cells, which express both surface IgM and IgD.

Collectively, the above data demonstrate that the majority of tonsillar SE B cells are resting cells characterized by a surface phenotype (CD19+, CD21±, CD23−, CD39−, CD10−, CD38±, CD44±, IgM+, IgD±, and IgA−) that is different from that of both FM B cells (CD39+, CD23+, CD44+, IgM+, IgD+) and GC B cells (CD10+, CD77+, CD38+, IgG+).

In situ analysis of the morphological features of SE B cells at both light and electron microscopy levels revealed that they are different from both FM and GC cells (FIGURES 2 and 3). Compared to the FM B cells, SE B cells are larger, with an extended cytoplasm containing numerous organelles and a prominent Golgi apparatus (FIGURE 2B). In addition, they have a characteristic distribution of the chromatin that confers a "speckled" morphology to the nuclei. GC B cells (FIGURES 3B and 3C) can be easily distinguished from both SE (FIGURE 2B) and FM (FIGURE 3A) B cells; centroblasts (FIGURE 3B) are larger cells, with blastlike features and a characteristic peripheral location of large nucleoli, and centrocytes display a typical indented nucleus (FIGURE 3C).

In situ analyses for the cytochemical localization of endogenous alkaline phosphatase (ALP) demonstrated that SE (but not GC or FM) B cells are positive for this enzyme activity. In this respect, SE B cells resemble the B cells of the splenic marginal zone that also express ALP activity.

PREPARATION OF PURIFIED SUSPENSIONS OF RESTING SE B CELLS

In our studies, the strategy used to purify B cell subset populations consisted of a first step in which human tonsillar B cells were fractionated on Percoll density gradients and a second step in which the different cell fractions were further separated by means of immune-rosetting methods with mAbs. The whole procedure is depicted

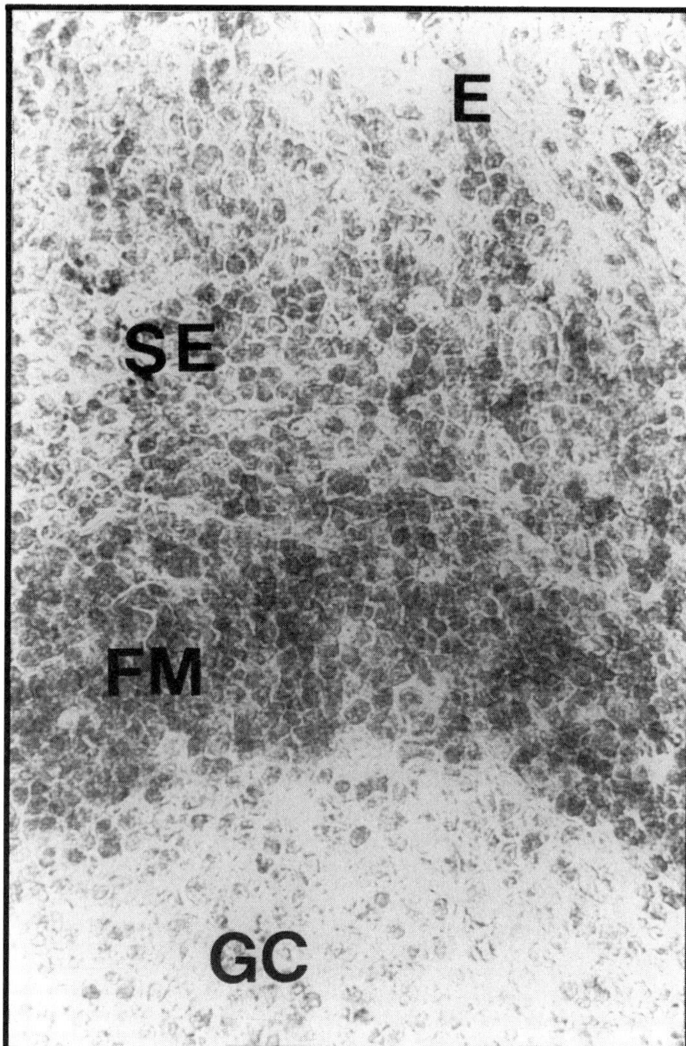

FIGURE 1. *In situ* expression of IgD of tonsillar SE regions. SE regions are localized between the epithelial lining of the cryptae (E) and the follicular mantle (FM) of a secondary follicle. The germinal center of the secondary follicle is indicated (GC). Staining for surface IgD demonstrates that virtually all of the FM B cells are positive, whereas only a proportion of SE B cells are stained. Magnification: ×300.

in FIGURE 4, which also provides the phenotypic features of the different cell subpopulations. Tonsillar B cells were fractionated into resting, activated, and large B cells on Percoll gradients (see FIGURE 4). The resting B cells were subsequently separated into CD5+ and CD5− B cells. GC B cells were found in the large cell

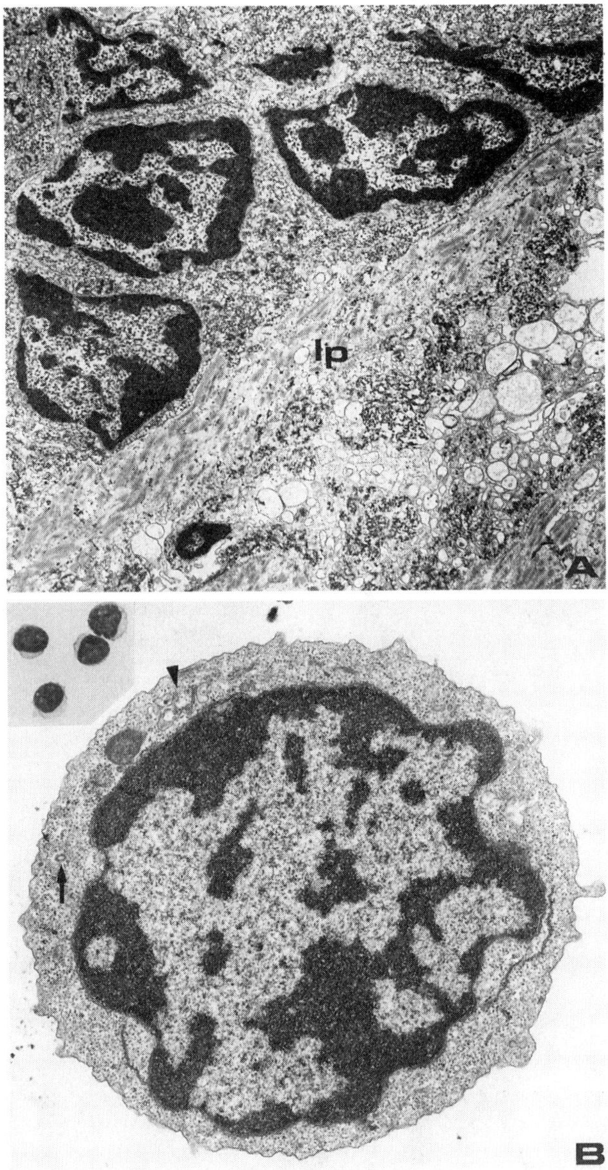

FIGURE 2. Ultrastructural features of tonsillar SE cells *in situ* and in suspension. (A) Several lymphocytes with characteristically "speckled" nuclei are found in the vicinity of collagen bundles in the tonsillar lamina propria (lp). (B) A lymphocyte in the tonsillar SE fraction shows a chromatin organization similar to that of the cells in panel A. Isolated strands of rough endoplasmic reticulum are detected in the cytoplasm, together with a coated vesicle (arrow) and smooth vesicles (arrowhead). (Inset) Morphology of SE B cells under light microscopy. Panels: A, ×6450; B, ×16,100. (Figure reduced to 67%.)

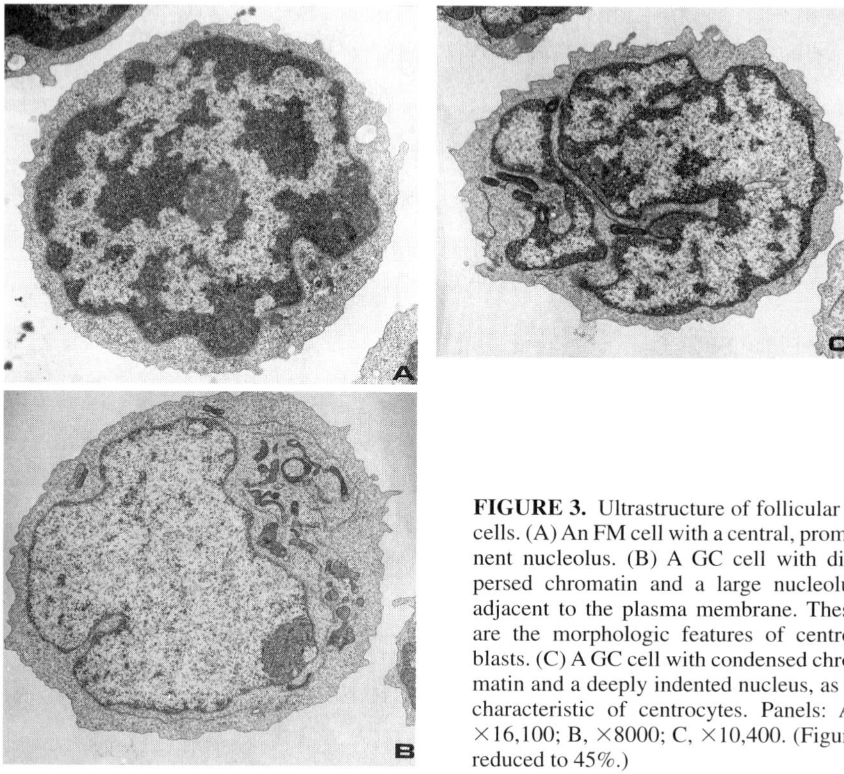

FIGURE 3. Ultrastructure of follicular B cells. (A) An FM cell with a central, prominent nucleolus. (B) A GC cell with dispersed chromatin and a large nucleolus adjacent to the plasma membrane. These are the morphologic features of centroblasts. (C) A GC cell with condensed chromatin and a deeply indented nucleus, as is characteristic of centrocytes. Panels: A, ×16,100; B, ×8000; C, ×10,400. (Figure reduced to 45%.)

fractions; however, they were contaminated by a variable number of IgD+ CD39+ B cells, which had to be removed by an immune-rosetting procedure.

Although the resting CD5+ B cells comprised almost exclusively FM B cells (CD39+, CD23+, CD10−, CD38−, IgM+, IgD+), CD5− B cells largely comprised SE B cells as demonstrated by their expression of abundant surface IgM and relatively scarce surface IgD, and by the low expression or absence of CD21, CD23, CD38, CD10, and CD77. Notably, SE B cells isolated in this manner comprised only resting SE B cells, as also documented by a lack of surface activation markers. Thus, these SE B cells represented only a part (albeit probably a major one) of the SE B cells characterized *in situ,* which comprised also a minority of activated cells. These *in vivo* activated cells were likely to copurify within the activated B cell fraction (see FIGURE 4). The majority of this fraction, in fact, consisted of cells with the features of FM B cells (IgM+, IgD+, CD23+, CD39+). It is possible, although not formally proven, that the SE B cells present in the activated cell fraction expressed surface IgG. In connection with this, it is of interest that Liu *et al.* recently isolated tonsillar memory B cells (defined on the basis of surface IgG expression) and found that these cells had features compatible with those of *in vivo* activated SE B cells.[29] In analyzing the data reported in FIGURE 4, it is important to note the following finding: although all of the

FM B cells from the resting cell fraction expressed CD5, only a proportion of the FM B cells from the activated cell fraction were CD5+. This finding raises questions about the possible heterogeneity of FM cells. Moreover, because CD5 expression often correlates with specific cellular functions, such as the capacity to produce polyspecific antibody or to respond to polyclonal B cell activators *in vitro,* these findings open up interesting avenues regarding a potential heterogeneity in the function of FM B cells.

FUNCTIONAL STUDIES ON PURIFIED SE B CELLS

Purified SE B cells were tested for a number of functional features *in vitro* and were compared with the B cells of the other subsets described above. Because these studies relate to different experimental procedures, they will be analyzed separately. TABLE 1 summarizes all of the functional data obtained in these experiments.

Response to Thymus-independent (TI) Antigens in Vitro

Response of the various B cell subsets to TI-1 antigens was analyzed by stimulating the cells with TNP-Ba (prototype of TI-1 antigens) or TNP-Ficoll (TI-2 antigen). The response to TNP was subsequently measured by a very sensitive ELI

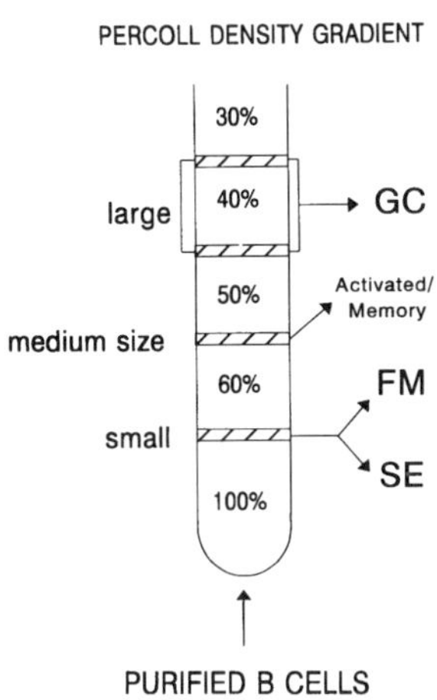

	CD21	CD10	CD38	CD39	CD23	CD44	IgM	IgD	IgG	IgA	ALP
GC	+	++	++	–	–	–	(–)	–	+	+	–
Activated/Memory	+	–	±	++	+	++	+	+	(+)	–	–
FM	+	–	–	+	++	++	+	+	–	–	–
SE	±	–	±	–	–	+	+	±	–	–	+

FIGURE 4. Schematic diagram of the procedure for the purification of different tonsillar B cell subsets and surface marker analyses. The procedure to purify the different B cell subsets is depicted on the left. Briefly, purified B cells were separated into fractions of different density by centrifugation through discontinuous Percoll gradients. SE and FM B cells were separated from the highest density fraction (60% Percoll) by an immune-rosetting procedure. GC B cells were isolated by depletion of IgD+ and CD39+ B cells from the large B cell fraction (30–40% Percoll). On the right, a summary of the phenotypical analyses of the purified SE, FM, activated/memory, and GC B cells detected by immunofluorescence is shown.

spot assay. SE B cells were able to mount a good response to TI-2 antigens, but not to TI-1 antigens. Their response was observed only in the presence of IL2 (and not of other cytokines such as IL3, IL4, IL5, IL6, or IL10) and did not require the simultaneous addition of T cells to the cultures. FM and GC B cells did not produce anti-TNP antibodies in response to TNP-Ba or TNP-Ficoll, even when the cytokines mentioned above were added to the cultures. In contrast, activated B cells formed a substantial number of ELI spots to TNP in response to IL2 alone and the proportion of these spots was increased upon exposure of the cells to TNP-Ba (and not to TNP-Ficoll). Collectively, these data indicate that the capacity of responding to TI-2 antigens is a unique feature of SE B cells. Moreover, the aforementioned observations in both humans and experimental animals indicate that the MZ of the spleen is the site of active response to TI-2 antigens.[17–19,26] These data are therefore in accord with these concepts and seem to stress further the notion that, in tonsils, the SE area represents the equivalent of the splenic MZ. Furthermore, these results obtained with

TABLE 1. Summary of the Major Functional Features of the Predominant B Cell Subsets from Human Tonsils

B Cell Subsets	Response to: TI-1 Ag	TI-2 Ag	Mitogens	Polyreactive Antibodies	Apoptosis	MLR	Recirculation
SE	−	++	−	−	−	++	−
FM	−	−	++	++	−	+/−	+
GC	−	−	+	−	++	nd[a]	?
activated/memory	+/−	−	++	+	−	nd	+

[a]nd = not determined.

purified B cell suspensions *in vitro* lend support to the hypothesis that the capacity of responding to TI-2 antigens is an intrinsic capacity of MZ B cells and of their equivalent B cells, rather than related to the presence of special accessory cells in the anatomical areas where these B cells home.

Capacity to Recirculate

Experiments in rats and mice have determined that the B cells of the splenic MZ are resident cells with scarce capacities to recirculate.[14,20,21] That this is the case also for the human B cells from the splenic MZ or the equivalent areas in other lymphoid tissues is suggested by observations on the mode of spreading of lymphoproliferative disorders originating from this subset of B cells.[30,31] It was, therefore, of interest to determine whether cells with the properties of tonsillar SE B cells could be found in the circulation. Two observations, however, appear to exclude this possibility. First, the large majority of peripheral blood B cells have a surface phenotype that resembles that of FM B cells because they express CD23, CD39, surface IgM and IgD, and high levels of CD44. In addition, there are very few, if any, B cells that express IgM only (i.e., in the absence of surface IgD). Second, peripheral blood B cells do not have the ability to respond to TI-2 antigens (i.e., TNP-Ficoll), although they can mount a substantial response to TI-1 antigens.

Production of Polyspecific Antibodies and Spontaneous Apoptosis in Vitro

When appropriately stimulated *in vitro,* FM B cells produce IgM antibodies to a variety of antigens, including self-antigens, such as human IgG, ssDNA, and dsDNA. GC B cells undergo spontaneous apoptosis *in vitro.* These features have been taken as functional hallmarks for FM and GC B cells, respectively. In order to collect further information on SE B cells, we have tested whether they had the capacity to produce polyspecific antibodies or to undergo spontaneous apoptosis *in vitro.*[8,12] However, it was found that, upon infection and transformation with EBV *in vitro,* the cell lines that originated from SE B cells failed to produce polyspecific antibodies. In contrast, the cell lines that originated from FM B cells under identical experimental conditions produced substantial titers of polyspecific antibodies. Likewise, SE B cells consistently failed to undergo apoptosis *in vitro* under circumstances in which GC B cells would undergo apoptosis readily. In this respect, they appear to constitute a distinct B cell subset.

Antigen Presentation

The anatomical localization of SE B cells in an area that is heavily exposed to antigens of pathogens penetrating through the epithelial lining of the tonsillar cryptae suggested that, perhaps, they are capable of efficiently presenting antigens to T cells. This notion could be possibly reinforced by some of the morphological features of SE B cells characterized by an extended endosomal compartment. Because the capacity to elicit a mixed leukocyte reaction (MLR) *in vitro* mimics the cell antigen-presenting capacities, we tested the ability of SE B cells to stimulate allogeneic T cells purified from both adult and cord blood. SE B cells were found to be good MLR stimulators of both responder T cell types. In order to exert this function, however, SE B cells had to be preactivated by exposure to anti-μ-ab. Under these experimental conditions, SE B cells proved to be MRL stimulators almost as efficient as dendritic cells (DC) prepared from peripheral blood monocytes. FM B cells were found to be poor MLR stimulators even when preactivated by exposure to anti-μ-ab. It is of interest, in connection with this, that stimulation with anti-μ-ab induced the expression of activation molecules such as CD80, CD86, CD69, and CD95 in both FM and SE B cells. Moreover, it was found that both CD86 and CD80 were involved in MLR stimulation as documented by the inhibition of MLR obtained by addition of the relevant mAbs to the culture. The failure of FM B cells to elicit an MLR despite their capacity to express activation molecules upon stimulation with CD80 and CD86 indicates that the sole expression of these structures may not be sufficient per se to confer antigen-presenting capacities *in vitro.*

Response to Polyclonal B Cell Activators

Initial studies on the capacity of tonsillar resting CD5− B cells demonstrated that they consistently failed to proliferate or to produce Ig molecules in response to polyclonal B cell activators including SAC, anti-μ-ab, and CD40 mAb, even in combination with several cytokines. In contrast, resting CD5+ B cells and the CD5+ and CD5− B cells from the activated B cell fraction were induced to proliferate and to produce Ig molecules in response to the same mitogens. These initial studies led one to suspect that the tonsillar CD5− B cells were indeed SE B cells, especially in view of similar studies on murine splenic MZ B cells showing that these cells were characterized by a poor-to-absent response to polyclonal activators. Further studies along this line confirmed the incapacity of SE B cells to respond to polyclonal B cell activators, including CD40 mAb presented by fibroblasts transfected with the appropriate Fc receptor. In striking contrast, it was found that SE B cells could be induced to mount a proliferative response and to differentiate into Ig-secreting plasma cells by coculture with activated T cells. These observations have a number of implications. For example, the *in vitro* system constituted by SE B cells and activated T cells represents a very useful tool to study T-B cell interactions. Moreover, the observation that SE B cells require a close interaction with T cells in order to be activated polyclonally, whereas responding readily to TI-2 antigens in the absence of T cells, raises the question of a possible heterogeneity of SE B cells. Finally, the incapacity to respond to polyclonal B cell activators may represent a hallmark of SE B cells that helps to distinguish them from other B cell subsets.

CONCLUDING REMARKS

In these studies, we have outlined several distinguishing features of a subset of resting tonsillar B cells that appear to home in the subepithelial areas. These are virgin B cells and can be distinguished from other virgin B cell subsets (i.e., FM B cells) or activated B cells (i.e., GC B cells and other low-density cells) based upon a variety of phenotypic, morphologic, and functional features. It is possible that these cells represent the prototypic cells of the so-called extrafollicular B cells of humans, which also include the splenic MZ B cells. Thus, they can be useful to further investigate functional features and especially the mode of response to antigens by this specialized B cell subset population.

REFERENCES

1. Hsu, S-M., J-W. Waldron, P-L. Hsu & J. Haugh. 1993. Prog. Pathol. **24:** 1040–1057.
2. Clark, E. A. & J. A. Ledbetter. 1994. Nature **367:** 425–428.
3. Stein, H., A. Bonk, G. Tolksdorf, K. Lennert, H. Rodt & J. Gerdes. 1980. J. Histochem. Cytochem. **28:** 746–760.
4. Möller, G., Ed. 1992. Germinal Centers in the Immune Response. Immunol. Rev. Volume 126.
5. Thorbecke, G. J., A. R. Amin & V. K. Tsiagbe. 1994. FASEB J. **8:** 832–840.
6. Kelsoe, G. 1994. J. Exp. Med. **180:** 5–6.

7. LIU, Y-J., G. D. JOHNSON, J. GORDON & I. C. M. MACLENNAN. 1992. Immunol. Today **13:** 17–21.
8. LIU, Y-J., D. E. JOSHUA, G. T. WILLIAMS, C. A. SMITH, J. GORDON & I. C. M. MACLENNAN. 1989. Nature **342:** 929–931.
9. ZUPO, S., E. RUGARI, M. DONO, G. TABORELLI, F. MALAVASI & M. FERRARINI. 1994. Eur. J. Immunol. **24:** 1218–1222.
10. PASCUAL, V., Y-J. LIU, A. MAGALSKI, O. DE BOUTEILLER, J. BANCHEREAU & D. CAPRA. 1994. J. Exp. Med. **180:** 329–339.
11. DONO, M., S. ZUPO, R. MASANTE, G. TABORELLI, N. CHIORAZZI & M. FERRARINI. 1993. Eur. J. Immunol. **23:** 873–881.
12. ZUPO, S., M. DONO, L. AZZONI, N. CHIORAZZI & M. FERRARINI. 1991. Eur. J. Immunol. **21:** 351–359.
13. MÖLLER, P. & B. MIELKE. 1989. Extrafollicular peripheral B cell report. *In* Leucocyte Typing IV. W. Knapp, B. Dörken, W. R. Gilks, E. P. Rieber, R. E. Schmidt, H. Stein & A. E. G. Kr. von dem Borne, Eds.: 213–214. Oxford University Press. London/New York.
14. MACLENNAN, I. & E. CHAN. 1993. Immunol. Today **14:** 29–34.
15. DUNN-WALTERS, D. K., P. G. ISAACSON & J. SPENCER. 1995. J. Exp. Med. **182:** 559–568.
16. TIMENS, W. & S. POPPEMA. 1985. Am. J. Pathol. **120:** 443–454.
17. MOSIER, D. E. & B. SUBBARAO. 1982. Immunol. Today **3:** 217–222.
18. AMLOT, P. L., D. GRENNAN & J. H. HUMPHREY. 1985. Eur. J. Immunol. **15:** 508–512.
19. MOSIER, D. E., J. J. MOND & E. A. GOLDINGS. 1977. J. Immunol. **119:** 1874–1881.
20. GRAY, D., I. C. M. MACLENNAN, H. BAZIN & H. KHAN. 1982. Eur. J. Immunol. **12:** 564–572.
21. KUMARARATNE, D. S. & I. C. M. MACLENNAN. 1981. Eur. J. Immunol. **11:** 865–869.
22. MORENTE, M., M. A. PIRIS, J. L. ORRADRE, C. RIVAS & R. VILLUENDAS. 1992. J. Clin. Pathol. **45:** 668–672.
23. VAN DER OORD, J. J., C. DE WOLF–PEETERS & V. J. DESMET. 1986. Am. J. Clin. Pathol. **86:** 475–479.
24. MÖLLER, P., B. MIELKE & W. J. HOFMANN. 1989. Immunophenotype of medullary thymic B cells. *In* Leucocyte Typing IV. W. Knapp, B. Dörken, W. R. Gilks, E. P. Rieber, R. E. Schmidt, H. Stein & A. E. G. Kr. von dem Borne, Eds.: 222–224. Oxford University Press. London/New York.
25. SPENCER, J., T. FINN, K. A. F. PULFORD, D. Y. MASON & P. G. ISAACSON. 1985. Clin. Exp. Immunol. **62:** 607–612.
26. AMLOT, P. L. & A. E. HAYES. 1985. Lancet **I:** 1008–1011.
27. KÄYHTY, H., V. KARANKO, H. PELTOLA & P. H. MÄKELÄ. 1984. Pediatrics **74:** 857–866.
28. SMITH, D. H., G. PETER, D. L. INGRAM, A. L. HARDING & P. ANDERSON. 1973. Pediatrics **52:** 637–643.
29. LIU, Y-J., C. BARTHELEMY, O. DE BOUTEILLER, C. ARPIN, I. DURAND & J. BANCHEREAU. 1995. Immunity **2:** 239–254.
30. WOTHERSPOON, A. C., C. DOGLIONI, T. C. DISS, L. PAN, A. MOSCHINI, M. DE BONI & P. G. ISAACSON. 1993. Lancet **342:** 575–577.
31. QIN, Y., A. GREINER, M. J. F. TRUNK, B. SCHMAUSSER, M. OTT & K. MÜLLER-HERMELINK. 1995. Blood **9:** 3528–3537.

Natural Autoantibodies, Tolerance, and Autoimmunity

G. DIGHIERO

Unité d'Immunohématologie et d'Immunopathologie
Institut Pasteur
75724 Paris Cedex 15, France

There is evidence indicating that autoreactive B cells constitute a substantial part of the B cell repertoire. This autoreactive repertoire secretes the so-called natural autoantibodies (NAA), characterized by their broad reactivity mainly directed against very well conserved public epitopes. They fulfill the definition of an autoantibody because they are self-reactive, but they are not self-specific. As yet, NAA directed against determinants of polymorphism have not been reported. Their germinal origin is suggested by their early appearance during ontogeny, by their expression of cross-reactive idiotopes, and by structural studies of their sequence.

As for the physiological role of this repertoire, we can assume that it may play a major role as a first barrier of defense. It is presently unknown whether these polyreactive B cells could constitute a preimmune template that, through an antigen-driven process, may be involved in the production of immune high-affinity antibodies.

The presence of this repertoire in normal conditions challenges the clonal deletion theory as a unique explanation for self-tolerance. However, if we take into account that this autoreactive B cell repertoire is not self-specific, this contradiction may not be a real opposition. This repertoire may be the price to pay for ensuring self-tolerance. It may escape clonal deletion and be induced into a compartment submitted to stringent regulation by its connectivity. In contrast, true anti-self-B cell clones may be submitted to very strict regulation through clonal deletion, receptor editing, or very stringent anergic mechanisms. However, it is important to keep in mind that pathogenic autoantibodies share binding specificities with NAA, in the sense that they are not self-specific and recognize public epitopes shared by all individuals of a given species and even shared by individuals belonging to phylogenetically distant species.

The relationship between NAA and pathological autoantibodies is also presently unclear. It has not been definitively established whether pathological autoantibodies are the consequence of polyclonal stimulation, resulting in increased levels of germline-encoded NAA, or whether they are derived via an antigen-driven somatic mutation process operating in these NAA precursors. Although there are convincing results, indicating that the generation of pathogenic autoantibodies may be the consequence of an antigen-driven process, this has not been firmly established in the case of human pathogenic autoantibodies. It cannot be excluded that both polyclonal activation and antigen-driven selection of the pathogenic antibody could synergize in the case of systemic autoimmune diseases. It also remains as yet unclear whether germline-encoded natural autoantibodies could serve as a template for pathogenic autoantibodies or whether these may derive from a different B cell.

HISTORICAL BACKGROUND

In the early 1900s, an important controversy between the German and French schools helped establish the notion of tolerance and autoimmunity. In 1900, the group of Metchnikoff suggested the concept of autoimmunization by demonstrating the presence of autoantibodies in normal conditions;[1,2] this was opposed to the concept of horror autotoxicus raised by Ehrlich.[3,4] Nearly at the same time, Landsteiner described the rules governing blood compatibility.[5] He showed that a subject belonging to group A will never be able to produce anti-A antibodies. These results provided strong support for Ehrlich's idea. The influence of Ehrlich's idea was so strong that the experiments from the Metchnikoff school were forgotten and, when Donath and Landsteiner described for the first time an autoantibody, namely, the biphasic hemagglutinin responsible for the paroxystic "Frigore" hemoglobinuria, they failed to call it an autoantibody.[6] In 1949, Burnet and Fenner proposed the clonal deletion theory.[7] This theory was strongly influenced by the experiments carried out by Owen with dizygotic calves sharing a single placenta.[8] These two calves were mixing their red blood cells, but—despite the fact that they were expressing different blood groups—they were unable to produce alloantibodies against the blood groups from the other calf. The interpretation of these experiments and the experiments from Medawar's group,[9] which demonstrated that injection of newborn mice with spleen or marrow cells from an unrelated strain of mice enables these animals to accept skin grafts from the second strain, led both groups to conclude that during embryonic life the immune system learns to tolerate self-antigens.[7,9,10] The clonal deletion theory was a magnificent theory explaining tolerance and autoimmunity in a simple way. Autoimmunity, according to this theory, will only arise in the case of somatic mutations, which are unusual phenomena.

However, in 1956, Witebsky and Rose[11] were able for the first time to induce an experimental autoimmune disease mediated by autoantibodies: autoimmune thyroiditis. They succeeded in inducing this disease by injecting thyroglobulin in the presence of Freund's adjuvant. During the last several years, considerable data have accumulated that raise doubts concerning the clonal deletion theory as a general explanation for tolerance because (1) autoimmune diseases have been induced by injecting organ extracts,[11] (2) numerous autoantibodies have been demonstrated under normal conditions,[12] (3) the presence of normal autoreactive B cells has also been demonstrated,[13] and (4) autoantibodies have been induced from normal B lymphocytes upon mitogenic stimulation.[14] Because they were able to produce autoantibodies, the precursor B cells producing these autoantibodies should exist.

NATURAL AUTOANTIBODIES ARE AN IMPORTANT COMPONENT OF THE NORMAL B CELL REPERTOIRE

In collaboration with Guilbert and Avrameas,[15] we immobilized nine different antigens (tubulin, actin, thyroglobulin, myoglobin, fetuin, albumin, transferrin, collagen, and cytochrome c) on ACA beads. Sera from normal donors were successively run through the nine immunoadsorbents, from which we constantly eluted Ig (IgG, 70%; IgM and IgA, 15% each) natural autoantibodies (NAA) directed against immobilized antigen. Lutz and Wipf,[16] nearly at the same time, were able to demonstrate the constant presence of NAA against spectrin. These results agree with those from other groups reporting the presence, in normal serum, of NAA directed against different autoantigens.[17–21]

The presence of NAA under normal conditions implies, of necessity, the presence of autoreactive B lymphocytes. In order to demonstrate the presence of these B cell precursors, we employed hybridoma technology to fuse unimmunized BALB/c splenocytes with nonsecreting myelomas. Results indicated the presence, with high frequency, of hybridomas with NAA specificity.[22,23] Subsequently, Monier *et al.*[24] reported similar results with BALB/c mice and Prabhakar *et al.*[25] reported hybridomas derived from B lymphocytes of SJL/J or BALB/cJ mice that showed multiple organ reactivity. Idiotypic studies showed that these NAA displayed a high degree of connectivity.[26–32] In humans, Shoenfeld *et al.*[33,34] reported, for the first time, this type of autoantibody from B lymphocytes of lupic patients. Soon after, Notkins' group reported the presence of multiple-organ-reactive human monoclonal autoantibodies derived from normal B lymphocytes.[35,36] These results have been confirmed and extended by several groups using hybridoma technology, EBV immortalization, or both.[37–39]

Overall, these results indicate that, in normal serum, a substantial proportion of circulating Ig's are indeed NAA and that the precursors of this autoreactive repertoire account for a substantial part of normal B cells. Because these autoantibodies express recurrent idiotopes, express V genes frequently in germinal configuration, and predominate early in life, they represent the expression of the germinal repertoire.[40] Interestingly, this repertoire has been found in species phylogenetically distant from mammals, such as fish and batracians.[41] They are autoantibodies because they bind autoantigens. However, they are not self-specific because nobody has been able to demonstrate these types of autoantibodies against very critical self-antigens like the A and B red blood cell groups. On the contrary, these autoantibodies bind public epitopes shared by all individuals belonging to a given species and even antigens that are well conserved during evolution. However, this is also characteristic of pathogenic autoantibodies observed in autoimmune diseases. For instance, anti–red blood cell autoantibodies recognize public antigens; anti-DNA from SLE patients recognize human, rat, and murine DNA; anti-AChR autoantibodies recognize human and even fish receptors; etc.[40]

Thus, we have evolved from Ehrlich's horror autotoxicus notion to Burnet's forbidden clones hypothesis to reach now the view that autoimmunity is a normal physiological phenomenon. However, how can we reconcile the experiments of

Metchnikoff with the experiments of Ehrlich and Landsteiner because all these results could never be challenged.

Experiments with transgenic mice allow the integration of all this experimental evidence. The group of Nemazee has created double-transgenic mice expressing H-2Kk and anti-H2k transgenes. This is a very critical situation because the transgene is recognizing a determinant of polymorphism, that is, a real self-antigen. According to Burnet's prediction, B cells expressing the anti-H2k transgene were stringently downregulated through programmed cell death (PCD) and receptor editing.[42,43] However, in the case of Ig transgenes with autoantibody activity, which is not directed against critical self-polymorphism, the transgene is not deleted; it is simply downregulated or anergized. In double-transgenic mice expressing HEL and anti-HEL transgenes, B cells were downregulated.[44,45] B cells were also downregulated through anergy and receptor editing in transgenic mice expressing pathogenic anti-DNA transgenes.[46]

These experiments allow us to understand the apparent discrepancy between Ehrlich, Landsteiner, and Metchnikoff. Indeed, a subject expressing the A or B group will never produce typical autoantibodies against these determinants and no autoimmune hemolytic anemias displaying autoantibodies with such specificities have been reported. However, the production of autoantibodies against public antigens like the I group is a common phenomenon. Hemolytic anemia autoantibodies are mainly directed against these public antigens. Hence, the B cell repertoire that is going to be directed against polymorphic determinants will be probably submitted to very stringent negative selection, that is, deletion or stringent receptor editing mechanisms, whereas the repertoire that is directed against public determinants is probably not deleted and is an important component of the normal immune repertoire.

POLYREACTIVITY OF NATURAL AUTOANTIBODIES

One interesting and puzzling characteristic of these polyreactive natural autoantibodies is their broad reactivity. The simultaneous binding of these antibodies to several different cytoskeleton proteins, DNA, and different haptens, or to multiple organs, has been clearly demonstrated.[15,21,22,25,26,35–37,47–53] This widespread reactivity raises the question of the epitope(s) recognized by these antibodies. Because no evident homologies exist between such dissimilar molecules as proteins, nucleic acids, and polysaccharides, which are simultaneously recognized by some NAA, no definitive explanation for these cross-reactivities is presently available. The possibility that the antibody site simultaneously accommodates several different antigens has been advanced on the basis of results derived from crystallographic studies.[54] It has also been speculated that the charge distribution within the antibody site could account for immunological cross-reactions with diverse and unrelated substances sharing similarities in charge distribution.[55] Finally, the possibility that antibodies and antigens could cooperate to establish a better interaction through conformational changes has also been hypothesized.[55] Understanding of the molecular principles that govern antibody specificity and cross-reactivity remains a major challenge. Data from crystallographic studies demonstrated that degenerate binding of a similar structural motif did not require the existence of sequence homology or other chemical similarities, nor did it need be associated with particular physicochemical features of the interacting molecular surfaces. Hence, despite the absence of amino acid sequence homology in the CDRs, two different antilysozyme antibodies could establish contacts with very close epitopes in lysozyme.[56] In addition, seven amino acids of the anti-HEL D1.3 antilysozyme antibody were involved in interactions with both lysozyme and anti-idiotope antibody.[57] In these and other models, cross-reacting molecular surfaces did not show obvious structural similarities. Indeed, molecular surface adaptability appears to be a general principle underlying promiscuity in protein-protein interactions and it is presently unclear whether polyreactivity can be explained through this mechanism.

FUNCTION OF NATURAL AUTOANTIBODIES

What is the role of this B cell repertoire that we know is a prevalent repertoire? It might constitute an archaic immune system that could play a role as a first line of defense. Interestingly, this NAA polyreactive repertoire has been found to be prevalent in fish and batracians. We know that these animals are unable to make somatic mutations and to produce highly specific, high-affinity antibodies. Hence, their repertoire is much less diverse.[58] When the possibility of high diversification is absent, probably the only possible strategy is to produce these polyreactive, low-affinity antibodies. The reason why they are conserved during evolution is probably to serve as a first barrier of defense. Even with a memory response to a foreign antigen, it takes 5 to 6 days to obtain high-affinity antibodies. This polyreactive NAA repertoire might be the system that is coping with aggression during this time. Agammaglobulinemic children, dying very early in life, were improved just by injecting polyvalent gamma globulins every 21 days. Injecting polyvalent gamma globulins into these children is probably providing them with NAA and thus a first barrier of defense.

In 1983,[22] while reporting our results with murine hybridomas displaying NAA B activity and derived from BALB/c mice, we postulated the following: "If correct, this hypothesis would imply that these B cells carry a polyspecific receptor capable of fixing several different antigens. During active immunization, the binding of a given antigen to this receptor would then induce the corresponding B cell by a series of divisions and mutations, which, under the selective pressure of the antigen, would lead to the production of highly specific antibodies for a given epitope of these antigens. In that case, these B cells and their receptors would then be encoded by the germline, and the natural polyspecific antibodies would constitute the synthesized products secreted by these cells." This provocative hypothesis assumed that NAA were the product of the germline repertoire and that they constituted a template upon which antigen-driven selection and somatic mutation could operate to derive highly specific immune antibodies.

The germline origin was substantiated during the following years because (1) polyreactive NAA appear to predominate early during ontogeny,[23] even in germ-antigen-free animals,[59] (2) NAA express recurrent idiotypes[26–29,31,32] and appear to be highly interconnected,[30] and (3) structural studies have demonstrated their germinal origin[55,60–63] and the fact that these autoantibodies are encoded by structural genetic elements similar to those employed by nonautoimmune antibodies.[64]

The template hypothesis is still awaiting an experimental verification. Only indirect evidence has been obtained as yet. Napastek *et al.*[65] have studied a set of antibodies that use the $V_H Id^{CR}$ gene, employed for the antiarsonate system. They have found that germline-encoded antibodies of this system do not bind arsonate, but display a polyreactive pattern of binding by reacting with DNA and cytoskeleton proteins. Upon immunization with arsonate, the $V_H Ig^{CR}$ gene undergoes somatic mutations, allowing it to become a high-affinity antiarsonate antibody. This process is accompanied by loss of NAA activity. Guilbert *et al.*[66] studied hybridomas derived from mice previously immunized with several different antigens and reported that, besides hybrids binding to specific immunizing antigen, they could obtain hybrids binding to not only specific antigen, but also to self-antigen, suggesting that the latter could be in an intermediate stage between the preimmune and the specifically immune repertoire.

RELATIONSHIP BETWEEN NATURAL AND PATHOGENIC AUTOANTIBODIES

The relationship between natural and pathogenic autoantibodies remains as yet elusive. Two alternative views have been advanced to explain autoantibody production in autoimmune diseases.[67] The first proposes that they are the consequence of uncontrolled polyclonal stimulation of normal autoreactive B cells, resulting in increased levels of autoantibodies.[68] The second view assumes that pathological autoantibodies result from an antigen-driven selection process of autoreactive B cells, which, under the selective pressure of the antigen, undergo somatic mutations leading to the obtaining of pathological autoantibodies.[69,70] A more eclectic view tries to reconcile both ideas by admitting that the early IgM autoantibodies are polyclonally activated and that antigen-driven selection occurs in a second step.

The polyclonal activation model is supported by the following facts: (a) spontaneous polyclonal stimulation is constantly observed during systemic autoimmune diseases;[71,72] (b) polyclonal B cell stimulation, upon mitogenic stimulation, induces production of autoantibodies against DNA, against the Fc of IgG, and against erythrocytes;[67,73–76] (c) chronic polyclonal stimulation can induce autoimmune disease in genetically nonprone mice;[73–76] and (d) autoantibodies derived by hybridoma technology from lupic mice and lupus patients are frequently encoded by germline genes.[64]

Pathogenic autoantibody induction through an antigen-driven process is supported by the work from several laboratories. Initial results from Shlomchik *et al.* on murine hybridomas with anti-DNA[70] and RF activity[69] derived from MRL-lpr/lpr lupic mice showed evidence of numerous somatic mutations predominating in the CDR regions, thus favoring the view of a positive selection process induced by the antigen. In addition, results from different laboratories have demonstrated in mice that mutations inducing the appearance of arginines in the CDR3 V_H region are highly selected among pathogenic anti-DNA autoantibodies.[77–82] Arginine generation in the CDR3 V_H

region may occur through four different mechanisms:[83] (a) *N* sequence addition at the V_H-D_H or D_H-J_H junction; (b) D_H-D_H recombination; (c) a shift in the normal reading frame related to either *N* additions or D_H-D_H recombination; and (d) somatic mutations through the CDR3. As regards light chains, arginines in position 29 and in position 96 have been recurrently found among pathogenic anti-DNA autoantibodies. In humans, evidence has been obtained favoring an antigen-driven selection process in the generation of pathogenic rheumatoid factors.[84] In addition, the role of V gene mutation in the induction of pathogenic autoantibodies in humans is more difficult to establish because studies of the V gene expressed in normal circulating B cells have revealed that 80% of the circulating B cells appear to contain mutated V genes.[85,86]

CONCLUDING REMARKS

In conclusion, there is consistent evidence indicating that NAA account for a substantial part of the normal B cell repertoire. As for their role, it appears logical to assign them a role as a first barrier of defense, which could be favored by their polyreactive binding pattern. This characteristic may explain why this archaic immune repertoire has been kept during evolution and is still a preeminent repertoire in species disposing of very sophisticated mechanisms of diversification, as it is the case for mammals.

The presence of this repertoire in normal conditions challenges the clonal deletion theory as a unique explanation for self-tolerance. However, if we take into account that this autoreactive B cell repertoire is not self-specific, this contradiction may not be a definitive one. This repertoire may be the price to pay for ensuring self-tolerance. It may escape clonal deletion and be induced into a compartment submitted to stringent regulation by its connectivity.[30] In contrast, true antiself-B cell clones may be submitted to very strict regulation through clonal deletion, receptor editing, or very stringent anergic mechanisms. However, it is important to keep in mind that pathogenic autoantibodies share binding specificities with NAA, in the sense that they are not self-specific and recognize public epitopes shared by all individuals of a given species and even shared by individuals belonging to phylogenetically distant species. Although there is evidence indicating that pathogenic autoantibodies may derive through an antigen-driven process, it remains as yet unclear whether NAA germline-encoded antibodies could serve as a template for pathogenic autoantibodies or whether these may derive from a different B cell.

REFERENCES

1. METCHNIKOFF, S. 1900. Etudes sur la spermatoxine. Ann. Inst. Pasteur **9:** 577.
2. BESREDKA, M. 1901. Les anti-hémolysines naturelles. Ann. Inst. Pasteur **15:** 785.
3. EHRLICH, P. & J. MORGENROTH. 1957. On haemolysins: third communication. *In* The Collected Papers of Paul Ehrlich. Volume 2, p. 205–212. Pergamon. London.
4. EHRLICH, P. & J. MORGENROTH. 1957. On haemolysins: fifth communication. *In* The Collected Papers of Paul Ehrlich. Volume 2, p. 246–255. Pergamon. London.
5. LANDSTEINER, K. 1900. The Specificity of Serological Reactions. Volume 27, p. 357–371. Harvard University Press. Cambridge, Massachusetts.

6. DONATH, J. & K. LANDSTEINER. 1904. Uber paroxysmale hamoglobinurie. Munch. Med. Wochenschr. **51:** 1590–1595.
7. BURNET, F. M. & F. FENNER. 1949. The Production of Antibodies. Macmillan & Co. London.
8. OWEN, R. D. 1945. Immunogenetic consequences of vascular anastomoses between bovine cattle twins. Science **102:** 400–404.
9. BILLINGHAM, R. E., L. BRENT & P. B. MEDAWAR. 1953. Actively acquired tolerance of foreign cells. Nature **172:** 603.
10. BURNET, F. M. 1959. The Clonal Selection Theory of Acquired Immunity. Cambridge University Press. London/New York.
11. ROSE, N. R. & E. WITEBSKY. 1956. Studies on organ specificity: V changes in the thyroid glands of rabbits following acute immunization with rabbit thyroid extracts. J. Immunol. **76:** 417–428.
12. HOOPER, B., S. WHITTINGHAM & J. D. MATHEWS. 1972. Autoimmunity in a rural community. Clin. Immunol. **12:** 79–87.
13. MACKAY, I. R. 1983. Natural autoantibodies to the fore—forbidden clones to the rear? Immunol. Today **4:** 340–342.
14. IZUI, S., P. H. LAMBERT & G. L. FOUNIE. 1977. Features of systemic lupus erythematosus in mice infected with bacterial lipopolysaccharides. J. Exp. Med. **145:** 1115–1128.
15. GUILBERT, B., G. DIGHIERO & S. AVRAMEAS. 1982. Naturally occurring antibodies against nine common antigens in normal humans. I. Detection, isolation, and characterization. J. Immunol. **128:** 2779–2787.
16. LUTZ, H. U. & G. WIPF. 1982. Naturally occurring auto-antibodies to skeletal proteins from human red blood cells. J. Immunol. **128:** 1695–1701.
17. MARTIN, S. E. & W. J. MARTIN. 1975. Interspecies brain antigen detected by naturally occurring mouse anti-brain auto-antibody. Proc. Natl. Acad. Sci. U.S.A. **72:** 1036–1041.
18. MARTIN, W. J. & S. E. MARTIN. 1975. Thymus reactive IgM auto-antibodies in normal mouse sera. Nature **254:** 716–718.
19. WALFORD, R. L. 1969. The Immunologic Theory of Aging. Munksgaard. Copenhagen.
20. SELA, B. A., J. L. WANG & G. M. EDELMAN. 1975. Antibodies reactive with cell surface carbohydrates. Proc. Natl. Acad. Sci. U.S.A. **72:** 1127–1132.
21. DIGHIERO, G., P. LYMBERI, B. GUILBERT, T. TERNYNCK & S. AVRAMEAS. 1986. Natural autoantibodies constitute a substantial part of normal circulating immunoglobulins. Ann. N.Y. Acad. Sci. **475:** 135–145.
22. DIGHIERO, G., P. LYMBERI, J. C. MAZIÉ, S. ROUYRE, G. S. BUTLER-BROWNE, R. G. WHALEN & S. AVRAMEAS. 1983. Murine hybridomas secreting natural monoclonal antibodies reacting with self antigens. J. Immunol. **131:** 2267–2272.
23. DIGHIERO, G., P. LYMBERI, D. HOLMBERG, I. LUNDQUIST, A. COUTINHO & S. AVRAMEAS. 1985. High frequency of natural autoantibodies in normal newborn mice. J. Immunol. **134:** 765–771.
24. MONIER, J. C., J. BROCHIER, A. MOREIRA, C. SAULT & B. ROUX. 1984. Generation of hybridoma antibodies to double-stranded DNA from non-autoimmune BALB/c strain: studies on anti-idiotype. Immunol. Lett. **8:** 61–68.
25. PRABHAKAR, B. S., J. SAEGUSA, T. ONODERA & A. L. NOTKINS. 1984. Lymphocytes capable of making monoclonal autoantibodies that react with multiple organs are a common feature of the normal B cell repertoire. J. Immunol. **133:** 2815–2817.
26. RAUCH, J., E. MURPHY, J. B. ROTHS, B. D. STOLLAR & R. S. SCHWARTZ. 1982. A high frequency idiotypic marker of anti-DNA autoantibodies in MR-lpr/lpr mice. J. Immunol. **129:** 236–241.
27. TRON, F., C. L. LE GUERN, P. A. CAZENAVE & J. F. BACH. 1982. Intrastrain recurrent idiotypes among anti-DNA antibodies of (NZB/NZW)F1 hybrid mice. Eur. J. Immunol. **12:** 761–766.
28. MARION, T. N., A. R. LAWTON, J. F. KEARNEY & D. E. BRILES. 1982. Anti-DNA autoantibodies in (NZB × NZW)F1 mice are clonally heterogeneous, but a majority share a common idiotype. J. Immunol. **128:** 668–674.
29. ISENBERG, D. A., Y. SHOENFELD, M. R. MADAIO, J. RAUCH, M. REICHLIN & B. D. STOLLAR. 1983. Z-DNA specific antibodies in human systemic lupus erythematosus. J. Clin. Invest. **71:** 314–321.

30. HOLMBERG, D., S. FORSGREN, F. IVARS & A. COUTINHO. 1984. Reactions among IgM antibodies derived from normal, neonatal mice. Eur. J. Immunol. **14:** 435–440.
31. LYMBERI, P., G. DIGHIERO, T. TERNYNCK & S. AVRAMEAS. 1985. A high incidence of cross-reactive idiotypes among murine natural autoantibodies. Eur. J. Immunol. **15:** 702–707.
32. MATTHES, T. & G. DIGHIERO. 1988. Detection of private and recurrent idiotopes on natural anti-tubulin antibodies by monoclonal anti-idiotopic antibodies. J. Immunol. **140:** 148–154.
33. SHOENFELD, Y., S. C. HSU-LIN, J. E. GABRIELS, L. E. SILBERSTEIN, B. C. FURIE, B. D. STOLLAR & R. S. SCHWARTZ. 1982. Production of autoantibodies by human-human hybridomas. J. Clin. Invest. **70:** 205–208.
34. SHOENFELD, Y., J. RAUCH, H. MASSICOTTE, S. K. DATTA, J. ANDRÉ-SCHWARTZ, B. D. STOLLAR & R. S. SCHWARTZ. 1983. Polyspecificity of monoclonal lupus autoantibodies produced by human-human hybridomas. N. Engl. J. Med. **308:** 414–420.
35. SATOH, J., B. S. PRABHAKAR, M. V. HASPEL, F. GINSBERG-FELLNER & A. L. NOTKINS. 1983. Human monoclonal autoantibodies that react with multiple endocrine organs. N. Engl. J. Med. **309:** 217–220.
36. HASPEL, M. V., T. ONODERA, B. S. PRABHAKAR, K. E. MCCLINTOCK, U. R. RAY, S. YAGIHASHI & A. L. NOTKINS. 1983. Multiple organ-reactive monoclonal autoantibodies. Nature **304:** 74–76.
37. CAIRNS, E., J. BLOCK & D. A. BELL. 1984. Anti-DNA autoantibody producing hybridomas of normal human lymphoid cell origin. J. Clin. Invest. **74:** 880–887.
38. DIGHIERO, G., P. PONCET, S. ROUYRE & J. C. MAZIÉ. 1986. Newborn Xid mice carry the genetic information for the production of natural autoantibodies. J. Immunol. **136:** 4000–4006.
39. HASKARD, D. O., V. GUL, A. MORGAN, P. KATAAHA, N. A. STAINES & J. R. ARCHER. 1985. Human monoclonal autoantibodies from patients with rheumatoid arthritis against cellular constituents. Clin. Exp. Immunol. **61:** 496–502.
40. DIGHIERO, G. 1995. Natural autoantibodies in humans: their relevance in autoimmunity and lymphoproliferative disorders. Forum Trends Exp. Clin. Med. **5:** 58–71.
41. GONZALES, R., J. CHARLEMAGNE, W. MAHANA & S. AVRAMEAS. 1988. Specificity of natural serum antibodies present in phylogenetically distinct fish species. Immunology **63:** 31–36.
42. NEMAZEE, D. & K. BURKI. 1989. Clonal deletion of B lymphocytes in a transgenic mouse bearing anti-MHC class antibody genes. Nature **337:** 562–566.
43. NEMAZEE, D. 1995. Does immunological tolerance explain the waste in the B-lymphocyte immune system? Experiment and theory. Ann. N.Y. Acad. Sci. **764:** 397–401.
44. GOODNOW, C. C., R. BRINK & E. ADAMS. 1991. Breakdown of self-tolerance in anergic B lymphocytes. Nature **352:** 532–536.
45. RATHMELL, J. C. & C. C. GOODNOW. 1995. Autoimmunity: the Fas track. Curr. Biol. **5**(11): 1218–1221.
46. ERIKSON, J., M. Z. RADIC, S. A. CAMPER, R. R. HARDY, C. CARMACK & M. WEIGERT. 1991. Expression of anti-DNA immunoglobulin transgenes in non-autoimmune mice. Nature **349:** 331–335.
47. LAFER, E. M., J. RAUCH, C. ANDRZEWSKI, D. MUDD, B. FURIE, R. S. SCHWARTZ & B. D. STOLLAR. 1981. Polyspecific monoclonal lupus autoantibodies reactive with both polynucleotides and phospholipids. J. Exp. Med. **153:** 897–909.
48. DIGHIERO, G., B. GUILBERT & S. AVRAMEAS. 1982. Naturally occurring antibodies against nine common antigens in human sera: II. High incidence of monoclonal Ig exhibiting antibody activity against actin and tubulin and sharing antibody specificities with natural antibodies. J. Immunol. **128:** 2788–2792.
49. DIGHIERO, G., B. GUILBERT, J. P. FERMANT, P. LYMBERI, F. DANON & S. AVRAMEAS. 1983. Thirty-six human monoclonal immunoglobulins (MIg) with antibody activity against cytoskeleton proteins, thyroglobulin, and native DNA: immunological studies and clinical correlations. Blood **62:** 264–270.
50. ANDRÉ-SCHWARTZ, J., S. K. DATTA, Y. SHOENFELD, D. A. ISENBERG, B. D. STOLLAR & R. S. SCHWARTZ. 1984. Binding of cytoskeletal proteins by monoclonal anti-DNA lupus autoantibodies. Clin. Immunol. Immunopathol. **31:** 261–271.

51. RAUCH, J., H. TANNENBAUM, B. D. STOLLAR & R. S. SCHWARTZ. 1984. Monoclonal anticardiolipin antibodies bind to DNA. Eur. J. Immunol. **14:** 529–534.
52. JACOB, L., F. TRON, J. F. BACH & D. LOUVARD. 1984. A monoclonal anti-DNA antibody also binds to cell surface proteins. Proc. Natl. Acad. Sci. U.S.A. **81:** 3843–3845.
53. PONCET, P., T. MATTHES, A. BILLECOCQ & G. DIGHIERO. 1988. Immunochemical studies of polyspecific natural autoantibodies: charge lipid reactivity, Fab′2 fragments activity, and complement fixation. Mol. Immunol. **25:** 981–989.
54. AMIT, A. G., R. A. MARIUZZA, S. E. PHILLIPS & R. J. POLJAK. 1986. Three-dimensional structure of an antigen-antibody complex at 2.8-A resolution. Science **233:** 747–753.
55. BACCALA, R., T. V. QUANG, M. GILBERT, T. TERNYNCK & S. AVRAMEAS. 1989. Two murine natural polyreactive autoantibodies are encoded by nonmutated germ-line genes. Proc. Natl. Acad. Sci. U.S.A. **86:** 4624–4628.
56. LESCAR, J., M. PELLEGRINI, H. SOUCHON, D. TELLO, R. J. POLJAK, N. PETERSON, M. GREENE & P. M. ALZARI. 1995. Crystal structure of a cross-reaction complex between Fab F9.13.7 and guinea fowl lysozyme. J. Biol. Chem. **270:** 18067–18073.
57. BENTLEY, G. A., G. BOULOT, M. M. RIOTTOT & R. J. POLJAK. 1990. Three-dimensional structure of an idiotope–anti-idiotope complex. Nature **348:** 254–260.
58. DU PASQUIER, L. 1993. Evolution of the immune system. *In* William Paul Fundamental Immunology. Third edition, p. 199–235. Raven Press. New York.
59. BOS, N. A., C. G. MEENSWEN, H. HOOIJKAAS, R. BENNER, B. S. WOSTMAN & J. R. PLEASANTS. 1987. Early development of Ig secreting cells in young of germ Balb mice fed a chemically defined ultrafiltered diet. Cell. Immunol. **105:** 235–245.
60. KOFLER, R., D. I. NOONARS, D. E. LEVY, M. C. WILSON, N. P. H. MOLLER, F. J. DIXON & A. N. THEOFILOPOULOS. 1985. Genetic elements utilized for a murine lupus anti-DNA autoantibody are closely related to those for antibodies to exogenous antigens. J. Exp. Med. **161:** 805–815.
61. TREPICCHIO, W., JR., A. MARUYA & K. J. BARRETT. 1987. The heavy chain genes of a lupus anti-DNA autoantibody are encoded in the germline of a nonautoimmune strain of mouse and conserved in strains of mice polymorphic for this gene locus. J. Immunol. **139:** 3139–3147.
62. AGUADO, M. T., R. S. BALDERAS, R. L. RUBIN, M. A. DUCHOSAL, R. KOFLER, B. K. BIRSHTEIN, D. S. SECHER, F. J. DIXON & A. N. THEOFILOPOULOS. 1987. Specificity and molecular characteristics of monoclonal IgM rheumatoid factors from arthritic and non-arthritic mice. J. Immunol. **139:** 1080–1089.
63. SANZ, I., P. CASALI, J. W. THOMAS, A. L. NOTKINS & J. O. CAPRA. 1989. Nucleotide sequences of eight human natural autoantibody V_H regions reveal apparent restricted use of V_H families. J. Immunol. **142:** 4054–4061.
64. KOFLER, R., F. J. DIXON & A. N. THEOFILOPOULOS. 1987. The genetic origin of autoantibodies. Immunol. Today **8:** 374–379.
65. NAPASTEK, Y., J. ANDRÉ-SCHWARTZ, T. MANSER, L. J. WYSOCKI, L. BREITMAN, B. D. STOLLAR, M. GEFTER & R. S. SCHWARTZ. 1986. A single germline V_H gene segment of normal A/J mice encodes autoantibodies characteristic of systemic lupus erythematosus. J. Exp. Med. **164:** 614–626.
66. GUILBERT, B., W. MAHANA, M. GILBERT, J. C. MAZIÉ & S. AVRAMEAS. 1985. Presence of natural autoantibodies in hyperimmunized mice. Immunology **56:** 401–408.
67. DZIARSKI, R. 1988. Autoimmunity: polyclonal activation or antigen induction? Immunol. Today **9:** 340–342.
68. KLINMAN, D. & A. D. STEINBERG. 1987. Systemic autoimmune disease arises from polyclonal B-cell activation. J. Exp. Med. **165:** 1755–1760.
69. SHLOMCHIK, M. J., A. MARSHAK-ROTHSTEIN, C. B. WOLFOWICZ, T. L. ROTHSTEIN & M. G. WEIGERT. 1987. The role of clonal selection and somatic mutation in autoimmunity. Nature **328:** 805–811.
70. SHLOMCHIK, M. J., A. H. AUCOIN, D. S. PISETSKY & M. G. WEIGERT. 1987. Structure and function of anti-DNA autoantibodies derived from a single autoimmune mouse. Proc. Natl. Acad. Sci. U.S.A. **84:** 9150–9154.
71. THEOFILOPOULOS, A. N. & F. J. DIXON. 1985. Murine models of systemic lupus erythematosus. Adv. Immunol. **37:** 269–290.

72. Schwartz, R. S. & B. D. Stollar. 1985. Origins of anti-DNA autoantibodies. J. Clin. Invest. **75:** 321–325.
73. Cunningham, A. J. 1974. Large numbers of cells in normal mice produce antibody components of isologous erythrocytes. Nature **252:** 749–751.
74. Izui, S., N. M. Zaldivar, I. Scher & P. H. Lambert. 1977. Mechanism for induction of anti-DNA antibodies by bacterial lipopolysaccharides in mice. I. Anti-DNA induction by LPS without significant release of DNA in circulating blood. J. Immunol. **119:** 2151–2160.
75. Playfair, J. H. 1982. Immunity to malaria. Br. Med. Bull. **38:** 153–156.
76. Kazyumba, G., M. Berney & G. Brighouse. 1986. Expression of the B cell repertoire and autoantibodies in human African trypanosomiasis. Clin. Exp. Immunol. **65:** 10–16.
77. Behar, S. M., D. L. Lustgarten, S. Corbet & M. D. Scharff. 1980. Characterization of somatically mutated S10è VH11-encoded anti-DNA autoantibodies derived from autoimmune (NZB × NZW) F1 mice. J. Exp. Med. **148:** 1198–1213.
78. Marion, T. N., A. L. M. Bothwell, D. E. Briles & C. J. Janeway. 1989. IgG DNA autoantibodies within an individual autoimmune mouse are the products of clonal selection. J. Immunol. **142:** 4269–4278.
79. Marion, T. N., D. M. Tillman & N. T. Jou. 1990. Interclonal and intraclonal diversity among anti-DNA antibodies from an (NZB × NZW) F1 mouse. J. Immunol. **145:** 2322.
80. O'Keefe, T. L., S. Bandyopadhyay, S. K. Datta & T. Imanishi-Kari. 1990. V region sequences of an idiotypically connected family of pathogenic anti-DNA autoantibodies. J. Immunol. **144:** 4275–4282.
81. Radic, M. Z., M. A. Mascelli, J. Erikson, H. Shan, M. Shlomchik & M. Weigert. 1989. Structural patterns in anti-DNA antibodies from MRL/*lpr* mice. Cold Spring Harbor Symp. Quant. Biol. **54:** 993–1001.
82. Smith, R. G. & E. W. Voss, Jr. 1990. Variable region primary structures of monoclonal anti-DNA autoantibodies from (NZB × NZW) F1 mouse. Mol. Immunol. **27:** 463–471.
83. Marion, T. N., D. M. Tillman, N. T. Jou & R. J. Hill. 1992. Selection of immunoglobulin variable regions in autoimmunity to DNA. Immunol. Rev. **128:** 123–150.
84. Randen, I., K. M. Thompson, S. J. Thorpe, O. Forre & J. B. Natvig. 1993. Human monoclonal IgG rheumatoid factors from the synovial tissue of patients with rheumatoid arthritis. Scand. J. Immunol. **37:** 668–672.
85. Stewart, A. K., C. Huang, A. A. Long, B. D. Stollar & R. S. Schwartz. 1992. VH-gene representation in autoantibodies reflects the normal human B-cell repertoire. Immunol. Rev. **128:** 101–122.
86. Huang, C., A. K. Stewart, R. S. Schwartz & B. D. Stollar. 1992. Immunoglobulin heavy chain gene expression in peripheral blood B lymphocytes. J. Clin. Invest. **89:** 1331–1343.

Human Peripheral B Cell Development

sIgM$^-$IgD$^+$CD38$^+$ Hypermutated Germinal Center Centroblasts Preferentially Express Igλ Light Chain and Have Undergone μ-to-δ Switch

CHRISTOPHE ARPIN, ODETTE DE BOUTEILLER, DIANE RAZANAJAONA, FRANCINE BRIÈRE, JACQUES BANCHEREAU, SERGE LEBECQUE, AND YONG-JUN LIU

Laboratory for Immunological Research
Schering-Plough
69571 Dardilly, France

INTRODUCTION

We have recently identified a subset of germinal center (GC) dark zone centroblasts that express only the sIgD immunoglobulin isotype and have accumulated up to 80 mutations per heavy-chain variable region (IgV_H) gene[1] (FIGURE 1). We hypothesized that these sIgM$^-$IgD$^+$CD38$^+$ GC centroblasts have undergone Cμ-deletion by nonhomologous recombination through $\sigma\mu$-$\Sigma\mu$ or Sμ-$\Sigma\delta$ sequences, as described in IgD-secreting plasmacytoma cells[2–4] or in hairy cell leukemia, respectively.[4] Here, we present molecular and functional evidence indicating that sIgM$^-$IgD$^+$CD38$^+$ GC centroblasts indeed have undergone Cμ-deletion. Moreover, these cells preferentially express the λ light chain, a second feature of IgD-secreting plasmacytoma cells.[5] We propose that sIgM$^-$IgD$^+$CD38$^+$ centroblasts represent the origin of IgD-secreting plasmacytoma cells.

HYPERMUTATED sIgM$^-$IgD$^+$CD38$^+$ CENTROBLASTS ALL EXPRESS λ LIGHT CHAINS

Thirteen independent EBV clones from sIgM$^-$IgD$^+$CD38$^+$ B cells and 9 independent EBV clones from sIgD$^-$CD38$^+$ germinal center B cells were generated in order to analyze, at the molecular level of the same cell, the following two points: (i) Cμ-deletion by nonhomologous recombination through Sμ-$\Sigma\delta$ sequences;[4] (ii) somatic mutation status of Ig heavy chain and light chain. Strikingly, all 13 EBV clones from the hypermutated sIgM$^-$IgD$^+$CD38$^+$ centroblasts express the Igλ light chain, whereas only 2 out of the 9 EBV clones from the sIgD$^-$CD38$^+$ germinal center B cells express the Igλ light chain (FIGURE 2).

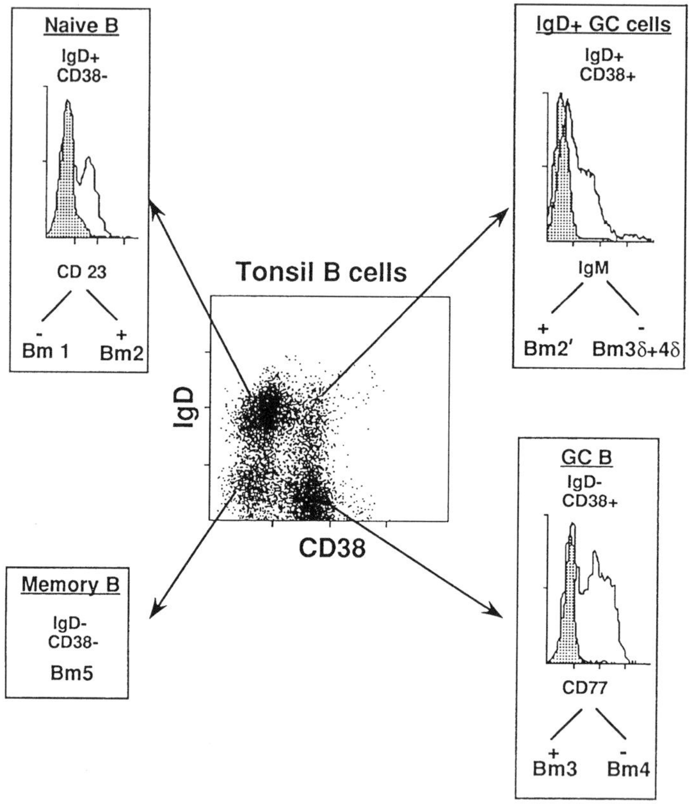

FIGURE 1. Identification of $sIgM^-IgD^+CD38^+$ tonsillar B cells. The tonsillar B cells can be sorted into four subsets based on anti-IgD and anti-CD38 double-immunofluorescence staining. Then, $sIgD^+CD38^-$ naive B cells are separated into a $CD23^-$ subset (Bm1) and a $CD23^+$ subset (Bm2). $sIgD^+CD38^+$ B cells can be further separated into an $sIgM^+$ subset (Bm2′) and an $sIgM^-$ subset (Bm3δ + 4δ). $sIgD^-CD38^+$ germinal center B cells are separated into $CD77^+$ centroblasts (Bm3) and $CD77^-$ centrocytes (Bm4). $sIgD^-CD38^-$ B cells (Bm5) represent memory B cells.

HYPERMUTATED $sIgM^-IgD^+CD38^+$ CENTROBLASTS HAVE UNDERGONE μ-TO-δ SWITCH

One obvious explanation for the $sIgM^-IgD^+$ phenotype is the nonhomologous recombination between regions containing pentameric repeats and localized upstream of Cμ (Sμ) and within the Cμ-Cδ intron (Σδ)[2,3] (FIGURE 3). Using a 5′-primer located to the left (5′) of the Sμ region and a 3′-primer within the Cμ-Cδ intron (FIGURE 3A), a PCR assay was performed on the EBV clones derived from $sIgM^-IgD^+CD38^+$ hypermutated centroblasts and from $sIgM^+IgD^+CD38^+$ germinal center founder

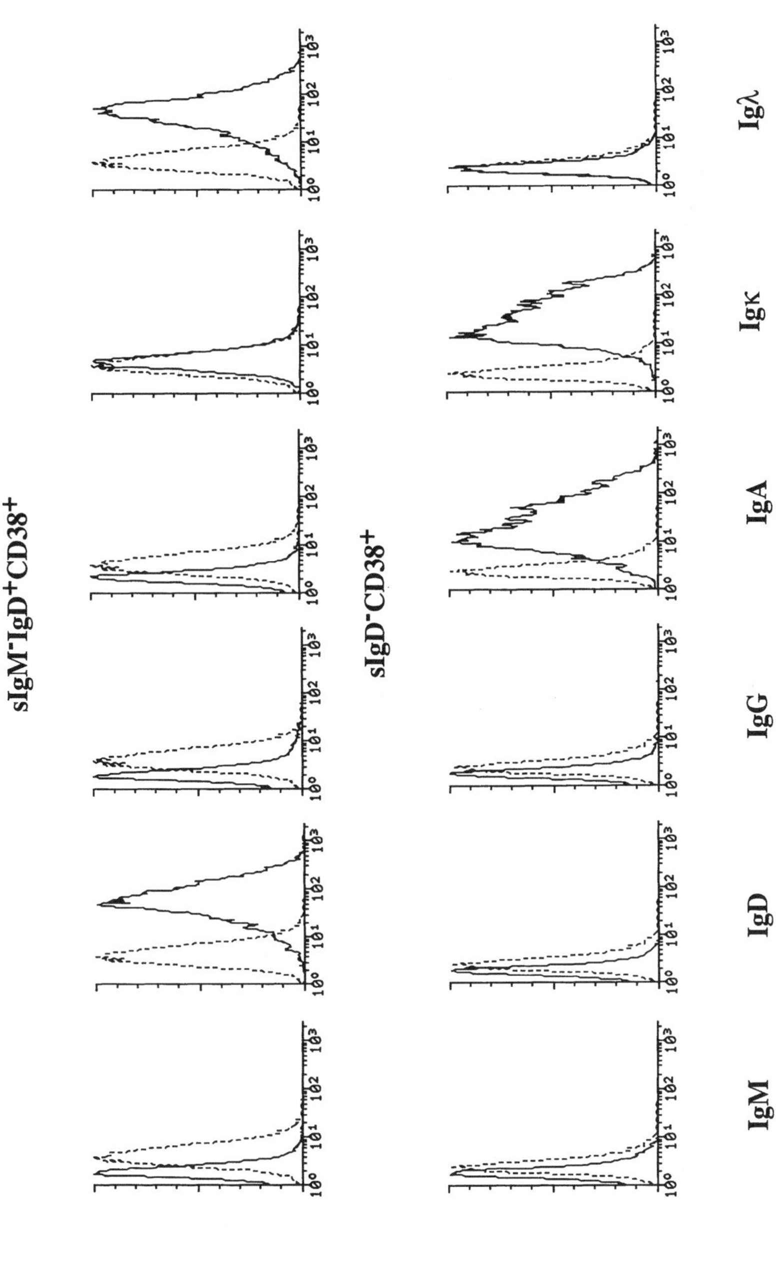

FIGURE 2. Surface expression of immunoglobulin heavy and light chains on a representative EBV cell clone from sIgM^{-}IgD^{+}CD38^{+} centroblasts (Bm3δ + 4δ) and from sIgD^{-}CD38^{+} germinal center cells (Bm3 + 4). Dashed histograms represent isotype-matched controls.

A

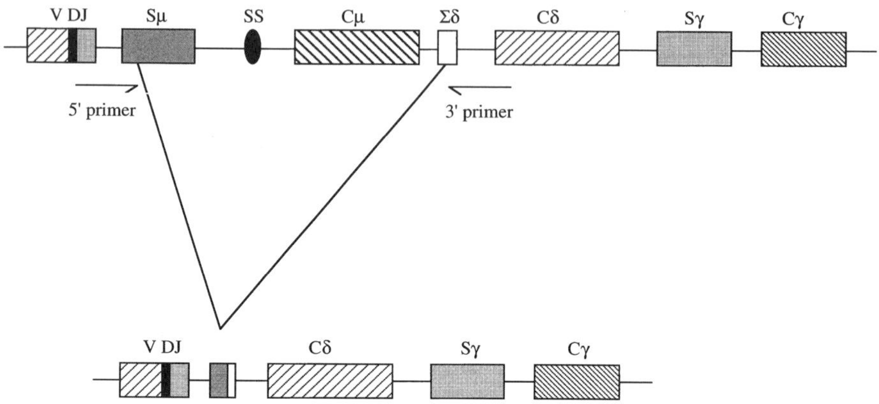

B

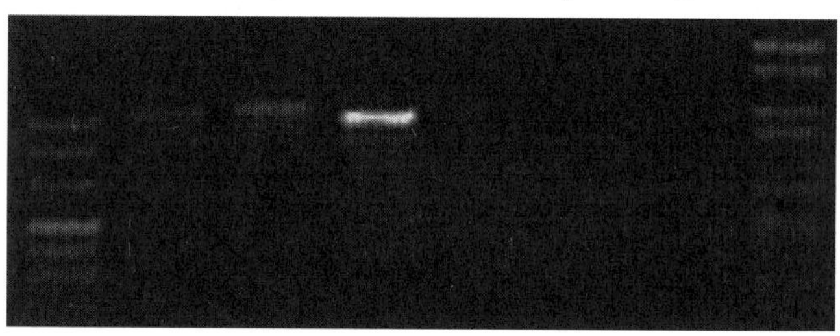

FIGURE 3. (A) Cμ-deletion mediated by nonhomologous recombination between Sμ and Σδ sequences located in the J_H-Cμ intron and the Cμ-Cδ intron, respectively. This recombination results in the deletion of four elements: (a) Cμ exons; (b) a putative somatic mutation silencer (SS) within the J_H-Cμ intron; (c) a part of the Cμ switch region (Sμ); and (d) a part of the 5.4-kb Cμ-Cδ intron. (B) PCR amplification of a 1-kb product generated by Cμ-deletion in three EBV clones from $sIgM^-IgD^+CD38^+$ centroblasts (Bm3δ + 4δ). Products of 11 kb could not be amplified by Taq polymerase in the two EBV clones from unswitched $sIgM^+IgD^+CD38^+$ GC founder cells.

cells. One-kb PCR products were obtained from the 3 EBV clones of $sIgM^-IgD^+$ cells, but not from the 2 EBV clones of $sIgM^+IgD^+$ cells (FIGURE 3B); this suggests that $sIgM^-IgD^+$ cells, but not $sIgM^+IgD^+$, have undergone Sμ-Σδ mediated deletion of about 10 kb, covering a part of Sμ, Cμ, and a part of both the J_H-Cμ intron and the Cμ-Cδ intron (FIGURE 3A).

$sIgM^-IgD^+CD38^+$ CENTROBLASTS SECRETE LARGE AMOUNTS OF IgD, BUT NOT OTHER Ig ISOTYPES, DURING TWO WEEKS OF CULTURE WITH CD40-LIGAND, IL-2, AND IL-10

The loss of a large part of the Sμ sequence by $sIgM^-IgD^+CD38^+$ centroblasts should render them unable to undergo further isotype switching. To functionally test this hypothesis, $sIgM^+IgD^+CD38^-$ naive B cells, $sIgM^+IgD^+CD38^+$ GC founder cells, $sIgD^-CD38^+$ GC cells, and $sIgM^-IgD^+CD38^+$ centroblasts were cultured with CD40-ligand-transfected L cells, IL-10, and IL-2, a culture condition under which naive B cells undergo an isotype switch to IgG.[6] After 10 days of culture, the IgM, IgD, IgG, and IgA levels in each of the culture supernatants were analyzed by ELISA. FIGURE 4 shows that the $sIgM^-IgD^+CD38^+$ centroblasts mostly produce IgD, whereas the three other B cell subsets produce IgM, IgG, and IgA. This indicates that the Sμ-Σδ mediated μ-to-δ switch results in a quasifrozen $sIgM^-IgD^+$ phenotype.

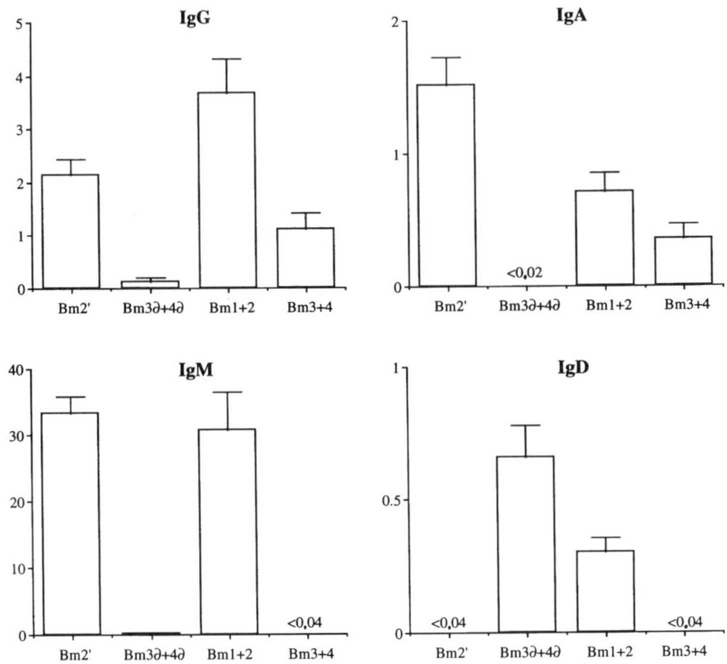

FIGURE 4. IgM, IgD, IgG, and IgA production from four subsets of B cells cultured with CD40-ligand-transfected L cells, IL-2, and IL-10. $sIgM^-IgD^+CD38^+$ centroblasts (Bm3δ + 4δ) were cultured in parallel with $sIgM^+IgD^+CD38^-$ naive B cells (Bm1 + 2), $sIgM^+IgD^+CD38^+$ GC founder cells (Bm2′), and $sIgD^-CD38^+$ GC cells (Bm3 + 4). After 14 days, supernatants were harvested and IgA, IgG, IgM, and IgD titers were measured by a classical ELISA sandwich assay.

CONCLUSIONS

A population of sIgM$^-$IgD$^+$CD38$^+$ GC centroblasts have been isolated. They have undergone extensive somatic mutation in their Ig variable region genes and an Sμ-Σδ mediated μ-to-δ switch, they preferentially express the Igλ light chain, and they mostly secrete IgD upon differentiation. Because IgD-secreting plasmacytoma cells were reported to have undergone a σμ-Σμ mediated μ-to-δ switch and only express the Igλ light chain, it is possible that sIgM$^-$IgD$^+$CD38$^+$ centroblasts represent the origin of these unique plasma cell tumors. The molecular mechanisms underlying the high somatic mutation activity, the biased light-chain expression, and the signals for triggering the σμ-Σμ or Sμ-Σδ mediated μ-to-δ switch in this peculiar population of B cells deserve further investigation.

REFERENCES

1. Liu, Y-J., O. de Bouteiller, C. Arpin, F. Brière, L. Galibert, S. Ho, H. Martinez-Valdez, J. Banchereau & S. Lebecque. 1996. Normal human IgD$^+$IgM$^-$ germinal center B cells can express up to 80 mutations in the variable region of their IgD transcripts. Immunity **4:** 603–613.
2. Gilliam, A. C., A. Shen, J. E. Richards, F. R. Blattner, J. F. Mushinski & P. W. Tucker. 1984. Illegitimate recombination generates a class switch from Cμ to Cδ in an IgD-secreting plasmacytoma. Proc. Natl. Acad. Sci. U.S.A. **81:** 4164–4168.
3. Yasui, H., Y. Akahori, M. Hirano, K. Yamada & Y. Kurosawa. 1989. Class switch from μ to δ is mediated by homologous recombination between σμ and Σμ sequences in human immunoglobulin gene loci. Eur. J. Immunol. **19:** 1399–1403.
4. Kluin, P. M., H. Kayano, V. J. Zani, H. C. Kluin-Nelemans, P. W. Tucker, E. Satterwhite & M. J. S. Dyer. 1995. IgD class switching; identification of a novel recombination site in neoplastic and normal B cells. Eur. J. Immunol. **25:** 3504–3508.
5. Van Nieuwkoop, J. A. & J. Radl. 1985. Light chain types of IgD in human bone marrow and serum. Clin. Exp. Immunol. **60:** 654.
6. Malisan, F., F. Brière, J-M. Bridon, N. Harindranath, F. C. Mills, E. E. Max, J. Banchereau & H. Martinez-Valdez. 1996. Interleukin-10 induces immunoglobulin G isotype switch recombination in human CD40-activated naive B lymphocytes. J. Exp. Med. **183:** 937–947.

Mutually Dependent T and B Cell Responses in Germinal Centers

ADAM GULBRANSON-JUDGE,
MONTSERRAT CASAMAYOR-PALLEJA,
AND IAN C. M. MACLENNAN[a]

Department of Immunology
University of Birmingham Medical School
Birmingham B15 2TT, United Kingdom

INTRODUCTION

Germinal centers are structures that develop in the B cell follicles of secondary lymphoid tissues during a wide range of antibody responses.[1] They are associated with massive oligoclonal expansion of B cells.[2,3] A hypermutation mechanism is activated in these cells that is selectively directed at the genes that encode the variable regions of their antigen-binding receptors, that is, their immunoglobulin variable-region genes (Ig V-region genes).[4] The resulting mutation can cause alteration of the affinity or specificity of the receptor for the antigen that is driving the response. In some cases, the altered receptor will be of higher affinity for antigen, but in others affinity may be lost; it is also possible that on occasions the receptors may acquire affinity for autoantigens. It is not surprising, therefore, that a stringent selection mechanism has evolved that acts upon germinal center B cells that have altered receptors for antigen.[5] The selection is based upon the ability of the B cells to take up antigen specifically from specialized antigen-retaining cells that are located in follicles[6] and then to make cognate interaction with local T cells.[1] These antigen-retaining cells are known as the follicular dendritic cells (FDC). The aim of this communication is to summarize experiments that probe the systems that initiate and control clonal expansion of B cells and those that select the B cells after they have altered their Ig V-region genes. Particular emphasis will be placed on the role of T cells in these processes.

THE T CELL–DEPENDENCE OF GERMINAL CENTERS

Germinal centers characteristically develop in response to T cell–dependent antigens within the B cell follicles that are found in all secondary lymphoid organs.[7] Classically, germinal centers are induced by protein-based antigens and the T cells involved have αβ T cell receptors. They are also seen sometimes in mice that do not respond to protein antigens; thus, germinal centers are occasionally found in congenitally athymic rodents[8] and in mice unable to generate αβ T cells.[9] This particularly applies to mice with deletion of the genes encoding the α T cell receptor genes. These

[a]To whom all correspondence should be addressed.

mice have large germinal centers in their secondary lymphoid tissues. Surprisingly, the T cells in these germinal centers express the β chain of the T cell receptor. This is not associated with pre-T α.[10] Very occasionally, germinal centers with γδ T cells have been observed in these mice[9] and this reflects the lack of germinal centers in conventionally housed mice that have their β T cell receptor genes deleted. These mice only have γδ T cells. In certain circumstances, germinal centers with γδ T cells can be induced in β T cell receptor knockout mice (Adrian Hayday, unpublished results). The role of non-αβ T cells in antibody responses against nonprotein antigens is an important area for future investigation, particularly as the α T cell receptor knockout mice develop autoantibodies, including antibodies against double-stranded DNA.[11] The necessity for these T cells in responses to nonprotein antigens is implied by the failure to find germinal centers in mice lacking any T cells.

BOTH T AND B CELLS UNDERGO ANTIGEN-SPECIFIC CLONAL EXPANSION IN FOLLICLES DURING GERMINAL CENTER FORMATION

In the absence of antigenic challenge, the B cell follicles in secondary lymphoid tissues contain small recirculating B cells that permeate the FDC network. Specific B cells appear in the FDC network after challenge with antigen and these start to grow exponentially.[3] The cell cycle time of these cells is of the order of 6–7 hours and at this rate the average of 3 B blasts that seed the germinal center expand to become 10^4 to 1.5×10^4 cells in three days.[3] The follicular dendritic cell network is then filled with the B blasts, and the small recirculating B cells that originally filled the follicle are confined to its periphery, forming the follicular mantle. At this stage, the compartments associated with mature germinal centers develop (FIGURE 1). The blasts migrate to one pole of the FDC network, generally the one nearest the T zones, and form the dark zone of the germinal center. These blasts are now termed centroblasts; they continue in cell cycle, but fail to increase in number, for they are continually giving rise to nondividing progeny—centrocytes—which pass into the follicle center with its dense antigen-laden FDC network.[12] This is known as the light zone of the germinal center. The relationship of this to the dark zone and the follicular mantle is depicted in FIGURE 1. It seems that Ig V-region gene–directed hypermutation occurs in the centroblast population and it is the centrocytes that are subject to selection. The selection mechanism relies on the centrocyte dying spontaneously by apoptosis unless antigen-specific selection signals are received.

Although T cells are less abundant than B cells in germinal centers, it has become clear that these cells play an important role in the germinal center response. In fully formed germinal centers, the T cells are located mainly in the light zone and particularly where this abuts the follicular mantle.[13,14] The T cells characteristically are CD4+ and CD45RO+ and lack intracellular Bcl-2; about half of these cells contain preformed CD40-ligand[14] and a substantial minority coexpress CD57.[15]

T cells in germinal centers appear to be driven there by antigen-specific activation.[16–19] Primary follicles that have never supported a germinal center reaction contain very few T cells. If the accumulation/growth of antigen-specific T cells is assessed during a response to a protein-based antigen, it becomes clear that the growth of antigen-specific T cells in the follicles is quantitatively as important as that in the T zones, which constitutively have vastly more T cells (FIGURE 2). This has been studied during the response of B10A mice to pigeon cytochrome c.[19] The reason for choosing this esoteric antigen is that mice that express the class-II MHC molecule IE^k on their antigen-presenting cells make a T cell response to this antigen that is dominated by cells with Vβ3/Vα11 T cell receptors.[20,21] Four days after intraperitoneal immunization, the number of cells with Vβ3/Vα11 T cell receptors starts to increase in the T zones of the spleen, and T cells with these receptors appear in the follicles for the first

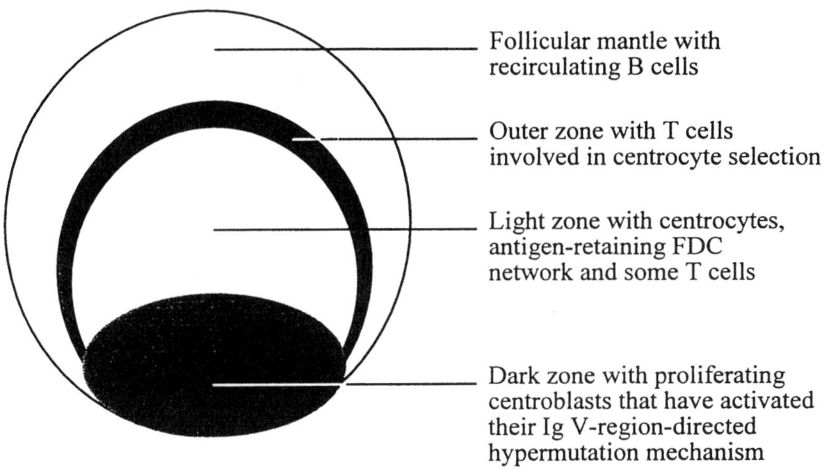

FIGURE 1. The compartments of secondary follicles. The outer zone, light zone, and dark zone are all part of the germinal center; centroblasts give rise to centrocytes; and centrocytes undergo selection as is depicted in FIGURE 3.

time. The number of T cells in the T zone peaks at the end of the first week and then falls to below preimmunization levels by day 10 (FIGURE 2a). This fall contrasts with an impressive rise in the number of cells with Vβ3/Vα11 T cell receptors in the follicles during the second week; this rise coincides with the development of germinal centers (FIGURE 2b). T cells in that site only decline as the germinal center reaction wanes, but small numbers persist in follicles for at least several weeks. As the germinal center reaction subsides, the number of cells with Vβ3/Vα11 T cell receptors in the T zone once again increases to levels modestly above those found before immunization. The increase in the number of T cells in the follicles is at least partially attributable to these cells proliferating within the follicles.[19] Analysis of the T cell receptor V-region gene structure indicates that many T cells within single follicles are

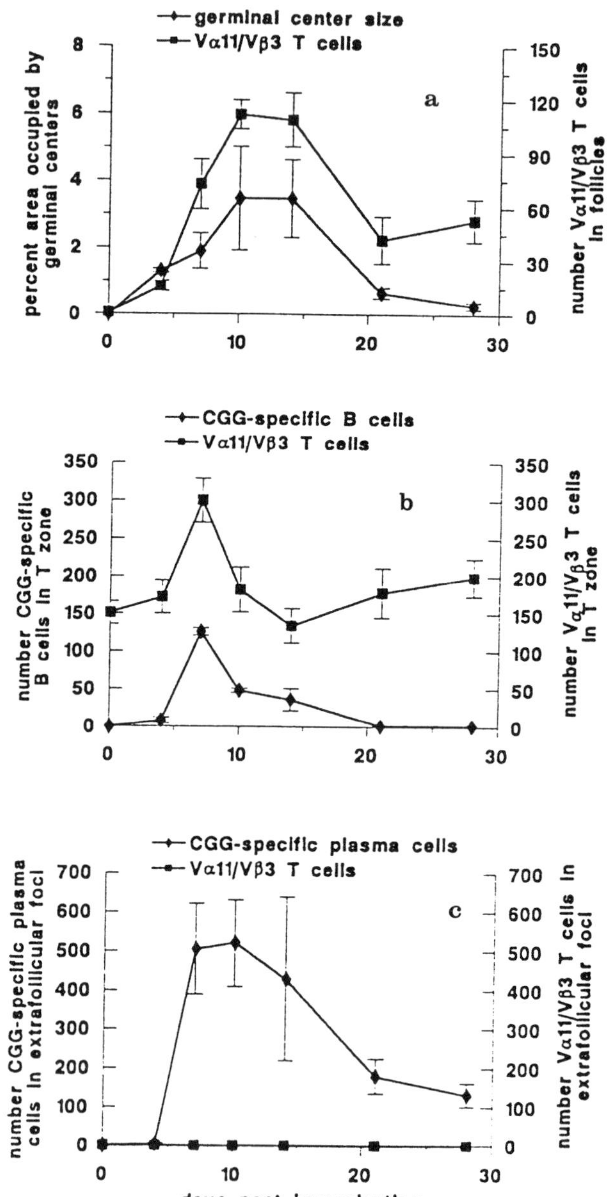

germinal center size
Vα11/Vβ3 T cells
percent area occupied by germinal centers
number Vα11/Vβ3 T cells in follicles
a
CGG-specific B cells
Vα11/Vβ3 T cells
number CGG-specific B cells in T zone
number Vα11/Vβ3 T cells in T zone
b
CGG-specific plasma cells
Vα11/Vβ3 T cells
number CGG-specific plasma cells in extrafollicular foci
number Vα11/Vβ3 T cells in extrafollicular foci
c
days post immunization

FIGURE 2

clonally related.[18] Once the T cell numbers in germinal centers reach stable levels, proliferation stops.[19] This fits with the finding that T cells typically do not express the proliferation-associated antigen Ki67 in the chronically stimulated germinal centers of Peyer's patches, the appendix, and tonsils. Although T cell numbers in follicles again increase during secondary responses, the proportion of proliferating cells is only about 10% of that seen during the primary follicular response. This presumably reflects the entry of memory cells generated in the primary response to germinal centers on reexposure to antigen. A similar effect is seen in studies of germinal center formation induced by the B lymphotrophic murine mammary tumor virus—MMTV (SW). The T cell response to this virus is driven by a Vβ6-binding superantigen; 10% of peripheral T cells in BALB/c mice are Vβ6+.[22] The numbers of T cells accumulating in the germinal centers that form in response to this virus are similar to those expected in response to a conventional protein antigen, but there is very little T cell proliferation in the germinal center (Luther, Gulbranson-Judge, Acha-Orbea, and MacLennan; unpublished observations). It seems likely that this reflects the large number of superantigen-reactive T cells available.

The extent of T cell proliferation in germinal centers induced in response to pigeon cytochrome c is considerably greater than is required to account for the increase in the number of these cells in the germinal center. It follows that either there is T cell death in the germinal center or there is emigration of T cells from the germinal center, or both of these. Evidence supporting both of these possibilities exists: (i) ipsiclonal T cells with the same mutations in their α T cell receptor genes have been found in different germinal centers;[18] (ii) apoptosis among germinal center T cells has been identified histologically (G. Kelsoe, personal communication).

The findings discussed in this section suggest that there is a relationship between primed helper T cells within and outside germinal centers, but mechanisms that regulate the location, movement, and size of clones of these cells are obscure. Nevertheless, follicles seem to be important sites where these clones grow. In this respect, it may be important that the FDC network provides the only known site where antigen can be taken up by B cells and presented to T cells after extrafollicular sources of antigen are dissipated. In the case of soluble protein antigens, extrafollicular sources of antigen are lost shortly after the start of antibody production against this antigen. This antibody is necessary to initiate the transport of antigen to follicular dendritic cells.

FIGURE 2. The numbers of antigen-specific T cells in the spleen at sites of B cell activation during primary responses to pigeon cytochrome c or chicken gamma globulin (CGG): (a) The percent of spleen section area occupied by germinal centers, and the number of follicular Vα11/Vβ3+ cells per 20 mm^2 of tissue section during primary response to pigeon cytochrome c. (b) The number of T zone Vα11/Vβ3+ cells per 20 mm^2 of tissue section during primary response to pigeon cytochrome c, compared with the number of T zone CGG-specific B cells during primary response to CGG. (c) The marked absence of Vα11/Vβ3+ cells in the extrafollicular foci of B cell proliferation during primary response to pigeon cytochrome c, compared with the number of CGG-specific B cells and plasma cells in the extrafollicular foci of B cell proliferation during primary response to CGG. The experiments represented in this figure are reported in full in reference 19.

CENTROCYTE SELECTION IN GERMINAL CENTERS

The death of cells in germinal centers is apparent from the condensed chromatin that makes up the characteristic tingible bodies found in germinal center macrophages. Fliedner showed that many of the cells in germinal centers that die have recently been in cell cycle.[23] It was proposed in 1986 that the death in germinal centers reflects cells that had failed to be selected after they had mutated their Ig V-region genes.[24] It seemed logical at that time that selection would involve the interaction of centrocytes with antigen held on FDC and this hypothesis is still sustainable. A way in which cell death could occur in the nonselected cells emerged when it became clear that isolated germinal center B cells died rapidly by apoptosis on culture; that is, the default for these cells is to die.[5] If this is to be meaningful for selection, then it should be possible to prevent the onset of apoptosis by antigen-specific signals. Initial experiments to test this met with only limited success. The onset of apoptosis could be delayed, but not prevented, if the surface Ig of centrocytes was cross-linked by treatment with red cells coated with anti-human Ig. Soluble anti-Ig was ineffective. Cytokines and antibodies against many other B cell surface molecules were tested. It was striking that antibody against CD40 had a remarkable ability to inhibit the onset of apoptosis of cultured centrocytes. CD40, a member of the tumor necrosis factor receptor family, is constitutively expressed by B cells. The likely significance of this effect of CD40-ligation to centrocyte selection started to become apparent when it was shown that a ligand for CD40 is expressed on the surface of appropriately activated T cells.[25] Recombinant human CD40-ligand was found to be just as effective at preventing germinal center cells from entering apoptosis as the antibody against CD40.[26] These findings opened the possibility that the selection of germinal center cells was a two-stage process: first, centrocytes have to interact with antigen held on FDC; second, they have to find a local T cell that recognizes processed peptides of this antigen presented on the centrocyte surface in association with class-II MHC molecules. This scheme for centrocyte selection is shown in FIGURE 3.

T CELL INVOLVEMENT IN CENTROCYTE SELECTION REDUCES THE CHANCE OF SURVIVAL OF AUTOREACTIVE CELLS

A theoretical advantage to T cell involvement in this process is that it reduces the chance of selecting cells that have acquired autoreactivity as the result of Ig V-region gene hypermutation. Although interaction with autoantigen may occur, it is unlikely that a T cell that recognizes self-peptide will be found within a germinal center. The latter possibility could occur by a passenger effect—thus, B cells that acquire rheumatoid factor activity might take up foreign antigen complexed with antibody from the surface of FDC. A protection against this eventuality seems to have been found because soluble antigen encountered rather than antigen on FDC seems to induce apoptosis in germinal center cells.[27,28] It is probable that the B cell with newly acquired specificity for self-Ig will encounter soluble Ig before Ig complexed with antigen on FDC and will consequently expire.

DIFFERENTIATION PATHWAYS OF CENTROCYTES SELECTED IN GERMINAL CENTERS

There are two main differentiation pathways for selected centrocytes resulting in the cells leaving the germinal center. They can become either memory B cells or plasma cells. There is some evidence that selected centrocytes can also be induced to

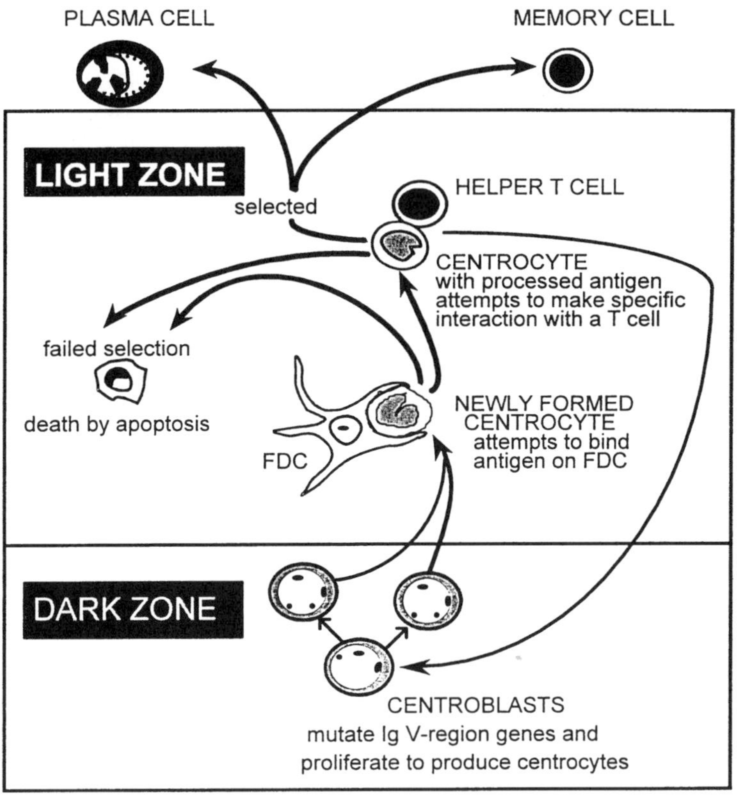

FIGURE 3. Cellular events during centrocyte selection in germinal centers. This figure is reproduced, with permission, from the *1995–1996 Handbook on the Physiology of the Immune System* produced for medical students at the University of Birmingham Medical School.

reenter the dark zone as a centroblast and undergo a further round of Ig V-region gene mutation and selection. Coico *et al.* showed memory cells could be derived from mouse germinal center cells transferred to another mouse.[29] The germinal center cells were isolated on the basis of their ability to bind peanut agglutinin. This conclusion is reinforced by the finding that most putative memory B cells have somatic mutations in their Ig V-region genes.[30] Evidence that germinal center cells give rise to plasma cells is again implied by the finding of somatic mutations in the long-lived plasma cells[31] that are found in epithelia and in the bone marrow.[32] Benner *et al.* showed that bone marrow plasma cells are derived from the spleen and peripheral lymph nodes during the established phase of T cell–dependent antibody responses.[33] More direct evidence for the germinal center origin was provided by Tew and colleagues.[34] Evidence that centrocytes might again become centroblasts was considered on the basis of mathematical modeling.[35] This is supported by the finding that CD40-ligand blockade causes the dissolution of established germinal centers.[36] This finding would not be expected if centroblasts were directly self-renewing rather than being replaced by differentiation of selected centrocytes. A caveat to this conclusion is the observation that CD40-ligand may be expressed by activated B cells.[37] If this is the case, then it is feasible that centroblasts maintain self-renewal by homotypic CD40-ligation. Evidence that centrocytes can be induced by T cells to differentiate to become centroblasts *in vitro* is discussed in the next section.

TRANSIENT CD40-LIGATION IS NECESSARY, BUT NOT SUFFICIENT, TO INDUCE CENTROCYTES TO DIFFERENTIATE TO BECOME PLASMA CELLS

Chronic CD40-ligation achieved by culturing centrocytes with CD40 monoclonal antibodies or recombinant CD40-ligand prevents centrocytes from entering apoptosis, but a nonphysiological phenotype develops in these cells.[38] This phenotype that has not been found to be expressed by any B cell *in vivo* is shown in TABLE 1. Studies have been published where memory B cell phenotypes have been reported to be generated from centrocytes cultured for several days with fibroblasts expressing CD40-ligand in the presence of cytokines.[39] The problem with this interesting result is that it is unlikely to reflect physiological memory formation. Two main reasons for coming to this conclusion are as follows: (i) the tempo of centroblast differentiation to centrocytes and then to memory B cells occurs in less than 24 hours *in vivo*;[40] (ii)

TABLE 1. The Phenotype of Freshly Isolated Human Tonsil B Cell Subsets and the Effect of CD40-Ligation *in Vitro* over 24 Hours[a]

	Surface Phenotype of Cells				
	Ig	CD77	CD44	CD23	CD38
centrocytes	+	+/++	+	−	+++
centroblasts	+	++/+++	−	−	+++
memory B cells	+++	−	+++	−	−
germinal center B cells cultured with CD40-L	++	+++	+++	++	++
memory B cells cultured with CD40-L	+++	−	+++	−	−

[a]The results shown in this table are based on data from reference 38.

TABLE 2. Centrocytes Are Prevented from Entering Apoptosis by Coculture with Preparations of Autologous Germinal Center T Cells Induced to Express CD40-Ligand; Naive T Cells Expressing CD40-Ligand Do Not Rescue Centrocytes from Entry to Apoptosis

Tonsil Cells Used in Cocultures		Culture Additive	Centrocyte Survival after 48 h
B Cells	T Cells		
centrocytes	activated[a] CD45RA$^-$	none	≈50%
centrocytes	activated[a] CD45RA$^-$	blocking Ab versus CD40-L	<5%
centrocytes	activated[a] CD45RA$^+$	none	<5%
centrocytes	none	none	<5%
centrocytes	none	recombinant CD40-L	≈50%

[a]T cells were activated by culture with phorbol dibutyrate and ionomycin for 4 hours at 37 °C. After this, the T cells were washed and added to the autologous centrocytes. CD40-ligand (L) expression was induced at equivalent levels in both CD45RA$^-$ and CD45RA$^+$ cells. In both preparations, the CD40-ligand was rapidly lost on coculture with the centrocytes. Full technical details are given in reference 38.

CD40-ligation *in vivo* is likely to be transient. CD40-ligand expression probably occurs only at the point of contact between primed T cells with preformed intracellular CD40-ligand and a B cell that carries processed antigen that these T cells recognize.[14] It is known that CD40-ligand expressed in such a situation is rapidly downregulated.[41] CD40-ligand is not found on freshly isolated CD45RO+, CD4+ T cells.

With these points in mind, we set out to investigate if transient CD40-ligation of centrocytes induced by autologous T cells would prevent centrocytes from killing

TABLE 3. Centrocytes Rapidly Acquire a Memory B Cell Phenotype on Coculture with Preparations Enriched for Autologous Germinal Center T Cells Induced to Express CD40-Ligand Transiently

	Surface Phenotype of Cells				
	Ig	CD77	CD44	CD23	CD38
freshly isolated centrocytes	+	+/++	+	−	+++
centrocytes cultured for 24 h with autologous activated[a] CD45RA$^-$ T cells	+++	−	+++	−	+++
memory B cells cultured for 24 h with autologous activated[a] CD45RA$^-$ T cells	+++	−	+++	−	++

[a]T cells were activated by culture for 4 hours with phorbol dibutyrate plus ionomycin, which induces them to express CD40-ligand. The stimulants were removed by washing before the activated cells were added to the B cells. Full details of this experiment are given in reference 38. Bcl-2 characteristically is expressed by memory B cells, but not by centrocytes. Centrocytes came to express Bcl-2 at levels associated with memory cells between 24 and 48 hours after the start of coculture with autologous phorbol dibutyrate plus ionomycin–activated CD45RA$^-$ T cells.

themselves by apoptosis and, if so, whether it would induce differentiation to memory B cells.[36] In order to induce CD40-ligand expression, T cells were cultured for 4 hours with phorbol dibutyrate and ionomycin and the activators were then removed by washing. This induced CD40-ligand expression by almost all tonsil T cells. It was confirmed that this was rapidly downregulated if these activated T cells were then cultured with autologous germinal center B cells. When germinal center T cell–enriched preparations were used for the coculture experiments, the centrocytes were prevented from entering apoptosis (TABLE 2) and within 24 hours had adopted a memory B cell phenotype[36] (TABLE 3). The requirement for CD40-ligation for prevention of apoptosis in this situation was apparent when blocking antibodies against CD40-ligand were introduced to these cultures; then, all the centrocytes died by apoptosis. It became clear that transient CD40-ligation alone is not sufficient to prevent apoptosis because it was found that activated CD45RA+ (naive) T cells that had been induced to express CD40-ligand could not inhibit centrocytes from dying by apoptosis (TABLE 2). Lagresle *et al.*[42] have also succeeded in inducing rapid differentiation of centrocytes to memory B cells by coculturing germinal center B cells with phytohemagglutinin-activated mitomycin C–treated allogeneic CD4+ T cells.

Memory B cells were the main differentiated product of centrocytes cultured with autologous activated T cells. Some cells with a centroblast phenotype—$CD77^{high}CD44^{low}$—were also generated.[38] These cells are difficult to analyze because they dissociate from T cells and then die by apoptosis. It will be interesting to determine if distinct T cell subsets are responsible for generating the diverse differentiated progeny of centrocytes. Germinal center T cell heterogeneity is demonstrated by the expression of preformed CD40-ligand and CD57, which are only expressed in a proportion of these T cells.[14]

REFERENCES

1. MACLENNAN, I. C. M. 1994. Germinal centers. Annu. Rev. Immunol. **12:** 117–139.
2. KROESE, F. G. M., A. S. WUBENNA, H. G. SEIJEN & P. NIEUWENHUIS. 1987. Germinal centers develop oligoclonally. Eur. J. Immunol. **17:** 1069–1072.
3. LIU, Y-J., J. ZHANG, P. L. J. LANE, E. Y-T. CHAN & I. C. M. MACLENNAN. 1991. Sites of specific B cell activation in primary and secondary responses to T cell–dependent and T cell–independent antigens. Eur. J. Immunol. **21:** 2951–2962.
4. JACOB, J., G. KELSOE, K. RAJEWSKY & U. WEISS. 1991. Intraclonal generation of antibody mutants in germinal centres. Nature **354:** 389–392.
5. LIU, Y-J., D. E. JOSHUA, G. T. WILLIAMS, C. A. SMITH, J. GORDON & I. C. M. MACLENNAN. 1989. Mechanisms of antigen-driven selection in germinal centres. Nature **342:** 929–931.
6. MANDEL, T. E., T. E. R. PHIPPS, A. ABBOT & J. TEW. 1980. The follicular dendritic cell: long-term antigen retention during immunity. Immunol. Rev. **53:** 29–59.
7. JACOBSEN, E. B., L. H. CORPORALE & G. J. THORBECKE. 1974. Effect of thymus cell injections on germinal center formation in lymphoid tissues of nude (thymusless) mice. Cell. Immunol. **13:** 416–430.
8. SCHUURMAN, H. J., E. B. BELL, K. GARTNER, H. J. HEDRICH, A. K. HANSEN, B. C. KRUIJT, P. DE-VREY, R. LEYTEN, S. J. MAEDER, R. MOUTIER, U. MOHNLE, D. PASS, J. VANKERKOM, R. BOOT, R. BROEKHUIZEN, J. DORMANS, H. VAN HERCK, P. G. C. HERMANS, J. HOEKMAN, J. VAN DER LOGT, M. VAN WIJK, J. G. VOS & L. F. M. VAN ZUTPHEN. 1992. Comparative evaluation of the immune status of congenitally athymic and euthymic rat strains bred and maintained at different institutes: 2. Athymic rats. J. Exp. Anim. Sci. **35:** 33–43.

9. DIANDA, L., A. GULBRANSON-JUDGE, W. PAO, A. C. HAYDAY, I. C. M. MACLENNAN & M. J. OWEN. 1996. Germinal center formation in mice lacking $\alpha\beta$ T cells. Eur. J. Immunol. **26:** 1603–1607.
10. BRUNO, L., B. ROCHA, A. ROLINK, H. VON BOEHMER & H-R. RODEWALD. 1995. Intra- and extra-thymic expression of the pre-T cell receptor α gene. Eur. J. Immunol. **25:** 1877–1882.
11. WEN, L., S. J. ROBERTS, J. L. VINEY, S. WONG, C. A. MALLICK, R. C. FINDLEY, J. P. CRAFT, M. J. OWEN & A. C. HAYDAY. 1994. Immunoglobulin synthesis and generalized autoimmunity in mice deficient in $\alpha\beta(+)$ T cells. Nature **369:** 654–658.
12. HANNA, M. G. 1964. An autoradiographic study of the germinal center in spleen white pulp during early intervals of the immune response. Lab. Invest. **13:** 95–104.
13. HARDIE, D. L., G. D. JOHNSON & I. C. M. MACLENNAN. 1993. Quantitative analysis of molecules which distinguish functional compartments in germinal centers. Eur. J. Immunol. **23:** 997–1004.
14. CASAMAYOR-PALLEJA, M., M. KHAN & I. C. M. MACLENNAN. 1995. A subset of $CD4^+$ memory T cells contains preformed CD40 ligand that is rapidly, but transiently expressed on their surface after activation through the T cell receptor complex. J. Exp. Med. **181:** 1293–1301.
15. VERLADI, A., M. C. MINGARI, L. MORETTA & C. E. GROSSI. 1986. Functional analysis of germinal center CD4+ cells with natural killer–related features: divergence from typical T helper cells. J. Immunol. **137:** 2808–2813.
16. FULLER, K. A., O. KANAGAWA & M. H. NAHM. 1993. T cells within germinal centers are specific for the immunizing antigen. J. Immunol. **151:** 4505–4512.
17. KEARNEY, K. R., K. A. PAPE, D. Y. LOH & M. K. JENKINS. 1994. Visualization of peptide-specific T cell immunity and peripheral tolerance induction *in vivo.* Immunity **1:** 327–339.
18. ZHENG, B., W. XUE & G. KELSOE. 1994. Locus-specific somatic hypermutation in germinal center T cells. Nature **372:** 556–559.
19. GULBRANSON-JUDGE, A. & I. C. M. MACLENNAN. 1996. Sequential antigen-specific growth of T cells in the T zones and follicles in response to pigeon cytochrome c. Eur. J. Immunol. **26:** 1830–1837.
20. HEDRICK, S. M., I. ENGEL, D. L. MCELLIGOTT, P. J. FINK, M-L. HSU, D. HANSBURG & L. A. MATIS. 1988. Selection of amino acid sequences in the beta-chain of the T cell antigen receptor. Science **239:** 1541–1544.
21. MCHEYZER-WILLIAMS, M. G. & M. DAVIS. 1995. Antigen-specific development of primary and memory T cells *in vivo.* Science **268:** 106–111.
22. ACHA-ORBEA, H. & H. R. MACDONALD. 1995. Superantigens of mouse mammary tumor virus. Annu. Rev. Immunol. **13:** 459–486.
23. FLIEDNER, T. M. 1967. On the origin of tingible bodies in germinal centers in immune responses. *In* Germinal Centers in Immune Responses. H. Cottier, Ed.: 218–224. Springer-Verlag. Berlin/New York.
24. MACLENNAN, I. C. M. & D. GRAY. 1986. Antigen-driven selection of virgin and memory B cells. Immunol. Rev. **91:** 61–85.
25. ARMITAGE, R. J., W. C. FANSLOW, L. STROCKBINE, T. A. SATO, K. N. CLIFFORD, B. M. MACDUFF, D. M. ANDERSON, S. D. GIMPLE, T. DAVIS-SMITH, C. R. MALISZEWISKI, E. A. CLARKE, C. A. SMITH, K. H. GRABSTEIN, D. COSMAN & M. K. SPRIGGS. 1992. Molecular and biological characterisation of a murine ligand for CD40. Nature **357:** 80–82.
26. HOLDER, M. J., H. WANG, A. E. MILNER, M. CASAMAYOR-PALLEJA, R. ARMITAGE, M. K. SPRIGGS, W. C. FANSLOW, I. C. M. MACLENNAN, C. D. GREGORY & J. GORDON. 1993. Suppression of apoptosis in normal and neoplastic human B lymphocytes by CD40 ligand. Eur. J. Immunol. **23:** 2368–2371.
27. PULENDRAN, B., G. KANNOURAKIS, K. NOURI, G. C. SMITH & G. J. V. NOSSAL. 1995. Soluble antigen can cause enhanced apoptosis of germinal center B cells. Nature **375:** 331–334.
28. SHOKAT, K. M. & C. C. GOODNOW. 1995. Antigen-induced B cell death and elimination during germinal center immune responses. Nature **375:** 334–338.
29. COICO, R. F., B. S. BHOGAL & G. J. THORBECKE. 1983. The relationship of germinal centers in lymphoid tissue to immunologic memory. VI. Transfer of B cell memory with lymph node

cells fractionated according to their receptors for peanut agglutinin. J. Immunol. **131:** 2254–2257.

30. PASCUAL, V., Y-J. LIU, A. MAGALSKI, O. DE BOUTEILLER, J. BANCHEREAU & J. D. CAPRA. 1994. Analysis of somatic mutation in 5 B cell subsets of human tonsil. J. Exp. Med. **180:** 329–339.
31. HO, F., J. E. LORTAN, M. KHAN & I. C. M. MACLENNAN. 1986. Distinct short-lived and long-lived antibody-producing cell populations. Eur. J. Immunol. **16:** 1297–1301.
32. BAKKUS, M. H. C., I. VANRIET, B. VANCAMP & K. THIELEMANS. 1994. Evidence that the clonogenic cell in multiple myeloma originates from a pre-switched, but somatically mutated B cell. Br. J. Haematol. **87:** 68–74.
33. BENNER, R., W. HIJMANS & J. J. HAAIJMAN. 1981. The bone marrow: the major source of immunoglobulins, but still a neglected site of antibody formation. Clin. Exp. Immunol. **46:** 1–8.
34. TEW, J. G., R. M. DILOSA, G. F. BURTON, M. H. KOSCO, L. I. KUPP, A. MASUDA & A. K. SZAKAL. 1992. Germinal centers and antibody production in bone marrow. Immunol. Rev. **126:** 99–112.
35. KEPLER, T. B. & A. S. PERELSON. 1993. Cyclic reentry of germinal center B cells and the efficiency of affinity maturation. Immunol. Today **14:** 412–415.
36. HAN, S. H., K. HATHCOCK, B. ZHENG, T. B. KEPLER, R. HODES & G. KELSOE. 1995. Cellular interaction in germinal centers: roles of CD40 ligand and B7-1 and B7-2 in established germinal centers. J. Immunol. **155:** 556–567.
37. GRAMMER, A., M. C. BERGMAN, Y. MIURA, K. FUGITA, L. S. DAVIS & P. E. LIPSKY. 1995. The CD40 ligand expressed by human B cells costimulates B-cell responses. J. Immunol. **154:** 4996–5010.
38. CASAMAYOR-PALLEJA, M., J. FEUILLARD, J. BALL, M. DREW & I. C. M. MACLENNAN. 1996. Centrocytes rapidly adopt a memory B cell phenotype on coculture with autologous germinal-center T cell–enriched preparations. Int. Immunol. **8:** 737–744.
39. ARPIN, C., J. DECHANET, C. VAN KOOTEN, P. MERVILLE, G. GROUARD, F. BRIÈRE, J. BANCHEREAU & Y-J. LIU. 1995. Generation of memory B cells and plasma cells *in vitro.* Science **268:** 720–722.
40. CHAN, E. & I. C. M. MACLENNAN. 1993. Only a small proportion of splenic B cells in adults are short-lived virgin cells. Eur. J. Immunol. **23:** 357–363.
41. YELLIN, M. J., K. SIPPEL, G. INGHIRAMI, L. R. COVEY, J. J. LEE, J. SINNING, E. A. CLARK, L. CHESS & S. LEDERMAN. 1994. CD40 molecules induce down-modulation and endocytosis of T cell surface T cell–B cell activating molecule/CD40L: potential role in regulating helper effector function. J. Immunol. **152:** 598–608.
42. LAGRESLE, C., C. BELLA, P. T. DANIEL, P. H. KRAMMER & T. DEFRANCE. 1995. Regulation of germinal center B cell differentiation: role of the human APO-1/Fas (CD95) molecule. J. Immunol. **154:** 5746–5756.

A Germinal Center–like Reaction in the Nonlymphoid Tissue of the Synovial Membrane[a]

C. BEREK AND A. E. SCHRÖDER

Deutsches Rheuma ForschungsZentrum Berlin
10117 Berlin, Germany

THE MATURATION OF THE IMMUNE RESPONSE IN GERMINAL CENTERS

The analysis of T-dependent immune responses to hapten carrier antigens like 2-phenyl-oxazolone (phOx) has demonstrated that, within two weeks after immunization, a maturation of the immune response takes place.[1] Antigen-activated B cells migrate into the primary follicles of the peripheral lymphatic organs. Rapid proliferation of these cells leads to the formation of large germinal centers (FIGURE 1). By day ten, mature germinal centers have developed in which a dark and a light zone can be distinguished.[2] In the dark zone, B cells are clonally expanded. During proliferation, a hypermutation mechanism becomes activated and the V gene repertoire is diversified. Stepwise somatic mutations are introduced into the variable regions of the H- and the L-chains.[3,4] In this way, B cell variants develop that differ in their affinity for the antigen. Those cells with a relatively high affinity are selected to differentiate into memory cells and presumably such variants also give rise to the plasma cells. In secondary and tertiary responses, further rounds of maturation through hypermutation and selection of variants with increased affinity for the antigen will take place.[1]

The mechanism of affinity selection is still poorly understood. It is believed that follicular dendritic cells (FDCs) that form the dense cellular network of the light zone play a crucial role. FDCs present antigen complexed with antibody to the B cells. Competition for the antigen may determine which B cells are selected to differentiate and which will die through apoptosis.[2] On the other hand, the analysis of germinal center–derived sequences has suggested that selection for affinity may have occurred already during proliferation of B cells in the dark zone.[5]

The analysis of tonsillar B cells and of human splenic B cells has demonstrated that these maturation processes take place during naturally induced immune responses.[6,7]

[a]This work has been supported through the financial help of the Senate for Research and Education of the city of Berlin.

FOLLICLE-LIKE STRUCTURES IN NONLYMPHOID TISSUE

In autoimmune diseases, extensive mononuclear cell infiltrates are observed in the inflamed tissue. It is thought that the infiltrating cells are predominantly CD4+ T cells. However, there is increasing evidence that B cells are also present in these clusters. In the synovial tissue (ST) of patients with rheumatoid arthritis (RA), the ratio of B to T cells seems to correlate with the size of the infiltrates, in that large cell aggregates consist mainly of B cells.[8] Follicle-like cell clusters have been described in various tissues. In myasthenia gravis one finds them in the thymus,[9] in Hashimoto's disease in the thyroid,[10] in Sjögren's syndrome in the salivary glands,[11] and in RA in the ST.[12] Often, these infiltrates form germinal center–like structures where FDCs as well as T and B cells are present.[8,10,12,13]

Whether B cells accumulate in the affected tissue due to an antigen-dependent process remains an open question. There are only a few cases of autoimmune diseases

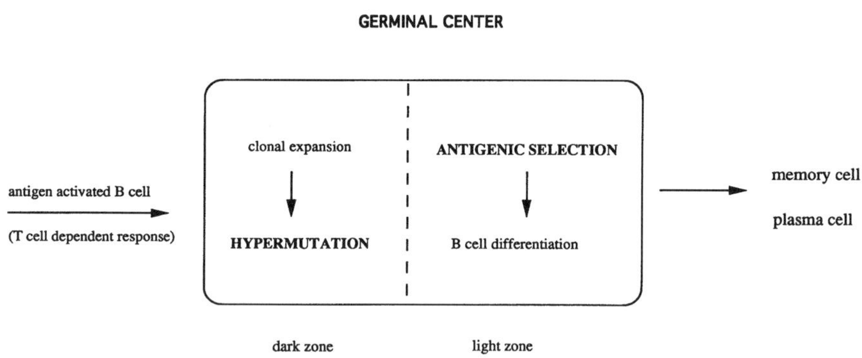

FIGURE 1. Schematic representation of B cell differentiation in germinal centers.

where it has been demonstrated that self-specific B cells are directly involved. One example is Graves' disease, where antibodies specific for the hormone receptor interfere with the production of thyroid hormones.[14] In the glands, lymphocytic infiltrates can be demonstrated and it has been shown that B cells secrete pathogenic autoantibodies.[15] However, even in this case, the etiology of the disease is not at all clear. It has been speculated that an acute virus infection may have triggered the response and a cross-reaction with the tissue-specific hormone receptor may have led to the induction of the autoimmune response.[14] In other cases, inflammation may cause a polyclonal, antigen-independent activation of B cells, which leads to an accumulation of cells in the affected tissue. Autoreactive cells may be activated locally and thus may be retained in the respective tissue. In addition, local destruction of tissue through an immune response against infected cells may release autoantigens that are normally not present. In this way, a humoral autoimmune response may be triggered and a perpetual autoreactive process may develop that is independent from the initiating agent.

In autoimmune diseases like rheumatoid arthritis, the role of autoreactive B cells and their antibodies is much less well defined. The majority of patients are positive for rheumatoid factors (RF), which are autoantibodies with specificity for self-Ig. Such antibodies are often found in low concentration in healthy people as well and may have a physiological function. It has been suggested that B cells expressing RF on their surface may take up antigens trapped in immune complexes.[16] In presenting processed antigen, helper T cells may be stimulated that may promote further activation of B cells. In this way, rheumatoid factors may enhance the inflammatory processes taking place in the ST.

A REPERTOIRE ANALYSIS OF SYNOVIAL B CELLS

To address the question of B cell involvement in autoimmunity, lymphocytic aggregates were directly isolated from frozen tissue sections derived from the synovial membrane of patients with RA.[8] DNA was prepared and the rearranged V regions of H- and L-chains were amplified by PCR. A repertoire analysis of the synovial B cells was performed. The results showed a restricted diversity. Certain V_H genes like DP47, DP75, or DP71 and certain V_L genes like DPL11, O12/O20, or B3 were found in multiple rearrangements, whereas other V regions frequently observed in peripheral blood cells were not seen.

A distinct population of B cells seems to accumulate in the ST of patients with RA. An analysis of control persons showed that, in peripheral blood B cells, Vλ1, Vλ2, and Vλ3 contribute equally to the repertoire. In order to assess V gene diversity in the synovial membrane, DNA was prepared from a total tissue section that contained several thousand plasma cells. Rearranged Vλ L-chains were amplified and cloned, and their diversity was determined. B cells expressed a surprisingly restricted repertoire, in that 44 out of 47 sequences used germline genes of the Vλ2 gene family. Sequences of the gene families Vλ1 and Vλ3 were significantly underrepresented, with there being only one Vλ1 and two Vλ3 rearrangements. In contrast, in the peripheral blood of the same patient, only Vλ1 and Vλ3 sequences were found. Even amplification with a Vλ2-specific primer resulted in no Vλ2 sequences. Thus, in the ST of this patient, a subset of B cells has accumulated that expresses a selected repertoire.

SOMATIC DIVERSITY OF SYNOVIAL B CELLS

The notion that B cells in the synovium are a population distinct from those in the peripheral blood is supported by a comparison of the number of somatic mutations seen in the two populations. Whereas the majority of peripheral B cells differ by no or only a few nucleotide exchanges from the putative germline genes, synovial B cells are highly mutated. In the sequences derived from lymphocytic infiltrates, 18 somatic mutations/variable region were found on average. Assuming a rate for hypermutation of 10^{-3}/base pair/generation, B cells must have divided at least 100 times in order to accumulate this high frequency of somatic mutations.[1]

Somatic mutations are nonrandomly distributed. They have accumulated in the CDR residues, which may indicate that B cells are selected for affinity. However, multiple replacement mutations are also seen in the FRW regions, particularly in FRWIII. In some of the sequences, there are so many amino acid exchanges that it becomes questionable whether a functional antibody can still be formed.

It is unlikely that the diversity is due to V gene polymorphism in the human population. For some of the sequences, an analysis of germline genes has been performed. In no cases were there more than two exchanges from the published germline sequences. Thus, B cells found in the lymphocytic infiltrates are long-term memory cells. They seem to be part of the chronic inflammation process taking place in the ST of patients with RA.

CLONAL EXPANSION OF MEMORY B CELLS

A single section of an infiltrate may contain several hundred B cells. When such a cell cluster was isolated, no more than seven different V_H or V_L rearrangements were found. Identical V (D) J joinings were isolated multiple times, suggesting that there is clonal expansion of B cells in the ST. This interpretation was confirmed by the finding of identical sequences in consecutive sections. The majority of these sequences had an identical pattern of somatic mutations. These data demonstrate that memory cells in the ST may proliferate without further accumulation of somatic mutations. Similar observations were made when hybridoma lines from the autoimmune-prone strain MRL/lpr were analyzed.[17] Whereas in general the number of somatic mutations increases from the primary to the secondary and tertiary immune response,[1] chronic activation may push B memory cells to a differentiation stage where the hypermutation mechanism can no longer be activated. Hence, B cells isolated from the ST of patients with chronic RA may represent long-term memory cells that still proliferate without further accumulation of somatic mutations. Another interpretation might be that the microenvironment of the ST promotes proliferation, but not the diversification of the B cell repertoire.

GERMINAL CENTER–LIKE REACTION IN NONLYMPHOID TISSUE

From one of the infiltrates, 8 sequences with an identical DP51 rearrangement were isolated that had 18 somatic mutations in common, but that differed by up to 12 nucleotides from each other.[8] The isolation of clonal variants from a single tissue section demonstrates that somatic mutations accumulated stepwise during proliferation in the synovial membrane. The clonal diversification is illustrated in the form of a genealogic tree (FIGURE 2a).

The somatic mutations common to these sequences may have been acquired in a germinal center in the peripheral lymphoid tissue. In this case, a memory B cell, upon migration into the ST, becomes reactivated and a further diversification can take place in the nonlymphoid tissue of the synovial membrane. Another interpretation might be

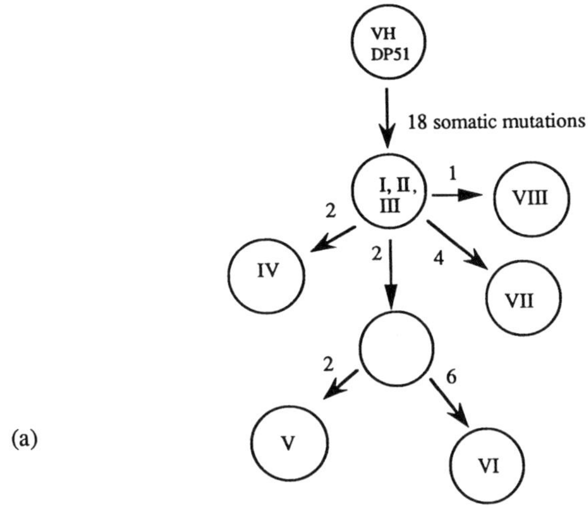

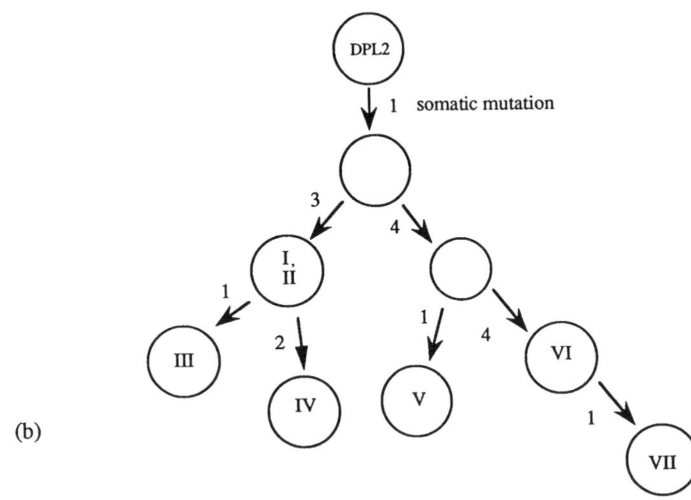

FIGURE 2. Intraclonal diversification of B cells in the ST. Genealogical trees of B cell clones isolated from the ST of a patient with RA (a) and with reactive arthritis (b) are shown. Roman numerals refer to isolated sequences; numbers alongside the arrows refer to the number of nucleotide exchanges that accumulated during clonal expansion. Hypothetical intermediates are included (circles without roman numerals).

that a newly activated B cell enters and the diversification of the V regions occurs locally in the ST. An analysis of B cell infiltrates from the ST of a patient with reactive arthritis has demonstrated that the hypermutation mechanism can be induced in newly activated B cells. Sequences were isolated from this patient that had only 1 somatic mutation in common, but that differed by up to 14 somatic mutations from each other (FIGURE 2b).

Thus, in autoimmune diseases, the local inflammation allows a microenvironment to build up that promotes the diversification of the B cell repertoire. A germinal center–like reaction may take place in the nonlymphoid tissue.

ANTIGEN-DEPENDENT DIFFERENTIATION OF B CELLS

A germinal center reaction is observed only in a T cell–dependent immune response and the hypermutation mechanism becomes activated only after antigenic stimulation of B cells.[1] The major unanswered question is as follows: what are the antigens that drive the germinal center–like reaction in the ST of patients with RA? Are these autoantigens, and if so are these tissue-specific or are foreign antigens involved? We now have the tools to isolate those B cells that go through an antigen-dependent differentiation in the ST. Molecular biologic techniques will enable us to express their Ig repertoire. In this way, it will be possible to search for the antigens that lead to a germinal center formation in the nonlymphoid tissue and this will be crucial for reaching an understanding of the origin of autoimmune responses.

ACKNOWLEDGMENTS

We thank S. A. Camacho for critical reading of the manuscript.

REFERENCES

1. BEREK, C. & C. MILSTEIN. 1987. Mutation drift and repertoire shift in the maturation of the immune response. Immunol. Rev. **96:** 23–41.
2. LIU, Y-J., G. D. JOHNSON, J. GORDON & I. C. M. MACLENNAN. 1992. Germinal centers in T-cell-dependent antibody responses. Immunol. Today **13:** 17–21.
3. BEREK, C., A. BERGER & M. APEL. 1991. Maturation of the immune response in germinal centers. Cell **67:** 1121–1129.
4. JACOB, J., G. KELSOE, K. RAJEWSKY & U. WEISS. 1991. Intraclonal generation of antibody mutants in germinal centres. Nature **354:** 389–392.
5. BEREK, C. & M. ZIEGNER. 1993. The maturation of the immune response. Immunol. Today **14:** 400–404.
6. VARADE, W. S. & R. A. INSEL. 1993. Isolation of germinal center–like events from human spleen RNA: somatic hypermutation of a clonally related V_H6DJ_H rearrangement expressed with IgM, IgG, and IgA. J. Clin. Invest. **91:** 1838–1842.
7. PASCUAL, V., Y-J. LIU, A. MAGALSKI, O. DE BOUTEILLER, J. BANCHEREAU & J. D. CAPRA. 1994. Analysis of somatic mutation in 5 B cell subsets of human tonsil. J. Exp. Med. **180:** 329–339.
8. SCHRÖDER, A. E., A. GREINER, C. SEYFERT & C. BEREK. 1996. Differentiation of B cells in the nonlymphoid tissue of the synovial membrane of patients with rheumatoid arthritis. Proc. Natl. Acad. Sci. U.S.A. **93:** 221–225.
9. GUIGOU, V., D. EMILIE, S. BERRIH-AKNIN, F. FUMOUX, M. FOUGERAU & C. SCHIFF. 1991. Individual germinal centers of myasthenia gravis human thymuses contain polyclonal activated B cells that express all the VH and Vk families. Clin. Exp. Immunol. **83:** 262–266.
10. BIGAZZI, P. E. 1993. Hashimoto's disease. *In* The Molecular Pathology of Autoimmune Diseases. C. Bona, K. A. Siminovitch, M. Zanetti & A. N. Theophilopoulos, Eds.: 493–510. Harwood Academic Pub. Chur, Switzerland.

11. FREIMARK, B. R., R. FANTOZZI, R. BONE, G. BORDIN & R. FOX. 1989. Detection of clonally expanded salivary gland lymphocytes in Sjögren's syndrome. Arthritis Rheum. **32:** 859–869.
12. YOUNG, C. L., T. C. ADAMSON, J. H. VAUGHAN & R. I. FOX. 1984. Immunohistologic characterization of synovial membrane lymphocytes in rheumatoid arthritis. Arthritis Rheum. **27:** 32–39.
13. RANDEN, I., J. MELLBYE, Ø. FØRRE & J. B. NATVIG. 1995. The identification of germinal centers and follicular dendritic cell networks in rheumatoid synovial tissue. Scand. J. Immunol. **41:** 481–486.
14. SONG, Y-H., L. YANGXIN & N. K. MACLAREN. 1996. The nature of autoantigens targeted in autoimmune endocrine diseases. Immunol. Today **17:** 232–238.
15. CHAZENBALK, G. D., S. PORTOLANO, D. RUSSO, J. S. HUTCHISON, B. RAPOPORT & S. MCLACHLAN. 1993. Human organ-specific autoimmune diseases. J. Clin. Invest. **92:** 62–74.
16. ROOSNEK, E. & A. LANZAVECCHIA. 1991. Efficient and selective presentation of antigen-antibody complexes by rheumatoid factor B cells. J. Exp. Med. **173:** 487–489.
17. SHLOMCHIK, M. J., A. MARSHAK-ROTHSTEIN, C. B. WOLFOWICZ, T. L. ROTHSTEIN & M. G. WEIGERT. 1987. The role of clonal selection and somatic mutation in autoimmunity. Nature **328:** 805–811.

Unique Site of Autoantibody Production in Fas-deficient Mice[a]

BRUCE A. JACOBSON, LINDA C. FOOTE, DAVID J. PANKA, SHYR-TE JU, THOMAS L. ROTHSTEIN, AND ANN MARSHAK-ROTHSTEIN[b]

Departments of Microbiology and Medicine
Boston University School of Medicine
Boston, Massachusetts 02118

INTRODUCTION

Fas and Fas-ligand (FasL) are prototypic members of the TNF receptor and TNF gene families, respectively. Reciprocal interactions among these family members trigger pathways that regulate lymphocyte death, survival, and/or differentiation. In many cases, the cell type or state of differentiation of the target population determines whether a particular receptor will transmit a positive or negative signal.[1] For example, CD40 signaling is usually associated with survival and differentiation, but cross-linking of CD40 on certain tumor populations has been shown to result in death.[2] By comparison, Fas engagement has been most frequently associated with apoptotic cell death,[3,4] but anti-Fas antibodies under certain experimental conditions have also been shown to provide costimulatory signals.[5]

Fas/FasL interactions impact the immune system in numerous ways. Both Fas and FasL are upregulated in activated $CD4^+$ Th1 cell lines and, by either fratricidal or suicidal interactions, account for the phenomenon of activation-induced cell death.[6–8] *In vitro* assay systems have demonstrated that FasL-expressing $CD4^+$ and $CD8^+$ cytotoxic effector populations also have the capacity to efficiently kill a variety of Fas^+ (but $FasL^-$) target populations, ranging from tumor cell lines to both T and B lymphoblast populations.[9–11] Such *in vitro* experiments indicate that Fas/FasL-mediated events are likely to have important *in vivo* regulatory correlates, consistent with the pleiotropic defects of the natural Fas and FasL mutant phenotypes, *lpr* and *gld*. Studies from our laboratories over the past several years have focused on a combination of *in vitro* and *in vivo* approaches aimed at specifically defining when and where FasL-expressing effector cells regulate B cell populations.

ABNORMAL FEATURES OF *lpr* B CELL IMMUNITY

To begin to understand the role of the Fas/FasL system in the regulation of B cell immunity, it is important to clearly delineate what is abnormal and what is normal

[a]This work was supported by USPHS Grant Nos. AR-35230 (to A. Marshak-Rothstein), AI-29690 (to T. L. Rothstein), and T32-CA-64070 (to B. A. Jacobson).

[b]To whom all correspondence should be addressed.

about B cell function in Fas-deficient (or FasL-deficient) mice. The most obvious defect is the excessive production of a wide range of autoantibodies, with specificities similar in many respects to the autoantibodies present in the sera of individuals suffering from systemic lupus erythematosus (SLE). MRL/*lpr* mice begin to produce detectable autoantibody titers at about 6–8 weeks of age and levels rapidly progress to remarkably high concentrations. Reactivities include DNA, SmRNP, autologous IgG, and a variety of other nuclear, cytoplasmic, and cell surface autoantigens.[12] Although the spectrum of autoantibody specificities is stochastically distributed among the individual mice in a colony, we found that the majority of MRL/*lpr* mice develop dramatically elevated levels of rheumatoid factor (RF) specific for autologous IgG2a.[13] When hybridoma cell lines were derived from the spleens of diseased *lpr* mice, most of the lines secreted IgG antibodies and at least 10% of the lines made antibodies with RF activity. This high frequency of RF^+ cell lines prompted a rigorous sequence analysis of the V region genes encoding the RF repertoire of individual mice. In studies carried out in collaboration with M. Weigert and colleagues, the RF response was found to exhibit isotype switching, extensive somatic mutation, and modest affinity maturation.[14–16] Similar results were subsequently obtained for other autoantibody specificities.[17] Thus, the *lpr* autoantibody response bears all the features of a prototypic T-dependent response to foreign antigen.

Not only do *lpr* mice actively produce endogenously encoded autoantibodies, but transgene-encoded autoantibodies were also found to be expressed in at least one model. The VH3H9 heavy-chain V region sequence has been repeatedly isolated from anti-DNA antibodies spontaneously arising in MRL/*lpr* mice. VH3H9 can pair with many different light-chain genes to give DNA-reactive antibodies.[18] MRL/*lpr* mice inheriting a VH3H9 transgene make Tg^+ autoantibodies with a homogeneous nuclear (HN) reactivity pattern, and hybridoma cell lines making Tg^+ anti-HN mAb's can readily be derived from the spleens of these mice. In contrast, Tg^+ anti-HN antibodies have never been isolated from transgene-positive wild-type mice.[19]

It is unlikely that autoantibody production in *lpr* mice is simply due to dysregulated T cell help. Evidence that the *lpr* mutation results in an intrinsic defect in B cell activity initially came from studies involving various kinds of [*lpr* + wild-type] hematopoietic chimeras; B cells derived from the *lpr* parent were routinely found to be the predominant source of serum IgG, even though in many cases relatively few *lpr*-derived B cells could be identified in the peripheral lymphoid tissues.[20–23] It is now known that resting B cells from wild-type mice express low levels of Fas, although the level of Fas can be dramatically upregulated by certain activation events, resulting in B lymphoblasts that in some cases are very sensitive to Fas-mediated effector mechanisms (see below). Together, the data suggest that Fas expression by B cells has significant *in vivo* consequences.

NORMAL FEATURES OF *lpr* B CELL IMMUNITY

B cell tolerance to self-antigens is established by a combination of mechanisms ranging from clonal deletion to varying levels of clonal anergy. Clonal deletion, or complete elimination of self-reactive B cells early in their development, is thought to be most important in the removal of B cells that bind self-antigen with relatively high avidity, whereas clonal anergy, or downregulation of the signaling capacity of the sIg receptor, is thought to control B cells with less avid recognition of self-antigen. Experimental models designed to study the induction of tolerance to self-antigen have been applied to *lpr* mice. For example, in the anti-hen egg lysozyme (HEL)/membrane HEL (mHEL) double-transgene system, *lpr* B cells are appropriately deleted in the bone marrow.[24] Furthermore, *lpr* B cells expressing the anti-HEL transgene can be anergized in the periphery by soluble HEL (sHEL), although a breakdown in tolerance is eventually detected in the HEL/sHEL *lpr* mice, as determined by elevated anti-HEL titers in random individuals. Similar results have been obtained in other systems as well and imply that, for B cells with germline-encoded autoreactive receptors, the induction of tolerance in *lpr* mice is intact and not regulated by Fas/FasL interactions.

However, not all autoreactive B cells express germline-encoded genes. B cells specific for foreign antigens can acquire the ability to bind self-antigen as a result of somatic mutation,[25] somatic mutation is known to take place in germinal centers, and Fas has been shown to be upregulated on germinal center B cells.[26–28] It is therefore important to consider the possibility that autoantibody production in *lpr* mice results from the failure to eliminate autoreactive B cells generated by somatic mutation during the course of T-dependent responses to conventional foreign antigens. If this were the case, then the response of *lpr* mice to challenge with T-dependent foreign antigens should be qualitatively, and perhaps quantitatively, different from that of wild-type mice challenged with the same antigen. For the most part, such differences have not been observed. Early studies demonstrated that the serological responses of young (prediseased) *lpr* mice to T-dependent foreign antigens were essentially normal with regard to titer and kinetics, and the antigen-specific responses did not increase even with the onset of the autoimmune disease process.[29,30] More recently, careful analysis at the cellular level has shown that the numbers of antigen-specific antibody-forming cells (AFC) and memory B cells elicited in response to a hapten-protein conjugate are comparable in *lpr* and wild-type mice.[27] Histological examination has further shown that there is nothing unusual about the size, cellular composition, or kinetics of the young *lpr* germinal center response. In addition, the number of apoptotic cells appears comparable in *lpr* and wild-type germinal centers, even when soluble antigen is injected during an ongoing response.[31] Moreover, based on sequence analysis of V region genes isolated from germinal center B cells, the pattern of somatic mutation and the extent of affinity maturation appear to be comparable in *lpr* and wild-type mice.[27]

In summary, *lpr* mice present an intriguing dichotomy: T-dependent responses to foreign antigens are essentially normal, whereas T-dependent responses to autoantigens are dramatically dysregulated. To explain this apparent inconsistency, we propose that autoantibody production in *lpr* mice results from an inability to appropriately maintain anergic B cells in an inactive state. It follows that the conditions leading to the production of antibodies specific for foreign antigen and the conditions leading to the production of antibodies specific for self-antigen are mechanistically distinct. Even though the foreign and self-reactive antibodies exhibit similarities with regard to molecular characteristics such as isotype switching and somatic mutation, there must be other functional and/or environmental criteria that distinguish one from the other. To try to address this issue, we have asked two specific questions: (1) what physiologic signals make B cells sensitive to Fas-mediated apoptosis?; (2) where are the autoantibody-producing B cells initially located?

B CELL SENSITIVITY TO FAS-MEDIATED APOPTOSIS

Early studies of Th1 cell–mediated cytotoxicity (CMC) demonstrated that B cell lines, as well as B cells activated with the mitogen LPS, could be killed in a Fas-dependent assay system.[10] We subsequently found that not all B cell activation pathways resulted in comparable sensitivity to Th1 effector populations. B cells activated by cross-linking CD40 with a soluble CD40L-CD8 fusion protein (followed by anti-CD8 antibody) were significantly more sensitive to Th1 CMC than were LPS blasts. In contrast, B cells activated by anti-IgM Fab′2 fragments were completely resistant to Th1 CMC. Costimulation with CD40L plus anti-IgM resulted in B cell blasts that were almost as resistant as the B cells activated with anti-IgM alone, indicating that sIgM signals not only fail to bring about sensitivity to Fas-mediated apoptosis, but actively suppress Fas apoptosis in otherwise sensitive B cells. B cell Fas resistance was reproducibly found in both lectin-dependent and antigen-specific assay systems (FIGURE 1).[32]

The dominant role of antigen receptor cross-linking was further demonstrated with the B cell receptor transgenic mouse line, 3-83, developed by David Nemazee. B cells from this line specifically recognize the MHC class I molecules K^k and K^b, but not K^d. When 3-83 B cells were activated with CD40L in culture wells containing mitomycin C–treated K^d spleen cells, they became exquisitely sensitive to Th1 CMC; however, when K^k or K^b cells were present in the cultures together with CD40L, the 3-83 B cell target populations acquired a resistant phenotype. These studies strongly suggest that antigen-specific receptor engagement essentially protects the B cell from FasL-induced apoptosis and they explain why T-dependent antibody responses (where the B cell receptors have been effectively engaged) are normal in young *lpr* mice.

The FasL-resistant phenotype of the dual-stimulated CD40L/anti-IgM normal B cells as well as the CD40L/K^k or K^b cocultured 3-83 cells was not simply due to lowered levels of Fas expression. Fas expression in both populations was comparable to that of B cells stimulated with CD40L alone, as detected by flow cytometry with the Jo2 mAb. The possibility that the resistant phenotype resulted from changes in the expression of other cell surface molecules that prevented appropriate conjugate formation between the target and effector populations was also ruled out by cold competition analysis. The possibility that specific T cell/B cell interactions contribute to Fas resistance was explored by screening CD40L and dual-treated target populations for sensitivity to soluble FasL (kindly provided by David Lynch, Immunex), as well as Th1 CMC. The Th1 effector population and the soluble FasL both killed the CD40L-stimulated, but not the CD40L/anti-IgM-stimulated, target populations (FIG-

URE 1), indicating that the resistant phenotype resulted from internal modification of the Fas signaling pathway and the inability to appropriately signal through the expressed Fas receptor. Parenthetically, both target populations were found to be sensitive to the Jo2 mAb, and this killing could be blocked with an anti-Fc receptor

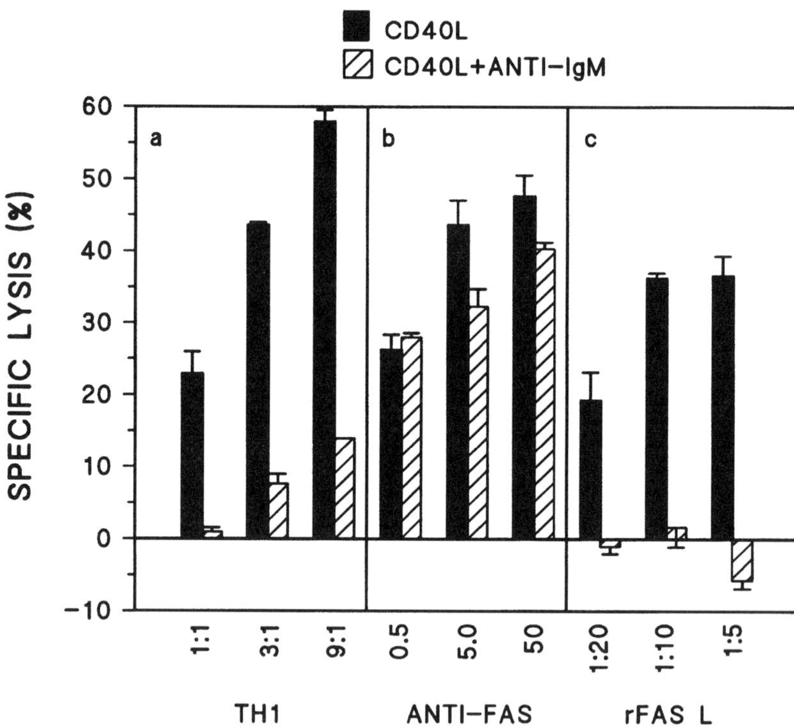

FIGURE 1. Antigen receptor engagement renders B cells resistant to both Th1-mediated and soluble rFasL-mediated cytotoxicity. Primary B cells were cultured either with CD40L alone (CD40L-CD8α fusion protein plus anti-CD8) for 48 h (solid bars) or with the combination of CD40L for 48 h and $F(ab')_2$ GaM IgM for the final 24 h (hatched bars). B cells were then tested for the susceptibility to Fas-dependent cytotoxicity mediated by (a) $CD4^+$ Th1 AE7 effector cells at the effector:target ratios indicated, (b) Jo2 monoclonal anti-Fas antibody at the concentrations indicated (ng/mL), or (c) soluble, recombinant Fas ligand at the dilutions of baculovirus supernatant indicated. For each condition, the mean percent specific lysis of triplicate wells from a ^{51}Cr release assay is shown, along with bars indicating the standard error of the mean.

antibody. Such results suggest that at least some monoclonal antibodies, by virtue of their potent cross-linking capacity, do not appropriately recapitulate the activity of the physiological ligand and also indicate that, even in FasL-resistant B cells, the Fas pathway leading to apoptosis is not completely deleted.

The major conclusion that can be drawn from these *in vitro* experiments is that activated B cells that have received a complete signal through their sIg antigen receptors are protected from FasL-induced apoptosis. The logical corollary is that Fas/FasL interactions *in vivo* serve to downregulate the activation of B cells that have not been effectively triggered through their antigen receptors, that is, either bystander or anergic B cells; B cells specifically responding to T-dependent antigens are not likely to be regulated in a Fas-dependent fashion.

INNER PALS LOCALIZATION OF *lpr* AUTOANTIBODY-PRODUCING CELLS

To further address the role of Fas/FasL interactions in the regulation of B cell immunity, we felt it was important to identify the microenvironment of cells that had escaped from FasL-expressing T cells, that is, *lpr* autoantibody-producing cells. We found that B cells that were actively producing antibodies could be readily identified in frozen sections of lymphoid tissue by *in situ* hybridization with antisense riboprobes specific for Ig constant region domains. In splenic sections from unimmunized wild-type mice, a Cμ probe readily distinguished between resting B cells present in the follicular region of the white pulp (around the T cell–rich inner PALS) and antibody-forming cells (AFC) present in the red pulp. Very few non-IgM AFC were present in these mice, but a small number of cells identified with a Cγ2a probe could also be found in the red pulp (FIGURES 2 and 3).[33]

Prediseased (6-week) MRL/*lpr* mice had a very similar staining pattern to the BALB/c mice, but a dramatically different distribution pattern was apparent by the time that the MRL/*lpr* mice reached 10–12 weeks of age. Many $C\mu^+$ AFC were still present in the red pulp and along the terminal arterioles; however, an increased frequency of $C\mu^+$ AFC was found in the T cell–rich inner PALS. T cells were identified by the staining of contiguous sections with monoclonal antibodies specific for CD4 and CD8. Most significantly, the inner PALS regions were now heavily stained with the Cγ2a probe, indicating that high numbers of IgG2a AFC were accumulating in this predominantly T cell region (FIGURES 2 and 3). Consistent with the presence of IgG2a AFC, many of the $C\gamma 2a^+$ regions could also be shown to contain cells producing rheumatoid factor, a prototypic autoantibody in MRL/*lpr* mice.[33] These results clearly demonstrate that autoantibody production in *lpr* mice occurs in a microenvironment distinct from that of B cells producing antibody in response to conventional foreign antigens.

This localization of AFC to the inner PALS in *lpr* mice further links Fas/FasL interactions to the regulation of anergic B cells. Elegant studies by Goodnow and collaborators, using the HEL/sHEL double-transgene model, have shown that the recirculation pattern of anergic (self-reactive) B cells is severely compromised in mice that also have reasonable numbers of nontransgenic B cells. The anergic cells are selectively retained in the periphery of the inner PALS, where they can be rapidly eliminated subsequent to recognition by FasL-expressing T cells. Recognition by FasL-deficient T cells leads to activation of the target anergic B cells.[34,35] Although these activated "anergic" cells did not differentiate to AFC, one can envision that

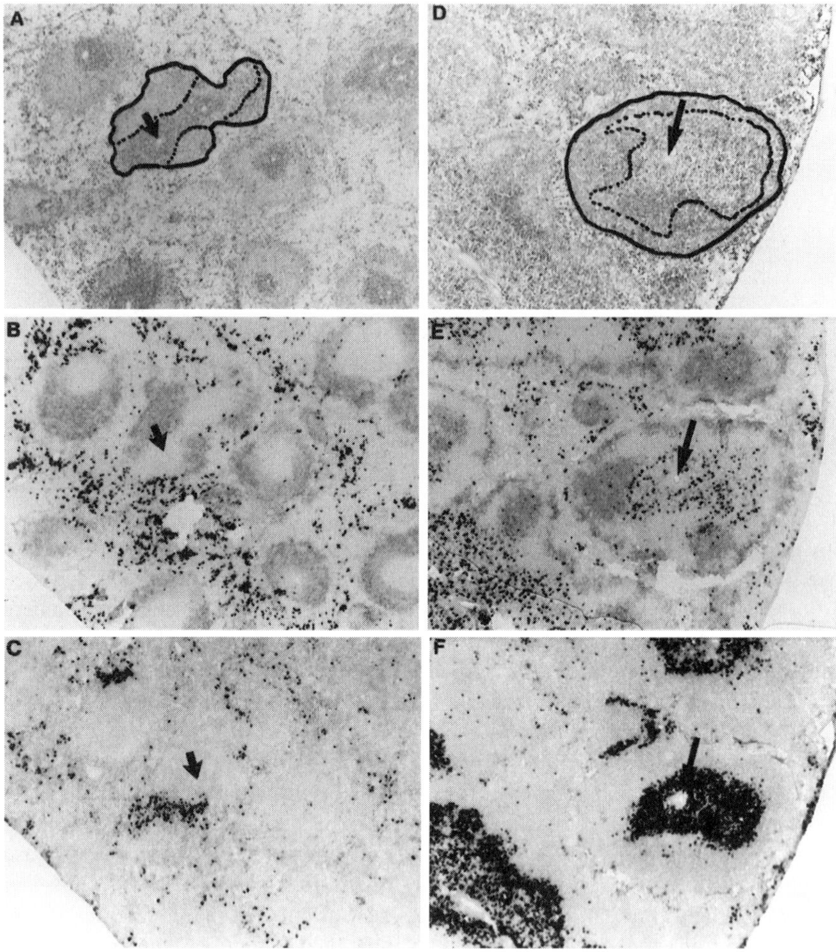

FIGURE 2. *In situ* hybridization of IgM and IgG2a antibody-forming cells in MRL/+ and MRL/*lpr* splenic tissue sections. IgM- and IgG2a-producing cells were detected by *in situ* hybridization and T cells and resting sIgM$^+$ B cells were identified by immunohistochemistry in the spleens of either an 18-week-old MRL/+ mouse (A, B, and C) or a 12-week-old MRL/*lpr* mouse (D, E, and F). Serial 6-μm splenic cryosections were double-stained with anti-CD4-digoxigenin (DIG) and anti-CD8-DIG and with anti-IgM-biotin (BIO) to identify T cells and IgM$^+$ B cells, respectively (A and D). DIG-labeled antibodies were detected with sheep-anti-DIG (gold) followed by silver enhancement. IgM$^+$ B cells were identified using an avidin-biotin alkaline phosphatase conjugate (ABC-AP) and the substrate Vector Red. Sections were also hybridized with the antisense DIG-labeled riboprobes Cμ (B and E) and Cγ2a (C and F) and detected with sheep-anti-DIG-alkaline phosphatase and the substrates nitroblue tetrazolium salt (NBT) and 5-bromo-4-chloro-3-indolyl phosphate toluidium salt (BCIP). NBT/BCIP produces a dark precipitate. Resting IgM$^+$ cells exhibit a faint dark stain, whereas IgM- and IgG2a-producing cells appear more darkly stained. In panels A and D, a white pulp region is outlined by a solid dark line. The region between the solid line and the dotted line is the B cell follicle. The region within the dotted line is the T-zone. In some areas, the T-zone borders the red pulp. Arrows denote central arterioles in contiguous sections. Original magnification: ×40. (Figure reduced to 58%.)

chronic activation of anergic cells with endogenously encoded lower-avidity (for self-antigen) receptors in Fas- or FasL-deficient mice could eventually lead to excessive autoantibody production.

INNER PALS LOCALIZATION OF AFC IN MICE WITH CHRONIC GVH DISEASE

As discussed elsewhere in this volume,[36] normal B cells exposed to a combination of CD40L and IL4 also become resistant to FasL-mediated cytolysis, suggesting that a breakdown in Fas/FasL regulatory events may be at least partially responsible for systemic diseases associated with a skewing toward $CD4^+$ Th2 helper activity. Autoantibody production has been shown to occur in individuals with chronic parasite infections[37] and also in mice that overexpress IL4 as a transgene.

Another experimental system in which Th2 activity has been correlated with autoantibody production is the model for chronic graft-versus-host (GVH) disease developed by Gleichmann and collaborators.[38–40] They showed that the inoculation of unmanipulated (DBA/2 × B6) F1 mice with DBA/2 lymphocytes led to a chronic

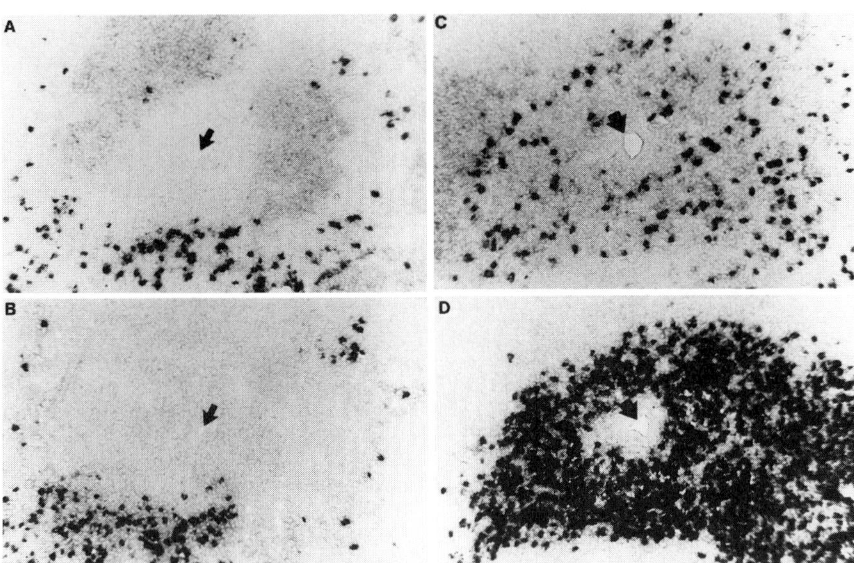

FIGURE 3. *In situ* hybridization of IgM and IgG2a antibody-forming cells in MRL/+ and MRL/*lpr* splenic tissue sections. IgM-forming (A and C) and IgG2a-forming (B and D) cells in MRL/+ (A and B) and MRL/*lpr* (C and D) splenic cryosections were identified by *in situ* hybridization as described in the legend to FIGURE 2. FIGURES 3A and 3C are higher magnifications of the white pulp region shown in FIGURES 2B and 2E, respectively. FIGURES 3B and 3D are higher magnifications of the white pulp region shown in FIGURES 2C and 2F, respectively. Arrows denote central arterioles in contiguous sections. Original magnification: ×160. (Figure reduced to 47%.)

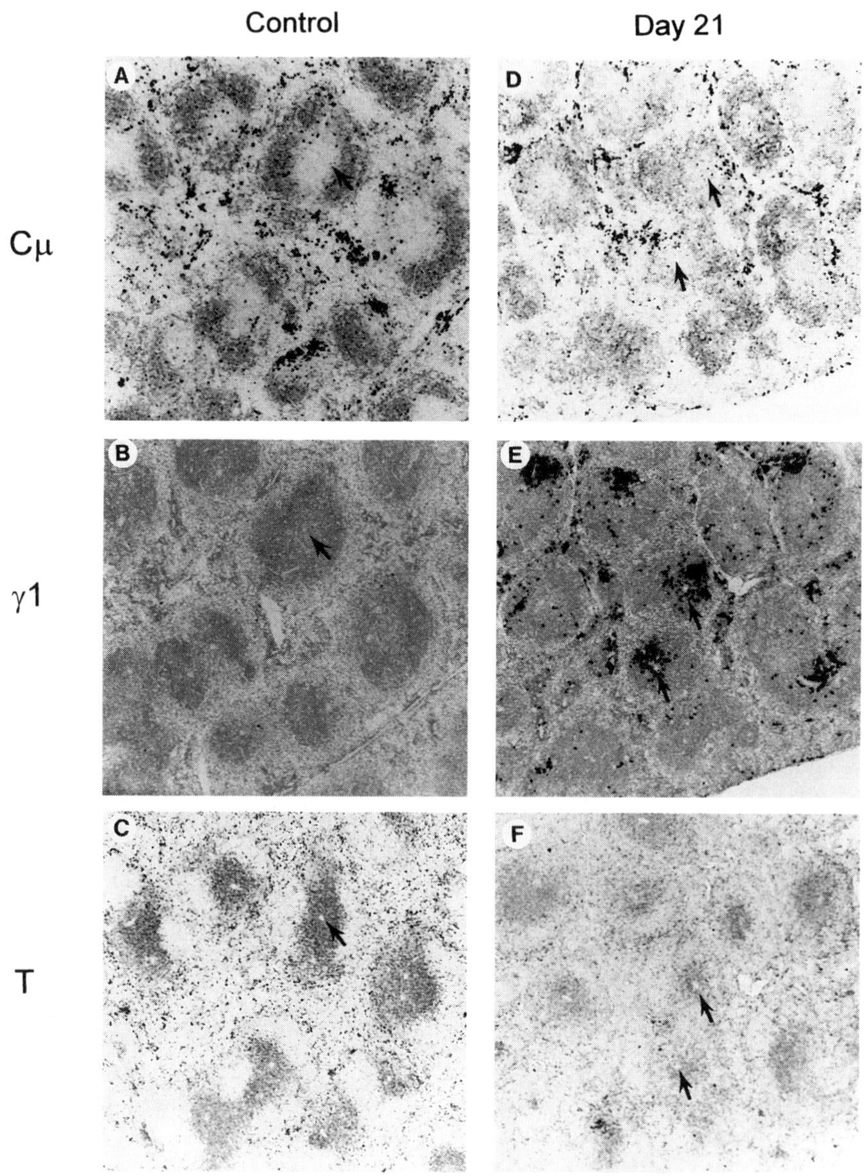

FIGURE 4. *In situ* hybridization of IgM and IgG1 antibody-forming cells in P → F1 chronic GVHD splenic cryosections. DBA/2 spleen and lymph node cells were injected iv into B6D2F1 mice to induce chronic graft-versus-host disease (GVHD). IgM-producing (A and D) and IgG1-producing (B and E) cells were detected by *in situ* hybridization and T cells (C and F) were identified by immunohistochemistry in spleen tissue from uninjected control F1 mice (A, B, and C) and F1 mice injected 21 days previously with parental cells (D, E, and F). See the legend to FIGURE 2 for details of the staining. Arrows denote central arterioles in contiguous sections. Original magnification: ×40. (Figure reduced to 85%.)

GVH disease associated with elevated IgG titers, excessive autoantibody production, and eventual glomerulonephritis. Autoantibodies were specific for nuclear, cytoplasmic, and cell surface antigens, similar to the autospecificities found in patients with SLE. The response was due to allorecognition of the class II disparate F1 B cells by the donor T helper cells.[41] Despite an entire MHC mismatch in this strain combination, it was subsequently shown that the chronic GVH, as opposed to acute GVH, syndrome was unique to the DBA donor population. CD8 cells in the DBA responder population produced negligible levels of IFNγ and the responding $CD4^+$ cells became rapidly skewed to a Th2-type phenotype.[42,43]

We examined the microenvironment of the AFC in this GVH model by *in situ* hybridization. Spleen sections from (DBA/2 × B6) F1 mice injected with 90×10^6 DBA/2 lymphocytes 21 days previously were compared to sections from F1 mice injected with PBS alone. In both control and GVH mice, single positive T cells could be identified in the inner PALS around the central arteriole, resting B cells could be seen in the follicular region, and $C\mu^+$ AFC could be found in the red pulp. However, staining with a Cγ1 riboprobe revealed clusters of IgG1 AFC in the inner PALS of the GVH, but not the control, F1 mice (FIGURE 4). This pattern is strongly reminiscent of the distribution of AFC described above in the *lpr* model and extends the correlation between inner PALS-localized AFC and autoantibody production.

SUMMARY

The inability of B and T lymphocytes from mice expressing the *lpr* mutation to express functional Fas on their cell surface leads to an immunoregulatory defect associated with excessive autoantibody production. Nevertheless, T-dependent antibody response to foreign antigens in these mice appears relatively normal. To better understand exactly how Fas/FasL interactions control autoantibody production, studies were undertaken to determine (1) what kind(s) of B cells are sensitive to Fas-mediated apoptosis and (2) where the autoantibody-producing cells in *lpr* mice are located. We found that B cells activated by CD40L are extremely sensitive as targets in assays of Th1 CMC. However, B cells that receive a complete signal through their sIgM antigen receptor acquire a FasL-resistant phenotype. *In situ* analysis of splenic sections from *lpr* mice demonstrated that autoantibody-producing cells were uniquely localized to the T cell–rich inner PALS. A similar distribution pattern of IgG AFC was found in mice with chronic GVH disease. These data are consistent with the premise that the inner PALS, and not the germinal center, is the major site of FasL regulation of B cell activity and that, as a result of genetic or inducible loss of sensitivity to Fas-mediated apoptosis, autoreactive B cells may survive and differentiate in this location to cause serological autoimmunity.

REFERENCES

1. ROTHSTEIN, T. L. 1996. Curr. Opin. Immunol. **8:** in press.
2. FUNAKOSHI, S., D. L. LONGO, M. BECKWITH, D. K. CONLEY, G. TSARFATY, I. TSARFATY, R. J. ARMITAGE, W. C. FANSLOW, M. K. SPRIGGS & W. J. MURPHY. 1994. Blood **83:** 2787–2794.

3. Trauth, B. C., C. Klas, A. M. J. Peters, S. Matzku, P. Moler, W. Falk, K-M. Debatim & P. Krammer. 1989. Science **245:** 301–305.
4. Yonehara, S., A. Ishii & M. Yonehara. 1989. J. Exp. Med. **169:** 1747–1756.
5. Alderson, M. R., R. J. Armitage, E. Maraskovsky, T. W. Tough, E. Roux, K. Schooley, F. Ramsdell & D. Lynch. 1993. J. Exp. Med. **178:** 2231–2235.
6. Ju, S-T., D. J. Panka, H. Cui, R. Ettinger, M. El-Khatib, D. H. Sherr, B. Z. Stanger & A. Marshak-Rothstein. 1995. Nature **373:** 444–448.
7. Dhein, J., H. Walczak, C. Baumer, K-M. Debatim & P. H. Krammer. 1995. Nature **373:** 438–441.
8. Brunner, T., R. J. Mogli, D. LaFace, N. J. Yoo, A. Mahboubi, F. Echeverri, S. J. Martin, W. R. Force, D. Lynch, C. F. Ware & D. R. Green. 1995. Nature **373:** 441–444.
9. Rouvier, E., M-F. Luciani & P. Goldstein. 1993. J. Exp. Med. **177:** 195–200.
10. Ju, S-T., H. Cui, D. J. Panka, R. Ettinger & A. Marshak-Rothstein. 1994. Proc. Natl. Acad. Sci. U.S.A. **91:** 4185–4189.
11. Stalder, T., S. Hahn & P. Erb. 1994. J. Immunol. **152:** 1127–1133.
12. Andrews, B. S., R. A. Eisenberg, A. N. Theofilopoulos, S. Izui, C. B. Wilson, P. J. McConahey, E. D. Murphy, J. B. Roths & F. J. Dixon. 1978. J. Exp. Med. **148:** 1198–1215.
13. Wolfowicz, C. B., P. Sakorafas, T. L. Rothstein & A. Marshak-Rothstein. 1988. Clin. Immunol. Immunopathol. **46:** 382–395.
14. Shlomchik, M. J., A. Marshak-Rothstein, C. B. Wolfowicz, T. L. Rothstein & M. G. Weigert. 1987. Nature **328:** 805–811.
15. Jacobson, B. A., J. Sharon, H. Shan, M. Shlomchik, M. G. Weigert & A. Marshak-Rothstein. 1994. J. Immunol. **152:** 4489–4499.
16. Shan, H., M. J. Shlomchik, A. Marshak-Rothstein, D. S. Pisetsky, S. Litwin & M. G. Weigert. 1994. J. Immunol. **153:** 5104–5120.
17. Shlomchik, M. J., A. H. Aucoin, D. S. Pisetsky & M. G. Weigert. 1987. Proc. Natl. Acad. Sci. U.S.A. **84:** 9150.
18. Radic, M. Z., J. Erikson, S. Litwin & M. Weigert. 1993. J. Exp. Med. **177:** 1165–1173.
19. Roark, J. H., C. L. Kuntz, K-A. Nguyen, A. J. Caton & J. Erikson. 1995. J. Exp. Med. **181:** 1157–1167.
20. Perkins, D. L., R. M. Glaser, C. A. Mahon, J. Michaelson & A. Marshak-Rothstein. 1990. J. Immunol. **145:** 549–555.
21. Nemazee, D., D. Guiet, K. Buerki & A. Marshak-Rothstein. 1991. J. Immunol. **147:** 2536–2539.
22. Sobel, E. S., T. Katagiri, K. Katagiri, S. C. Morris, P. L. Cohen & R. A. Eisenberg. 1991. J. Exp. Med. **173:** 1441–1449.
23. Glaser, R. M., C. A. Mahon & A. Marshak-Rothstein. 1992. Cell. Immunol. **142:** 313–325.
24. Rathmell, J. C. & C. C. Goodnow. 1994. J. Immunol. **153:** 2831–2842.
25. Ray, S. K., C. Putterman & B. Diamond. 1996. Proc. Natl. Acad. Sci. U.S.A. **93:** 2019–2024.
26. Lagresle, C., C. Bella, P. T. Daniel, P. H. Krammer & T. Defrance. 1995. J. Immunol. **154:** 5746–5756.
27. Smith, K. G. C., G. J. V. Nossal & D. M. Tarlinton. 1995. Proc. Natl. Acad. Sci. U.S.A. **92:** 11628–11632.
28. Watanabe, D., S. Takashi & S. Nagata. 1995. Int. Immunol. **7:** 1949–1956.
29. Park, C. L., T. L. Balderas, T. M. Fieser, J. H. Slack, G. J. Prud'homme, F. J. Dixon & A. N. Theofilopoulos. 1987. J. Immunol. **138:** 466–469.
30. Very, D. L., D. J. Panka, D. Weissman, L. Wysocki, T. Manser & A. Marshak-Rothstein. 1993. Immunology **80:** 518–526.
31. Han, S., B. Zheng, J. Dal Porto & G. Kelsoe. 1995. J. Exp. Med. **182:** 1635–1644.
32. Rothstein, T. L., J. K. M. Wang, D. J. Panka, L. C. Foote, Z. Wang, B. Stanger, H. Cui, S-T. Ju & A. Marshak-Rothstein. 1995. Nature **374:** 163–165.

33. JACOBSON, B. J., D. J. PANKA, K-A. NGUYEN, J. ERIKSON, A. K. ABBAS & A. MARSHAK-ROTHSTEIN. 1995. Immunity **3:** 509–519.
34. CYSTER, J. G. & C. C. GOODNOW. 1995. Immunity **3:** 691–701.
35. RATHMELL, J. C., M. P. COOKE, W. Y. HO, J. GREIN, S. E. TOWNSEND, M. M. DAVIS & C. C. GOODNOW. 1995. Nature **376:** 181–184.
36. FOOTE, L. C., A. MARSHAK-ROTHSTEIN & T. L. ROTHSTEIN. 1997. This volume.
37. SHAKIB, F., D. I. PRITCHARD, E. A. WALSH, S. J. SMIT, A. POWELL-RICHARDS, S. KUMAR & P. EDMONDS. 1993. Parasite Immunol. **15:** 1547–1553.
38. GLEICHMANN, E. & H. GLEICHMANN. 1976. Eur. J. Immunol. **6:** 899.
39. VAN DER VEEN, J. P. W., A. G. ROLINK & E. GLEICHMANN. 1981. Clin. Exp. Immunol. **46:** 589–596.
40. GLEICHMANN, E., E. H. VAN ELVEN & J. P. W. VAN DER VEEN. 1982. Eur. J. Immunol. **12:** 152–159.
41. PALS, S. T., T. RADASKIEWICZ & E. GLEICHMANN. 1984. J. Immunol. **132:** 1669–1678.
42. GOLDMAN, M., P. DRUET & E. GLEICHMANN. 1991. Immunol. Today **12:** 223–232.
43. RUS, V., A. SVETIC, P. NGUYEN, W. C. GAUSE & C. S. VIA. 1995. J. Immunol. **155:** 2396–2406.

Microbial Antigens Can Elicit Autoantibody Production

A Potential Pathway to Autoimmune Disease

PHILIP KUO, CZESLAWA KOWAL, BOAZ TADMOR, AND BETTY DIAMOND

Departments of Microbiology/Immunology and Medicine
Albert Einstein College of Medicine
Yeshiva University
Bronx, New York 10461-1602

A major unresolved question regarding the etiology of the autoimmune disease, systemic lupus erythematosus (SLE), is the nature of the antigen that triggers the anti-DNA response.[1,2] Although it is clear that a dominant serum response in SLE is directed to double-stranded DNA, it is not clear whether this represents a response to an immunogenic form of DNA or some different cross-reactive self-antigen or whether the anti-DNA response represents an unwanted by-product of the response to a foreign, non-DNA, antigen.

We have been interested in determining whether anti-DNA antibodies can arise by somatic mutation during the response to foreign antigen. The hypothesis that somatic mutation of protective antibodies might lead to autoreactivity was derived from the observation that somatic mutation in an *in vitro* culture system could convert an antipneumococcal antibody to an antibody with specificity for double-stranded (ds) DNA.[3] The S107 antibody binds phosphorylcholine (PC), the dominant hapten on the pneumococcal cell wall. U4 is an *in vitro*–derived variant with a glutamic acid to alanine substitution at residue 35 in the first complementarity determining region of the heavy chain. U4 has lost binding to PC, but has acquired binding to dsDNA and other phosphorylated macromolecules (such as cardiolipin), which are also significant autoantigens in patients with systemic lupus. This observation led us to ask in both murine and human studies whether potentially pathogenic autoantibodies arise routinely during the response to foreign antigen and, if so, what mechanisms of tolerance induction are used to prevent autoimmunity and tissue injury.

MURINE STUDIES

Based on the S107-U4 observation, we had reasoned that somatic mutation might frequently generate U4-like antibodies. Efforts to isolate anti-dsDNA hybridomas from PC-immunized nonautoimmune mice proved frustrating, however, and only rare cross-reactive anti-PC, anti-dsDNA hybridomas could be obtained.[4] One possibility was that autoreactivity was an infrequent consequence of somatic mutation and that only a very small percent of B cells binding foreign antigen mutated to antiself reactivity. Alternatively, the autoreactive B cells arising during the response to PC were subject to deletion or anergy and were not recoverable as viable hybridomas.

To test the latter possibility, we elected to transfect the NSO fusion partner with cDNA encoding the antiapoptotic gene bcl-2.[5] Although most germinal center B cells undergo apoptosis, the bcl-2 protein is known to be upregulated in those germinal center B cells that move into a survival pathway.[6] Furthermore, mice transgenic for constitutive bcl-2 expression in the B cell compartment display a marked increase in B cell number and, in certain genetic backgrounds, display autoantibody production as well.[7,8]

R4A transgenic mice express the heavy chain of a pathogenic anti-DNA antibody.[9,10] The R4A heavy chain pairs with some light chains to form an anti-DNA antibody and with other light chains to form an antibody with no specificity for DNA.[11] Sera of R4A transgenic nonautoimmune BALB/c mice display no elevation in titers of anti-DNA antibody, yet LPS stimulation of splenocytes *in vitro* leads to secretion of transgene-encoded anti-DNA antibody.[11] Thus, there is a population of anti-DNA B cells present in the spleens of R4A transgenic mice. Fusion of unstimulated splenocytes with NSO cells repeatedly failed to yield anti-DNA hybridomas. Fusion with $NSO^{bcl\text{-}2}$, in contrast, yielded anti-DNA hybridomas representing approximately 10% of the hybridomas expressing the R4A transgene. Thus, $NSO^{bcl\text{-}2}$ could be shown to form viable hybridomas with anergic or preapoptotic cells, that is, cells that would not routinely form viable hybridomas[5] (FIGURE 1).

We now had a tool to examine the B cell repertoire that does not contribute to serum antibody responses, that is, B cells that do not undergo positive selection or that are subject to mechanisms of negative selection.[12–14] Armed with this tool, we again analyzed hybridomas derived from PC-immunized nonautoimmune mice, this time fusing primary splenocytes to $NSO^{bcl\text{-}2}$.[15] Fusions performed on days 2 and 5 after immunization yielded no anti-PC, anti-DNA cross-reactive hybridomas. Fusions performed on days 10 and 11 following immunization yielded a high frequency of cross-reactive hybridomas (TABLE 1). Approximately 30–40% of the day 10 and day 11 anti-PC hybridomas displayed cross-reactivity with dsDNA. This study suggested that anti-DNA reactivity is generated frequently during the response to foreign antigen. Furthermore, the survival of cross-reactive hybridomas following fusion to $NSO^{bcl\text{-}2}$ suggested that such cross-reactive cells are routinely regulated by apoptosis.

Molecular analysis of cross-reactive antibodies revealed that the immunoglobulin variable-region genes had undergone somatic mutation and for one antibody, b9-5, mutation was shown to be responsible for the acquisition of dsDNA binding.[15] b9-5 is encoded by the heavy- and light-chain variable-region genes that encode S107 and differs from the S107 antibody by only two amino acids, one in the heavy chain and one in the light chain. S107 displays no reactivity with dsDNA; therefore, the two amino acid differences confer dsDNA binding on b9-5. b9-5 is an *in vivo* analogue of U4.

Several cross-reactive anti-PC, anti-DNA antibodies were tested for pathogenicity in an *in vivo* model in which hybridoma cells were grown in the peritoneal cavity of SCID mice.[4,15] Whereas some antibodies displayed minimal glomerular deposition,

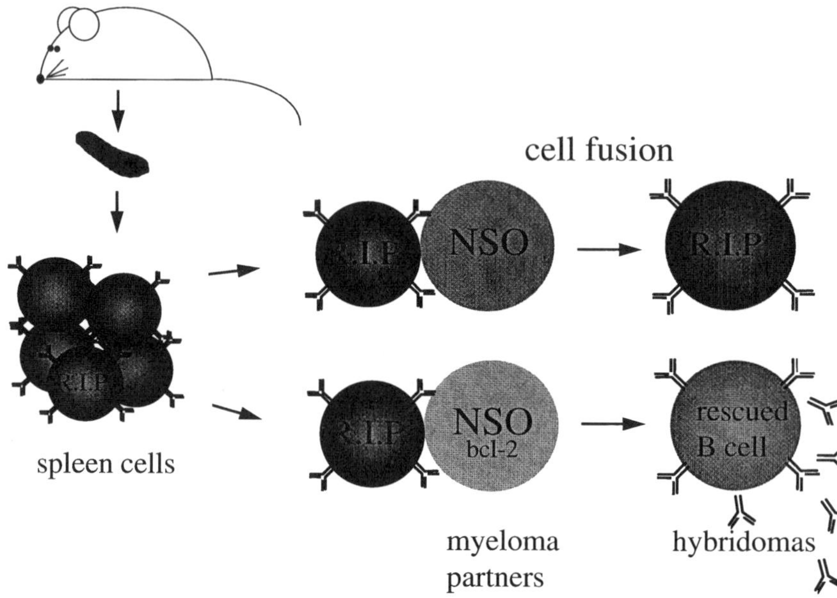

FIGURE 1. Schematic of hybridoma formation with $NSO^{bcl\text{-}2}$. Primary B cells that are programmed for cell death can be rescued by fusion with $NSO^{bcl\text{-}2}$.

others led to extensive glomerular and tubular deposition similar to anti-DNA antibodies derived from lupus-prone mice.

These studies demonstrated that potentially pathogenic autoreactivity arises at high frequency among B cells responding to foreign antigen. Because the frequency of cross-reactive B cells displaying both antiself and antiforeign specificities is so great, there must be mechanisms to regulate their activation *in vivo.* Recent studies clearly demonstrate that signaling from both antigen and T cells is necessary to prevent B cell apoptosis in germinal centers.[16–19] B cells producing antibodies that have specificity only for self are thought to be excluded from a survival pathway because they lack T cell help. In the absence of antigen-specific T cells, autoreactive B cells would receive only an antigen signal and would undergo apoptosis. Cross-reactive B cells present a different hazard to the organism. Unlike antiself B cells, they will receive T cell help because they are able to contact, process, and present foreign antigen.[20] Cross-reactive B cells should then undergo positive selection within germinal centers. The elimination of these B cells must therefore occur by a mechanism that is spatially and/or temporally removed from the process of positive selection. Because bcl-2 rescues cross-reactive B cells, it appears that programmed cell death is the mechanism routinely responsible for their elimination. We have speculated that the negative selection of these cells occurs after positive selection, probably outside of germinal centers, when the cells have entered a pool of recirculating memory cells. Circulating cross-reactive B cells might encounter self-antigen in the absence of foreign antigen and therefore in the absence of T cell help. Signaling of these B cells through

TABLE 1. Cross-reactive Hybridomas from PC-immunized Mice[a]

	Anti-PC	Cross-reactive Anti-PC, Anti-DNA
fusions 1, 2	20	0
fusions 3, 4, 5	34	13 (38%)

[a]Fusions 1 and 2 were performed on days 2 and 5 following PC immunization; fusions 3, 4, and 5 were performed on days 10 and 11.

membrane immunoglobulin alone without T cell signals would induce anergy or deletion.

HUMAN STUDIES

Studies of human antibodies also have led us, by a convergent path, to the hypothesis that anti-DNA antibodies may be clonally related to antimicrobial, specifically antipneumococcal, antibodies. 3I is an idiotypic specificity on a high percentage of anti-DNA antibodies present in the serum of most patients with systemic lupus.[21,22] Furthermore, among the population of $3I^+$ antibodies, a subset of pathogenic antibodies are found deposited in kidneys of patients with lupus nephritis.[22]

In order to analyze whether $3I^+$ antibodies could also be part of a protective antibody repertoire, we analyzed the serum response of nonautoimmune individuals vaccinated with pneumococcal polysaccharide.[23] All postvaccination sera contained $3I^+$ antipneumococcal antibodies, demonstrating a structural relationship between anti-DNA antibodies in lupus patients and antipneumococcal antibodies in nonautoimmune individuals. We did not observe any $3I^+$ anti-DNA antibodies following vaccination. Presumably, if such B cells arise, they undergo negative selection in nonautoimmune individuals.

In order to further explore a possible clonal relationship between anti-DNA and antimicrobial antibodies, we decided to generate a combinatorial library from spleen cells of a patient with systemic lupus (SLE) who displayed elevated serum titers of $3I^+$ anti-DNA antibodies.[24] The patient had been vaccinated with pneumococcal polysaccharide prior to splenectomy; therefore, both antipneumococcal and anti-DNA B cells should be present among the splenic lymphocytes. The combinatorial library technique provides for a random association of heavy and light chains. Although this approach, in principle, will generate antibodies that do not exist in splenic B cells, it should also generate a complete representation of the splenic B cell repertoire.

We elected to isolate Fab bearing the 3I idiotype and to analyze these for pneumococcal and DNA binding. Of all $3I^+$ Fab examined, approximately 36% bound pneumococcal polysaccharide and 21% bound DNA (TABLE 2). Of the antipneumococcal antibodies obtained, 40% cross-reacted with dsDNA. Although these antibodies have not yet been sequenced to determine if those that show specificity uniquely for bacterial polysaccharide are clonally related either to those that cross-react with dsDNA or to those that bind uniquely to dsDNA, the antibodies displayed a range of antigenic specificities similar to those seen in B cells of PC-immunized mice. Furthermore, only 6 of 19 Fab with specificity for dsDNA did not cross-react with pneumococcal polysaccharide, suggesting that a major portion of the anti-DNA response in the spleen may have been triggered by bacterial antigen.

During the course of a response to foreign antigen in a human spleen, there arise antibodies that bind uniquely to foreign antigen and antibodies that bind to both foreign antigen and self-antigen. Because extensive studies of immunoglobulin variable-region genes in the mouse and in humans have revealed no lupus-associated polymorphisms, it is highly unlikely that only a patient with SLE would produce autoreactive B cells.[25,26] Rather, it is far more likely that all individuals have the capacity to generate lupuslike antibodies. Even nonautoimmune individuals during the course of a response to bacterial antigen may generate some antibodies specific to that antigen and other antibodies that recognize both the eliciting bacterial antigen and self-antigen.

The capacity to generate cross-reactive antiforeign, antiself antibodies represents an important potential hazard for the immune system. According to our current understanding of B cell activation, B cells making such antibodies ought to routinely receive the signals that mediate positive selection and stimulate differentiation to

TABLE 2. Antigenic Specificity: $3I^+$ Fab from a Combinatorial Library

number of clones tested	90
number of clones binding pneumococcal polysaccharide	33
number of antipneumococcal clones cross-reactive with dsDNA	6
number of clones binding dsDNA only	19

plasma cells and memory cells. Cross-reactive B cells that become plasma cells may thus be responsible for producing the autoantibodies that are so often associated with microbial infection.[27–29] When foreign antigen is eradicated, B cells specific for that antigen return to a resting state. However, cross-reactive B memory cells, once the foreign antigen has been eliminated, may receive an antigen signal without accompanying T cell help and so be targeted for anergy or apoptosis. In nonautoimmune individuals, the autoantibody response that is activated by infection would disappear with the resolution of the infection, presumably as autoreactive B cells are subjected to anergy induction or deletion. In individuals with some defect in B cell regulation, there may be a failure to eliminate cross-reactive B cells. Should this occur, it might lead to prolonged secretion of autoantibodies and, in susceptible individuals, to autoimmune pathology.

REFERENCES

1. Diamond, B., J. B. Katz, E. Paul, C. Aranow, D. Lustgarten & M. D. Scharff. 1992. The role of somatic mutation in the pathogenic anti-DNA response. Annu. Rev. Immunol. **10:** 731–757.

2. Radic, M. Z. & M. Weigert. 1994. Genetic and structural evidence for antigen selection of anti-DNA antibodies. Annu. Rev. Immunol. **12:** 487–520.
3. Diamond, B. & M. D. Scharff. 1984. Somatic mutation of the T15 heavy chain gives rise to an antibody with autoantibody specificity. Proc. Natl. Acad. Sci. U.S.A. **81:** 5841–5844.
4. Putterman, C., W. Limpanisithikul & B. Diamond. 1996. The double-edged sword of the immune response: mutational analysis of a murine anti-pneumococcal, anti-DNA antibody. J. Clin. Invest. **97:** 2251–2259.
5. Ray, S. & B. Diamond. 1994. Generation of a novel fusion partner to sample the repertoire of splenic B cells destined for apoptosis. Proc. Natl. Acad. Sci. U.S.A. **91:** 5548–5551.
6. Liu, Y. J., D. Y. Mason, G. D. Johnson, S. Abbot, C. D. Gregory, D. L. Hardie, J. Gordon & I. C. MacLennan. 1991. Germinal center cells express bcl-2 protein after activation by signals which prevent their entry into apoptosis. Eur. J. Immunol. **21:** 1905–1910.
7. Strasser, A., S. Whittingham, D. L. Vaux, M. L. Bath, J. M. Adams, S. Cory & A. W. Harris. 1991. Enforced BCL2 expression in B-lymphoid cells prolongs antibody responses and elicits autoimmune disease. Proc. Natl. Acad. Sci. U.S.A. **88:** 8661–8665.
8. Strasser, A., A. W. Harris, D. L. Vaux, E. Webb, M. L. Bath, J. M. Adams & S. Cory. 1990. Abnormalities of the immune system induced by dysregulated bcl-2 expression in transgenic mice. Curr. Top. Microbiol. Immunol. **166:** 175–181.
9. Shefner, R., G. Kleiner, A. Turken, L. Papazian & B. Diamond. 1991. A novel class of anti-DNA antibodies identified in BALB/c mice. J. Exp. Med. **173:** 287–296.
10. Katz, J. B., W. Limpanisithikul & B. Diamond. 1994. Mutational analysis of an autoantibody: differential binding and pathogenicity. J. Exp. Med. **180:** 925–932.
11. Offen, D., L. Spatz, H. Escowitz, S. Factor & B. Diamond. 1992. Induction of tolerance to an IgG autoantibody. Proc. Natl. Acad. Sci. U.S.A. **89:** 8332–8336.
12. Jacob, J., G. Kelsoe, K. Rajewsky & U. Weiss. 1991. Intraclonal generation of antibody mutants in germinal centres. Nature **354:** 389–392.
13. Rajewsky, K. 1996. Clonal selection and learning in the antibody system. Nature **381:** 751–758.
14. Paul, E., A. Manheimer-Lory, A. Livneh, A. Solomon, C. Aranow, C. Ghossein, R. Shefner, D. Offen, M. Pillinger & B. Diamond. 1990. Pathogenic anti-DNA antibodies in SLE: idiotypic families and genetic origins. Int. Rev. Immunol. **5:** 295–313.
15. Ray, S., C. Putterman & B. Diamond. 1996. Pathogenic autoantibodies are routinely generated during the response to foreign antigen: a paradigm for autoimmune disease. Proc. Natl. Acad. Sci. U.S.A. **93:** 2019–2024.
16. Pulendran, B., G. Kannourakis, S. Nouri, K. G. C. Smith & G. J. V. Nossal. 1995. Soluble antigen can cause enhanced apoptosis of germinal-centre B cells. Nature **375:** 331–334.
17. Shokat, K. M. & C. C. Goodnow. 1995. Antigen-induced B-cell death and elimination during germinal-centre immune responses. Nature **375:** 334–338.
18. Foy, T. M., J. D. Laman, J. A. Ledbetter, A. Aruffo, E. Claassen & R. J. Noelle. 1994. gp39-CD40 interactions are essential for germinal center formation and the development of B cells memory. J. Exp. Med. **180:** 157–163.
19. Ku, J., T. M. Foy, J. D. Laman, E. A. Elliott, J. J. Dunn, T. J. Waldschmidt, J. Elsemore, R. J. Noelle & R. A. Flavell. 1994. Mice deficient for the CD40 ligand. Immunity **1:** 423–431.
20. Lanzavecchia, A. 1987. Antigen uptake and accumulation in antigen-specific B cells. Immunol. Rev. **99:** 39–51.
21. Solomon, G., J. Schiffenbauer, H. D. Keiser & B. Diamond. 1983. The use of monoclonal antibodies to identify shared idiotypes on human antibodies to native DNA from patients with systemic lupus erythematosus. Proc. Natl. Acad. Sci. U.S.A. **80:** 850–854.
22. Davidson, A., R. Halpern & B. Diamond. 1986. Speculation on the role of somatic mutation in the generation of anti-DNA antibodies. Ann. N.Y. Acad. Sci. **475:** 174–180.
23. Grayzel, A., A. Solomon, C. Aranow & B. Diamond. 1991. Antibodies elicited by pneumococcal antigens bear an anti-DNA associated idiotype. J. Clin. Invest. **87:** 842–846.

24. SCOTT, J. K. & G. P. SMITH. 1990. Searching for peptide ligands with an epitope library. Science **249:** 386–390.
25. PAUL, E., A. LIVNEH, A. MANHEIMER-LORY & B. DIAMOND. 1991. Characterization of the human immunoglobulin VλII gene family and analysis of VλII and Cλ polymorphism in systemic lupus erythematosus. J. Immunol. **147:** 2771–2776.
26. MANHEIMER-LORY, A., R. MONHIAN, A. SPLAVER, B. GAYNOR & B. DIAMOND. 1995. Analysis of the V_kI family: germline gene and expressed antibodies. Autoimmunity **20:** 259–265.
27. CUNHA-NETO, E., M. DURANTI, A. GRUBER, B. ZINGALES, I. DEMESSIAS, N. STOLF, G. BELLOTTI, M. E. PATARROYO, F. PILLEGGI & J. KALIL. 1995. Autoimmunity in Chagas' disease cardiopathy: biological relevance of a cardiac myosin-specific epitope cross-reactive to an immunodominant *Trypanosoma cruzi* antigen. Proc. Natl. Acad. Sci. U.S.A. **92:** 3541–3545.
28. EL-ROIEY, A., O. SELA, D. A. ISENBERG, R. FELDMAN, B. C. COLACO, R. C. KENNEDY & Y. SHOENFELD. 1987. The sera of patients with *Klebsiella* infections contain a common anti-DNA idiotype (16/6) Id and anti-polynucleotide activity. Clin. Exp. Immunol. **67:** 507–515.
29. VASHISHTHA, A. & A. FISCHETTI. 1993. Surface-exposed conserved region of the streptococcal M protein induces antibodies cross-reactive with denatured forms of myosin. J. Immunol. **150:** 4693–4701.

Positive and Negative Selection of Human B Lymphocytes *in Vitro*

JACQUES BANCHEREAU, LAURENT GALIBERT,
CHRISTOPHE ARPIN, NICOLAS BURDIN,
YONG-JUN LIU, AND PIERRE GARRONE

Laboratory for Immunological Research
Schering-Plough
69571 Dardilly, France

INTRODUCTION

The function of B lymphocytes is to produce antibodies (humoral immune response) that bind, inactivate, and eventually eliminate invading antigens/pathogens. Naive B lymphocytes, generated within the bone marrow, migrate into the secondary lymphoid organs where they either die or are recruited into the recirculating B cell pool. Without antigenic encounter, these naive B cells recirculate through the blood, secondary lymphoid organs, and lymph and back to the blood. However, once antigens/pathogens are localized within a secondary lymphoid organ, the recirculating naive B lymphocytes (and naive T lymphocytes) bearing specific antigen receptors are retained. The secondary lymphoid organs (tonsils, lymph nodes, spleen, and mucosal-associated lymphoid tissues) are organized into B cell–rich follicles and T cell–rich extrafollicular areas. Whereas B cell follicles contain follicular dendritic cells (FDCs) that trap native antigen in the form of immune complexes for long periods of time, T cell–rich extrafollicular areas contain interdigitating dendritic cells, that is, antigen-presenting cells, that can activate naive T cells.

During T cell–dependent immune responses, naive B cells that carry specific antigen receptors are activated in association with antigen-specific T cells and interdigitating dendritic cells within the extrafollicular areas. The activated B blasts either undergo terminal differentiation towards plasma cells or become germinal center founder cells that will migrate into the primary follicles or the dark zone of established germinal centers of secondary follicles.

The germinal center founder cells undergo clonal expansion and differentiation into centroblasts that form and sustain the dark zones. At the same time, point mutations are introduced into the IgV region genes in a stepwise fashion during the course of the clonal proliferation of centroblasts. Three types of mutants can be generated, including high-affinity, low-affinity, and autoreactive mutants, which compose the basal light zone of the germinal center. The survival of these somatic mutants depends on their binding to the low levels of antigen-antibody immune complexes on the surface of follicular dendritic cells. High-affinity mutants pick up antigen, process it, and present it to germinal center T cells that are mainly localized within the apical light zone. Autoreactive mutant clones and low-affinity mutants are deleted. The selected high-affinity centrocytes present processed antigen to antigen-specific T cells that are induced to express CD40-ligand and secrete cytokines including IL-4 and IL-10, all being key elements for B cell survival, proliferation, and isotype switching. This cognate T cell–B cell interaction results in the expansion and isotype switch of high-affinity centrocytes. Finally, the high-affinity, isotype-switched centrocytes differentiate into memory B cells in the presence of prolonged CD40-ligand signaling and into plasma cells when CD40-ligand signaling is removed. During secondary humoral immune responses, recirculating memory B cells can be activated in extrafollicular areas, giving rise to plasma cells and germinal center founder cells.

The availability of mice with transgenic antigen-specific B or T cell receptors represents a considerable revolution for the understanding of positive and negative selection of B lymphocytes[1,2] (also see other papers in this volume). However, for an eventual therapeutic use of the observation, there is a need to determine whether they may or may not apply to humans. Consequently, this requires a thorough scrutinizing of the B cell response to T cell–dependent antigens. This requires both an *ex vivo* analysis of the various B cell maturation stages as well as an *in vitro* analysis of their response to signals delivered by other cell types.

Over the past decade, numerous studies have been performed aimed at understanding the role of cytokines in the growth and differentiation of human B cells activated *in vitro* through different means. The present report will summarize the *in vitro* effects of recombinant cytokines on purified human B lymphocytes triggered through (i) their antigen receptors, (ii) CD40 antigen, and (iii) Fas antigen.

FUNCTIONAL CONSEQUENCES OF ANTIGEN RECEPTOR ENGAGEMENT

Purified mature B lymphocytes undergo limited DNA synthesis when activated through their antigen receptors (BCR) using immobilized anti-Ig antibodies.[3] Particles of *Staphylococcus aureus* strain Cowan (SAC) also act as a strong polyclonal activator of B cells, involving BCR cross-linking and possibly the engagement of other B cell surface molecules.

IL-2, IL-4, IL-10, IL-13,[4] IFNγ, TNFα and β, and high-molecular-weight BCGF (IL-14?)[5] have been shown to enhance to some extent the DNA synthesis of BCR-activated B cells. IL-2 represents one of the most efficient cytokines, particularly after several days of culture. IL-2 and IL-10 can induce SAC-activated B cells to secrete IgG, IgA, and IgM, whereas IL-4 only induces the production of low levels of IgM and IgG. Under these conditions, B cells triggered through their BCR do not undergo isotype switch in response to cytokines.

FUNCTIONAL CONSEQUENCES OF CD40 ENGAGEMENT

Historical Considerations

The limited B cell growth and differentiation observed following BCR cross-linking led to the proposal that the engagement of BCR may essentially represent an activation and/or a selection signal for B cells. Such a hypothesis implies that other B cell surface molecules are involved in the massive expansion and differentiation of the rare antigen-specific B cells *in vivo.* In particular, models were established in which activated T cells were shown to induce considerable B cell proliferation and Ig secretion.[6] Although cytokines produced by activated T cells play a key role in the growth and differentiation of B cells, the contact between T cells and B cells cannot be replaced by T cell supernatants. Thus, fixed activated T cells or their membranes can induce B cells to proliferate, and addition of cytokines can further enhance growth and can induce Ig secretion. These studies led to the identification of CD40 as a key antigen involved in B cell growth and differentiation. CD40, a member of the TNFα receptor family, is a receptor for CD40-L, an activation antigen of T cells and a member of the TNFα family.[7–9]

Proliferation of B Lymphocytes

Anti-CD40 antibodies were identified by their ability to costimulate with either anti-IgM antibodies or phorbol esters for the proliferation of purified B cells. Culture of resting B cells in the CD40 system (anti-CD40 antibody presented by a fibroblastic cell line transfected with FcγRII/CD32) or on CD40-L-transfected cells results in strong and long-lasting B cell proliferation. These culture conditions allow the proliferation of various B cell subpopulations, including naive $sIgD^+$ $sIgM^+$ B cells, germinal center B cells, and memory B cells.

Addition of IL-4/IL-13 to B cells cultured in the CD40 system, or over CD40-L-transfected cells, results in their sustained proliferation and allows the generation of factor-dependent long-term normal B cell lines. B cell clones of several hundred cells can be obtained under these conditions. Cells cultured in the CD40 system with IL-4 express CD19, CD20, CD40, sIg, CD23, and HLA class II antigens and interestingly retain their sIgD.

IL-10 enhances the proliferation of CD40-activated B cells and the combination of IL-4 and IL-10 results in additive proliferation. B cells cultured in IL-10 differ microscopically from those cultured in IL-4 in that loose aggregates are observed early on, which then yield cultures mostly composed of single large cells. IL-10 upregulates the expression of CD25/Tac on anti-CD40-activated B cells and, accordingly, addition of IL-2 strongly enhances B cell proliferation, although IL-2 itself does not enhance proliferation of CD40-activated B cells.[10]

CD40 Triggering Turns on Expression of Functional Fas/APO-1/CD95

Whereas all germinal center (GC) B cells express Fas at a high level, memory B cells express it at a low level and naive B cells do not express it at all. After ligation of their CD40 antigen, resting B cell populations, which are composed of both naive and memory B cells, readily express Fas, and GC B cells express enhanced levels of Fas.[11–14] Addition of a functional anti-Fas antibody to cultures of CD40-activated B cells results in an inhibition of cell proliferation that can be seen after three to four days of culture. This late inhibition is due to a delayed acquisition of sensitivity to Fas-mediated programmed cell death (apoptosis). Neither recombinant cytokines (IL-2, IL-4, IL-10, IFNγ) nor activated T cell supernatants could counteract the Fas-induced death of human CD40-activated B cells and downregulate CD40-induced Fas expression. The delayed functional response to Fas ligation after CD40 activation may represent a way to limit the size of a specific B cell clone that is generated during antigen-driven, T cell/B cell interactions that occur either during the extrafollicular reaction or during the germinal center reaction after high-affinity centrocytes have been generated. In contrast, engagement of the BCR does not turn on Fas expression on B cells and, interestingly, decreases the sensitivity of CD40-activated B cells to Fas-induced apoptosis.[11,14] Therefore, in the absence of positive signaling through the BCR, concomitant CD40–CD40-L and Fas–Fas-L interactions would result in B cell apoptosis, thus censoring bystander B cell activation[15] and tolerant/anergic B cell expansion.[16] Alternatively, this may represent a mechanism through which centrocytes that have lost antigen reactivity following somatic mutations are eliminated following noncognate interaction with activated T cells expressing Fas-L. In keeping with this, the upper light zone is filled with activated T cells. These cells may express Fas-L and thus may represent an ultimate selection gate to kill nonselected germinal center B cells in a Fas/Fas-L-dependent interaction.

Differentiation of B Lymphocytes

B cells cultured in the CD40 system or with CD40-L-transfected cells produce marginal amounts of immunoglobulins, but further addition of SAC particles results in the secretion of large amounts of IgM, IgG, and IgA as a consequence of B cell differentiation without any isotype switch.[17] The surface antigen that is specifically engaged by SAC particles to turn on the differentiation of CD40-activated B cells remains unidentified.

Addition of IL-4 or IL-13 to CD40-activated B cells results in a slight increase in the production of IgM and IgG and in the secretion of IgE following isotype switching. Addition of IL-10 to CD40-activated B lymphocytes results in the production of considerable amounts of IgM, IgG, and IgA without IgE as a result of a differentiation into plasma cells. IL-10 induces CD40-activated naive sIgD$^+$ sIgM$^+$ B cells to secrete essentially IgM, but also IgG$_1$ and IgG$_3$, indicating that this cytokine acts as a switch factor for certain IgG subclasses.[17,18] CD40-activated naive sIgD$^+$ sIgM$^+$ B cells cultured with IL-10 also produce low levels of IgA, and addition of TGFβ induces large amounts of IgA while inhibiting IgM and IgG production.[19] TGFβ is likely to be an IgA-switch factor both in humans and in mice.[20,21] Thus, the engagement of CD40 on B cells turns on their isotype-switching machinery, the specificity of which is subsequently provided by cytokines.

CD40 Triggering Directs the Differentiation of Germinal Center B Cells towards Memory B Cells rather than Plasma Cells

Inasmuch as GC B cells are CD38$^+$CD20$^+$, memory B cells are CD38$^-$CD20$^+$, and plasma cells are CD38$^+$CD20$^-$, the levels of CD38 and CD20 can be used to follow the *in vitro* differentiation of GC B cells into either plasma cells or memory B cells. Germinal center B cells can be successfully cultured on CD40-L-transfected L cells with IL-2 and IL-10, a system that mimics the *in vivo* situation when high-affinity GC B cells have picked up antigen from follicular dendritic cells and are presenting it to CD40-L-expressing GC T cells.[22,23] GC B cells, rescued from apoptotic cell death, grow in exponential phase after three days of culture as $CD38^+CD20^+$ B cell blasts. These $CD38^+CD20^+$ B blast cells acquire a $CD38^-CD20^+$ memory B cell phenotype after a further three days of culture on CD40-L-transfected L cells with IL-2 and IL-10. These cells secrete little Ig and have the ability to proliferate in response to triggering through antigen receptor and CD40. In contrast, the $CD38^+CD20^+$ B blasts become terminally differentiated plasma cells after a further three days of culture with IL-2 and IL-10 in the absence of CD40-L signal. Thus, CD40-L plays a key role in directing germinal center B cells towards the memory B cell pathway rather than the plasma cell pathway.

COMBINATION OF CD40 AND BCR TRIGGERING YIELDS B CELLS WITH PARTIAL GERMINAL CENTER PHENOTYPE

A combination of CD40 triggering and BCR triggering synergizes for strong B cell proliferation/expansion over short-term cultures (up to five days). The observed cellular expansion is comparable to that observed with CD40 triggering and IL-4.[24,25] However, after five days of culture, all activated B cells quickly enter into apoptosis and they do not downregulate Bcl-2. Phenotypic analysis, at this time point, shows that many IgD^+ B cells have acquired some germinal center B cell markers, including CD38, Fas, and carboxypeptidase-M;[25,26] unlike GC B cells, though, they lack CD10 and express CD44. Whereas resting (naive + memory) B cells secrete IL-6 in response to either BCR or CD40 triggering, they fail to do so when receiving dual activation. This observation is consistent with the inability of germinal center B cells to secrete IL-6 in response to activation.[27] The B cell death observed after prolonged dual BCR and CD40 triggering is unlikely to be due to autocrine or paracrine Fas/Fas-L-dependent interactions because (i) the effect of BCR triggering is direct inasmuch as anti-λ antibody only kills λ^+ cells without affecting the surrounding κ^+ cells, (ii) cross-linked anti-κ and anti-λ antibodies partially protect CD40-activated B cells from Fas-mediated apoptosis, and (iii) Fas-L mRNA could not be detected by RT-PCR in such activated B cells (FIGURE 1). Interestingly, IL-4, but neither IL-2 nor IL-10, can significantly prevent the entry of these cells into apoptosis. Thus, the combination of CD40 and BCR triggering may represent the basic signals allowing differentiation of naive/memory B cells into germinal center B cells. Once the resting B cells have acquired some germinal center features, their survival and proliferation depend on T cell cytokines such as IL-4, a finding consistent with the presence of IL-4 and $CD40\text{-}L^+$ T cells in germinal centers.[28,29]

BCR TRIGGERING INDUCES APOPTOSIS OF CD40-ACTIVATED CENTROBLASTS

$CD44^-$ germinal center B cells (centroblasts) are rescued from apoptosis and reexpress CD44 and sIg following CD40 ligation. However, triggering BCR with anti-immunoglobulin κ and λ light-chain antibodies or anti-Igβ/CD79b quickly blocks proliferation and induces apoptosis of CD40-activated centroblasts, while enhancing the proliferation of CD40-activated naive and memory B cells.[30] BCR-mediated killing of CD40-activated centroblasts can be partially antagonized by the

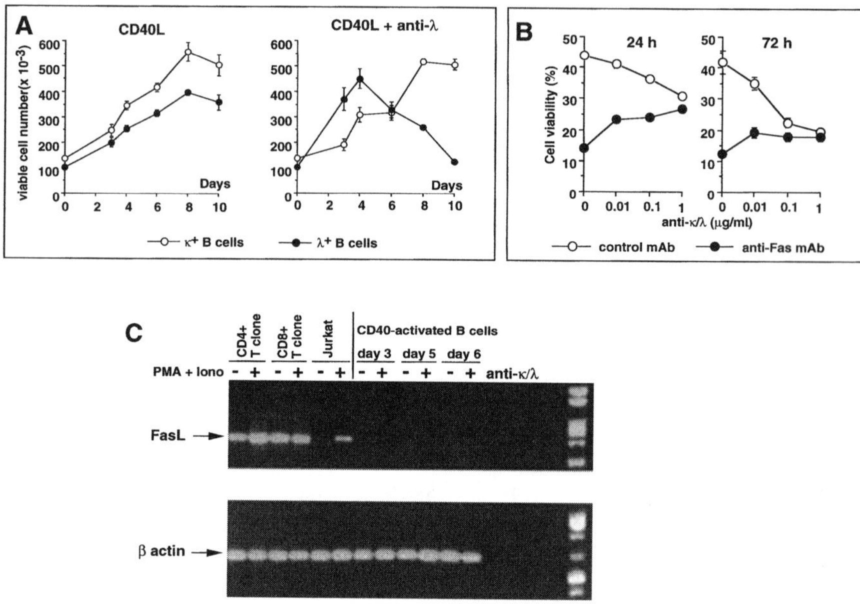

FIGURE 1. Prolonged BCR triggering induces the Fas-independent death of CD40-activated B cells. (A) Both positive and negative effects of BCR cross-linking are selectively induced in B cells receiving the dual CD40 and BCR triggering. Purified resting tonsil B cells were cultured over CD40-L/CD32 double-transfected L cells in the absence (left) or presence (right) of 1 μg/mL of anti-λ mAb. The number of viable B cells expressing either the κ or λ light chain was calculated at different time points according to the cell viability determined by trypan blue dye exclusion and according to the percentage of κ-expressing cells determined by FACS analysis. (B) BCR cross-linking partially inhibits Fas-dependent killing while inducing death of CD40-activated B cells. Resting B cells were cultured over CD40-L/CD32-transfected L cells with or without increasing concentrations of anti-κ/λ mAbs. Anti-Fas or control mAb was then added after 5 days of culture, and cell viability was further determined after 24 or 72 h by propidium iodide staining and FACS analysis. (C) B cells activated through CD40 and BCR cross-linking fail to express Fas-L mRNA. Resting B cells were activated on CD40-L/CD32 L cells with or without 1 μg/mL of anti-κ/λ mAbs. Total RNA was extracted from activated B cells at different time points and then reverse-transcribed, and generated cDNA was amplified by PCR with primers specific for either human Fas-L or β-actin. Positive controls were performed with cDNA from activated (PMA + ionomycin, 4 h) T cell clones or the T cell line Jurkat.

addition of IL-4. This observation may indeed represent an *in vitro* model that mimics the window for tolerance induction happening in germinal centers and that permits the deletion of autoreactive B cell clones incidentally generated by somatic mutations in the absence of antigen-specific T cells. The partial rescue by IL-4 may represent the

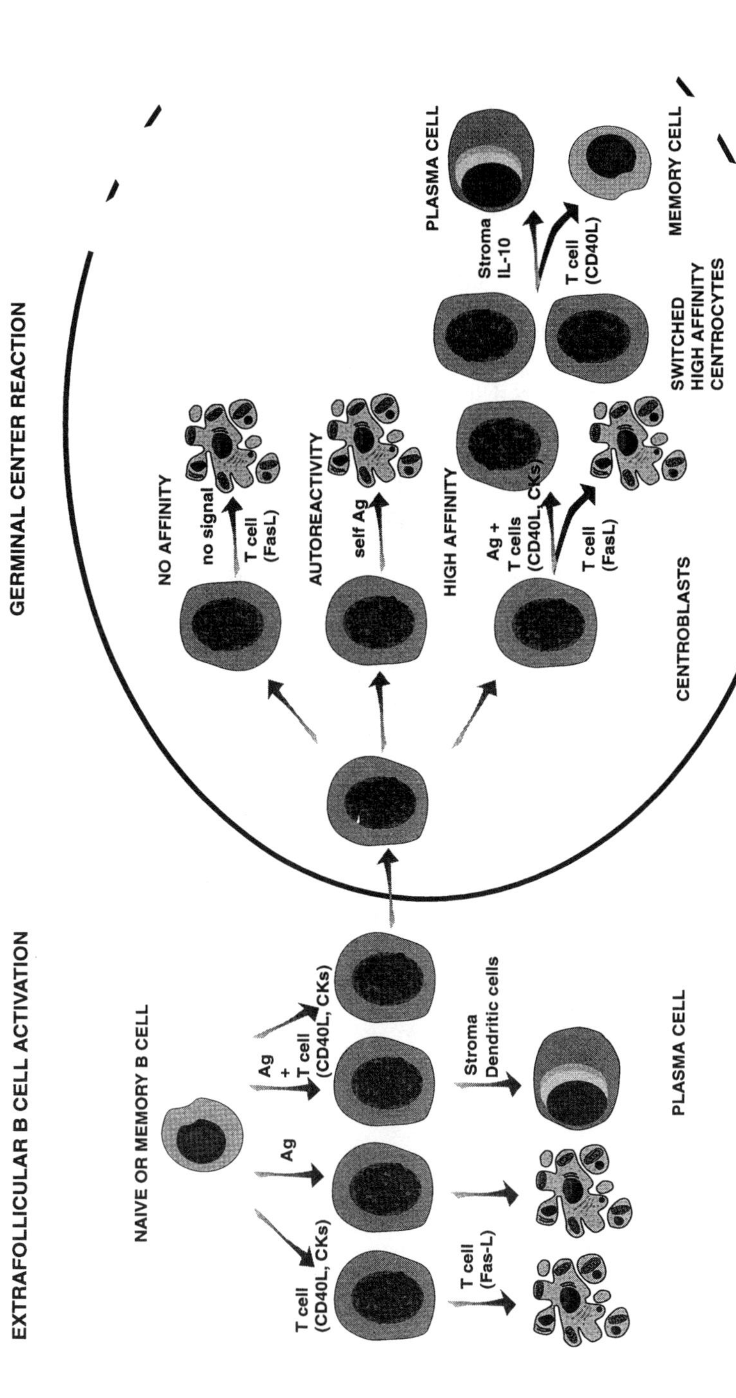

FIGURE 2. Schematic representation of antigen-driven T cell–dependent extrafollicular B cell activation and germinal center reaction in secondary lymphoid organs (for details, see text).

contribution of antigen-specific T cells that colonize germinal centers together with antigen-specific B cells. It is also likely that follicular dendritic cells retaining the Ag in the form of immune complexes contribute to the rescue of selected B cells through mechanisms that need to be identified.

CONCLUSIONS AND PERSPECTIVES

Considerable progress has been made during the past few years with regard to the understanding of human B cell immunopoiesis. As described herein, subpopulations of B cells, which represent the discrete stages of the maturation of B cell experience following an encounter with a T cell–dependent antigen, have been characterized and can be obtained in a highly purified fashion. Furthermore, *in vitro* culture systems have been set up that permit B cells to grow, switch isotype, and be positively and negatively selected, as well as to transit through some of the discrete maturation stages, and therefore have permitted the identification and analysis of signals regulating B cell maturation during Ag-driven T cell–dependent humoral responses (FIGURE 2). Whereas CD40-L, Ag, IL-2, IL-4, IL-10, and TGFβ have been identified as critical paracrine molecules affecting B cell immunopoiesis, others clearly remain to be identified. They include (1) the T cell molecule that permits CD40/CD40-L-independent activation, proliferation, and differentiation of naive B cells as observed in the hyper-IgM syndrome, (2) the molecules involved in interactions of B cells with dendritic cells, (3) the molecule(s) controlling the massive proliferation of B cell blasts and centroblasts in the dark zone, and (4) the cell surface trigger whose engagement leads to the activation of the somatic mutation machinery.

In vitro models should soon permit the analysis of the intracellular molecular pathways controlling the key events occurring at each step (growth, death, somatic mutation, isotype switch) as well as those that open the gate to the next maturation stage. This analysis should be greatly facilitated by a concomitant study of the genes expressed/repressed in each discrete B cell subset. This should ultimately permit the elucidation of the nature of (1) the molecular complex that controls the somatic mutation machinery and (2) the complex that controls isotype switching. When considering B cell tolerance, the determination of whether death induced by Fas ligation utilizes the same pathways as death induced by BCR triggering should be addressed as well. Identifying these pathways should ultimately permit the design of small molecules that can alter them, thus eventually leading to specific therapies of B cell malignancies and/or autoimmunity.

ACKNOWLEDGMENTS

We wish to thank C. Barthélémy, F. Brière, D. Capra, O. de Bouteiller, I. Durand, E. Garcia, F. Malisan, E. M. Neidhardt, and V. Pascual for their contributions to the project; J. Chiller for support; and S. Bonnet-Arnaud and D. Lepot for editorial assistance.

REFERENCES

1. GOODNOW, C. C. 1996. Proc. Natl. Acad. Sci. U.S.A. **93:** 2264–2271.
2. NOSSAL, G. J. V. 1996. J. Exp. Med. **183:** 1953–1956.

3. BANCHEREAU, J. & F. ROUSSET. 1992. Adv. Immunol. **52:** 125–251.
4. MCKENZIE, A. N. J., J. A. CULPEPPER, R. DE WAAL MALEFIJT, F. BRIÈRE, J. PUNNONEN, G. AVERSA, A. SATO, W. DANG, B. G. COCKS, S. MENON, J. E. DE VRIES, J. BANCHEREAU & G. ZURAWSKI. 1993. Proc. Natl. Acad. Sci. U.S.A. **90:** 3735–3739.
5. AMBRUS, J. L., J. PIPPIN, A. JOSEPH, C. XU, D. BLUMENTHAL, A. TAMAYO, K. CLAYPOOL, D. MCCOURT, A. SRIKIATCHATOCHORN & R. J. FORD. 1993. Proc. Natl. Acad. Sci. U.S.A. **90:** 6330–6334.
6. PARKER, D. C. 1993. Annu. Rev. Immunol. **11:** 331–360.
7. BANCHEREAU, J., F. BAZAN, D. BLANCHARD, F. BRIÈRE, J. P. GALIZZI, C. VAN KOOTEN, Y-J. LIU, F. ROUSSET & S. SAELAND. 1994. Annu. Rev. Immunol. **12:** 881–922.
8. VAN KOOTEN, C. & J. BANCHEREAU. 1996. Adv. Immunol. **61:** 1–77.
9. FOY, T. M., A. ARUFFO, J. BAJORATH, J. E. BUHLMANN & R. J. NOELLE. 1996. Annu. Rev. Immunol. **14:** 591–617.
10. FLUCKIGER, A. C., P. GARRONE, I. DURAND, J. P. GALIZZI & J. BANCHEREAU. 1993. J. Exp. Med. **178:** 1473–1481.
11. GARRONE, P., E. M. NEIDHARDT, E. GARCIA, L. GALIBERT, C. VAN KOOTEN & J. BANCHEREAU. 1995. J. Exp. Med. **182:** 1265–1273.
12. SCHATTNER, E. J., K. B. ELKON, D-H. YOO, J. TUMANG, P. H. KRAMMER, M. K. CROW & S. M. FRIEDMAN. 1995. J. Exp. Med. **182:** 1557–1565.
13. LAGRESLE, C., C. BELLA, P. T. DANIEL, P. H. KRAMMER & T. DEFRANCE. 1995. J. Immunol. **154:** 5746–5756.
14. LAGRESLE, C., P. MONDIÈRE, C. BELLA, P. H. KRAMMER & T. DEFRANCE. 1996. J. Exp. Med. **183:** 1377–1388.
15. ROTHSTEIN, T. L., J. K. M. WANG, D. J. PANKA, L. C. FOOTE, Z. WANG, B. STANGER, H. CUI, S-T. JU & A. MARSHAK-ROTHSTEIN. 1995. Nature **374:** 163–165.
16. RATHMELL, J. C., M. P. COOKE, J. GREIN, W. HO, M. M. DAVIS & C. C. GOODNOW. 1995. Nature **376:** 181–184.
17. MALISAN, F., F. BRIÈRE, J. M. BRIDON, N. HARINDRANATH, F. C. MILLS, E. E. MAX, J. BANCHEREAU & H. MARTINEZ-VALDEZ. 1996. J. Exp. Med. **183:** 937–947.
18. BRIÈRE, F., C. SERVET-DELPRAT, J. M. BRIDON, J. M. SAINT-REMY & J. BANCHEREAU. 1994. J. Exp. Med. **179:** 757–762.
19. DEFRANCE, T., B. VANBERVLIET, F. BRIÈRE, I. DURAND, F. ROUSSET & J. BANCHEREAU. 1992. J. Exp. Med. **175:** 671–682.
20. COFFMAN, R. L., D. A. LEBMAN & B. SHRADER. 1989. J. Exp. Med. **170:** 1039–1045.
21. ISLAM, K. B., L. NILSSON, P. SIDERAS, L. HAMMARSTRÖM & C. I. E. SMITH. 1991. Int. Immunol. **3:** 1099–1106.
22. ARPIN, C., J. DÉCHANET, C. VAN KOOTEN, P. MERVILLE, G. GROUARD, F. BRIÈRE, J. BANCHEREAU & Y-J. LIU. 1995. Science **268:** 720–722.
23. LAGRESLE, C., C. BELLA & T. DEFRANCE. 1993. Int. Immunol. **5:** 1259–1268.
24. WHEELER, K., J. D. POUND, J. GORDON & R. JEFFERIS. 1993. Eur. J. Immunol. **23:** 1165–1168.
25. GALIBERT, L., N. BURDIN, B. DE SAINT–VIS, P. GARRONE, C. VAN KOOTEN, J. BANCHEREAU & F. ROUSSET. 1996. J. Exp. Med. **183:** 77–85.
26. DE SAINT–VIS, B., L. CUPILLARD, D. PANDRAU-GARCIA, S. HO, N. RENARD, G. GROUARD, V. DUVERT, X. THOMAS, J. P. GALIZZI, J. BANCHEREAU & S. SAELAND. 1995. Blood **86:** 1098–1105.
27. BURDIN, N., L. GALIBERT, P. GARRONE, I. DURAND, J. BANCHEREAU & F. ROUSSET. 1996. J. Immunol. **156:** 4107–4113.
28. BUTCH, A. W., G-H. CHUNG, J. W. HOFFMANN & M. H. NAHM. 1993. J. Immunol. **150:** 39–47.
29. CASAMAYOR-PALLEJA, M., M. KHAN & I. C. M. MACLENNAN. 1995. J. Exp. Med. **181:** 1293–1301.
30. GALIBERT, L., N. BURDIN, C. BARTHÉLÉMY, G. MEFFRE, I. DURAND, E. GARCIA, P. GARRONE, F. ROUSSET, J. BANCHEREAU & Y-J. LIU. 1996. J. Exp. Med. **183:** 2075–2085.

Anti–Red Blood Cell Immunoglobulin Transgenic Mice

An Experimental Model of Autoimmune Hemolytic Anemia

SAZUKU NISITANI, MASAO MURAKAMI,
AND TASUKU HONJO[a]

Department of Medical Chemistry
Faculty of Medicine
Kyoto University
Kyoto 606, Japan

The onset of autoimmune diseases is affected by at least two factors: genetic factors and environmental factors. To understand the molecular mechanisms of B cell tolerance and autoimmunity, anti-self Ig-transgenic (Tg) mice have been generated by several groups (TABLE 1). In only a few cases, however, the Tg mice developed autoimmune diseases because self-reactive B cells were either anergized or deleted. Fortunately, in our anti–red blood cell (RBC) Ig H+L Tg mice (HL mice), about half developed autoimmune hemolytic anemia, although self-reactive B cells in the bone marrow and peripheral lymphatic organs were clonally deleted.[1] In marked contrast, there is a normal level of self-reactive B lymphocytes in the peritoneal cavity, in which B cells being sequestrated, without exposure to self-antigens (RBCs) and therefore escaping from the deletion process, can expand. Peritoneal self-reactive B cells are activated by environmental antigens in the gut lumen and differentiate into antibody-producing cells,[2] resulting in autoimmune hemolytic anemia (FIGURE 1). Autoimmune hemolytic anemia can be cured by elimination of self-reactive B cells after injection of RBCs into the peritoneal cavity. HL mice are thus an ideal model to analyze the mechanisms of B cell tolerance as well as autoimmunity.

B CELL TOLERANCE AND AUTOIMMUNITY IN HL MICE

We established HL mice by introducing the H- and L-chain genes isolated from NZB-derived anti-RBC autoantibody-producing hybridoma[3] into fertilized mouse eggs. The presence of the anti-RBC autoantibodies causes autoimmune hemolytic anemia. Interestingly, the individual HL mice showed variable phenotypes ranging from severe autoimmune hemolytic anemia to a lack of the disease. This may be due to the fact that autoimmune symptoms are induced by environmental factors. Indeed, HL mice do not manifest autoimmune symptoms under germ-free or SPF conditions (unpublished observation).

[a]To whom all correspondence should be addressed.

Almost all B cells in the peritoneal cavity of HL mice belong to the B-1 lineage[4] and have strong self-replenishing capacity. A critical role of peritoneal B-1 cells in autoimmune anemia is supported by the fact that HL × *xid* male mice lack self-reactive peritoneal B cells and are free from the autoimmune disease.[5] Because peritoneal B-1 cells are responsible for autoimmune symptoms in HL mice, we thought that autoimmune hemolytic anemia could be cured by eliminating peritoneal self-reactive B-1 cells. Indeed, after intraperitoneal injection of RBCs, the peritoneal B-1 cells of anemic HL mice were deleted.[2] After five weekly injections, the hematocrit values recovered to the normal value and the amount of anti-RBC antibody associated with circulating RBCs decreased drastically. In contrast, oral administration of LPS into asymptomatic HL mice induced autoimmune anemia by activating self-reactive B-1 cells in the peritoneal cavity and in the lamina propria of the gut.[5] HL mice under conventional conditions are exposed to environmental antigens such as intestinal bacteria, and the antigens induce differentiation of peritoneal self-reactive B-1 cells into anti-RBC autoantibody-producing cells.[5] HL mice thus serve as a

TABLE 1. B Cell Tolerance and Autoimmunity in Ig Transgenic Mice

Transgene	Ag Specificity	B Cell Tolerance	Autoimmune Symptoms	Investigators	Reference
IgM	anti-HEL/HEL (soluble)	anergy	increased Ig under lpr/lpr background	Goodnow (1988)	11
IgM	anti-H-2K^k/ H-2K^k	deletion	anti-DNA Ab under lpr/lpr background	Nemazee (1989)	12
IgM	anti-CD8.2	deletion	not reported	Köhler (1991)	13
IgM	anti-HEL/HEL (membranous)	deletion	not reported	Goodnow (1991)	14
IgM	anti-ssDNA	anergy	not reported	Weigert (1991)	15
IgM	anti-RBC	deletion	autoimmune anemia	Honjo (1992)	1
IgG_{2a}	anti-dsDNA	deletion	no nephritis; slightly increased anti-dsDNA	Diamond (1992)	16
IgG_{2a}	anti-ds + ssDNA (nephritogenic mAb)	absent	mild nephritis	Tsao (1992)	17
IgM	anti-dsDNA	absent	not reported	Weigert (1993)	18
IgM	human RF	absent	increased RF under lpr/lpr background	Tighe (1993)	19
IgM	anti-PtC	absent	not reported	Clarke (1994)	20
IgM	anti-OVA	deletion (*in vitro*)	not reported	Loh (1995)	21

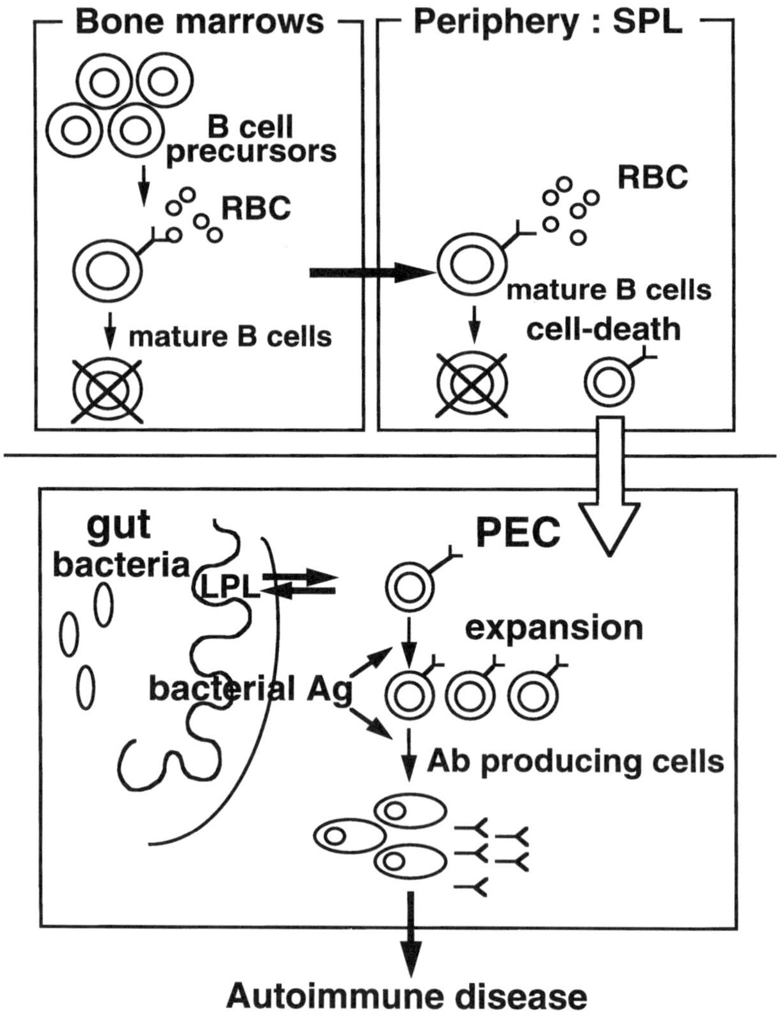

FIGURE 1. Schematic diagram of B cell tolerance and onset of autoimmunity in HL mice. Self-reactive B cells in the bone marrow and in the peripheral lymphatic organs are clonally deleted upon interaction with RBCs. Self-reactive B cells in the peritoneal cavity (PEC) are sequestrated from RBCs and do not undergo clonal deletion. Upon interaction with environmental antigens such as intestinal bacteria, peritoneal self-reactive B-1 cells are triggered to differentiate into anti-RBC autoantibody-producing cells, resulting in autoimmune hemolytic anemia.

unique "reversible model of autoimmunity," in which we can assess the mechanisms of onset and treatment of the autoimmune disease (FIGURE 2).

DEFECT OF B-1 CELL ACTIVATION BY DEPLETION OF T CELLS IN HL MICE

Self-reactive B cells are clonally deleted upon interaction with self-antigens. In contrast, stimulation of B cells by foreign antigens together with T helper (Th) cell–derived signals induce proliferation and differentiation of B cells into antibody-producing cells. The ability of T cells to prevent tolerance induction in immature B cells, which are more susceptible to tolerance, argues for this possibility.[6] However, it is not yet clear how T helper cell–derived signals induce antibody production from B-1 cells *in vivo*. RAG-$2^{-/-}$ mice lack mature T and B cells, but the B cell deficiency can be complemented by introduction of transgenic Ig genes. A normal number of B cells and a normal level of spontaneous IgM production are observed in RAG-$2^{-/-}$ × μλ Tg mice.[7] To assess the effect of Th2 cell help to peritoneal self-reactive B-1 cells, we have mated HL mice with RAG-$2^{-/-}$ mice (RAG-$2^{-/-}$ × HL mice). Bone marrow and spleen B cells in RAG-$2^{-/-}$ × HL mice are completely deleted (manuscript in

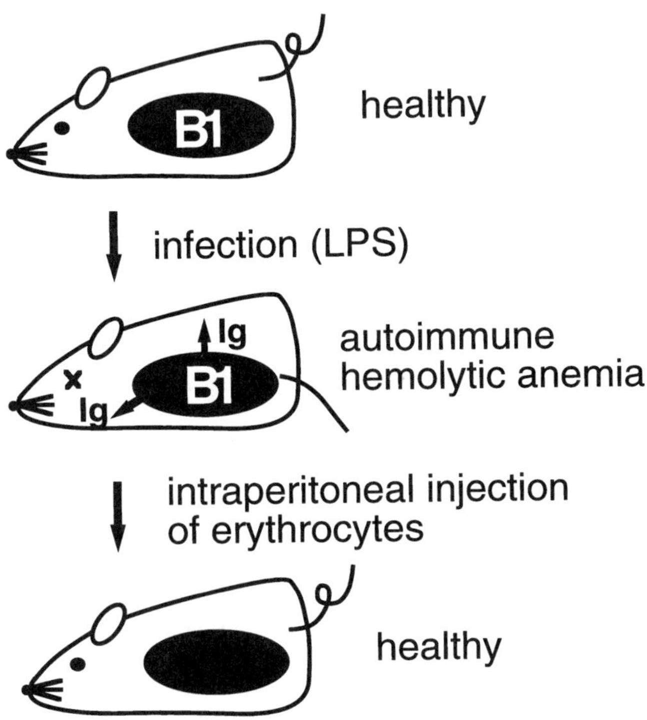

FIGURE 2. HL mice as a reversible model of autoimmunity. See text for details.

preparation). The most interesting feature of RAG-$2^{-/-}$ × HL mice is that neither B-1 cells nor anti-RBC antibody-producing cells are found in the peritoneal cavity. Consequently, RAG-$2^{-/-}$ × HL mice did not manifest autoimmune hemolytic anemia. The result strongly indicates that Th2 cells play a pivotal role in the expansion and activation of self-reactive B-1 cells in the peritoneal cavity of HL mice (FIGURE 3).

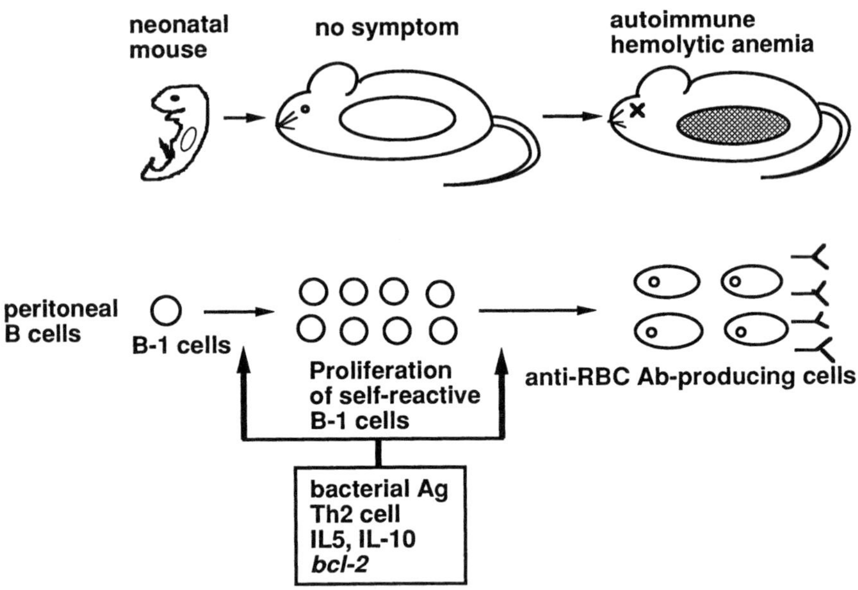

FIGURE 3. Factors involved in the proliferation and activation of peritoneal self-reactive B-1 cells in HL mice.

IL-5 AND IL-10 PRODUCED BY TH2 CELLS ENHANCE AUTOIMMUNE SYMPTOMS IN HL MICE

To assess the mechanisms of Th2 cell–derived help to B cells, we administrated the Th2 cell–derived cytokines IL-4, IL-5, and IL-10 into HL mice.[8] Ten daily administrations of IL-5 or IL-10 induced differentiation of peritoneal self-reactive B-1 cells and autoimmune anemia in asymptomatic HL mice. In contrast, IL-4 induced neither activation of peritoneal B-1 cells nor anemia. It was proposed that the self-reactive B-1 cells travel between the peritoneal cavity and GALT.[5] Self-reactive B cells in the GALT may be activated by IL-5 or IL-10 produced by GALT-Th2 cells. Activated B-1 cells then move to the peritoneal cavity. Oral administration of LPS increased the number of peritoneal B-1 cells and induced their differentiation into antibody-producing cells, resulting in autoimmune anemia in RAG-$2^{-/-}$ × HL mice. Although LPS appears to complement the roles of Th2 cells, it is not clear whether or not LPS stimulates B-1 cells in GALT directly. LPS may stimulate other cytokine-producing cells like dendritic cells to secrete cytokines that can activate B-1 cells.

GENETIC CONTROL OF AUTOANTIBODY PRODUCTION IN HL MICE

In addition to the genes encoding lymphocyte receptors, other genes must be involved in the onset of autoimmune diseases. Dysregulation of apoptosis may play a role in autoimmunity.[9] Bcl-2 is unique among oncogene products in that it appears to enhance lymphocyte survival by interfering with apoptosis rather than promoting cell proliferation. Therefore, we have studied the effect of the *bcl-2* gene on the appearance of autoimmune hemolytic anemia by introducing the *bcl-2* gene into HL mice (*bcl-2* × HL mice).[10] Analysis of *bcl-2* × HL mice showed that the *bcl-2* gene product inhibits clonal deletion of self-reactive mature B cells, but not that of bone marrow immature B cells. Autoimmune hemolytic anemia was aggravated in *bcl-2* × HL mice possibly because of prolonged survival of peritoneal anti-RBC antibody-producing cells. Thus, HL mice may be also useful for searching other background genes that might play a role in the onset of the autoimmune disease and the increasing incidence of autoimmunity.

REFERENCES

1. OKAMOTO, M., M. MURAKAMI, A. SHIMIZU, S. OZAKI, T. TSUBATA, S. KUMAGAI & T. HONJO. 1992. A transgenic model of autoimmune hemolytic anemia. J. Exp. Med. **175:** 71–79.
2. MURAKAMI, M., T. TSUBATA, M. OKAMOTO, A. SHIMIZU, S. KUMAGAI, H. IMURA & T. HONJO. 1992. Antigen-induced apoptotic death of Ly-1 B cells responsible for autoimmune disease in transgenic mice. Nature **357:** 77–80.
3. OZAKI, S., R. NAGASAWA, H. SATO & T. SHIRAI. 1984. Hybridoma autoantibodies to erythrocytes from NZB mice and the induction of hemolytic anemia. Immunol. Lett. **8:** 115–119.
4. KANTOR, A. B. & L. A. HERZENBERG. 1993. Origin of murine B cell lineages. Annu. Rev. Immunol. **11:** 501–538.
5. MURAKAMI, M., T. TSUBATA, R. SHINKURA, S. NISITANI, M. OKAMOTO, H. YOSHIOKA, T. USUI, S. MIYAZAKI & T. HONJO. 1994. Oral administration of lipopolysaccharides activates B-1 cells in the peritoneal cavity and lamina propria of the gut and induces autoimmune symptoms in an autoantibody transgenic mouse. J. Exp. Med. **180:** 111–121.
6. METCALF, E. S. & N. R. KLINMAN. 1976. *In vitro* tolerance induction of neonatal murine B cells. J. Exp. Med. **143:** 1327–1340.
7. YOUNG, F., B. ARDMAN, Y. SHINKAI, R. LANSFORD, T. K. BLACKWELL, M. MENDELSOHN, A. ROLINK, F. MELCHERS & F. W. ALT. 1994. Influence of immunoglobulin heavy- and light-chain expression on B-cell differentiation. Genes Dev. **8:** 1043–1057.
8. NISITANI, S., T. TSUBATA, M. MURAKAMI & T. HONJO. 1995. Administration of interleukin 5 or 10 activates peritoneal B-1 cells and induces autoimmune hemolytic anemia in anti-erythrocyte autoantibody transgenic mice. Eur. J. Immunol. **25:** 3047–3052.
9. ROSE, L. M., D. S. LATCHMAN & D. A. ISENBERG. 1994. Bcl-2 and Fas, molecules which influence apoptosis: a possible role in systemic lupus erythematosus? Autoimmunity **17:** 271–278.
10. NISITANI, S., T. TSUBATA, M. MURAKAMI, M. OKAMOTO & T. HONJO. 1993. The *bcl-2* gene product inhibits clonal deletion of self-reactive B lymphocytes in the periphery, but not in the bone marrow. J. Exp. Med. **178:** 1247–1254.

11. GOODNOW, C. C., J. CROSBIE, S. ADELSTEIN, T. B. LAVOIE, S. J. SMITH-GILL, R. A. BRINK, H. PRITCHARD-BRISCOE, J. S. WOTHERSPOON, R. H. LOBLAY, K. RAPHAEL, R. J. TRENT & A. BASTEN. 1988. Altered immunoglobulin expression and functional silencing of self-reactive B lymphocytes in transgenic mice. Nature **334:** 676–682.
12. NEMAZEE, D. A. & K. BÜRKI. 1989. Clonal deletion of B lymphocytes in a transgenic mouse bearing anti-MHC class I antibody genes. Nature **337:** 562–566.
13. BROMBACHER, F., G. KÖHLER & H. EIBEL. 1991. B cell tolerance in mice transgenic for anti-CD8 immunoglobulin μ chain. J. Exp. Med. **174:** 1335–1346.
14. HARTLEY, S. B., J. CROSBIE, R. BRINK, A. B. KANTOR, A. BASTEN & C. C. GOODNOW. 1991. Elimination from peripheral lymphoid tissues of self-reactive B lymphocytes recognizing membrane-bound antigens. Nature **353:** 765–769.
15. ERIKSON, J., M. Z. RADIC, S. A. CAMPER, R. R. HARDY, C. CARMACK & M. WEIGERT. 1991. Expression of anti-DNA immunoglobulin transgenes in non-autoimmune mice. Nature **349:** 331–334.
16. OFFEN, D., L. SPATZ, H. ESCOWITZ, S. FACTOR & B. DIAMOND. 1992. Induction of tolerance to an IgG autoantibody. Proc. Natl. Acad. Sci. U.S.A. **89:** 8332–8336.
17. TSAO, B. P., K. OHNISHI, H. CHEROUTRE, B. MITCHELL, M. TEITELL, P. MIXTER, M. KRONENBERG & B. H. HAHN. 1992. Failed self-tolerance and autoimmunity in IgG anti-DNA transgenic mice. J. Immunol. **149:** 350–358.
18. GAY, D., T. SAUNDERS, S. CAMPER & M. WEIGERT. 1993. Receptor editing: an approach by autoreactive B cells to escape tolerance. J. Exp. Med. **177:** 999–1008.
19. TIGHE, H., P. P. CHEN, R. TUCKER, T. J. KIPPS, J. ROUDIER, F. R. JIRIK & D. A. CASON. 1993. Function of B cells expressing a human immunoglobulin M rheumatoid factor autoantibody in transgenic mice. J. Exp. Med. **177:** 109–118.
20. ARNOLD, L. W., C. A. PENNELL, S. K. MCCRAY & S. H. CLARKE. 1994. Development of B-1 cells: segregation of phosphatidyl choline–specific B cells to the B-1 population occurs after immunoglobulin gene expression. J. Exp. Med. **179:** 1585–1595.
21. DUSTIN, L. B., E. D. BULLOCK, Y. HAMADA, T. AZUMA & D. Y. LOH. 1995. Antigen-driven differentiation of naive Ig-transgenic B cells *in vitro*. J. Immunol. **154:** 4936–4949.

Functional Properties and Molecular Characteristics of Autoantibodies Associated with Tight Skin Syndrome[a]

K. KASTURI,[b] T. MURYOI,[c] S. SHIBATA,[c]
A. HATAKEYAMA,[c] C. MURAI,[b] Y. SIMAKOSHI,[c]
AND C. BONA[b,d]

[b]*Department of Microbiology*
Mount Sinai School of Medicine
New York, New York 10029

[c]*Second Department of Internal Medicine*
Tohoku University School of Medicine
Sendai 980, Japan

INTRODUCTION

Studies carried out during the past decade suggest that the tight skin (TSK) mouse represents an excellent experimental model for human scleroderma[1,2] and congenital fascial dystrophy.[3] TSK syndrome is due to an autosomal dominant mutation located on chromosome 2 at about 2 cm distal to the pallid mutation, close to β2 microglobulin, IL-1a, and fibrillin-1 loci.[4] In homozygous state, the mutants die *in utero*. The TSK syndrome is characterized by cutaneous hyperplasia, tightness of the skin, cardiac hypertrophy, pulmonary emphysema, and hypertrophy of the skeleton.[4] The histopathological alterations seen in the skin are due to an increase in the expression of type I and III procollagen genes,[5] excessive accumulation of collagens,[6] glycosaminoglycans,[7] and increased propyl hydroxylase enzyme activity.[8]

Human scleroderma is a polymorphic disease manifested as localized scleroderma (morphea) progressive systemic sclerosis (PSS) or as CREST syndrome. All these syndromes are associated with the production of autoantibodies displaying a variety of specificities against cellular autoantigens. Our studies were aimed at characterizing the autoantibodies associated with tight skin syndrome, as well as determining their pathogenic properties.

[a]This study was supported by Grant No. AI24671 from the National Institutes of Health.
[d]To whom all correspondence should be addressed.

PROPERTIES OF AUTOANTIBODIES ASSOCIATED WITH TSK SYNDROME

Antinuclear Antibodies

Antinuclear antibodies (ANAs) are commonly detectable in the sera of scleroderma patients and approximately 25% of the antinuclear antibodies are specific for Scl 70 or topoisomerase I.[9] ANAs were also found in the sera of more than 40% of 8-month-old TSK/+ mice, whereas the mice younger than 8 months were negative. In positive staining of HEP-2 cells, a fine speckled pattern was detected at 1:40 or higher dilutions of the sera.[10,11] ANAs found in the sera of old TSK/+ mice did not bind to dsDNA, as assessed by the lack of reactivity against native DNA in a *Crithidia* luciferase fluorescence test.[10]

Anticellular Autoantibodies

Muryoi *et al.*[11] analyzed the fine binding specificity of a large panel of monoclonal antibodies produced by hybridomas obtained from young and old TSK/+ mice. Among 29 hybridomas that bound to various cytoplasmic antigens such as keratin, vimentin, Golgi, and mitochondria, 1 monoclonal antibody stained the nucleoli and 4 stained the nucleoli and mitochondria in immunofluorescence staining. In double-staining experiments, the mitochondrial pattern of TSK/+ autoantibodies was superimposable with the staining of human antimitochondrial antibodies. Studying the binding properties of TSK mouse antinuclear and anticytoplasmic autoantibodies with a large panel of self and foreign antigens showed that these antibodies are not polyspecific as many natural antibodies are.[11]

Anti–Heparan Sulfate (HS) Autoantibodies

An important difference between TSK mouse disease and human PSS is the absence of vascular lesions in the animal model. As a component of the cell surface and extracellular matrix, heparan sulfate (HS) proteoglycans play an important role in the function of most organs, including the vasculature. Therefore, from our large panel of monoclonal antibodies, we selected those that bind to HS employing solid-phase RIA. Our studies showed that there is an increase in the clonal frequency of hybridomas secreting anti-HS antibody in TSK/+ mice compared to that of C57BL/6 pa/pa (control) mice. These mAbs exhibited little or no cross-reactivity with other glycosaminoglycans. Anti-HS antibodies inhibited the binding of HS to antithrombin III and prevented the formation of thrombin-antithrombin complexes.[12] Thus, anti-HS antibodies may promote the procoagulation state by preventing accelerated formation of thrombin–antithrombin III complexes, which may explain the absence of vascular lesions in TSK mice.

Anti-FcR Autoantibodies

During the screening of sera from mice prone to develop various autoimmune diseases, we observed that TSK mice had high levels of anti-FcR autoantibodies.[13] Following this initial observation, we studied the frequency of anti-FcR autoantibodies produced among our panel of hybridomas obtained from TSK mice. We found that TSK mouse hybridomas with FcγR specificity comprised a large subset of TSK hybridomas producing polyspecific mAbs.[14] These antibodies caused degranulation of neutrophils accompanied by significant morphological changes as shown by scanning and transmission electron microscopy. The degranulation process is accompanied by the release of hydrolases from both azurophils and specific granules of human neutrophils. Anti-FcR mAbs bind to FcγRIII, but not to FcγRII. Organ injury resulting from inflammatory processes is a fundamental sign in many autoimmune diseases. Anti-FcR autoantibodies, similar to the binding of immune complexes to FcγR on effector cells, can contribute to the inflammatory processes by releasing hydrolases, activated oxygen intermediates, and cytokines. Based on these preliminary observations made in TSK mice, we extended our studies to human disease. We found that 16 of 40 patients with PSS (40%) had anti-FcR autoantibodies.[15] From a patient with PSS and heart block, we obtained anti-FcR mAbs exhibiting the same specificity as TSK mAbs.[16] The presence of anti-FcγRIII autoantibodies was reported previously in patients with juvenile neutropenia[17] and in patients with SLE.[18]

Anti–RNA Polymerase I Autoantibodies

Anti–RNA polymerase I autoantibodies are not specific for scleroderma because these antibodies have been described in SLE, RA, and MCTD.[19] Mammalian RNA polymerase I (pol I) is a complex enzyme composed of six to eight subunits.[20] Autoantibodies produced in various autoimmune diseases are specific for different subunits of the enzyme. Production of antibodies specific for the 190-kDa subunit appears to be characteristic of patients with PSS.[21] Shibata *et al.*[22] demonstrated that the TSK mice produced high titers of anti–RNA pol I autoantibodies. Analysis of the fine specificity of mAbs produced by the hybridomas obtained from TSK mice showed some similarities, as well as differences, when compared with human and TSK serum anti–RNA pol I autoantibodies. Scleroderma anti–RNA pol I antibodies gave speckled-type nucleolar staining as well as staining of fibrillar regions of drug-induced segregated nucleoli.[19,21] TSK autoantibodies gave a similar speckled nucleolar staining pattern, namely, bright fluorescent dots in colcemid- or actinomycin D–treated Vero cells, but did not show necklace-type nucleolar staining in actinomycin D–treated cells as scleroderma antibodies.

TSK autoantibodies bound not only to the 190-kDa subunit of rat and murine RNA pol I, but also to viral (T7) enzyme and to two large subunits (115 and 150 kDa) of the bacterial (*E. coli*) enzyme. Like scleroderma autoantibodies, the TSK antibodies bound better to the phosphorylated enzyme than to the native enzyme. Another important property of human autoantibodies is their ability to inhibit the enzymatic activity.[22] By contrast, TSK autoantibodies displayed three different properties:

(1) autoantibodies that inhibit the enzyme activity like human autoantibodies;
(2) antibodies that enhance the enzyme activity;
(3) a group that will not have any effect on the enzyme activity.

These results clearly show that the inhibiting and enhancing activities are due to the interaction of TSK autoantibodies with distinct epitopes. In summary, our studies demonstrate that TSK mice spontaneously developed anti–RNA pol I autoantibodies similar to those found in scleroderma patients.

Antitopoisomerase I Autoantibodies

Autoantibodies specific for Scl 70 antigen, which was shown later to be topoisomerase I[9] (topoI), were described only in patients with diffuse scleroderma, but not in patients with morphea or CREST syndrome. Thus, one of the major aims of our studies was to determine whether TSK mice spontaneously produce anti-topoI autoantibodies. Muryoi *et al.*[23] first demonstrated that TSK mice exhibited an age-dependent increase in the serum anti-topoI antibodies of both IgM and IgG isotypes. These antibodies bound to 70-kDa purified topoisomerase I as well as a 70-kDa protein found in Scl 70 commercial antigen. Competitive inhibition RIA studies using scleroderma and TSK mAbs showed that human and murine anti-topoI autoantibodies recognized identical epitopes. This conclusion was strengthened by the results obtained using fusion proteins encompassing the entire topoI polypeptide. Both human and TSK mAbs bound strongly to fusion protein C encompassing the NH_2-terminal portion of the enzyme and weakly to fusion proteins F and G containing the regions close to the COOH-terminal.[24]

Binding to F and G proteins can be related to a tripeptide EDD shared by C, F, and G fusion proteins that may represent the core of a dominant epitope. Recently, Hatakeyama *et al.*[25] showed that there is a good correlation between the titer of anti-topoI autoantibodies, the thickness of the skin, and the content of soluble collagen I and hydroxyproline. Thus, this study indicated that the concentration of antitopoisomerase I autoantibodies is a useful marker to identify the TSK phenotype as it is an important clinical marker for the diagnosis of PSS. Like human autoantibodies, TSK antitopoisomerase antibodies inhibited the enzymatic activity of the enzyme. TABLE 1 summarizes the characteristics of TSK mouse autoantibodies.

It is generally accepted that the spontaneous occurrence of autoantibodies is due to an increased frequency of autoantibody-producing B cells. The precursors of these cells either have escaped the negative selection in bone marrow during development or alternatively have emerged subsequent to breaking the peripheral tolerance (anergy).

Transfer of TSK bone marrow cells or purified splenic B cells into C57BL/6 pa/pa mice was followed by the appearance of autoantibodies in the recipient mice. Anti–RNA pol I autoantibodies (IgM and IgG) were observed one month after infusion of purified B cells.[26] These observations strongly indicate the existence of memory autoreactive B cells in TSK mice, which continue to produce autoantibodies after the transfer. This observation is in agreement with the demonstration that NZB B cells are capable of transferring anti-DNA production into H-2 compatible recipients.[27]

MOLECULAR CHARACTERISTICS OF TSK MOUSE AUTOANTIBODIES

Antibody diversity is generated by somatic recombination of diverse germline gene segments coding for heavy- and light-chain variable regions, somatic mutation,

TABLE 1. Autoantibodies Associated with Human Scleroderma and Tight Skin Syndrome[a]

Specificity	PSS	CREST	TSK	Characteristics of TSK Antibodies
Topoisomerase I	+	−	+	High frequency in old mice Bind to 1–139 aa N-terminal epitope
Centromere CENP A, B, C	−	+	−	
RNA pol I	+	−	+	Increased frequency in TSK mice Bind to murine, rat, viral, and bacterial enzymes Dephosphorylation of enzymes decreases binding activity Inhibit enzyme activity
Fibrillarin	+	+	ND	
FcR	+	+	+	Bind to FcγRIII and RII recombinant proteins Trigger degranulation of PMNs Trigger release of lysosomal enzymes
ANA	+	+	+	Increased frequency in old mice (44%)
Mitochondria	−	−	+	Bind to nucleoli and occasionally to Golgi
Heparan sulfate	ND	ND	+	Increased frequency in TSK mice Inhibit binding of HS to antithrombin III
PM-Scl	+	−	ND	
Nor 90	+	−	ND	
Nucleoli	+	+	+	High frequency in TSK mice

[a]ND = not done.

insertion or deletion of nucleotides, D-D fusions, inversion, and gene conversions that occur during the recombination process. Based on DNA homology, the V genes of heavy and light chains were classified into gene families.[28,29] The mouse genome contains 100–1000 V_H, 200 V_K, and 3 $V\lambda$ functional germline genes. Whereas the

3′-end V_H gene families are preferentially expressed in early pre-B cells and adult bone marrow pre-B cells,[30] the expression of the V_H gene families in adult animals is random, corresponding to their respective genomic complexities.[30,31] Analysis of the usage of V_H and V_K gene families in TSK autoantibodies with various specificities showed the following features:[32]

(a) high usage of V_H genes derived from the V_HJ558 family;
(b) stochastic pairing of V_H and V_K family genes;
(c) most of the autoantibody-producing cells belonged to a conventional B cell (B2) subset.

Because the V_HJ558 gene family is preferentially used by TSK monoclonal autoantibodies, we have studied the molecular characteristics of V_HJ558 genes. The V_HJ558 gene family is the largest of the murine V_H gene families. Based on nucleotide homology, the murine V_HJ558 family was divided into eight subfamilies.[33] Sequence analysis of V_HJ558 genes expressed in TSK autoantibodies showed some interesting features:

(a) The usage of subfamilies resembles the pattern of V gene expression in the pre-B cell repertoire[33] and there is no bias in the usage of any V_HJ558 subfamilies in TSK autoantibodies.[34] Two new germline genes that may represent the prototypes for a new subfamily of V_HJ558 genes are repeatedly used in TSK autoantibodies. The increased frequency of expression of some V_HJ558 subfamily genes may be due to V_H gene–mediated selection of autoreactive memory B cells as an increase in the expression of some V_HJ558 subfamilies was observed in "persistent" B cells.
(b) A majority of TSK autoantibodies use unmutated germline J558 genes. Hybridomas expressing similar V_H genes assembled with distinct D and/or J segments exhibit different binding specificities.
(c) Several V_HJ558 genes expressed in TSK autoantibodies share a conserved heptapeptide sequence that is highly represented in the CDR2 of various V_HJ558 subfamilies as well as in anti-GAT and antiphenyl arsonate antibodies, but not in anti-α(1-3)-dextran and oxazalone mAbs. It is possible that this motif represents a regulatory sequence recognized by T cells. It has been shown in other systems that T_H cells specific for regulatory idiotypes can play a role in the emergence of clonal dominance.[35,36]
(d) The frequency of insertion of *N* nucleotides at D-J_H junctions is rare, whereas the frequency of D-D fusions and D-inversions is higher in both autoantibodies and the V_HJ558 repertoire of TSK mice. The molecular characteristics of TSK autoantibodies[32,34] are summarized in TABLE 2. In summary, our results suggest that the establishment of the autoimmune repertoire in TSK mice is mediated by V_H gene–dependent selection of conventional B cells.

AUTOANTIBODIES IN TSK MICE REPRESENT AN EPIPHENOMENON

Self-reactive antibodies can be divided into three major categories:

(1) natural antibodies that are characterized by low binding affinities to a variety of self and foreign antigens;

(2) pathogenic autoantibodies that cause the primary injury and can induce disease when transferred into a normal animal;
(3) nonpathogenic autoantibodies specific for a variety of antigens released subsequent to primary injury; this category of autoantibodies can be considered as an epiphenomenon.

To determine the role of autoantibodies associated with TSK syndrome, we have studied the frequency of occurrence of this syndrome in backcross progeny obtained from crossing TSK/+ Ig+/− F_1 with +/+ Ig−/− mice. Ig knockout mice lack mature B cells and Ig in the serum.[37] Because only TSK/+ mice are viable, we expect

TABLE 2. Molecular Characteristics of V_HJ558 Genes Expressed in TSK Autoantibodies[a]

Prototype of J558 Subfamily	TSK Hybridoma	% Homology
V_H186.2	L2-4	99
	L185-3	97
	L365-11	95
V3 (CH10)	M31-1	99
G4D11 (VpW32)	M51-0	97.5
V130	L238-3	99
L350-7	34A1-26	99.6
	L229-26	98
	GM63-3	99.6
	L99-18	99.6
	113A4-1	97.6
	GM5-7	96.5

[a]Genes derived from the V_HJ558 family are expressed in 70% of the hybridomas producing autoantibodies with various specificities. TSK autoantibodies are encoded by V_HJ558 genes belonging to various J558 subfamilies. TSK autoantibodies are encoded by germline genes. TSK autoantibodies share a conserved peptide in CDR2, YNE(Q)KFKG; this peptide is shared by various V_HJ558 subfamily genes and by some anti-GAT and phenyl arsonate antibodies, but not by anti-α(1-3)-dextran antibodies. The frequency of *N* nucleotide addition at D-J_H regions is rare. The frequency of the DFL1.16 D segment is higher in TSK autoantibodies than in MRL/lpr, NZB × NZW F_1, or DBA/1 autoantibodies. The frequency of D-D fusions and D-inversions in autoantibodies and the TSK repertoire is higher than in MRL/lpr or NZB autoantibodies.

from this cross to obtain four genotypically different progenies: TSK/+ Ig−/−, TSK/+ Ig+/−, +/+ Ig−/−, and +/+ Ig+/−. An accurate correlation between the mice bearing the TSK mutation and the occurrence of TSK syndrome was possible by the recent demonstration of a defect in the fibrillin-1 gene that may represent a TSK mutation.[38,39] In mice, the fibrillin-1 gene is composed of 61 exons and encodes an 11-kb mRNA.

In TSK mice, the fibrillin-1 gene has a duplication of 17–41 exons and encodes a transcript of 14 kb. TSK mice exhibit a unique polymorphic DNA band when the DNA is digested with Bam HI and EcoRI and hybridized with a 4720–5446 bp probe of

Fbn-1 cDNA.[39] Study of the F_1 progeny obtained from crossing TSK/+ with RAG2−/− or C57BL/6 vit/vit mice showed an excellent correlation between the presence of a defective Fbn-1 gene and thickness of the skin.[39] Thus, we took advantage of the presence of a distinctive Fbn-1 gene polymorphism and the lack of Ig production to identify four genotypically different progenies obtained from the crossing of TSK/+ Ig+/− F_1 with +/+ Ig−/− mice. Histopathological and electron microscopic analysis of the skin, quantitation of soluble collagen type I, and the content of hydroxyproline in the skin showed that an equal number of backcross progeny exhibited the TSK/+ Ig−/− and TSK/+ Ig+/− genotypes[39] (TABLE 3). From this experiment, two major conclusions can be drawn:

(a) the autoimmunity associated with TSK syndrome is mediated by T cells;
(b) the autoantibodies associated with TSK syndrome represent an epiphenomenon.

Note that they are not pathogenic because TSK syndrome occurs in mice devoid of mature B cells and immunoglobulins. Thus, the cause or causes of production of autoantibodies specific for systemic autoimmune diseases such as anti-Sm autoantibodies in SLE, anti-tRNA synthetase antibodies in polymyositis, antipyruvate dehydrogenase complex in primary biliary cirrhosis, anti-HK-ATPase in pernicious anemia, and antitopoisomerase I in scleroderma and tight skin are still unknown. Unraveling this mystery is a challenge for scientists trying to understand autoimmunity.

TABLE 3. Frequency of the Occurrence of TSK Syndrome in 54 Backcross Progeny Obtained from Crossing TSK/+ J_H+/− with J_H−/− Mice

Genotype of Backcross	Expected (n)	Number of Mice Developing TSK Syndrome[a]	χ^2
TSK/+ J_H−/−	8.5	9	0.11
+/+ J_H−/−	8.5	8	
TSK/+ J_H+/−	8.5	8	
+/+ J_H+/−	8.5	9	

[a]TSK syndrome was determined by measuring the thickness of the skin in histological sections under light microscopy, the percentage of soluble collagen type I hydroxyproline content present in the skin, and the concentration of serum anti-topoI autoantibodies in TSK/+ J_H+/− and +/+ J_H+/− mice.

REFERENCES

1. JIMENEZ, S. A. & P. CHRISTNER. 1994. Animal models of systemic sclerosis. Clin. Dermatol. **12:** 425–436.
2. KASTURI, K. N., S. SHIBATA, T. MURYOI & C. A. BONA. 1994. Tight-skin mouse: an experimental model for scleroderma. Int. Rev. Immunol. **11:** 253–271.
3. JABLONSKA, S., H. SCHUBERT & I. KIKUCHI. 1989. Congenital fascial dystrophy: stiff skin syndrome—a human counterpart of the tight-skin mouse. J. Am. Acad. Dermatol. **21:** 943–950.

4. GREEN, M. C., H. O. SWEET & L. E. BUNKER. 1976. Tight-skin, a new mutation of the mouse causing growth of connective tissue and skeleton. Am. J. Pathol. **82:** 493–512.
5. JIMENEZ, S. A., C. J. WILLIAMS, J. C. MEYERS & R. BASHEY. 1986. Increased collagen biosynthesis and increased expression of type I and type III procollagen genes in tight-skin (TSK) mouse fibroblasts. J. Biol. Chem. **261:** 657–662.
6. OSBORN, T. G., R. I. BASHEY, T. L. MOORE & V. W. FISCHER. 1987. Collagenous abnormalities in the heart of tight-skin mouse. J. Mol. Cell. Cardiol. **19:** 581–587.
7. ROSENBERG, G. T., S. C. ROSS & T. G. OSBORN. 1984. Glycosaminoglycan content in the lung of the tight-skin mouse. J. Rheumatol. **11:** 318–320.
8. SHIKATA, H., M. HIRMATSU, M. KAHIMATA, M. NOGUCHI, T. MASUMIZU, D. FUJIMOTO & N. UTSUMI. 1986. Enzyme activities involved in connective tissue metabolism in the skin of tight-skin (TSK) mice. Arch. Dermatol. Res. **278:** 510–512.
9. SHERO, J. H., B. BORDWELL, N. F. ROTHFIELD & W. C. EARNSHAW. 1986. High titers of auto-antibodies to topoisomerase I (Scl-70) in sera from scleroderma patients. Science **231:** 737–740.
10. BOCCHIERI, M. H., P. D. HEURIKSEN, K. N. KASTURI, T. MURYOI, C. A. BONA & S. A. JIMENEZ. 1991. Evidence for autoimmunity in the tight skin (TSK/+) mouse model of progressive systemic sclerosis. Arthritis Rheum. **34:** 599–605.
11. MURYOI, T., J. ANDRE-SCHWARTZ, Y. SAITOH, C. DAIAN, B. HALL, A. DIMITRIU-BONA, R. S. SCHWARTZ, C. BONA & K. N. KASTURI. 1992. Self-reactive repertoire of tight skin mouse: immunochemical and molecular characterization of anti-cellular antibodies. Cell. Immunol. **143:** 43–55.
12. SHIBATA, S., P. HARPEL, C. BONA & H. FILLIT. 1993. Monoclonal antibodies to vascular heparan sulfate inhibit heparan sulfate binding to antithrombin III and the formation of thrombin–antithrombin III complexes. Clin. Immunol. Immunopathol. **67:** 264–272.
13. BOROS, P., J. CHEN, C. BONA & J. C. UNKELESS. 1990. Autoimmune mice make anti-FcR antibodies. J. Exp. Med. **171:** 1581–1595.
14. BOROS, P., J. A. ODIN, T. MURYOI, S. K. MASUR, C. BONA & J. C. UNKELESS. 1991. IgM anti-FcR autoantibodies trigger neutrophil degranulation. J. Exp. Med. **173:** 1473–1482.
15. SZEGEDI, A., P. BOROS, C. BONA, M. KAFINA & J. C. UNKELESS. 1993. An FcγRIII (CD16)–specific autoantibody from a patient with progressive systemic sclerosis. Immunol. Lett. **33:** 69–76.
16. BOROS, P., T. MURYOI, H. SPIERA, C. BONA & J. C. UNKELESS. 1993. Autoantibodies directed against different classes of FcγR are found in sera of autoimmune patients. J. Immunol. **150:** 2018–2025.
17. LALEZARI, P., M. KHORSHIDI & M. PETROSOVA. 1986. Autoimmune neutropenia of infancy. J. Pediatr. **109:** 764.
18. SIPOS, A., C. CSORTOS, S. SIPKA, P. GERGELY, I. SONKOLY & A. SZEGEDI. 1988. The antigen/receptor specificity of antigranulocyte antibodies in patients with SLE. Immunol. Lett. **19:** 329.
19. STETLER, D. A., K. M. ROSE, M. E. WENGER, C. M. BERLIN & S. T. JACOB. 1982. Antibodies to distinct polypeptides of RNA polymerase I in sera from patients with rheumatic diseases. Proc. Natl. Acad. Sci. U.S.A. **79:** 6499–6503.
20. BURGESS, R. R. 1971. RNA polymerase. Annu. Rev. Biochem. **40:** 711–740.
21. REIMER, G., K. M. ROSE, U. SCHEER & E. M. TAN. 1987. Autoantibody to RNA polymerase I in scleroderma sera. J. Clin. Invest. **79:** 65–72.
22. SHIBATA, S., T. MURYOI, Y. SAITOH, T. D. BRUMEANU, C. BONA & K. N. KASTURI. 1993. Immunochemical and molecular characterization of anti–RNA polymerase I autoantibodies produced by tight-skin mice. J. Clin. Invest. **92:** 984–995.
23. MURYOI, T., K. KASTURI, O. USUBA, J. PERLISH, R. FLEISCHMAJER & C. BONA. 1991. Anti-topoisomerase antibodies produced by tight skin (TSK) mice exhibit similar immunochemical and functional properties to those produced by patients with diffuse scleroderma. Autoimmunity **9:** 109–117.
24. MURYOI, T., K. N. KASTURI, M. KAFINA, B. S. CRAM, L. C. HARRISON, T. SASAKI & C. BONA. 1992. Antitopoisomerase I monoclonal autoantibodies from scleroderma patients and tight skin mouse interact with similar epitopes. J. Exp. Med. **175:** 1109.

25. HATAKEYAMA, A., K. N. KASTURI, I. WOLF, R. G. PHELPS & C. BONA. 1996. Correlation between the concentration of serum antitopoisomerase I autoantibodies and histological and biochemical alterations in the skin of tight skin mice. Cell. Immunol. **167:** 135–140.
26. PHELPS, R. G., C. DAIAN, S. SHIBATA, R. FLEISCHMAJER & C. A. BONA. 1993. Induction of skin fibrosis and autoantibodies by infusion of immunocompetent cells from tight-skin mice into C57BL/6 pa/pa mice. J. Autoimmun. **6:** 701–718.
27. KLINMAN, D. M. & A. D. STEINBERG. 1986. Proliferation of anti-DNA producing NZB B cells in a non-autoimmune environment. J. Immunol. **137:** 69–75.
28. BLANKENSTEIN, T. & U. KRAWINKEL. 1987. Immunoglobulin V_H region genes of the mouse are organized in overlapping clusters. Eur. J. Immunol. **17:** 1351–1357.
29. D'HOOSTELAERE, L. A. & D. M. KLINMAN. 1990. Characterization of new mouse V_K groups. J. Immunol. **145:** 2706–2712.
30. MALYNN, B., G. D. YANCOPOULOS, J. E. BARTH, C. A. BONA & F. ALT. 1990. Biased expression of J_H proximal V_H genes occurs in the newly generated repertoire of neonatal and adult mice. J. Exp. Med. **171:** 843–861.
31. KAUSHIK, A., D. H. SCHULZE, F. A. BONILLA, C. A. BONA & G. KELSOE. 1990. Stochastic pairing of V_H and V_K families occurs in polyclonally activated B cells. Proc. Natl. Acad. Sci. U.S.A. **87:** 4932–4936.
32. KASTURI, K. N., C. DAIAN, Y. SAITOH, T. MURYOI & C. BONA. 1993. Tight-skin mouse autoantibody repertoire: analysis of V_H and V_K gene usage. Mol. Immunol. **30:** 969–978.
33. GU, H., D. TARLINTON, W. MULLER, K. RAJEWSKY & I. FORSTER. 1991. Most peripheral B cells in mice are ligand selected. J. Exp. Med. **173:** 1357–1371.
34. KASTURI, K. N., X. Y. YIO & C. A. BONA. 1994. Molecular characterization of J558 genes encoding tight-skin mouse autoantibodies: identical heavy-chain variable genes code for antibodies with different specificities. Proc. Natl. Acad. Sci. U.S.A. **91:** 8067–8071.
35. RUBINSTEIN, L. J., M. YEH & C. A. BONA. 1982. Idiotype-antiidiotype network. II. Activation of silent clones by treatment at birth with idiotopes is associated with the expansion of idiotype-specific helper T cells. J. Exp. Med. **156:** 506–521.
36. GLEASON, K. & H. KOHLER. 1982. Regulatory idiotope T helper cells recognized a shared V_H idiotype on phosphorylcholine-specific antibodies. J. Exp. Med. **156:** 539–549.
37. CHEN, J., M. TROUNSTINE, F. ALT, F. YOUNG, C. KURAHARA, J. F. LORING & D. HUSZAR. 1993. Immunoglobulin gene rearrangement in B cell deficient mice generated by targeted deletion of the J_H locus. Int. Immunol. **5:** 647–656.
38. SIRACUSA, L., R. MCGRATH, Q. MOSKWO, J. J. MANNE, P. J. CHRISTNER, A. M. BUCKBERG & S. A. JIMENEZ. 1996. A tandem duplication within the fibrillin 1 gene is associated with the mouse tight skin mutation. Genome Res. **6:** 300–313.
39. KASTURI, K. N., A. HATAKEYAMA, C. MURAI, R. G. PHELPS & C. BONA. 1996. Development of cutaneous hyperplasia in mouse is associated with defective fibrillin-1 gene. Submitted.

Nuclear Localization of Autoantibodies

Novel Insights into Protein Translocation and Cellular Function[a]

MICHAEL P. MADAIO,[b] KUMIKO YANASE,[b]
MARY H. FOSTER,[b] ROBERT M. SMITH,[b]
THOMAS KIEBER EMMONS,[b] MARINA FABBI,[c]
ANTONIO PUCCETTI,[c] AND LEONARD JARETT[b]

[b]*Departments of Medicine and Pathology and Laboratory Medicine*
University of Pennsylvania
Philadelphia, Pennsylvania 19104

[c]*Advanced Biotechnology Center*
Genoa, Italy

The production of high quantities of autoantibodies that react with DNA and other intranuclear antigens is characteristic of individuals with systemic lupus erythematosus and other autoimmune diseases. Although penetration and localization of serum antibodies within intracellular compartments were initially recognized two decades ago, the capacity of lupus autoantibodies to penetrate cells and induce functional perturbations *in vivo* has been debated.[1–11] Recent accounts of localization of monoclonal antibodies within living cells have rekindled interest in the pathophysiology and cell biology underlying this phenomenon. In this regard, during the search for pathologic autoantibodies, we discovered a subgroup of monoclonal anti-DNA antibodies derived from MRL-lpr/lpr and (NZB × SWR)F1 mice[12] that, following administration to normal mice, produced intranuclear immune deposits *in vivo* in multiple organs. Intranuclear Ig deposits were also observed after cross-linking the tissue prior to direct immunofluorescence, indicating that the phenomenon had occurred *in vivo* and was not an artifact due to the fixation process per se. This phenomenon was highly reproducible and its specificity was supported by the finding that intranuclear localization was unique to this subset of anti-DNA antibodies and not observed with others. Additionally, after iv injection of F(ab′) fragments derived from the relevant anti-DNA antibodies to normal animals, intranuclear deposits were present, further supporting specificity and indicating that penetration and localization were dependent on the antigen-binding region of the molecules.[12]

Animals that had received these immunoglobulins were found to display morphologic and functional abnormalities, including the following: glomerular hypercellularity; epithelial foot process fusion; new fiber bundle formation within the mesangium, suggestive of new collagen synthesis; and proteinuria.[12] Collectively, these results

[a]This work was supported by PHS Grant Nos. DK33694, AI27915, DK07006, and DK45191; the DCI-RED Fund; and an award from the Lupus Foundation of Philadelphia.

indicated that a subset of autoantibodies penetrated cells *in vivo* to influence normal cellular functions; this observation suggested that intranuclear autoantibodies contribute to the functional and pathologic abnormalities in individuals with systemic lupus.

To examine the mechanisms responsible for these phenomena, the capacity of these monoclonal anti-DNA antibodies to penetrate living cells was further evaluated. Using cultured living cell lines, multiple experimental approaches were employed to evaluate nuclear localization of these anti-DNA antibodies, including immunofluorescence, confocal microscopy, immunoelectron microscopy, and quantitative analysis of cellular and nuclear uptake of radiolabeled antibodies.[13] In the latter group of experiments, the requirements for nuclear localization were evaluated in nuclei isolated from cells following coculture with radiolabeled antibodies under varying experimental conditions.

The results provided useful information. Nuclear localization was observed with the same subset of anti-DNA antibodies that localized within nuclei in whole animal experiments, whereas anti-DNA antibodies that did not produce intranuclear deposits in animals did not do so in cultured cells.[13] Furthermore, similar to the whole animal experiments, nuclear localization was dependent on the antigen-binding region of the molecule. The specificity of these events was further supported by the observation that cellular uptake of radiolabeled immunoglobulin was significantly inhibited by unlabeled nuclear localizing antibody, but not by unlabeled anti-DNA antibodies that did not enter cells. Nuclear uptake of radiolabeled antibody (measured in nuclei isolated after coculture of radiolabeled antibodies) was also significantly inhibited by unlabeled nuclear localizing anti-DNA antibodies, but not by anti-DNA antibodies that did not localize within nuclei.

To more precisely examine these events, ultrastructural analyses of cells after incubation with tagged antibodies were performed. Following coculture of gold-labeled antibodies with cells, after varying and progressive intervals, the cells were visualized by electron microscopy. Immunoglobulins were observed: at the cell surface, within the cytoplasm, clustered at the nuclear pore, and within the nucleus.[13] Once internalized, these immunoglobulins transited through the cytoplasm, clustered at the nuclear pore, and entered the nucleus in an energy-dependent manner. Of interest, a fraction of internalized immunoglobulins were recycled and reappeared on the cell surface. Similar time-dependent migration of the antibodies through the cell was also observed by confocal microscopy. Cellular and nuclear localizations of Ig were also determined to be temperature-dependent processes; at 4 °C, these processes were inhibited.

As was observed in the whole animal experiments, cellular entry and nuclear localization of F(ab′) fragments of the anti-DNA antibodies were observed, indicating that both cellular entry and nuclear localization were dependent on the antigen-binding region of the Ig.[12,13] In further support of this conclusion, other anti-DNA antibodies that did not localize within nuclei in the cells in organs of animals did not localize in cultured cells.[13] Of particular relevance, nucleotide sequence analysis of the Ig indicated that nuclear localization–like motifs were present in the CDR3 of the heavy chain in these antibodies.[14] Although an identical consensus sequence was not found, the antibodies shared a tertiary conformation not present among nonnuclear localizing anti-DNA antibodies. All contained multiple positively charged amino acids in their CDR3 regions, resembling nuclear localization signals that direct protein import. Furthermore, two of the three antibodies that allowed modeling shared a conformational motif in the heavy-chain CDR3 region with this nuclear localization motif. This analysis was consistent with the notion that this region participated in nuclear import, and recent preliminary results support this hypothesis.

These experiments represented the first demonstration that monoclonal autoantibodies traversed both the cell and nuclear membranes to localize within the nuclei of cultured cells. Furthermore, nuclear localization of Ig was regulated in a manner analogous to that of other large cytoplasmic proteins that cross membranes and enter the nucleus. More recent results indicate that cellular entry is initiated by the binding of these antibodies to a 110-kDa cell surface protein that was immunoprecipitated from cells following ligation of this antibody.[15] Identification of this protein is in progress and its identity should provide clues to the cellular translocation of these antibodies from the extracellular region into the cytoplasm.

Finally, of potential relevance to the *in vivo* observations of glomerular hypercellularity, these anti-DNA antibodies were found to cross-react with DNase 1 and to inhibit functional activity of the enzyme *in vitro.*[16] Given the postulated role of DNase 1 during apoptosis, these preliminary observations provide the rationale for further examination of the functional consequences of this interaction *in vivo.* This finding is especially provocative in light of the observation that intranuclear antibodies were associated with glomerular hypercellularity. Taken together, these results implicate a novel pathogenic role for lupus autoantibodies. They also provide the means to examine the mechanism of transit of large proteins across cell and nuclear membranes, and they should be useful tools to further assess the functional role of DNase 1 in apoptosis.

REFERENCES

1. McCoy, R. C. 1972. Nuclear localization of immunoglobulins in renal biopsies of patients with lupus nephritis. Am. J. Pathol. **68:** 469–478.
2. Baart de la Faille–Kuyper, E. H. 1974. *In vivo* nuclear localization of immunoglobulins in clinically normal skin in systemic and procainamide-induced lupus erythematosus. Neth. J. Med. **17:** 58.
3. Gilliam, J. N. 1975. The significance of cutaneous immunoglobulin deposits in lupus erythematosus and NZB × NZW/F1 hybrid mice. J. Invest. Dermatol. **65:** 154–161.
4. Izuno, G. T. 1978. Observations on the *in vivo* reaction of antinuclear antibodies with epidermal cells. Br. J. Dermatol. **98:** 391–398.
5. Andersen, I., P. Anderson, P. Elling & H. Graudal. 1983. Epidermal nuclear immunoglobulin deposits in some connective tissue diseases: correlations with ENA antibodies. Ann. Rheum. Dis. **42:** 163–167.
6. Chen, Z. Y., R. L. Dobson, S. K. Ainsworth, R. M. Silver & H. R. Maricq. 1985. Epidermal nuclear immunofluorescence: serological correlations supporting an *in vivo* reaction. Br. J. Dermatol. **112:** 15–22.
7. Alarcon-Segovia, D., A. Ruiz-Arguelles & E. Fishbein. 1978. Antibody to nuclear ribonucleoprotein penetrates live human mononuclear cells through Fc receptors. Nature **271:** 67–69.

8. Alarcon-Segovia, D. & L. Lorente. 1983. Antibody penetration into living cells. IV. Different effects of anti-native DNA and anti-ribonucleoprotein IgG on the cell cycle of activated T cells. Clin. Exp. Immunol. **52:** 365–371.

9. Alarcon-Segovia, D., A. Ruiz-Arguelles & L. Lorente. 1979. Antibody penetration into living cells. II. Antiribonucleoprotein IgG penetrates into T lymphocytes, causing their deletion and the abrogation of suppressor function. J. Immunol. **122:** 1855–1862.

10. Okudaira, K., R. P. Searles, K. Tanimoto, K. Y. Horiuchi & R. C. Williams, Jr. 1982. T lymphocyte interaction with immunoglobulin G antibody in systemic lupus erythematosus. J. Clin. Invest. **69:** 1026–1038.

11. Okudaira, K., Y. Hisayoshi & R. C. Williams, Jr. 1987. Monoclonal anti-DNA antibody interacts with living mononuclear cells. Arthritis Rheum. **30:** 669–678.

12. Vlahakos, D. V., M. H. Foster, A. A. Ucci, K. J. Barrett, S. K. Datta & M. P. Madaio. 1992. Murine monoclonal anti-DNA antibodies penetrate cells, bind to nuclei, and induce glomerular proliferation and proteinuria *in vivo.* J. Am. Soc. Nephrol. **2:** 1345–1354.

13. Yanase, K., R. M. Smith, B. Cizman, M. H. Foster, L. D. Peachey, L. Jarett & M. P. Madaio. 1994. A subgroup of murine monoclonal anti-DNA antibodies traverse the cytoplasm and enter the nucleus in a time- and temperature-dependent manner. Lab. Invest. **71:** 52–60.

14. Foster, M. H., T. Kieber Emmons, M. Ohliger & M. P. Madaio. 1994. Molecular and structural analysis of nuclear localizing anti-DNA lupus antibodies. Immunol. Res. **13:** 172–185.

15. Yanase, K., R. M. Smith, M. H. Foster, L. Jarett & M. P. Madaio. 1996. A specific plasma membrane receptor initiates cellular internalization and nuclear translocation of murine anti-DNA antibodies. Submitted.

16. Madaio, M. P., M. Fabbi, M. Tiso, A. Daga, R. Millo & A. Puccetti. 1996. Nuclear localizing anti-DNA antibodies inhibit internucleosomal DNA degradation *in vivo.* Eur. J. Immunol. In press.

Complement Deficiency and Autoimmunity[a]

M. J. WALPORT, K. A. DAVIES, B. J. MORLEY, AND M. BOTTO

Rheumatology Unit
Department of Medicine
Royal Postgraduate Medical School
Hammersmith Hospital
London W12 0NN, United Kingdom

There are three unexplained paradoxes that characterize the association between the complement system and systemic lupus erythematosus (SLE). The first is that complement participates in the inflammatory lesions of SLE and yet inherited homozygous deficiency of certain complement proteins is powerfully associated with the development of SLE. The second is that C1q deficiency shows the strongest association with the development of SLE and yet, in patients with SLE who do not have C1q deficiency, autoantibodies to C1q commonly develop. The third paradox is that complement deficiency is associated with an impaired primary and secondary antibody response to T lymphocyte–dependent antigens, yet SLE is characterized by high levels of autoantibodies to many intracellular and cell surface antigens. In this report, we shall review the data related to these three paradoxes and some hypotheses to explain them.

THE CLINICAL OBSERVATIONS

Hereditary Homozygous Deficiency

Homozygous complement deficiency is rare. The commonest homozygous complement deficiency in white Caucasian populations is of C2, with a gene frequency of approximately 0.007,[1] which results in a prevalence of homozygous C2 deficiency of approximately 1 in 20,000 individuals. Homozygous complement deficiency is found in, at most, approximately 1% of patients with SLE. In spite of its rarity, the study of the association of homozygous complement deficiency with SLE is important. Homozygous complement deficiency is a very powerful disease-susceptibility gene for the development of SLE. As will be reviewed below, more than 90% of patients with C1q deficiency develop SLE, which is frequently severe and of early onset.

Although homozygous complement deficiency is rare, acquired complement deficiency in SLE is extremely common, with reduced levels of classical pathway proteins and of C3, a marker for active disease.[2–6] It is possible that this acquired

[a]This study was supported by the Arthritis and Rheumatism Council and the MRC.

hypocomplementemia acts as a factor perpetuating disease activity. If the mechanism of the association of inherited complement deficiency with SLE can be understood, the results may be relevant to the majority of SLE patients with acquired hypocomplementemia. We also may learn something of the role of complement in the maintenance of B cell tolerance to autoantigens.

There is a hierarchy of severity and susceptibility to SLE according to the position of the missing complement protein in the activation pathway of the classical pathway of complement. C1q deficiency is associated with the highest prevalence of disease, which tends to be severe and of early onset.[7] Combined C1r and C1s deficiency and C4 deficiency are similarly associated with a very high prevalence of severe disease. C2 deficiency is probably only associated with the development of SLE in a maximum of 33% of cases and the spectrum of disease is similar to that observed for idiopathic SLE as a whole.[8] By contrast, only a minority of patients with C3 deficiency develop clinical features associated with autoimmune disease, and mild, lupuslike illness has only been reported in three families (reviewed below).

The disparity between the clinical associations of C1q and C3 deficiency is surprising because C3 is quantitatively the most important complement protein, present in plasma at up to 1.5 g per liter, and subserves many of the physiological activities of the complement system. C3 is the precursor of several of the major opsonins of the complement system and of the anaphylatoxin C3a; C3 cleavage is also largely essential for the cleavage of C5, which is the source of the anaphylatoxin, C5a, and the first step in the formation of the membrane attack complex of complement. Although C4 can to a very minor extent substitute for C3 in the formation of a C5 convertase enzyme,[9] this is unlikely to be of significance *in vivo.* In the next few paragraphs, we will review in some more detail the differences between C1q and C3 deficiency. Those interested in deficiencies of other classical and alternative pathway complement deficiencies are referred to the following reviews: complement deficiency in general;[10–12] C1r and C1s;[13,14] C4;[15] C2;[8] factor I and factor H.[16]

C1q Deficiency

Hereditary homozygous C1q deficiency is a rare state. It was first described in a 10-year-old Turkish boy by Berkel and colleagues in 1977.[17] Since then, a total of 34 cases of C1q deficiency associated with recurrent skin lesions, chronic infections, systemic lupus erythematosus (SLE) or SLE-like diseases, and mesangial proliferative glomerulonephritis have been reported (reviewed in references 7, 14, 18, and 19). Only 1 healthy subject with C1q deficiency has been identified, the healthy sibling of 3 patients with C1q deficiency and SLE. Seven other families have been reported with more than 1 sibling with C1q deficiency and, in each case, all the siblings suffered from SLE. Disease onset is typically early, with a median age of 7 years. Nineteen of 25 patients with C1q deficiency in whom a result was reported had ANA detected. The results of autoantibodies to extractable nuclear antigens have been reported in 19 subjects (reviewed in references 7 and 18). Five results were negative and 14 patients had one or more positive test results [anti-RNP in 6; anti-Sm in 7 (including 2 reported as having high-titer RNase-resistant ENA); anti-Ro in 6]. Anti-dsDNA antibodies appear to be uncommon and have been reported in only 4 subjects with C1q deficiency.

C1q is composed of 18 polypeptide chains of three different chain types: A, B, and C. The A-, B-, and C-chain genes are tandemly arranged 5′ to 3′ in the order of A, C, B at chromosome 1p34.1–1p36.3.[5–7] The molecular basis of C1q deficiency has been described in 8 cases and these are summarized in reference 18. Mutations causing C1q deficiency have been described in each of the three genes and, in every case so far, have been point-changes; in 3 cases there were premature stop codons, in 1 case a single base deletion, and in 2 cases a glycine-to-arginine amino acid substitution at codon 6 of the C-chain, causing expression of a dysfunctional protein (summarized in reference 18).

C3 Deficiency

Twenty-four humans with C3 deficiency from 16 families from all over the world have been described and we have previously reviewed 20 of these patients.[20] Two further families have been reported since that review.[21,22] There are two major clinical associations of C3 deficiency, namely, increased susceptibility to pyogenic bacterial infections and "immune complex"–type disease, the latter particularly characterized by glomerulonephritis. Homozygous C3-deficient individuals in general are markedly susceptible to life-threatening bacterial infections caused by encapsulated bacteria such as *Neisseria meningitidis, Streptococcus pneumoniae,* and *Haemophilus influenzae.* Recurrent otitis media, meningitis, and pneumonia are particularly characteristic infections. Patients tend to become ill early in life and the median age of the first episode of infection is younger than that seen in other complement deficiencies. These repeated and severe infections emphasize the important physiological role of C3 as an opsonin for bacteria, especially in early childhood, when protective antibodies and anamnestic responses have not yet developed.

Two patterns of inflammatory illness have been described in patients with C3 deficiency. The first is rash, which typically follows closely after pyogenic sepsis. In 1 case, skin biopsy showed a dense neutrophilic infiltrate.[23] The second pattern of illness is glomerulonephritis, not overtly associated with pyogenic infection, typically with membranoproliferative histology. Very similar disease has been reported in dogs with C3 deficiency (reviewed below). Five patients from 3 families were reported to have lupuslike symptoms. In 3 patients from 2 Japanese families, ANA and LE cells were not detected (reviewed in reference 20). In a further 2 sisters from a Swedish family in which a dysfunctional C3 molecule was detected, antinuclear antibodies were detected in both and anti-dsDNA antibodies were detected in 1 sister.[21]

Partial Inherited Complement Deficiency

Given the strong association of homozygous complement deficiency with SLE, a number of studies have been undertaken to examine whether heterozygous complement deficiency also increases susceptibility to develop SLE. Such studies are difficult to perform because of the difficulty in phenotypic identification of heterozygous deficiency states. This difficulty is for two reasons. First, the range of complement protein levels expressed by normal homozygous individuals is large and there is overlap between the levels of expressed protein concentrations between homozygotes and heterozygotes. Second, the difficulty is compounded in SLE where consumption of classical pathway proteins is increased by the disease process. These difficulties can be overcome if the molecular basis of common null alleles of complement proteins can be identified and simple and reliable molecular assays can be applied to genotype individuals. Using this approach in the case of C2 deficiency, it has become apparent that approximately 1% of white Caucasian SLE patients have homozygous C2 deficiency, but there is no increase in the prevalence of heterozygotes for C2 deficiency.[1,24] Similarly, there is evidence that heterozygous C1q deficiency is not a significant disease-susceptibility allele for the development of SLE.[19]

The situation is much more complicated in the case of partial C4 deficiency. There are two isotypes of C4, namely, C4A and C4B, encoded by closely linked and highly polymorphic genes in the MHC. The polymorphisms of both of these genes include common null alleles associated with no expressed protein. These null alleles are candidate disease-susceptibility genes for the development of SLE.

There have been many studies to examine the associations of the polymorphic products of particular MHC genes in patients with SLE. These have mainly concentrated on HLA class II, complement, and TNF genes. All are difficult to interpret because of the problem of linkage disequilibrium between the many different genes encoded in the MHC. A number of studies have shown an excess of C4A null alleles in patients with SLE,[25,26] although some large studies have not found such an excess.[27–29] The most frequently reproduced of these associations is with a deleted C4A null allele found in the most-common white Caucasian haplotype: HLA-A1, -B8, -DRB1*0103, -DQA1*0501, -DQB1*0201, Bf*S, C2*C, C4A*Q0, C4*B1, TNFA*1, TNFB*2. This haplotype is associated with a number of autoimmune diseases, and candidate disease-susceptibility genes in this haplotype include MHC class II, complement, and TNF genes.

One approach to trying to narrow down the true disease-susceptibility gene is to study MHC associations with SLE in different ethnic groups. This approach is important because MHC haplotypes in different populations show different patterns of linkage between the polymorphic alleles of the different genes. For this reason, an association between a polymorphic marker of one gene and a particular disease is more likely to be relevant if the same association is found in different ethnic groups. Several such studies in different ethnic groups have tended to confirm associations of SLE with an excess of C4A null alleles: Chinese,[30] Korean,[31] African-American,[32,33] and Japanese.[34]

However, because of the difficulties of accurate ascertainment of C4 null alleles in patients with SLE, the role of C4A null alleles as disease-susceptibility genes for SLE is likely to remain unresolved until reliable genotyping methods are developed that can be applied to the common C4A null alleles in different ethnic populations.

Acquired Complement Deficiency

Further support for a pathogenic role of complement deficiency in inducing the development of SLE comes from observations in patients who have acquired complement deficiency. Patients with heterozygous deficiency of C1 inhibitor, associated with the disease hereditary angioedema, have chronically low levels of C4 and C2 because of dysregulated C1s activity. Approximately 1% of patients with hereditary angioedema develop SLE[35–37] and up to 4% develop glomerulonephritis.[37,38]

Patients with C3 nephritic factor, an autoantibody that stabilizes the complement amplification loop C3 convertase enzyme, C3bBb, have chronically low C3 levels. Several patients with this autoantibody have been reported to develop SLE, in each case many years after the initial development of nephritic factor.[39]

Artifactual Associations of Complement Deficiency with SLE—Ascertainment Artifact or Linked Genes

The first two subjects with hereditary deficiency of complement to be characterized were immunologists, who both suffered from C2 deficiency.[40,41] The simple interpretation of this finding is that C2 deficiency predisposes humans to become immunologists! This is an example of a common ascertainment artifact that should be considered as the explanation for any apparent causal association between a test result and a disease. The reason that the first complement-deficient humans to be described were immunologists is that they experimented on their own serum. If any particular analyte is only measured in a particular subset of individuals, then any abnormal results will be found in that subset.

Using the same reasoning, it could be argued that the association of complement deficiency with SLE may also be an ascertainment artifact. Given that complement measurements are routinely made in clinical laboratories as a marker of disease activity in SLE, there is a high likelihood of uncovering primary abnormalities of the complement system in these patients. Evidence that this is not the case comes from two large studies of healthy individuals, approximately 4000 recruits into the Swiss army[42] and 150,000 Japanese blood donors.[43,44] In neither of these groups were any examples of inherited deficiencies of classical pathway proteins or of C3 found; however, among the Japanese blood donors, 154 healthy individuals with homozygous deficiency of one of the proteins of the membrane attack complex of complement were found.

C1q AUTOANTIBODIES IN SLE

In view of the very strong association of homozygous C1q deficiency with SLE, it is of great interest that anti-C1q autoantibodies are commonly found in patients with SLE who do not have primary complement deficiencies. These antibodies[45–47] react with a neoepitope in the collagenous region of C1q that is exposed following activation of the C1 complex, with dissociation of C1r and C1s from C1q. These antibodies were first identified as C1q precipitins,[48] present in patients with hypocomplementemic vasculitis and in 23 out of 30 patients with SLE and hypocomplementemia. It was subsequently demonstrated that C1q precipitins were IgG autoantibodies to C1q.[49,50]

Anti-C1q antibodies show a number of specific clinical and serological associations. They are strongly associated with complement classical pathway activation, often with very low levels of C1q, C4, and C3. The most-striking clinical association of these antibodies is with hypocomplementemic urticarial vasculitis syndrome (HUVS),[51] characterized clinically by a variable combination of urticarial vasculitis, arthritis, obstructive bronchitis, and glomerulonephritis. The association of anti-C1q antibodies with HUVS is very specific and these are often the only autoantibodies identified in this disease, which points to the hypothesis that the antibodies may cause the disease. However, anti-C1q antibodies are also associated with hypocomplementemia and glomerulonephritis in patients with lupus[47] and occur in some patients with membranoproliferative glomerulonephritis in the absence of other features of SLE.[52]

The question of whether anti-C1q antibodies are pathogenic remains unresolved. It seems likely that they may augment activation of the complement system by immune complexes in tissues. In favor of this idea are experiments showing that anti-C1q antibodies, purified from two patients with systemic lupus erythematosus, deposited in mouse glomeruli in the presence of human C1q.[53]

The mechanism for the development of anti-C1q antibodies is not understood. They may be part of the primary autoimmune response found in SLE, but that begs the question as to what is the explanation for the range of antigens to which autoantibodies are formed in this disease—a question to which there is no answer at present. There is substantial evidence that the autoantibody response in SLE is antigen-driven (reviewed in reference 54). It is possible that anti-C1q antibodies are driven by C1q released from the C1 complex by complement activation following immune complex formation. However, anti-C1q antibodies do not always follow intense and prolonged C1 activation; for example, they are not found in patients with mixed essential cryoglobulinemia.

WHAT ARE THE HYPOTHESES?

The hypothesis that emerges from the clinical data reviewed in the first part of this paper is that an activity of the early classical pathway of complement protects against the development of SLE. This activity could be one of the known physiological activities of complement or one that is yet to be discovered. Three candidate activities of complement that could protect against the development of autoimmunity are host defense against infection, the processing of immune complexes, and the presentation of antigen. Each of these activities will now be dealt with in turn.

Complement and Infection

Complement is part of the innate immune system and, as such, plays an important role in host defense against infectious disease. The study of complement-deficient humans and animals is one of the most powerful approaches for determining the spectrum of infections against which complement is a major component of host defense. The evidence, reviewed above, shows an important role for complement in protection against encapsulated pyogenic bacteria. No other apparent infectious complications have been associated with complement deficiencies. In particular, complement does not seem to be important in defense against common viral infections. There are *in vitro* data to show that complement may play a part in defense against retroviruses, which are enveloped by a lipid bilayer cell membrane derived from host cells. However, the efficiency of lysis of retroviruses by complement is determined in part by the species origin of the host cell membrane and its constituent proteins[55] and there are no definite data that show that complement is important *in vivo* in protection against retroviral infection.

It is difficult to attribute the association between complement deficiency and lupus to the effects of infection. Other diseases associated with impaired host defense against pyogenic infection, such as bronchiectasis, are not associated with the development of SLE. Nor would the pattern of bacterial infections associated with complement deficiency explain why C1q deficiency is more strongly associated with SLE than C3 deficiency. The possibility cannot be excluded that an unknown and otherwise asymptomatic retroviral infection is associated with development of SLE. This is a hypothesis that is difficult to refute; however, there is no positive evidence in support of it.

Complement and the Physiology of Immune Complex Processing

There is some evidence to support the hypothesis that the role of complement in the processing of immune complexes helps in protection against the development of SLE. It has been known since experiments by Heidelberger in the 1940s[56] that complement maintains immune complexes in solution. The classical pathway of complement inhibits the formation of large immune-complex lattices and promotes uptake of immune complexes by the mononuclear phagocytic system. It does this by inhibiting Fc-Fc interactions and by disrupting antigen-antibody binding by the incorporation of C4b and C3b into the lattice. C1q, C3b, and C4b bound to immune complexes in turn promote binding of immune complexes to carrier molecules of CR1 on circulating red cells and to C1q and C3 receptors on cells of the mononuclear phagocytic system. These phagocytes take up immune complexes, catabolize them, and present the peptides derived from the antigens to T cells, which in turn drive a humoral immune response. We have recently reviewed the physiology and pathophysiology of the interactions between complement and immune complexes.[57]

Breakdown of these mechanisms provides a plausible explanation for the development of autoimmunity (reviewed in reference 58). Defective processing of immune complexes could result in large immune complexes escaping the mononuclear phagocytic system and depositing in tissues throughout the body. Inflammation may ensue, with the release of autoantigens ultimately driving an autoimmune response.

In support of such a model are studies showing that immune complexes are cleared with a very abnormal pattern in the presence of either acquired hypocomplementemia[59–61] or hereditary complement deficiency.[62,63] The two most-striking abnormalities of immune complex processing in complement-deficient humans are the impaired uptake of immune complexes into the mononuclear phagocytic system of the liver and the complete absence of uptake of immune complexes into the spleen.[63] This last observation leads into the third hypothesis linking complement deficiency with development of SLE, abnormal mechanisms of antigen presentation, and B cell peripheral tolerance.

Complement and Antigen Presentation

Although the complement system is mainly viewed as a component of the innate immune system, there is evidence that complement plays an important role in enhancing adaptive immune responses. Receptors for the major split fragments of C3 are found on B lymphocytes (CR1 and CR2) and on follicular dendritic cells (CR1, CR2, and CR3). On B lymphocytes, ligation of CR2 lowers the threshold for B cell activation[64,65] and there is recent evidence that oligomers of C3dg coupled to antigen may act as an adjuvant,[66] markedly enhancing antibody responses. Complement appears to play an essential role in the localization of antigens in the form of immune complexes to the surface of follicular dendritic cells.

The evidence that supports these statements may be briefly summarized as follows. Pepys[67] used cobra venom factor to deplete C3 activity *in vivo* and found an important role for complement in the induction of antibody responses and in the generation of B lymphocyte memory in germinal centers (reviewed in reference 68). Cobra venom factor only allows temporary depletion of C3 because it is antigenic and can only be given for a limited period. The identification of C3-deficient animals and patients offered the opportunity to investigate antibody responses thoroughly both in experimental animals and in humans with persistent deficiency of C3. Immunization of both C3-deficient guinea pigs and dogs with ΦX174, an experimental thymus-dependent immunogen, gave similar results: at low doses of antigen (1×10^9 PFU per kg), both the primary and secondary responses were markedly impaired; at high doses of antigen ($>5 \times 10^9$ PFU per kg), the titers of the primary and secondary antibody responses approached normal, but the normal switch from IgM to IgG did not occur as part of the secondary response and the IgG anti-ΦX174 antibody response was markedly impaired.[69,70] Impairment of primary and secondary responses was also seen in dogs in response to another T cell–dependent antigen, sheep red blood cells.[70] A similar abnormality was observed in dogs in response to the thymus-independent-2 antigen, DNP-Ficoll.

Experimental studies of immunization of complement-deficient patients are few and far between. A typical example was the South African patient studied by Alper and colleagues,[71] who showed a normal anamnestic response to diphtheria toxoid and a normal primary antibody response to the polyribose phosphate antigen of *H. influenzae* in terms of quantitative antibody response. Two C3-deficient subjects were immunized with ΦX174 and these patients demonstrated normal titers of antibody following both primary and secondary immunization, but also failure to switch the antibody response from IgM to IgG, a result similar to that seen in complement-deficient guinea pigs and dogs.[72] The majority of patients with C3 deficiency have had total IgG levels within normal limits. However, it has been observed that patients deficient in the classical pathway proteins of complement show reduced levels of IgG_4 and, to a lesser extent, IgG_2.[73]

In summary, it is clear that the antibody response in humans and animals with classical pathway complement deficiencies is abnormal with impaired primary and secondary responses, failure of the switch from IgM to IgG, and reduced IgG_2 and IgG_4 production. However, immunization with high doses of antigen overcomes these defects to a large extent.

It is striking that ligation of complement receptors on B cells lowers their threshold for activation and that complement deficiency is associated with impaired antibody responses to foreign antigens with impaired B cell memory, yet (by complete contrast) complement deficiency is associated with the production of high levels of autoantibodies. Can any hypothesis be developed to explain these apparently contradictory observations?

There are several mechanisms for the induction of B cell tolerance and these are discussed elsewhere in this volume. An important mechanism for censoring self-reactive B lymphocytes is by competitive exclusion from primary lymphoid follicles (reviewed in reference 74). In the presence of autoantigen, autoreactive B lymphocytes are excluded from primary follicles in the presence of B lymphocytes reactive with foreign antigens. The mechanism for this is not known. If complement were involved in the process, complement deficiency might modify the balance of the competition between B cells, allowing autoreactive B cells to enter primary follicles. This hypothesis is testable now that mice with targeted gene deletions of C1q and other complement proteins are available, as described below.

COMPLEMENT-DEFICIENT ANIMALS

Although the initial observations showing a link between complement deficiency and SLE have all come from humans, it may be necessary to turn to animal models in order to perform the experiments that will provide an explanation for the link. There are a number of spontaneous models of inherited deficiency of classical pathway complement proteins and of C3 in animals, although none of these are in mice. With the advent of techniques for targeted gene disruption in mice, a number of mouse strains have now been developed with classical and alternative pathway complement deficiencies and some preliminary data are now available. We will now review some results that have come from the study of animals with complement deficiency.

Spontaneous Deficiency

Colonies of guinea pigs have been identified with C2,[75] C4,[76] and C3[77] deficiencies (reviewed in references 78 and 79), as well as dogs with C3 deficiency[80] and, recently, pigs with factor H deficiency.[81] No spontaneous disease has been identified in any of the complement-deficient strains of guinea pigs. It may be relevant that guinea pigs, in contrast to humans, dogs, and mice, have not been reported to spontaneously develop lupus. However, some serological signs of autoimmunity were detected in the blood of C4- and C2-deficient guinea pigs, which spontaneously developed elevated levels of IgM and of rheumatoid factor, which was not seen in C3-deficient animals.[82]

In contrast, dogs with C3 deficiency develop a glomerulonephritis that is very similar to that reported in humans,[83] and pigs with factor H deficiency develop a severe early-onset lethal glomerulonephritis[81] that is more severe than the pathology reported in the small number of cases of humans with factor H or factor I deficiency (reviewed in reference 16).

Targeted Deficiency in Mice

The genes for C3, C4,[84] CR1/2,[85,86] FB, and C1q[87] have each been successfully targeted in mice. No spontaneous phenotype has been observed for any of these mice, with the exception of C1q-deficient mice on a mixed genetic background of 129 and C57BL/6. Our own preliminary data (unpublished) indicate that 5 out of a colony of 31 of these mice have died with crescentic nephritis at an age of approximately six months and antinuclear, anti-ssDNA, and anti-dsDNA antibodies have developed in up to 50% of this group of mice. These findings suggest that these mice may be a valuable model to explore the links between complement deficiency and SLE.

REFERENCES

1. Sullivan, K. E., M. A. Petri, B. J. Schmeckpeper, R. H. McLean & J. A. Winkelstein. 1994. Prevalence of a mutation causing C2 deficiency in systemic lupus erythematosus. J. Rheumatol. **21:** 1128–1133.
2. Lloyd, W. & P. H. Schur. 1981. Immune complexes, complement, and anti-DNA in exacerbations of systemic lupus erythematosus (SLE). Medicine (Baltimore) **60:** 208–217.
3. Swaak, A. J., J. Groenwold & W. Bronsveld. 1986. Predictive value of complement profiles and anti-dsDNA in systemic lupus erythematosus. Ann. Rheum. Dis. **45:** 359–366.
4. Koffler, D., V. Agnello, R. Thoburn & H. G. Kunkel. 1971. Systemic lupus erythematosus: prototype of immune complex nephritis in man. J. Exp. Med. **134**(suppl.): 169s.
5. Cameron, J. S., M. H. Lessof, C. S. Ogg, B. D. Williams & D. G. Williams. 1976. Disease activity in the nephritis of systemic lupus erythematosus in relation to serum complement concentrations: DNA-binding capacity and precipitating anti-DNA antibody. Clin. Exp. Immunol. **25:** 418–427.
6. Valentijn, R. M., H. van Overhagen, H. M. Hazevoet, J. Hermans, A. Cats, M. R. Daha & L. A. van Es. 1985. The value of complement and immune complex determinations in monitoring disease activity in patients with systemic lupus erythematosus. Arthritis Rheum. **28:** 904–913.
7. Bowness, P., K. A. Davies, P. J. Norsworthy, P. Athanassiou, J. Taylor-Wiedeman, L. K. Borysiewicz, P. A. Meyer & M. J. Walport. 1994. Hereditary C1q deficiency and systemic lupus erythematosus. QJM **87:** 455–464.

8. RUDDY, S. 1986. Component deficiencies. 3. The second component. Prog. Allergy **39:** 250–266.
9. MASAKI, T., M. MATSUMOTO, R. YASUDA, R. P. LEVINE, H. KITAMURA & T. SEYA. 1991. A covalent dimer of complement C4b serves as a subunit of a novel C5 convertase that involves no C3 derivatives. J. Immunol. **147:** 927–932.
10. COLTEN, H. R. & F. S. ROSEN. 1992. Complement deficiencies. Annu. Rev. Immunol. **10:** 809–834.
11. ROSS, S. C. & P. DENSEN. 1984. Complement deficiency states and infection: epidemiology, pathogenesis, and consequences of neisserial and other infections in an immune deficiency. Medicine (Baltimore) **63:** 243–273.
12. MORGAN, B. P. & M. J. WALPORT. 1991. Complement deficiency and disease. Immunol. Today **12:** 301–306.
13. REID, K. B. M. 1989. Deficiency of the first component of human complement. Immunodefic. Rev. **1:** 247–260.
14. LOOS, M. & H-P. HEINZ. 1986. Component deficiencies. 1. The first component: C1q, C1r, C1s. Prog. Allergy **39:** 212–231.
15. HAUPTMANN, G., G. TAPPEINER & J. A. SCHIFFERLI. 1988. Inherited deficiency of the fourth component of human complement. Immunol. Rev. **1:** 3–22.
16. VYSE, T. J., P. J. SPATH, K. A. DAVIES, B. J. MORLEY, P. PHILIPPE, P. ATHANASSIOU, C. M. GILES & M. J. WALPORT. 1994. Hereditary complement factor I deficiency. QJM **87:** 385–401.
17. BERKEL, A. J., O. SANAL, R. THESEN & M. LOOS. 1977. A case of selective C1q deficiency. Turk. J. Pediatr. **19:** 101–108.
18. TOPALOGLU, A., A. BAKKALOGLU, J. H. SLINGSBY, M. J. MIHATSCH, M. PASCUAL, P. NORSWORTHY, B. J. MORLEY, U. SAATCI, J. A. SCHIFFERLI & M. J. WALPORT. 1996. Molecular basis of hereditary C1q deficiency associated with SLE and IgA nephropathy in a Turkish family. Kidney Int. **50:** 635–642.
19. SLINGSBY, J. H., P. NORSWORTHY, G. PEARCE, A. K. VAISHNAW, H. ISSLER, B. J. MORLEY & M. J. WALPORT. 1996. Homozygous hereditary C1q deficiency and systemic lupus erythematosus: a new family and the molecular basis of C1q deficiency in three families. Arthritis Rheum. **39:** 663–670.
20. BOTTO, M. & M. J. WALPORT. 1993. Hereditary deficiency of C3 in animals and humans. Int. Rev. Immunol. **10:** 37–50.
21. NILSSON, U. R., B. NILSSON, K. E. STORM, G. SJOLIN-FORSBERG & R. HALLGREN. 1992. Hereditary dysfunction of the third component of complement associated with a systemic lupus erythematosus–like syndrome and meningococcal meningitis. Arthritis Rheum. **35:** 580–586.
22. PELEG, D., H. HARIT-BUSTAN, Y. KATZ, S. PELLER, M. SCHLESINGER & S. SCHONFELD. 1992. Inherited C3 deficiency and meningococcal disease in a teenager. Pediatr. Infect. Dis. J. **11:** 401–404.
23. WEISS, R. M. & E. J. SCHULZ. 1989. Complement deficiency in Sweet's syndrome. Br. J. Dermatol. **121:** 413–415.
24. TRUEDSSON, L., G. STURFELT & O. NIVED. 1993. Prevalence of the type I complement C2 deficiency gene in Swedish systemic lupus erythematosus patients. Lupus **2:** 325–327.
25. FIELDER, A. H. L., M. J. WALPORT, J. R. BATCHELOR, R. I. RYNES, C. M. BLACK, I. A. DODI & G. R. V. HUGHES. 1983. Family study of the major histocompatibility complex in patients with systemic lupus erythematosus: importance of null alleles of C4A and C4B in determining disease susceptibility. Br. Med. J. **286:** 425–428.
26. CHRISTIANSEN, F. T., R. L. DAWKINS, G. UKO, J. MCCLUSKEY, P. H. KAY & P. J. ZILKO. 1983. Complement allotyping in SLE: association with C4A null. Aust. N. Z. J. Med. **13:** 483–488.
27. HARTUNG, K., M. P. BAUR, R. COLDEWEY, M. FRICKE, J. R. KALDEN, H. J. LAKOMEK, H. H. PETER, D. SCHENDEL, P. M. SCHNEIDER, S. A. SEUCHTER, W. STANGEL & H. R. G. DEICHER. 1992. Major histocompatibility complex haplotypes and complement C4 alleles in systemic lupus erythematosus. J. Clin. Invest. **90:** 1346–1351.

28. SCHUR, P. H., D. MARCUS-BAGLEY, Z. AWDEH, E. J. YUNIS & C. A. ALPER. 1990. The effect of ethnicity on major histocompatibility complex complement allotypes and extended haplotypes in patients with systemic lupus erythematosus. Arthritis Rheum. **33:** 985–992.
29. GOLDSTEIN, R. & D. P. SENGAR. 1993. Comparative studies of the major histocompatibility complex in French Canadian and non–French Canadian Caucasians with systemic lupus erythematosus. Arthritis Rheum. **36:** 1121–1127.
30. DUNCKLEY, H., P. A. GATENBY, B. HAWKINS, S. NAITO & S. W. SERJEANTSON. 1987. Deficiency of C4A is a genetic determinant of systemic lupus erythematosus in three ethnic groups. J. Immunogenet. **14:** 209–218.
31. HONG, G. H., H. Y. KIM, F. TAKEUCHI, K. NAKANO, H. YAMADA, K. MATSUTA, H. HAN, K. TOKUNAGA, K. ITO & K. S. PARK. 1994. Association of complement C4 and HLA-DR alleles with systemic lupus erythematosus in Koreans. J. Rheumatol. **21:** 442–447.
32. WILSON, W. A., M. C. PEREZ & P. E. ARMATIS. 1988. Partial C4A deficiency is associated with susceptibility to systemic lupus erythematosus in black Americans. Arthritis Rheum. **31:** 1171–1175.
33. OLSEN, M. L., R. GOLDSTEIN, F. C. ARNETT, M. DUVIC, M. POLLACK & J. D. REVEILLE. 1989. C4A gene deletion and HLA associations in black Americans with systemic lupus erythematosus. Immunogenetics **30:** 27–33.
34. YAMADA, H., A. WATANABE, A. MIMORI, K. NAKANO, F. TAKEUCHI, K. MATSUTA, K. TANIMOTO, T. MIYAMOTO, Y. YUKIYAMA, K. TOKUNAGA *et al.* 1990. Lack of gene deletion for complement C4A deficiency in Japanese patients with systemic lupus erythematosus. J. Rheumatol. **17:** 1054–1057.
35. DONALDSON, V. H., E. V. HESS & A. J. MCADAMS. 1977. Lupus-erythematosus-like disease in three unrelated women with hereditary angioneurotic edema [letter]. Ann. Intern. Med. **86:** 312–313.
36. KOHLER, P. F., J. PERCY, W. M. CAMPION & C. J. SMYTH. 1974. Hereditary angioedema and "familial" lupus erythematosus in identical twin boys. Am. J. Med. **56:** 406–411.
37. BRICKMAN, C. M., G. C. TSOKOS, J. E. BALOW, T. J. LAWLEY, M. SANTAELLA, C. H. HAMMER & M. M. FRANK. 1986. Immunoregulatory disorders associated with hereditary angioedema. I. Clinical manifestations of autoimmune disease. J. Allergy Clin. Immunol. **77:** 749–757.
38. PAN, C. G., C. F. STRIFE, M. K. WARD, R. E. SPITZER & A. J. MCADAMS. 1992. Long-term follow-up of nonsystemic lupus erythematosus glomerulonephritis in patients with hereditary angioedema: report of four cases. Am. J. Kidney Dis. **19:** 526–531.
39. WALPORT, M. J., K. A. DAVIES, M. BOTTO, M. A. NAUGHTON, D. A. ISENBERG, D. BIASI, R. J. POWELL, N. T. CHEUNG & G. R. STRUTHERS. 1994. C3 nephritic factor and SLE: report of four cases and review of the literature. QJM **87:** 609–615.
40. SILVERSTEIN, A. M. 1969. Essential hypocomplementemia: report of a case. Blood **16:** 1338–1341.
41. KLEMPERER, M. R., H. C. WOODWORTH, F. S. ROSEN & K. F. AUSTEN. 1966. Hereditary deficiency of the second component of complement (C2) in man. J. Clin. Invest. **45:** 880–890.
42. HASSIG, A., J. F. BOREL & P. AMMANN. 1964. Essentielle hypocomplementemia. Pathol. Microbiol. **27:** 542–547.
43. FUKUMORI, Y., K. YOSHIMURA, S. OHNOKI, H. YAMAGUCHI, Y. AKAGAKI & S. INAI. 1989. A high incidence of C9 deficiency among healthy blood donors in Osaka, Japan. Int. Immunol. **1:** 85–89.
44. INAI, S., Y. AKAGAKI, T. MORIYAMA, Y. FUKUMORI, K. YOSHIMURA, S. OHNOKI & H. YAMAGUCHI. 1989. Inherited deficiencies of the late-acting complement components other than C9 found among healthy blood donors. Int. Arch. Allergy Appl. Immunol. **90:** 274–279.
45. WENER, M. H., S. UWATOKO & M. MANNIK. 1989. Antibodies to the collagen-like region of C1q in sera of patients with autoimmune rheumatic diseases. Arthritis Rheum. **32:** 544–551.
46. UWATOKO, S., S. AOTSUKA, M. OKAWA, Y. EGUSA, R. YOKOHARI & C. AIZAWA. 1984. Characterization of C1q-binding IgG complexes in systemic lupus erythematosus. Clin. Immunol. Immunopathol. **30:** 104–116.

47. SIEGERT, C., M. DAHA, M. L. WESTEDT, E. VAN DER VOORT & F. BREEDVELD. 1991. IgG autoantibodies against C1q are correlated with nephritis, hypocomplementemia, and dsDNA antibodies in systemic lupus erythematosus. J. Rheumatol. **18:** 230–234.

48. AGNELLO, V., D. KOFFLER, J. W. EISENBERG, R. J. WINCHESTER & H. G. KUNKEL. 1971. C1q precipitins in the sera of patients with systemic lupus erythematosus and other hypocomplementemic states: characterization of high and low molecular weight types. J. Exp. Med. **134**(3): 228–241.

49. MARDER, R. J., L. A. POTEMPA, J. V. JONES, D. TORIUMI, F. R. SCHMID & H. GEWURZ. 1984. Assay, purification, and further characterization of 7S C1q-precipitins (C1q-p) in hypocomplementemic vasculitis urticaria syndrome and systemic lupus erythematosus. Acta Pathol. Microbiol. Immunol. Scand. [C] **92:** 25–34.

50. UWATOKO, S. & M. MANNIK. 1988. Low-molecular-weight C1q-binding immunoglobulin G in patients with systemic lupus erythematosus consists of autoantibodies to the collagen-like region of C1q. J. Clin. Invest. **82:** 816–824.

51. WISNIESKI, J. J., A. N. BAER, J. CHRISTENSEN, T. R. CUPPS, D. N. FLAGG, J. V. JONES, P. L. KATZENSTEIN, E. R. MCFADDEN, J. J. MCMILLEN, M. A. PICK *et al.* 1995. Hypocomplementemic urticarial vasculitis syndrome: clinical and serologic findings in 18 patients. Medicine (Baltimore) **74:** 24–41.

52. STRIFE, C. F., A. E. LEAHY & C. D. WEST. 1989. Antibody to a cryptic, solid-phase C1q antigen in membranoproliferative nephritis. Kidney Int. **35:** 836–842.

53. UWATOKO, S., V. J. GAUTHIER & M. MANNIK. 1991. Autoantibodies to the collagen-like region of C1q deposit in glomeruli via C1q in immune deposits. Clin. Immunol. Immunopathol. **61:** 268–273.

54. WALPORT, M. J. 1993. Systemic lupus erythematosus. *In* Clinical Aspects of Immunology. Fifth edition. P. J. Lachmann, D. K. Peters, F. S. Rosen & M. J. Walport, Eds.: 1161–1204. Blackwell. Oxford.

55. TAKEUCHI, Y., F. L. COSSET, P. J. LACHMANN, H. OKADA, R. A. WEISS & M. K. COLLINS. 1994. Type C retrovirus inactivation by human complement is determined by both the viral genome and the producer cell. J. Virol. **68:** 8001–8007.

56. HEIDELBERGER, M. 1941. Quantitative chemical studies on complement or alexin: IA method. J. Exp. Med. **73:** 691–694.

57. DAVIES, K. A., J. A. SCHIFFERLI & M. J. WALPORT. 1994. Complement deficiency and immune complex disease. Springer Semin. Immunopathol. **15:** 397–416.

58. LACHMANN, P. J. & M. J. WALPORT. 1987. Deficiency of the effector mechanisms of the immune response and autoimmunity. *In* Autoimmunity and Autoimmune Diseases. J. Whelan, Ed.: 149–171. Wiley. New York.

59. LOBATTO, S., M. R. DAHA, F. C. BREEDVELD, E. K. PAUWELS, J. H. EVERS-SCHOUTEN, A. A. VOETMAN, A. CATS & L. A. VAN ES. 1988. Abnormal clearance of soluble aggregates of human immunoglobulin G in patients with systemic lupus erythematosus. Clin. Exp. Immunol. **72:** 55–59.

60. DAVIES, K. A., A. M. PETERS, H. L. BEYNON & M. J. WALPORT. 1992. Immune complex processing in patients with systemic lupus erythematosus: *in vivo* imaging and clearance studies. J. Clin. Invest. **90:** 2075–2083.

61. WAXMAN, F. J., L. A. HEBERT, J. B. COMACOFF, M. E. VAN AMAN, W. L. SMEAD, E. H. KRAUT, D. J. BIRMINGHAM & J. M. TAGULAM. 1984. Complement depletion accelerates the clearance of immune complexes from the circulation of primates. J. Clin. Invest. **74:** 1329–1340.

62. HALMA, C., M. R. DAHA, J. A. J. CAMPS, J. H. EVERS-SCHOUTEN, E. K. J. PAUWELS & L. A. VAN ES. 1992. Deficiency of complement component C3 is associated with accelerated removal of soluble ^{123}I-labelled aggregates of IgG from the circulation. Clin. Exp. Immunol. **90:** 394–400.

63. DAVIES, K. A., K. ERLENDSSON, H. L. BEYNON, A. M. PETERS, K. STEINSSON, H. VALDIMARSSON & M. J. WALPORT. 1993. Splenic uptake of immune complexes in man is complement-dependent. J. Immunol. **151:** 3866–3873.

64. CARTER, R. H. & D. T. FEARON. 1992. CD19: lowering the threshold for antigen receptor stimulation of B lymphocytes. Science **256:** 105–107.

65. FEARON, D. T. & R. H. CARTER. 1995. The CD19/CR2/TAPA-1 complex of B lymphocytes: linking natural to acquired immunity. Annu. Rev. Immunol. **13:** 127–149.
66. DEMPSEY, P. W., M. E. ALLISON, S. AKKARAJU, C. C. GOODNOW & D. T. FEARON. 1996. C3d of complement as a molecular adjuvant: bridging innate and acquired immunity. Science **271:** 348–350.
67. PEPYS, M. B. 1974. Role of complement in induction of antibody production *in vivo*: effect of cobra factor and other C3-reactive agents on thymus-dependent and thymus-independent antibody responses. J. Exp. Med. **140:** 126–145.
68. ERDEI, A., G. FUST & J. GERGELY. 1991. The role of C3 in the immune response. Immunol. Today **12:** 332–337.
69. BOTTGER, E. F., S. METZGER, D. BITTER-SUERMANN, G. STEVENSON, S. KLEINDIENST & R. BURGER. 1986. Impaired humoral immune response in complement C3–deficient guinea pigs: absence of secondary antibody response. Eur. J. Immunol. **16:** 1231–1235.
70. O'NEIL, K. M., H. D. OCHS, S. R. HELLER, L. C. CORK, J. M. MORRIS & J. A. WINKELSTEIN. 1988. Role of C3 in humoral immunity: defective antibody production in C3-deficient dogs. J. Immunol. **140:** 1939–1945.
71. ALPER, C. A., H. R. COLTEN, J. S. S. GEAR, A. R. RABSON & F. S. ROSEN. 1976. Homozygous human C3 deficiency: the role of C3 in antibody production, C1s-induced vasopermeability, and cobra venom–induced passive hemolysis. J. Clin. Invest. **57:** 222–229.
72. OCHS, H. D., R. J. WEDGWOOD, S. R. HELLER & P. G. BEATTY. 1986. Complement, membrane glycoproteins, and complement receptors: their role in regulation of the immune response. Clin. Immunol. Immunopathol. **40:** 94–104.
73. BIRD, P. & P. J. LACHMANN. 1988. The regulation of IgG subclass production in man: low serum IgG4 in inherited deficiencies of the classical pathway of C3 activation. Eur. J. Immunol. **18:** 1217–1222.
74. GOODNOW, C. C., J. G. CYSTER, S. B. HARTLEY, S. E. BELL, M. P. COOKE, J. I. HEALY, S. AKKARAJU, J. C. RATHMELL, S. L. POGUE & K. P. SHOKAT. 1995. Self-tolerance checkpoints in B lymphocyte development. Adv. Immunol. **59:** 279–368.
75. GOLDBERGER, G., F. S. COLE, L. P. EINSTEIN, H. S. AUERBACH, D. BITTER-SUERMANN & H. R. COLTEN. 1982. Biosynthesis of a structurally abnormal C2 complement protein by macrophages from C2-deficient guinea pigs. J. Immunol. **129:** 2061–2065.
76. WHITEHEAD, A. S., G. GOLDBERGER, D. E. WOODS, A. F. MARKHAM & H. R. COLTEN. 1983. Use of a cDNA clone for the fourth component of human complement (C4) for analysis of a genetic deficiency of C4 in guinea pig. Proc. Natl. Acad. Sci. U.S.A. **80:** 5387–5391.
77. BURGER, R., J. GORDON, G. STEVENSON, G. RAMADORI, B. ZANKER, U. HADDING & D. BITTER-SUERMANN. 1986. An inherited deficiency of the third component of complement, C3, in guinea pigs. Eur. J. Immunol. **16:** 7–11.
78. FRANK, M. M. 1995. Animal models for complement deficiencies. J. Clin. Immunol. **15:** 113S–121S.
79. BITTER-SUERMANN, D. & R. BURGER. 1986. Guinea pigs deficient in C2, C4, C3, or the C3a receptor. Prog. Allergy **39:** 134–158.
80. WINKELSTEIN, J. A., L. C. CORK, D. E. GRIFFIN, J. W. GRIFFIN, R. J. ADAMS & D. L. PRICE. 1981. Genetically determined deficiency of the third component of complement in the dog. Science **212:** 1169–1170.
81. HOGASEN, K., J. H. JANSEN, T. E. MOLLNES, J. HOVDENES & M. HARBOE. 1995. Hereditary porcine membranoproliferative glomerulonephritis type II is caused by factor H deficiency. J. Clin. Invest. **95:** 1054–1061.
82. BOTTGER, E. C., T. HOFFMANN, U. HEDDING & D. BITTER-SUERMANN. 1986. Guinea pigs with inherited deficiencies of complement components C2 or C4 have characteristics of immune complex disease. J. Clin. Invest. **78:** 689–695.
83. CORK, L. C., J. M. MORRIS, J. L. OLSON, S. KRAKOWKA, A. J. SWIFT & J. A. WINKELSTEIN. 1991. Membranoproliferative glomerulonephritis in dogs with a genetically determined deficiency of the third component of complement. Clin. Immunol. Immunopathol. **60:** 455–470.
84. WESSELS, M. R., P. BUTKO, M. MA, H. B. WARREN, A. L. LAGE & M. C. CARROLL. 1995. Studies of group B streptococcal infection in mice deficient in complement component C3 or

C4 demonstrate an essential role for complement in both innate and acquired immunity. Proc. Natl. Acad. Sci. U.S.A. **92:** 11490–11494.

85. AHEARN, J. M., M. B. FISCHER, D. CROIX, S. GOERG, M. MA, J. XIA, X. ZHOU, R. G. HOWARD, T. L. ROTHSTEIN & M. C. CARROLL. 1996. Disruption of the Cr2 locus results in a reduction in B-1a cells and in an impaired B cell response to T-dependent antigen. Immunity **4:** 251–262.

86. MOLINA, H., V. M. HOLERS, B. LI, Y. FUNG, S. MARIATHASAN, J. GOELLNER, J. STRAUSS-SCHOENBERGER, R. W. KARR & D. D. CHAPLIN. 1996. Markedly impaired humoral immune response in mice deficient in complement receptors 1 and 2. Proc. Natl. Acad. Sci. U.S.A. **93:** 3357–3361.

87. BOTTO, M., J. NASH, P. TAYLOR, A. BYGRAVE, P. P. PANDOLFI, M. LOOS, K. A. DAVIES & M. J. WALPORT. 1996. Immune complex processing in a murine model of C1q deficiency. Mol. Immunol. **33**(suppl. 1): 71 (abstract).

Clinical Relevance of Fcγ Receptor Polymorphisms

ASTRID RASCU,[a] ROLAND REPP,[a,b]
NOMDO A. C. WESTERDAAL,[c] JOACHIM R. KALDEN,[a]
AND JAN G. J. VAN DE WINKEL[c]

[a]*Department of Medicine III*
University Hospital Erlangen
91054 Erlangen, Germany

[c]*Department of Immunology*
University Hospital Utrecht
3508 GA Utrecht, the Netherlands

INTRODUCTION

Human immunoglobulin G receptors (FcγR) provide an important link between the humoral and cellular branches of the immune response. FcγR engagement may result in a plethora of biological responses, including phagocytosis, endocytosis, antibody-dependent cellular cytotoxicity (ADCC), release of inflammatory mediators, facilitation of antigen presentation, and clearance of immune complexes (IC).[1,2] FcγR belong to the Ig supergene family and three classes of leukocyte FcγR are currently distinguished, encoding 12 receptor isoforms. These molecules differ in affinity and specificity for IgG isotypes, cell distribution patterns, capacity to trigger intracellular signals, and molecular weights. In addition to the FcγR heterogeneity in each person, genetic polymorphisms introduce further variations between individuals.

Recent data support a role of importance for some FcγR polymorphisms in susceptibility to infections and autoimmune diseases. In this report, we focus on the clinical relevance of the different FcγR polymorphisms.

GENERAL CHARACTERISTICS OF HUMAN FcγR

FcγRI (CD64) is a 72-kDa high-affinity receptor for IgG ($K_a \approx 10^8$–10^9 M^{-1}), constitutively expressed on monocytes, macrophages, myeloid progenitor cells, and dendritic cells, and inducible on neutrophils by interferon-γ (IFN-γ) or granulocyte colony-stimulating factor (G-CSF).[3–5] Three highly homologous genes, FcγRIA, FcγRIB, and FcγRIC, encode members of the class-I FcγR and are localized on chromosome 1 (q21.1). FcγRIa and FcγRIb2 are transmembrane molecules with their extracellular regions composed of three (FcγRIa) or two (FcγRIb2) C2-set Ig-like domains, respectively. The full-length transcripts of FcγRIB (FcγRIb1) and FcγRIC

[b]To whom all correspondence should be addressed.

encode soluble molecules as predicted from cDNA analysis. FcγRI binds monomeric human (h) IgG1, hIgG3, and hIgG4 in decreasing order and interacts with mouse (m) IgG2a and mIgG3, as well as rat IgG2b antibodies.[1,2]

A family of 40-kDa FcγRII (CD32) molecules represent the most broadly distributed Fcγ receptor class. FcγRII members are expressed on most types of blood leukocytes, Langerhans' cells, different populations of endothelial cells, dendritic cells, macrophages, and platelets. Three genes, FcγRIIA, FcγRIIB, and FcγRIIC, located on chromosome 1 (q23–24) encode six isoforms (FcγRIIa1, IIa2, IIb1, IIb2, IIb3, and IIc), which differ profoundly in their cytoplasmic tails (TABLE 1). The extracellular region of FcγRII molecules contains two Ig-like domains. FcγRII is a low-affinity receptor ($K_a < 10^7$ M^{-1}), interacting only with complexed or aggregated IgG, and is the sole FcγR class that can bind hIgG2 (TABLE 1).[6,7]

FcγRIII (CD16) is a glycoprotein with a molecular weight ranging from 50 to 80 kDa. Two genes, FcγRIIIA and FcγRIIIB, located on chromosome 1 (q23–24), within 200 kb from the FcγRII genes, specify this receptor class. The FcγRIIIA gene product is a transmembrane receptor with two Ig-like domains, whereas FcγRIIIb is linked to the outer leaflet of the plasma membrane via a glycosyl phosphatidylinositol (GPI) anchor.[8,9] FcγRIIIa is present on natural killer (NK) cells, macrophages, subpopulations of T cells and freshly isolated blood monocytes, immature thymocytes, and placental trophoblasts and binds IgG with medium affinity ($K_a \approx 3 \times 10^7$ M^{-1}). FcγRIIIb is selectively expressed on neutrophils and is a low-affinity receptor for IgG ($K_a \approx < 10^7$ M^{-1}). Both isoforms effectively bind hIgG1 and hIgG3 and interact with mouse IgG in the following decreasing order: mIgG2a > mIgG2b ≫ mIgG1 (TABLE 1).

FcγR subunits: Most FcγR exist as hetero-oligomeric complexes and, as such, belong to the family of multichain immune recognition receptors (MIRR). The ligand-binding α-chains can associate with a number of signaling components named FcR γ-, β-, or ζ-chains. These signaling chains were originally defined as components of other MIRR. The FcR β- and γ-chains were identified as subunits of the high-affinity FcεRI and the ζ-chain as part of the TCR-CD3 complex. FcR γ- and ζ-chains form disulfide-linked homodimers or heterodimers (γ-γ, ζ-ζ, γ-ζ). In NK cells, FcγRIIIa molecules complex with one of these three types of dimers, which is crucial for cell surface expression. FcγRIa can be transiently expressed in transfectant systems in the absence of γ-chain. Stable surface expression of this receptor, however, requires the presence of γ-chain, both *in vivo* and *in vitro*.[10] FcγRIIa molecules have also been shown capable of interacting with FcR γ-γ-chain dimers, affecting their functional capacity.[11,12] The FcR β-chain is present in FcγRIIIa complexes on mast cells.[1,2]

The three FcR signaling chains and the α-chain of FcγRIIa bear a unique ≈26-amino-acid immunoreceptor tyrosine-based activation motif (ITAM) in their cytoplasmic domain. Phosphorylation of tyrosine residues within this ITAM by Src family protein tyrosine kinases (PTK) occurs after cross-linking of at least two FcγR α-chains. A subsequent association of Syk family PTK with the phosphorylated ITAM leads to activation of the Syk PTK. The next steps in signal transduction leading to cell activation are not clearly delineated at present. The FcγRIIb members contain a unique 13-amino-acid immunoreceptor tyrosine-based inhibitor motif (ITIM) involved in downmodulation of cellular functions.[1]

Soluble (s) forms are known for all FcγR classes, generated by alternative mRNA splicing (sFcγRIIa2),[13,14] proteolytic cleavage of membrane-bound FcγR (sFcγRIIIa, IIIb),[15–18] or translation of stop codons in the FcγR coding regions (sFcγRIb, Ic).[19] Elevated levels of sFcγRIIIb and sFcγRIIIa were detected in human serum, synovial fluid, and bronchio-alveolar lavage in a broad spectrum of inflammatory disorders, including systemic lupus erythematosus (SLE), primary Sjögren's syndrome, rheumatoid arthritis, and gout, as well as adult respiratory distress syndrome and HIV

TABLE 1. General Characteristics of Leukocyte FcγR

	FcγRI (CD64)	FcγRII (CD32)	FcγRIII (CD16)
Molecule	72 kDa	40 kDa	50–80 kDa
Affinity for IgG	high (10^8–10^9 M^{-1})	low (<10^7 M^{-1})	IIIa: medium (~3 × 10^7 M^{-1}) IIIb: low (<10^7 M^{-1})
Associated subunits	γ-chain	IIa: γ-chain	IIIa: γ-chain, ζ-chain, β-chain
Distribution			
constitutive	CD34+ myeloid progenitors, monocytes, macrophages, dendritic cells	monocytes, macrophages, B cells, platelets, basophils, neutrophils, Langerhans' cells, eosinophils, endothelial cells (subpopulation), T cells (subpopulation), dendritic cells	IIIa: macrophages, NK cells, monocytes (subpopulation), T cells (subpopulation) IIIb: neutrophils
induced	neutrophils (IFN-γ, G-CSF)		IIIa: monocytes (TGFβ)
Isotype specificity			
murine IgG	2a > 3 >>> 1,2b	1,2b >> 2a	2a > 2b >> 1
human IgG	3 > 1 > 4 >>> 2	3 > 1[a]	1 = 3 >>> 2,4
Monoclonals	10.1, 32, 22, 197, 44, 62	IV.3, KB61, AT10, Ku79, 41H16, CIKM5	3G8, CLB-Gran, GRM1, Leu11b/c, B73.1, 1D3, VEP13

[a]The three subclasses of FcγRII have distinct affinities for human IgG—FcγRIIa-R131: 3 > 1 >>> 2,4; FcγRIIa-H131: 3 > 1 = 2 >>> 4; FcγRIIb: 3 > 1 > 4 >> 2.

infection.[16,20–24] Although the biologic role of soluble FcγR is incompletely understood, different immunomodulatory effects like inhibition of Ig production by B cells[25] and reduction of a reverse passive Arthus inflammatory response have been demonstrated experimentally.[26]

POLYMORPHISMS OF FcγR

FcγRIa is not polymorphic, although a single family has been identified in Belgium, lacking phagocyte expression of FcγRIa.[27] This absence was recently linked to a single nucleotide (nt) difference between wild-type FcγRIa and the Belgian family members lacking this receptor (TABLE 2).[28] Interestingly, in spite of the absence of FcγRIa, the four members of this family were apparently healthy, lacking evidence for any autoimmune, infectious, or inflammatory disorder.

A well-studied polymorphism represents allelic variation within the myeloid FcγRIIa (CD32). A point mutation (G into A) results in an arginine (R131) or histidine (H131) at amino acid (aa) position 131 in the second Ig-like domain of FcγRIIa.[13] This variation has been shown to be critical for the binding of hIgG2 and hIgG3, as well as mIgG1 and rat IgG2b (TABLE 2 and FIGURE 1).[6,7,13,29] An independent polymorphic amino acid is located at aa position 27 (either glutamine or tryptophan), which is not known to affect the ligand binding of FcγR.[13]

The FcγRIIa-R-H131 polymorphism was originally identified in T lymphocyte proliferation assays, where 70% of Caucasian donors ("high-responders"—FcγRIIa-R/R131 and IIa-R/H131) supported T cell mitogenesis in PBMC with a murine IgG1 anti-CD3 mAb and where 30% lacked this capacity ("low-responders"—FcγRIIa-H/H131). These findings were confirmed in other functional assays such as EA-rosetting, phagocytosis and ADCC of mIgG1-opsonized targets, binding of mIgG1 aggregates, mIgG1-induced release of tumor necrosis factor-α (TNF-α), and adherence of PMN to mIgG1-coated endothelial cells.[30] Notably, the FcγRIIa-H131 allotype was shown to effectively bind hIgG2 dimers, hIgG2 anti-CD3 antibodies, and hIgG2-opsonized bacteria, in contrast to the FcγRIIa-R131-expressing cells.[1,2] Similarly, rat IgG2b-opsonized red blood cells (RBC) and rat IgG2b anti-CD3 mAb were much more effectively bound by FcγRIIa-H131-expressing cells.[29]

At present, three types of methods are available to assess the FcγRIIa polymorphism: (I) functional assays (see above), (II) immunofluorescence assays using both a pan-CD32 mAb (such as AT10[31]) and mAb 41H16 that specifically binds to the FcγRIIa-R131 allotype,[32] and (III) PCR-based allotyping methods. At present, two such assays are readily available. The first one employs amplification of an FcγRIIa-genomic region (containing EC2; step I), followed by hybridization with allele-specific oligonucleotides.[33] The other one uses the same step I, but combines this with a (second) allotype-specific PCR instead (A. Greinacher and J. G. J. van de Winkel, unpublished data). Notably, the distributions of the two FcγRIIa allotypic forms differ considerably between various ethnic groups (TABLE 3).

The FcγRIIb subclass has also been shown to exhibit genetic heterogeneity based on a single aa difference at position 11 in the cytoplasmic region, where a tyrosine is

TABLE 2. Human FcγR Polymorphisms

Receptor Class	Name	Allelic Variation	Functional Implications
FcγRI			
FcγRIa	Belgian family lacking FcγRIa	Termination codon instead of arginine at position 92 in EC1[a]	?
FcγRII			
FcγRIIa	R-H131 polymorphism	Arginine or histidine at position 131 in EC2[b]	Differential binding of hIgG2 and 3, mIgG1, and rat IgG2b
	Glu/Trp-27 polymorphism	Glutamine or tryptophan at position 27 in EC1	?
FcγRIIb		Tyrosine or aspartic acid at position 11 in CYT[c]	Differences in receptor internalization and capping characteristics
FcγRIII			
FcγRIIIa	48L-H-R polymorphism	Leucine, histidine, or arginine at position 48 in EC1	Differences in IgG binding between FcγRIIIa allotypes
		Higher number (~14,000/cell) or lower number (~5500/cell) of FcγRIII on cells	Differences in ADCC capacity between high- and low-expressing cells
	158V/F polymorphism	Phenylalanine or valine at position 158 in EC2	Differential binding of hIgG1 and hIgG3
FcγRIIIb	IIIb-NA1-NA2	Amino acids at positions 65 and 82 create two extra glycosylation sites in IIIb-NA2	Differences in hIgG1 and hIgG3 binding, and phagocytosis between NA1 and NA2
	NF(+)[d]	Alanine or aspartic acid at position 78	?

[a]EC1: first extracellular Ig-like domain.
[b]EC2: second (membrane proximal) Ig-like domain.
[c]CYT: cytoplasmic tail.
[d]NF(+) is associated with the IIIb-NA2 allele.

substituted by an aspartic acid.[34] Notably, distinct differences were observed in receptor internalization and capping characteristics between both receptor allotypes.[35]

At present, no null-alleles for FcγRIIA or FcγRIIB molecules are known. However, de Haas *et al.* studied 21 individuals who lacked both the FcγRIIC and

FcγRIIIB genes.[36] The cell distribution and biological relevance of FcγRIIC, though, is still unclear.[1,2]

Recently, a triallelic polymorphism of FcγRIIIa has been identified, based on single nucleotide differences (position 230), leading to a leucine, histidine, or arginine at position 48 in the first Ig-like domain of FcγRIIIa.[37] Notably, differences were reported in human IgG-binding characteristics between the three FcγRIIIa allotypes. Another polymorphism of FcγRIIIa was described by Ravetch and Perussia (1989. J. Exp. Med. **170:** 481–498). A nucleotide substitution at position 559 of FcγRIIIA predicts either a valine or a phenylalanine at amino acid position 158 of FcγRIIIa. Recently, Koenen *et al.* (manuscript in preparation) found functional differences in IgG binding, which also explains the IgG binding differences of the linked triallelic polymorphism at position 48. The third type of interindividual variation in FcγRIIIa represents an expression difference reported by Vance *et al.*[38] Individuals were identified with either a high (~14,000/cell) or a low (~5500/cell) level of CD16 expression on NK cells, supportive of a polymorphism. Functional differences were furthermore noted in NK-cell ADCC activity and binding of monomeric hIgG. However, a genetic basis for this heterogeneity remains to be established.

The neutrophilic FcγRIIIb bears a codominant, biallelic polymorphism originally identified in analyses of alloimmune and autoimmune neutropenias and blood transfu-

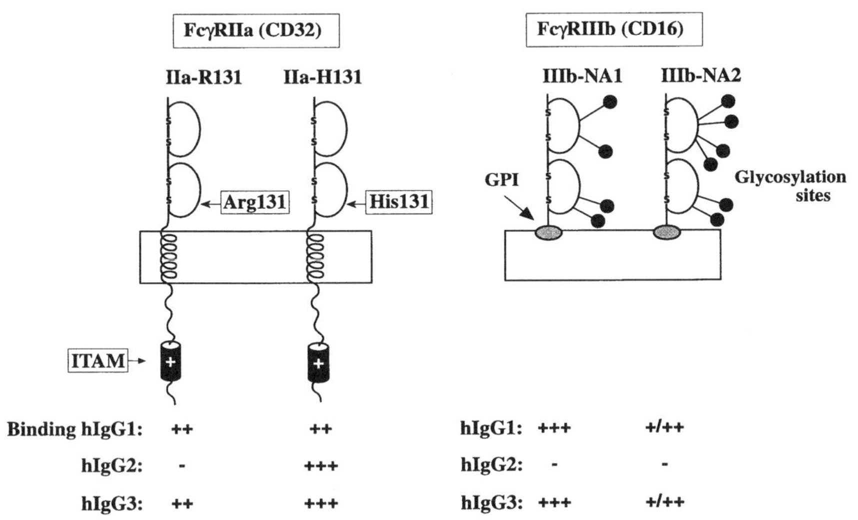

FIGURE 1. Schematic representation of human FcγR polymorphism. Two allotypic forms of human FcγRIIa have been distinguished by the presence of either an arginine (IIa-R131) or histidine (IIa-H131) at amino acid position 131. The FcγRIIIb-NA1 and IIIb-NA2 allotypic forms differ by five nucleotides, leading to two extra glycosylation sites in IIIb-NA2. The class IIa Fc receptor bears a well-defined signal transduction motif, named ITAM (immunoreceptor tyrosine-based activation motif), in its cytoplasmic tail, whereas the IIIb Fc receptor is a GPI-linked molecule selectively expressed on PMN. The FcγRIIa allotypic forms interact differentially with human IgG2 and human IgG3, whereas both human IgG1 and IgG3 are bound more readily by IIIb-NA1 than IIIb-NA2.

sion reactions. The allotypes are referred to as neutrophil antigen 1 (NA1) and 2 (NA2). Both FcγRIIIb allotypes differ by several aa, with changes at aa positions 65 and 82 resulting in two extra glycosylation sites (six instead of four) in the IIIb-NA2 allotypic form (FIGURE 1). This variation underlies differential electrophoretic mobility (and molecular weights) between IIIb-NA1 and IIIb-NA2.[39,40] PMN from IIIb-NA2 individuals were consistently found to exhibit lower levels of phagocytosis of erythrocytes either sensitized with hIgG1 and IgG3 anti–Rhesus D mAb or treated with concanavalin A compared to IIIb-NA1-PMN.[41,42] Furthermore, phagocytosis of hIgG1-opsonized bacteria by IIIb-NA2-PMN was also reduced in comparison to IIIb-NA1-PMN, whereas no difference was found using hIgG2-opsonized bacteria.[42]

At present, the FcγRIIIb NA1-NA2 polymorphism can be typed by (I) biochemical means (based on different electrophoretic mobilities) and (II) immunofluorescence assays using both IIIb-NA1-specific antibodies (such as CLB-Gran11) and IIIb-NA2-specific mAb (i.e., GRM1).[1,2] In addition, sensitive PCR-based methods are available to allotype for IIIb-NA1 and NA2.[36,43,44] In healthy Caucasian donors, the IIIb-NA2/NA2 phenotype is expressed more often,[45,46] whereas the IIIb-NA1/NA1 phenotype predominates in Japanese individuals[47] (TABLE 3). In a number of NA-null individuals, evidence for a complete absence of the FcγRIIIb gene has been provided.[48–51] The NA-null gene frequency was assessed to 0.03 in a French population.[51] Finally, FcγRIIIb expression is markedly reduced in patients with paroxysmal nocturnal hemoglobinuria (PNH) due to a defect in the GPI-anchor synthesis.[8,9]

TABLE 3. Phenotypic Distribution of FcγRIIa and FcγRIIIb Allotypes in Different Ethnic Populations

Ethnic Groups	FcγRIIa (%)[a]				FcγRIIIb (%)[a]				References
	n^b	R/R131	R/H131	H/H131	n^b	NA1/NA1	NA1/NA2	NA2/NA2	
Caucasians									
Dutch	123	23	48	29					46
German	187	27	45	28					—[c]
American	35	23	54	23	67	15	45	40	33, 73
French					3377	12	43	45	51
Asians									
Japanese	27	6	33	61	303	42	39	9	33, 47
Chinese	18	6	44	50					33
Indian	16	31	56	13					33
African-Americans	100	23	50	27					69

[a]Percent of individuals.
[b]Total number of individuals.
[c]R. Wassmuth *et al.*, manuscript in preparation.

In a recent case of alloimmune neonatal neutropenia, alloantibodies in the maternal serum were shown to recognize a new antigen on FcγRIIIb, which was termed NF1.[52] Nucleotide sequence analysis of NF1(+) individuals revealed a single base mutation (C into A, nt 266), resulting in either an alanine or an aspartic acid at position 78. NF1(+) was shown to be associated with the FcγRIIIb-NA2 allele, suggesting an additional polymorphism of FcγRIIIb.

CLINICAL RELEVANCE OF FcγR POLYMORPHISM

Infectious Diseases

Human IgG2 antibodies play a crucial role in immune defense to encapsulated bacterial infection. A clear correlation has been shown between low/absent levels of hIgG2 and the occurrence of recurrent upper/lower respiratory tract and encapsulated bacterial infections.[53] The biologic mechanisms of hIgG2-mediated immunity have long remained a mystery. This was so because hIgG2 is a poor activator of complement and was not known to interact with any Ig receptor.[54,55] Recently, however, this subclass was documented to interact with the FcγRIIa-H131 allotype on myeloid cells.[6,7] IIa-H/H131 homozygous neutrophils, furthermore, phagocytose hIgG2-opsonized bacteria significantly better than IIa-R/R131 cells.[56] These observations triggered the initiation of several pilot studies evaluating the possible relevance of the FcγRIIa polymorphism for encapsulated bacterial infections. The frequency of the IIa-H/H131 allotype in 48 children with recurrent bacterial respiratory tract infections was shown to be less than half (12.5% IIa-H/H131, 56% IIa-R/H131, and 31% IIa-R/R131) compared to controls (29% IIa-H/H131, 48% IIa-R/H131, and 23% IIa-R/R131).[46] Furthermore, it was suggested that the FcγRIIa polymorphism may be more critical when IgG2 levels are relatively low (as in children).[46] Notably, the IIIb-NA1-NA2 distribution did not differ significantly between these children and healthy controls. In an independent study, Bredius *et al.* found that children who survived fulminant meningococcal septic shock expressed the IIa-R/R131 allotype more frequently (44%) compared to normal donors (23%).[57] No skewed distribution of the FcγRIIIb allotypes was noted in these children. Notably, Fijen *et al.* found a highly significant association between the combined IIa-R/R131 and IIIb-NA2/NA2 phenotype and meningococcal infections in patients with terminal pathway of complement deficiency.[58]

Human IgG2 plays a critical role in the host response against *Actinobacillus actinomycetemcomitans*, an important pathogen in localized juvenile periodontitis (LJP). Black people are at greater risk for this disease and Wilson and Kalmar hypothesized the increased susceptibility for LJP in blacks to be linked to an overrepresentation of the FcγRIIa-R131 allotype in these individuals.[59] Noteworthy are also epidemiological studies showing a very low incidence of infections with encapsulated bacteria, like *Neisseria meningitidis* or *Haemophilus influenzae*, in the Japanese population,[1] where the IIa-H/H131 allotype predominates, compared to Caucasians (TABLE 3).

Autoimmune Diseases

Systemic Lupus Erythematosus

Abnormal clearance of IgG-sensitized erythrocytes in patients with systemic lupus erythematosus (SLE), the prototype of IC-mediated autoimmune diseases, was already described more than ten years ago.[60,61] FcγR dysfunction was furthermore correlated with disease activity, lupus nephritis, and IC levels.[61–63] Impaired Fc-mediated IC clearance was speculated to be caused by saturation/downmodulation of FcγR, leading to enhanced tissue deposition and inflammation. However, Fries *et al.* failed to demonstrate decreased FcγR numbers on blood monocytes of SLE patients.[64] Alternatively, FcγR, uncoupled from the signal transduction cascade, were also considered to lead to altered IC clearance,[60,65] and dissociation of receptor-ligand binding and receptor-mediated internalization was postulated to occur in SLE.[65] Two SLE patients were identified lacking FcγRIIIb expression, based on either a transport defect of one of the receptor alleles[66] or an abnormal/absent gene.[48]

It was tempting to speculate that FcγR polymorphism may underlie the impaired FcγR-mediated phagocytosis described in SLE patients. Indeed, Blasini *et al.* described an increased proportion (82%) of T cell responders to Leu4 (mIgG1 anti-CD3 mAb), expressing the IIa-R/R131 or IIa-R/H131 allotypes, in Venezuelan SLE patients, compared to patients with other autoimmune diseases.[67] No correlation between the mitogenic responder status and SLE disease activity was demonstrated. Recently, Duits *et al.* found a significant association between the IIa-R/R131 allotype and lupus nephritis (38% IIa-R/R131, 48% IIa-R/H131, and 14% IIa-H/H131) as compared to either SLE patients without nephritis (18% IIa-R/R131, 58% IIa-R/H131, and 24% IIa-H/H131) or healthy Caucasian donors.[68] No differences were found for the FcγRIIIb polymorphism between SLE patients with/without nephritis. In accordance with this study, Salmon *et al.* also reported a skewed distribution of the IIa-H/H131 genotype (9%) in African-American SLE patients compared to normal donors (30%).[69] These differences were even more striking in a larger collective of 214 SLE patients, where 37% expressed the IIa-R/R131 allotype compared to 23% IIa-R/R131 homozygotes in normal donors. The highest frequency of the IIa-R/R131 allotype was observed in SLE patients with nephritis (42% IIa-R/R131 and 12% IIa-H/H131).

SLE is a multisystemic disease with a marked variability of clinical manifestations. In order to evaluate the influence of the FcγRIIa polymorphism on the frequency of diverse clinical symptoms in SLE patients, we analyzed the clinical course of 116 German SLE patients (IIa-R/R131, 30%; IIa-R/H131, 35%; IIa-H/H131, 35%) with a medium follow-up time of 8.3 years. We observed an increased frequency of the manifestation of autoimmune hemolytic anemia (AIHA) and a more pronounced hypocomplementemia in IIa-R/R131 patients compared to IIa-H/H131 patients. The central immunologic disturbance in SLE patients is autoantibody production with high titers of anti-dsDNA antibodies as well as Sm antibodies, which are associated with the clinical course. Sm antibodies could be demonstrated more often in IIa-R/R131 patients. Furthermore, the onset of SLE is 4 years earlier in IIa-R/R131 patients compared to IIa-H/H131 patients and the manifestation of some clinical symptoms, such as discoid rash, occurs earlier after disease onset in IIa-R/R131 patients (TABLE 4; and K. Manger *et al.*, manuscript in preparation).

Morbus Wegener

Porges *et al.* demonstrated murine IgG anti-neutrophil cytoplasmic antibodies (ANCA), which are associated with Wegener's granulomatosis and systemic vasculitis, to engage and activate human neutrophils via FcγRIIa.[70] The production of reactive oxygen intermediates after incubation with mIgG1 ANCA was significantly increased in individuals expressing the IIa-R/R131 phenotype. These data are in accordance with those of Mulder *et al.*, who concluded ANCA-induced activation of neutrophils to be FcγRIIa-dependent,[71] and are correlated with hIgG3 ANCA titers in patients with Wegener's granulomatosis.[72] Depending on the ANCA IgG subclass

TABLE 4. Clinical Symptoms in 116 Caucasian SLE Patients in Relation to Their FcγRIIa Allotypes

More Frequent in IIa-R/R131 Patients	More Frequent in IIa-H/H131 Patients
Sm autoantibodies	Serositis (especially pericarditis)
Autoimmune hemolytic anemia (AIHA)	Livedo racemosa
Low C4	
Arthritis	
Earlier occurrence of discoid rash	
Younger age at disease onset	

specificity, FcγRIIa alleles may thus represent heritable disease risk factors in ANCA-triggered inflammation in patients with Wegener's granulomatosis and systemic vasculitis. Notably, evidence in support of a role for FcγRIIIb in Wegener's disease has also been obtained.[73]

Heparin-induced Thrombocytopenia

Heparin-induced thrombocytopenia (HIT) is characterized by FcγR-mediated platelet activation in the presence of patient serum and heparin and is diagnosed by evaluating the effect of patient plasma on the aggregation of normal donor platelets. Brandt *et al.* showed that platelets from donors bearing the IIa-H/H131 phenotype were largely unresponsive to plasma from patients with HIT or to murine IgG1 antiplatelet mAb.[74] The frequency of the IIa-H/H131 allotype was significantly increased in patients with HIT (34.4%) compared to nonthrombocytopenic patients (19%), suggesting a pathophysiologic role of the FcγRIIa polymorphism in HIT.[74]

Clinical Use of Monoclonal Antibodies

Wee *et al.* described marked differences in the clearance of T cells in kidney-transplant recipients, treated with mIgG1 anti-CD8 mAb (Leu2a), between IIa-R/R131 and IIa-H/H131 patients.[75] In addition, treatment with mIgG1 anti-CD3 mAb resulted in a "first dose cytokine response" only in kidney-transplant patients with the IIa-R/R131 allotype and not in IIa-H/H131 patients.[76]

Several mouse IgG1 mAb against tumor-associated antigens were tested in clinical trials. Because *in vitro* studies with mIgG1-opsonized tumor cells and myeloid effector cells clearly show a correlation between the FcγRIIa polymorphism and the rate of tumor cell lysis (Stockmeyer *et al.*, manuscript in preparation), typing of patients before administration of mouse IgG1 mAb seems relevant.

SUMMARY

Human IgG receptors are very heterogeneous and we currently distinguish three Fcγ receptor classes specifying at least 12 receptor isoforms. On top of this complexity, FcγR are further found to differ between different individuals. Polymorphisms have been identified for all three FcγR classes. The best-studied ones represent allelic variation of FcγRIIa (CD32) and FcγRIIIb (CD16). The FcγRIIa polymorphism is now considered to be a heritable risk factor for autoimmune and infectious diseases, and support for a relevant role of the IIIb polymorphism has also been obtained. A detailed analysis of the exact contribution of each of these FcγR polymorphisms in relation to previously implicated risk factors should unravel the pathophysiological importance of FcγR polymorphisms in the near future.

REFERENCES

1. van de Winkel, J. G. J. & P. J. A. Capel, Eds. 1996. Human IgG Fc Receptors. Landes Co. Austin, Texas.
2. van de Winkel, J. & P. J. A. Capel. 1993. Immunol. Today **14:** 215–221.
3. Guyre, P. M., P. M. Morganelli & R. Miller. 1983. J. Clin. Invest. **72:** 393–397.
4. Repp, R., T. Valerius, A. Sendler, M. Gramatzki, H. Iro, J. R. Kalden & E. Platzer. 1991. Blood **78:** 885–889.
5. Kerst, J. M., J. G. J. van de Winkel, A. H. Evans, M. de Haas, I. C. Slaper-Cortenbach, T. P. de Wit, A. E. von dem Borne, C. E. van der Shoot & R. H. van Oers. 1993. Blood **81:** 1457–1464.
6. Warmerdam, P. A. M., J. G. J. van de Winkel, A. Vlug, N. A. C. Westerdaal & P. J. A. Capel. 1991. J. Immunol. **147:** 1338–1343.
7. Parren, P. W. H. I., P. A. M. Warmerdam, L. C. M. Boeije, J. Arts, N. A. C. Westerdaal, A. Vlug, P. J. A. Capel, L. A. Aarden & J. G. J. van de Winkel. 1992. J. Clin. Invest. **90:** 1537–1546.
8. Selvaraj, P., W. F. Rosse, R. Silber & T. A. Springer. 1988. Nature **333:** 565–567.
9. Huizinga, T. W. J., C. E. van der Schoot, C. Jost, R. Klaassen, M. Kleijer, A. E. G. Kr. von dem Borne, D. Roos & P. A. T. Tetteroo. 1988. Nature **333:** 667–669.
10. van Vugt, M. J., I. A. F. M. Heijnen, P. J. A. Capel, S. Y. Park, C. Ra, T. Saito, J. S. Verbeek & J. G. J. van de Winkel. 1996. Blood **87:** 3593–3599.

11. MASUDA, M. & D. ROOS. 1993. J. Immunol. **151:** 7188–7195.
12. VAN DEN HERIK-OUDIJK, I. E., M. W. TER BEKKE, M. J. TEMPELMAN, P. J. CAPEL & J. G. J. VAN DE WINKEL. 1995. Blood **86:** 3302–3307.
13. WARMERDAM, P. A. M., J. G. J. VAN DE WINKEL, E. J. GOSSELIN & P. J. A. CAPEL. 1990. J. Exp. Med. **172:** 19–25.
14. RAPPAPORT, E. F., D. L. CASSEL, D. O. WALTERHOUSE, S. E. MCKENZIE, S. SURREY, M. A. KELLER, A. D. SCHREIBER & E. SCHWARTZ. 1993. Exp. Hematol. **21:** 689–696.
15. LANIER, L. L., J. H. PHILLIPS & R. TESTIS. 1989. Eur. J. Immunol. **19:** 775–778.
16. HUIZINGA, T. W. J., M. DE HAAS, M. KLEIJER, J. H. NUIJENS, D. ROOS & A. E. G. KR. VON DEM BORNE. 1990. J. Clin. Invest. **86:** 416–423.
17. LEVY, P. C., M. J. UTELL, H. B. FLEIT, N. J. ROBERTS, D. H. RYAN & R. J. LOONEY. 1991. Am. J. Respir. Cell Mol. Biol. **5:** 307–314.
18. HARRISON, D., J. H. PHILLIPS & L. L. LANIER. 1991. J. Immunol. **147:** 3459–3465.
19. ERNST, L. K., J. G. J. VAN DE WINKEL, I-M. CHIU & C. L. ANDERSON. 1992. J. Biol. Chem. **267:** 15692–15700.
20. KHAYAT, D., C. SOUBRANE, J. M. ANDRIEU, S. VISONNEUA, D. EME, J. M. TOURANI, K. BELDJORD, M. WEIL, E. FERNANDEZ & C. JACQUILLAT. 1990. J. Infect. Dis. **161:** 430–435.
21. FLEIT, B., C. D. KOBASIUK, C. DALY, R. FURIE, P. C. LEVY & R. O. WEBSTER. 1992. Blood **79:** 2721–2728.
22. LAMOUR, A., C. SOUBRANE, M. ICHEN, Y. L. PENNEC, D. KHAYAT & P. YOUINOU. 1993. Eur. J. Clin. Invest. **23:** 97–101.
23. HUTIN, P., A. LAMOUR, Y. L. PENNEC, C. SOUBRANE, G. DIEN, D. KHAYAT & P. YOUINOU. 1994. Int. Arch. Allergy Immunol. **103:** 23–27.
24. DE HAAS, M., M. KLEIJER, R. M. MINCHINTON, D. ROOS & A. E. G. VON DEM BORNE, JR. 1994. J. Immunol. **152:** 900–907.
25. SAUTES, C., N. VARIN, P. M. HOGARTH, J. C. UNKELESS, C. TEILLAUD, J. EVEN, A. LYNCH & W. H. FRIDMAN. 1990. Mol. Immunol. **27:** 1201–1207.
26. IERINO, F. L., M. S. POWELL, F. C. MCKENZIE & P. M. HOGARTH. 1993. J. Exp. Med. **178:** 1617–1628.
27. CEUPPENS, J. L., M. L. BAROJA, F. VAN VAECK & C. L. ANDERSON. 1988. J. Clin. Invest. **82:** 571–578.
28. VAN DE WINKEL, J. G. J., T. P. M. DE WIT, L. K. ERNST, P. J. A. CAPEL & J. L. CEUPPENS. 1995. J. Immunol. **154:** 2896–2903.
29. HAAGEN, I-A., A. J. G. GEERARS, M. R. CLARK & J. G. J. VAN DE WINKEL. 1995. J. Immunol. **154:** 1852–1860.
30. VAN DE WINKEL, J. G. J. & C. L. ANDERSON. 1991. J. Leukocyte Biol. **49:** 511–524.
31. GREENMAN, J., A. L. TUTT, A. J. T. GEORGE, K. A. F. PULFORD, G. T. STEVENSON & M. J. GLENNIE. 1991. Mol. Immunol. **28:** 1243–1254.
32. GOSSELIN, E. J., M. F. BROWN, C. L. ANDERSON, T. F. ZIPF & P. M. GUYRE. 1990. J. Immunol. **144:** 1817–1822.
33. OSBORNE, J. M., G. W. CHAKO, J. T. BRANDT & C. L. ANDERSON. 1994. J. Immunol. Methods **173:** 207–217.
34. WARMERDAM, P. A. M., I. E. VAN DEN HERIK-OUDIJK, P. W. H. I. PARREN, N. A. C. WESTERDAAL, J. G. J. VAN DE WINKEL & P. J. A. CAPEL. 1993. Int. Immunol. **5:** 239–247.
35. VAN DEN HERIK-OUDIJK, I. E., N. A. C. WESTERDAAL, N. V. HENRIQUEZ, P. J. A. CAPEL & J. G. J. VAN DE WINKEL. 1994. J. Immunol. **152:** 574–585.
36. DE HAAS, M., M. KLEIJER, R. VAN ZWIETEN, D. ROOS & A. E. G. KR. VON DEM BORNE. 1995. Blood **86:** 2403–2413.
37. DE HAAS, M., H. R. KOENE, M. KLEIJER, E. DE VRIES, S. SIMSEK, M. J. D. VAN TOL, D. ROOS & A. E. G. KR. VON DEM BORNE. 1996. J. Immunol. **156:** 2948–2955.
38. VANCE, B. A., T. W. HUIZINGA, K. WARDWELL & P. M. GUYRE. 1993. J. Immunol. **151:** 6429–6439.
39. ORY, P. A., I. M. GOLDSTEIN, E. E. KWOH & S. B. CLARKSON. 1989. J. Clin. Invest. **83:** 1676–1681.

40. HUIZINGA, T. W. J., M. KLEIJER, P. A. T. TETTEROO, D. ROOS & A. E. G. KR. VON DEM BORNE. 1990. Blood **75:** 213–217.
41. SALMON, J. E., J. C. EDBERG & R. P. KIMBERLY. 1990. J. Clin. Invest. **85:** 1287–1295.
42. BREDIUS, R. G. M., C. A. P. FIJEN, M. DE HAAS, E. J. KUIJPER, R. S. WEENING, J. G. J. VAN DE WINKEL & T. A. OUT. 1994. Immunology **83:** 624–630.
43. SATOH, T., M. KOBAYASHI, M. KANEDA, M. TANIHIRO, K. OKADA & K. UEDA. 1994. Blood **83:** 3312–3315.
44. STEIN, E. L., J. BUX, S. SANTOSO & C. MUELLER-ECKHARDT. 1994. Br. J. Haematol. **87:** 428–430.
45. LALEZARI, P., C. P. ENGELFRIET, J. J. VAN LOGHEM & A. E. G. KR. VON DEM BORNE, Eds. 1984. Immunohaematology, p. 33. Elsevier. Amsterdam/New York.
46. SANDERS, L. A. M., J. G. J. VAN DE WINKEL, G. T. RIJKERS, M. M. VOORHORST-OGINK, M. DE HAAS, P. J. A. CAPEL & B. J. M. ZEGERS. 1994. J. Infect. Dis. **170:** 854–861.
47. OHTO, H. & Y. MATSUO. 1989. Transfusion **29:** 654.
48. CLARK, M. R., L. LIU, S. B. CLARKSON, P. A. ORY & I. M. GOLDSTEIN. 1990. J. Clin. Invest. **86:** 341–346.
49. HUIZINGA, T. W. J., R. W. A. M. KUIPERS, T. W. J. SCHULPEN, T. M. CUYPERS, D. ROOS & A. E. G. KR. VON DEM BORNE. 1990. Blood **76:** 1927–1932.
50. STRONCEK, D., K. M. SKUBITZ, L. B. PLACHTA, R. A. SHANKAR, M. E. CLAY, J. HERMANN, H. B. FLEIT & J. MCCULLOUGH. 1991. Blood **77:** 1572–1580.
51. FROMONT, P., A. BETTAIEB, H. SKOURI, C. FLOCH, E. POULET, N. DUEDARI & P. BIERLING. 1992. Blood **79:** 2131–2134.
52. BUX, J., E-L. STEIN, M. CLAY, D. STRONCEK & S. SANTOSO. 1996. Submitted.
53. JEFFERIS, R. & D. S. KUMARARATNE. 1990. Clin. Exp. Immunol. **81:** 357–367.
54. FERRANTE, A., L. J. BEARD & R. G. FELDMAN. 1990. Pediatr. Infect. Dis. J. **9:** S16–S24.
55. PREUD'HOMME, J-L. & L. A. HANSON. 1990. Immunodefic. Rev. **2:** 129–149.
56. SANDERS, L. A. M., R. G. FELDMAN, M. M. VOORHORST-OGINK, M. DE HAAS, G. T. RIJKERS, P. J. A. CAPEL, B. J. M. ZEGERS & J. G. J. VAN DE WINKEL. 1995. Infect. Immun. **63:** 73–81.
57. BREDIUS, R. G. M., B. H. F. DERKX, C. A. P. FIJEN, T. P. M. DE WIT, M. DE HAAS, R. S. WEENING, J. G. J. VAN DE WINKEL & T. A. OUT. 1994. J. Infect. Dis. **170:** 848–853.
58. FIJEN, C. A. P., R. G. M. BREDIUS & E. J. KUIJPER. 1993. Ann. Intern. Med. **119:** 636.
59. WILSON, M. E. & J. R. KALMAR. 1996. J. Periodontol. **67:** 323–331.
60. FRANK, M. M., M. I. HAMBURGER, T. J. LAWLEY, R. P. KIMBERLY & P. H. PLOTZ. 1979. N. Engl. J. Med. **300:** 518–523.
61. HAMBURGER, M. I., T. J. LAWLEY, R. P. KIMBERLY, P. H. PLOTZ & M. M. FRANK. 1982. Arthritis Rheum. **25:** 48–54.
62. KABBASH, L., S. BRANDWEIN, J. ESDAILE, D. DANOFF, A. FUKS & J. SCHUSTER. 1982. J. Rheumatol. **9:** 374–379.
63. KIMBERLY, R. P., T. M. PARRIS, R. D. INMAN & J. S. MCDOUGAL. 1983. Clin. Exp. Immunol. **51:** 261–268.
64. FRIES, L. F., C. M. BRICKMAN & M. M. FRANK. 1984. J. Immunol. **132:** 695–700.
65. SALMON, J. E., R. P. KIMBERLY, A. GIBOFSKY & M. FOTINO. 1984. J. Immunol. **133:** 2525–2531.
66. ENENKEL, B., D. JUNG & J. FREY. 1991. Eur. J. Immunol. **21:** 659–663.
67. BLASINI, M., I. L. STEKMAN, M. LEON-PONTE, D. CALDERA & M. A. RODRIGUEZ. 1993. Clin. Exp. Immunol. **94:** 423–428.
68. DUITS, A. J., H. BOOTSMA, R. H. W. M. DERKSEN, P. E. SPRONK, L. KATER, C. G. M. KALLENBERG, P. J. A. CAPEL, N. A. C. WESTERDAAL, G. T. SPIERENBURG, F. H. GMELIG-MEYLING & J. G. J. VAN DE WINKEL. 1996. Arthritis Rheum. **39:** 1832–1836.
69. SALMON, J. E., S. MILLARD, L. A. SCHACHTER, F. C. ARNETT, E. M. GINZLER, M. F. GOURLEY, R. RAMSEY-GOLDMAN, M. G. E. PETERSON & R. P. KIMBERLY. 1996. J. Clin. Invest. **97:** 1348–1354.
70. PORGES, A. J., R. B. REDECHA, W. T. KIMBERLY, E. CSERNOK, W. L. GROSS & R. P. KIMBERLY. 1994. J. Immunol. **153:** 1271–1280.

71. MULDER, A. H., P. HEERINGA, E. BROUWER, P. C. LIMBURG & C. G. KALLENBERG. 1994. Clin. Exp. Immunol. **98:** 270–278.
72. MULDER, A. H., C. A. STEGEMAN & C. G. KALLENBERG. 1995. Clin. Exp. Immunol. **101:** 227–232.
73. WAINSTEIN, E., J. C. EDBERG, D. DOW, E. CSEMINK, M. SNELLER, E. KEYSTONE, W. GROSS, G. HOFFMAN & R. P. KIMBERLY. 1995. Arthritis Rheum. **38:** 1333.
74. BRANDT, J. T., C. E. ISENHART, J. M. OSBORNE, A. AHMED & C. L. ANDERSON. 1995. Thromb. Haemostasis **74:** 1564–1572.
75. WEE, S. L., R. B. COLVIN, J. M. PHELAN, F. I. PREFFER, T. A. REICHER, D. BERD & A. B. COSIMI. 1989. Transplantation **48:** 1012–1017.
76. TAX, W. J. M., L. A. M. FRENKEN, A. F. M. GLAUDEMANS, W. P. M. TAMBOER & R. A. P. KOENE. 1995. Transplant. Proc. **27:** 867–868.

Rheumatoid Factor Autoantibodies in Health and Disease[a]

RIZGAR A. MAGEED,[b] MARIE BØRRETZEN,[c]
SASHA P. MOYES,[b] KEITH M. THOMPSON,[c]
AND JACOB B. NATVIG[c]

[b]*Kennedy Institute of Rheumatology*
Hammersmith, London W6 7DW, United Kingdom

[c]*Institute of Immunology and Rheumatology*
The National Hospital
0172 Oslo, Norway

INTRODUCTION

Since their discovery, a vast amount of work has been done on the incidence, specificity, and genetics of human rheumatoid factors (RF) in a great many laboratories. In the main, these studies were inspired by the association of RF with RA and the hope that understanding mechanisms of their production may help define disease pathogenesis. However, studies of RF production and incidence have shown that RF are not restricted to patients with RA and that genes encoding RF are inherited in the normal human population. Furthermore, the documentation that RF specificity can be part of the natural antibody repertoire during early fetal life and that normal adults can produce RF following immunization are important indications for their physiological role in normals and in understanding mechanisms of B cell regulation in health and disease.

The initial attempts to define RF structure and genetics benefited from serological analysis with anti-idiotypic reagents and amino acid sequence analysis of RF paraproteins, or "M" components, from patients with mixed cryoglobulinemia, Waldenström's macroglobulinemia, and chronic lymphocytic leukemia.[1,2] More recently, nucleotide sequence analysis of RF genes isolated from immortalized human B cell hybridomas from normals and RA patients in our laboratories, and others, provided significant insight into how RF are produced and likely to be regulated.[3–5] Here, we show that RF produced in normal individuals are different from those found in the synovium of RA patients. RF in normals are frequently encoded by a limited set of IgV genes, do not appear to switch isotype, and have few replacement mutations in the CDRs. These observations support the concept that RF are under strict control to prevent the emergence of high-affinity RF in normals.

[a]Support for this work was provided by the Arthritis and Rheumatism Council of Great Britain (to R. A. Mageed and S. P. Moyes) and by the Norwegian Women's Health Organization (NKS) and the Norwegian Research Council (to M. Børretzen, K. M. Thompson, and J. B. Natvig).

Although the existence of tolerance mechanisms that regulate the emergence of autoreactive B lymphocytes in the bone marrow is now firmly established,[6] mechanisms that suppress the production of high-affinity autoreactive B cells in secondary lymphoid organs remain speculative. Recent studies, using transgenic animals, have shown that tolerance is dependent on both deletion and functional inactivation (anergy) of autoreactive B lymphocytes and that clonal deletion occurs in both immature and mature lymphocytes that have emigrated from the bone marrow.[7] Despite these advances, however, little is known about the regulation of RF production in healthy individuals and RA patients.

The presence of RF in normals is presumed to be for physiological reasons, yet the mechanisms that regulate affinity maturation and pathogenicity remain unknown.[8] Although it is suggested that T cells specific for IgG Fc are normally deleted, rendering RF-producing B cells incapable of undergoing somatic hypermutation and affinity maturation,[9] the ability of these cells to capture immune complexes and present antigens to T cells may provide a means to bypass the need for specific T cell help.[10] Nevertheless, our studies, and those using an RF transgenic mouse, attest to the fact that subtle regulatory elements may play a role in maintaining RF at low affinity in normals.[11]

We have compared the structure of RF produced in immunized normals and in RA synovia in order to determine whether there are any abnormalities in the regulation of RF production in RA. To achieve this, we isolated RF-secreting hybridomas from the peripheral blood of five healthy donors immunized with mismatched red blood cells (RBC).[12] The five donors responded to hyperimmunization with a specific anti-RBC response. In addition, IgM RF antibody levels increased twofold to fourfold. The rise and fall in specific anti-RBC and RF levels after immunization closely followed each other in each donor.[5] All fusions from the five donors yielded IgM RF-secreting hybridomas, but no IgA RF. In contrast, three fusions from nonimmunized donors yielded no RF-secreting hybridomas. This strongly suggests that the immortalized monoclonal RF-producing hybridomas are representative of those involved in the specific immune response.

PATHOLOGY OF SYNOVIAL INFLAMMATION IN RA

The synovium is the main site affected by the inflammatory processes characteristic of patients with RA. The synovial inflammation is characterized by infiltration of macrophages and T and B lymphocytes that form ectopic lymphoid tissues.[13] The synovial-lining layer proliferates extensively, leading to a thickening of the membrane and a striking vascularization. In typical cases, there is a clear development of ectopic lymphoid follicles with germinal center–like structures. The hallmark of immune cells in these structures is the presence of large numbers of T and B lymphocytes and plasma cells, which actively produce IgM and IgG immunoglobulins including RF.[14] These cells appear to be activated and are able to spontaneously secrete immunoglobulins *in vitro*.[15] The RF produced by these local B cells are thought to play a pathogenic role in RA through their ability to form immune complexes that bind complement, perpetuating the inflammatory processes and contributing to tissue damage.[16] The production of IgG RF is particularly important due to the ability of IgG RF to self-associate and form large aggregates with high complement-fixing potential.

The involvement of T cells in the synovial inflammation and the interaction with B cells have been the focus of numerous studies. T cell involvement in RA is suggested by the presence of T cell infiltrates in the synovium and by the genetic association with HLA-DR1 and DR4 haplotypes.[17,18] Synovial T cell infiltrates seem to be activated, but lack specificity for any particular autoantigen.[19] Only specificity for mycobacterial antigens has clearly been demonstrated.[20] Furthermore, investigation of possible clonal dominance within T cell populations in rheumatoid synovium has shown little evidence for interclonal similarity or dominance of T cell populations, suggesting that the synovial T cell population may have been selected by their activation state rather than by specificity.[21]

STRUCTURE-FUNCTIONAL ASPECTS OF HUMAN RF

The term RF is common for antibodies with specificities for determinants within the Fc region of IgG. Antibodies with these specificities are detectable in a variety of autoimmune and infectious diseases at varying levels and frequencies.[22–24] Many different specificities have been described for different RF. In general, IgG determinants recognized by RF can be categorized into the following groups: (1) subclass-specific antigens, or isotypic antigens, found on all or some of the four subclasses of human IgG; (2) genetically defined alloantigens of the Gm type; (3) cross-reactive antigens shared by human and animal IgG; (4) species-specific antigens found in human IgG, but not animal IgG; (5) neoantigens expressed on aggregated, denatured, or enzymatically digested IgG; and (6) determinants expressed on the Fab region of IgG (antibodies with specificity for these determinants are often referred to as antiglobulins, not RF). Extensive studies have shown that reactivity with an isotypic antigen expressed on IgG1, 2, and 4, but not IgG3 (the Ga determinant) is the main specificity known for RF.[25–28] Despite some minor differences, the overall conclusion has been that most RF, including RF established from normal individuals, bind sites related to the Ga determinant.[29] This site appears to be related to or overlaps with the site of staphylococcal protein A (SPA) binding.[30] Furthermore, pH titration and chemical modification studies implicate histidine and tyrosine residues on the IgG Fc in the binding of RF to the Ga determinant.[31] The epitope is situated in the Cγ2–Cγ3 interface region of IgG and involves three polypeptide loops, two from the Cγ2 and one from the Cγ3 domain, which come together in close proximity in the Cγ2–Cγ3 interface region. The amino acids involved in the binding are likely to include histidine at positions 310, 433, and 435 and tyrosine at 436. Despite the differing causes of RF production, the specificity to this region appears to be generally preserved.

IDIOTYPIC AND GENETIC BASIS OF HUMAN RF PRODUCTION

Idiotypic Analysis

The main questions addressed in studying the RF idiotype have been whether natural RF found in patients with lymphoproliferative disorders and pathogenic RF in RA patients are related and whether they are direct copies of germline genes or products of somatic mutations. The first set of human RF to be extensively studied were IgM paraproteins (or "M" components) isolated from the serum of patients with lymphoproliferative disorders (Waldenström's macroglobulinemia and cryoglobulinemia).[1] Anti-idiotypic antisera to these monoclonal antibodies were obtained following absorption of rabbit antisera with paraproteins from different individuals and with polyclonal IgG. This approach allowed the definition of three cross-reactive idiotypic families, or groups, designated Wa, Po, and Bla.[1,32] A decade later, practically similar protocols were followed in the selection of mouse monoclonal antibodies identifying cross-reactive idiotopes expressed by RF paraproteins.[33] A rapidly growing library of antibody sequences (derived from mRNA or DNA) from hybridomas whose protein products reacted with the antibodies has enabled the determination of the contribution of germline genes to RF production and has established the range of genes whose protein products were recognized by the monoclonal anti-idiotypic antibodies.[34]

We investigated the expression of V gene markers and cross-reactive idiotopes (CRI) using various murine monoclonal anti-idiotypic antibodies. These included G6 and G8, which recognize V_H1-associated CRI;[33,35] B6 and D12, which recognize V_H3-associated CRI;[36] and LC1, which recognizes protein products of the V_H4 family of genes.[37] V_κ gene family products were determined by C7 (specific for the $V_\kappa3$ family) and C6 (specific for the V 3b subfamily).[38] 17.109 was used to identify a CRI that was encoded by the $V_\kappa3$b-subfamily variable region gene, Kv325.[39] The majority of the RF paraproteins and RF from immunized donors expressed at least one of these markers (TABLE 1). Within individual donors, particularly the normal immunized donor, MR, groups of RF were found that shared identical patterns of V gene markers, suggesting a restricted response.[5]

Analyses of the monoclonal RF paraproteins showed a high degree of CRI expression.[40] The most-striking feature was the predominant use of the $V_\kappa3$-associated light-chain subgroup and CRI, with more than 90% expressing the $V_\kappa3$ light-chain subgroup.[2,38] Furthermore, it transpired that at least 60% of all IgMκ RF express light chains encoded by two $V_\kappa3$ genes whose protein products are recognized by the monoclonal anti-idiotypic antibodies 17.109 and 6B6.6.[40] Similarly, albeit to a lesser extent, the RF paraproteins were also shown to widely react with the G6 and G8 monoclonal anti-idiotypic antibodies. When the V_L and V_H genes were considered together, three different combinations of V_H–V_L could be identified. The largest group of these RF were those that expressed kappa light chains reactive with the monoclonal antibody 17.109 in association with V_H genes whose products were reactive with the monoclonal antibody G6, which was subsequently shown to be a serological marker for the DP-10 and hv1263 genes.[40] A second group of these RF expressed a $V_\kappa3$ light

TABLE 1. Incidence of V_κ and V_H Chain–associated Cross-reactive Idiotype (CRI) Expression in RF Paraproteins and Monoclonal RF Established from Peripheral Blood of Immunized Normals and the Synovial Membrane of RA Patients[a]

Source of RF	% RF with κ Chain Expressing κ3	% RF Reactive with 17.109	% RF Reactive with 6B6.6	% RF Reactive with G6/G8	% RF Reactive with B6/D12	% RF Reactive with LC1
paraproteins	90	27	32	35	30	25
HID PBL	90	15	ND	33	13	ND
RA SM	32	18	5	10	30	ND

[a]The data are based on references 5, 33–36, and 38–41. In most cases, the data have been added up from different studies, taking into account the total numbers studied, for the purpose of entirety. Only IgM RF-producing lines/hybridomas that have been extensively characterized are given. IgG and IgA RF-producing lines/hybridomas are not given. HID PBL and RA SM indicate that the original sources of the RF-producing cells used to establish the lines/hybridomas were from the peripheral blood lymphocytes of normal human immunized donors and the synovial membrane of RA patients, respectively. ND = not determined.

chain that was recognized by the 6B6.6 monoclonal antibody in association with V_H4 genes reactive with the LC1 monoclonal anti-idiotypic antibody.[41] The third group of RF (~30%) used V_H3 genes, many of which reacted with B6 and D12 antibodies, in association with a variety of light chains, including $V_\kappa1$, 2, 3, and lambda light chains.[36]

The pattern of CRI expression in the monoclonal IgM RF produced by B cell hybridomas from normals immunized with mismatched red blood cells revealed similarities, but also differences, with the RF paraproteins. A majority (90%) of these RF expressed $V_\kappa3$ light chains, similar to the percentage found in paraproteins. Similarly, about 33% of these RF expressed heavy chains recognized by the G6 and/or G8 monoclonal antibodies. However, RF reactive with the B6 and/or D12 antibodies were far less frequent, at 13%, than RF paraproteins (30%).[5,36]

The frequency of CRI expression by 22 IgM RF-producing hybridomas established from RA synovial membrane is also shown in TABLE 1. Only 6 (27%) of these RF were encoded by V_H1 genes, whereas 13 (59%) were encoded by genes from the V_H3 family, of which ~30% reacted with the B6/D12 monoclonal anti-CRI antibodies. The light chains were from the $V_\kappa1$, 3a, 3b, and λ1.

Analysis of V Gene Use by Nucleotide Sequencing

RF established from RA synovial tissues were found to use many diverse germline V gene segments to encode both the heavy and light chains. Comparison of the nucleotide sequences of V genes expressed in the RF-producing hybridomas established from RA synovial tissues and from immunized donors also showed different preferences in the two conditions (TABLE 2). The most-striking difference was in the use of light-chain segments from the $V_\kappa3$ family, which are used by 90% of RF from immunized donors, but only 32% of RF from synovial tissues. This overexpression of

$V_κ3$ in the RF from normals, together with a distribution of V_H gene segments of the V_H1, V_H3, and V_H4 families, closely resembled the distribution seen among the RF paraproteins. In contrast, RF from the synovial membrane of RA patients predominantly used heavy-chain segments encoded by genes from the V_H3 family. These data imply that RF paraproteins may be representative of RF used in normal physiological responses, but that have undergone neoplastic transformation. The overall conclusion from these studies is that RF produced in the synovial tissue of RA patients are encoded by a wider range of IgV genes than the RF paraproteins and RF in normal

TABLE 2. Frequency of V_H Gene Expression by RF Paraproteins and Monoclonal IgM RF Produced by Hybridomas Established from Peripheral Blood of Immunized Normals and Synovial Membrane of RA Patients[a]

V_H Family Used	Individual V_H Gene Used	No. of Paraproteins Expressing the Gene	No. of RF from Normals Expressing the Gene	No. of RF from RA SM Expressing the Gene	Total
1	DP-10	7	3	1	11
	DP-75	0	2	0	2
	HG3	0	0	1	1
	1-13	0	0	1	1
total		7	5	3	15
3	DP-54	1	3	0	4
	DP-49	0	1	3	4
	DP-46	1	0	2	3
	b18	0	1	0	1
	DP-35	0	1	1	2
	DP-47	1	0	1	2
	DP-42	0	1	0	1
	V3-53	0	1	0	1
	DP-31	0	0	1	1
total		3	8	8	19
4	4.18	0	0	1	1
	DP-71	0	1	0	1
	$V_H4.35$	0	1	0	1
	DP-65	0	1	0	1
	DP-66	0	0	1	1
total		0	3	2	5
7	DP-21	0	1	1	2
Overall total		10	17	14	41

[a]Summary of the data on V_H gene use in RF-producing B cell hybridomas generated in our laboratories. For the sake of simplicity, data generated in other laboratories are not included. Only IgM RF paraproteins and IgM RF-producing lines/hybridomas that have been well characterized are included. IgG and IgA RF-producing lines/hybridomas are not given. Normal PBL and RA SM indicate the original sources of the RF-producing cells used to establish the lines/hybridomas.

human immunized donors (HID). Furthermore, there is an increase in the representation of V_H3 genes in the synovial RF hybridomas.

Interestingly, when the values of RF expressing the CRI detected by the monoclonal antibodies G6, G8, B6, D12, and LC1 were assessed in monozygotic twins, concordant or discordant for RA, it appeared that the absolute levels of the CRI markers were higher than in normals and that the values were very similar within twins, irrespective of disease status, but different between unrelated twins.[42] These findings were taken to imply that there may be additional regulatory mechanisms, possibly genetic or idiotypic, that control the level of natural RF and that some of these regulatory mechanisms may be inherently abnormal in individuals with a genetic predisposition to develop RA.[42]

NATURE OF SOMATIC MUTATION IN RF

The increase in the affinity of antibodies to antigen and isotype switching is often referred to as maturation of the immune response. This maturation requires that the Ag-binding site of the antibody molecule be structurally different from antibodies in the primary response. This is typically achieved by somatic mutation and repertoire shift. Sequence analysis of IgV gene mRNA from a large collection of B cell hybridomas with specificity for a variety of different antigens has shown that such structural changes are often achieved through mutations leading to amino acid replacements in the CDRs.[43] In such responses, hypermutation of IgV genes is followed by both positive and negative selection pressures through which B cells with high-affinity receptors are selected for expansion. B cells with no mutations or with limited mutated receptors that have low affinity for antigen die, presumably by apoptosis. Besides an increase in affinity, positively selected B cells show a characteristic elevation of the ratio of R:S in the CDRs.[44] Surprisingly, RF produced in the healthy immunized normals also show evidence in their IgV genes of extensive somatic mutations (9–16 mutations per V_H gene). There was, however, evidence for selection against replacement mutations in the CDRs, suggesting that high-affinity variants were negatively selected. Without any selective pressures, random mutations in CDR1+2 of the DP-10 gene segment would generate R:S ratios of 4.4.[45] The overall R:S ratio of the CDR1+2 in the V_H region of the RF from the immunized donor MR, who had 10 RF encoded by the DP-10 gene, was significantly lower at 0.4 ($p < 0.0027$, Fisher's exact test, two-sided) (TABLE 3). In contrast, RF from RA synovia, bone marrow, and peripheral blood did not show a similar counterselection of replacement mutations in the CDRs as seen in RF from the normal immunized donors. RF from RA patients had between 2 and 18 nucleotide mutations compared with 9–16 in immunized normals (TABLE 3 and FIGURE 1).

Nucleotide sequencing of the light chains of 5 of the RF established from the normal immunized donor, MR, confirmed the clonal relatedness and showed that all used the Kv325 light-chain germline gene rearranged to the $J_\kappa 1$ gene segment with identical V_κ-J_κ junctions (RF-MR2, RF-MR13, RF-MR16, RF-MR28, and RF-MR30). Hypermutation was also evident in the light chains, but to a lesser degree than in the heavy chains. Four of the 5 related clones had 1 shared replacement mutation in the light chain. These data confirmed that RF from immunized donors clearly undergo somatic hypermutation.

ISOTYPE SWITCH IN RF-PRODUCING B CELLS

Following the initial interaction between virgin B cells and Ag, germline gene–encoded antibodies of the IgM isotype are produced. The ability of the immune system to adapt to combat antigenic challenge is manifested by further differentiation of Ag-specific B cells to produce antibodies with high affinity and of different isotypes.[43] Individual B cells with specificity for Ag can switch isotype while retaining the same recombined IgV genes and antibody specificity. These features of the immune system have been widely used to assess the nature and mechanisms of induction of immune responses to self-antigens in murine models of autoimmune diseases.[46,47] Specifically,

TABLE 3. Total Number of Nucleotide Changes Observed in the V_H Genes of RF Derived from Peripheral Blood of Immunized Normals, Synovial Membrane of RA Patients, and IgM Anti–Red Blood Cell Rh(D) Antigen from Immunized Normals

Source of Antibody	No. of Antibodies Included in the Analysis	Average No. of Nucleotide Changes from the Germline Gene	Total No. of Nucleotide Changes Seen in FR 1, 2, and 3		R:S Ratio	Total No. of Nucleotide Changes Seen in CDR 1 and 2		R:S Ratio
			R	S		R	S	
RF from immunized normals	10	12.0	17	16	1.1	7	16	0.4
RA SM	7	16.1	30	34	0.9	33	14	2.4
anti-Rh(D)	7	4.3	8	12	0.7	8	1	8.0

the ability to detect autoantibodies of the IgG, and to a lesser extent IgA, isotypes with increased affinity and similar specificity to autoantigens has been used as an indicator of specific autoantigen-driven immune responses in autoantibody production.

One of the most-characteristic serological features of RA patients with severe active disease and extra-articular symptoms is high levels of IgG RF.[48] High levels of IgG RF are often associated with circulating immune complexes and complement activation. The finding of large-size immune complexes is particularly important in RA synovial inflammation because such complexes can contribute to pathogenesis through complement activation, cell recruitment, and cartilage and bone damage.[16] In addition to the finding of high levels of IgG RF in the serum of a high proportion of RA patients, IgG RF-producing B cell hybridomas were also isolated from three RA patients in our studies.[49] In contrast, none of the immunized normal donors produced IgG RF or IgA RF, implying that the switch of isotype to IgG and IgA is a more common feature of RF-producing B cells in RA, but not normal, individuals.

	FR1								*******CDR1*******					FR2		*********CDR2*********					
	4	13	24	26	27	28	29	30	31	32	33	34	35	37	43	53	54	56	57	59	63
DP-10	CTG	AAG	CCT	GGA	GGC	ACC	TTC	AGC	AGC	TAT	GCT	ATC	AGC	GTG	ACA	CCT	ATC	GGT	ACA	AAC	AAG
RA-SM RF																					
RF-TS1	---	---	---	---	---	---	---	---	-C-	---	---	---	---	---	---	---	---	---	--G	---	---
RA-BM and PBL RF																					
YES8c	---	---	---	---	---	---	GG-	---	---	---	C--	---	---	---	---	---	C--	---	---	---	-G-
Re12	---	---	---	---	---	---	---	-A-	--G	C--	---	---	---	---	---	---	---	--a	---	---	--A
Ro47	---	---	--c	---	---	---	---	---	-C-	---	---	T--	---	---	---	--a	---	--g	--t	-G-	---
Ro7	---	---	---	---	---	--t	---	GA-	--A	---	A--	--a	-A-	---	---	---	---	--c	--g	---	---
HID-PBL RF																					
RF-MR2	---	---	---	---	---	--t	--t	--t	--t	---	A--	---	---	---	---	---	---	---	---	---	---
RF-MR13	---	---	---	---	---	---	--t	--t	--t	---	A--	--t	---	---	---	---	--t	---	---	---	---
RF-MR14	t--	---	---	---	---	---	--t	--t	--t	---	A-a	---	---	---	---	---	--t	--a	---	---	-C-
RF-MR30	---	-G-	---	---	---	---	---	--t	--t	--c	A--	---	---	---	---	---	---	--c	---	---	---
RF-MR33	---	---	---	--g	---	---	--t	--t	--t	---	A--	---	---	---	--g	---	G-t	--c	---	---	---
RF-MR37	---	---	--c	---	---	---	--t	--t	--t	---	A--	---	---	---	---	---	--t	---	---	---	---
RF-MR1	---	-C-	---	---	-A-	---	---	---	--t	---	A-c	---	---	---	---	---	---	---	--t	---	--c

	FR3													
	69	70	74	77	79	80	82	83	84	88	89	93	94	95
DP-10	ACG	ATT	GAA	AGC	GCC	TAC	GAG	CTG	AGC	TCT	GAG	GTG	TAT	TAC
RA-SM RF														
RF-TS1	---	---	---	---	---	---	---	---	---	---	---	--a	---	---
RA-BM and PBL RF														
YES8c	---	---	---	C--	---	---	---	G--	---	---	--a	--c	---	---
Re12	---	---	---	---	-G-	---	---	---	---	---	---	--c	---	--t
Ro47	---	---	---	--A	---	--t	---	t--	---	---	---	A-a	---	---
Ro7	G--	---	A--	-C-	---	---	--a	A--	---	---	---	---	---	---
HID-PBL RF														
RF-MR2	---	---	---	-A-	---	---	---	---	-A-	---	---	---	--c	--t
RF-MR13	---	---	---	-A-	---	---	--a	---	---	---	--a	A-a	---	--t
RF-MR14	---	---	---	-A-	-T-	---	---	---	---	---	---	A-a	---	--t
RF-MR30	---	---	---	-A-	---	-G-	---	t--	---	---	---	---	---	--t
RF-MR33	---	---	---	-A-	---	---	---	---	---	---	---	A-a	---	--t
RF-MR37	---	---	AC-	-A-	---	---	---	---	---	---	---	A-a	---	--t
RF-MR1	---	---	---	---	---	---	---	---	---	C--	---	--c	---	---

FIGURE 1. Nucleotide sequences of the rearranged DP-10 V_H genes of IgM RF-producing hybridomas established from the synovial membrane (SM) of an RA patient, from bone marrow (BM) and peripheral blood lymphocytes (PBL) of other RA patients, and from PBL of a normal human immunized donor (HID), MR, in comparison with the DP-10 germline gene sequence. Nucleotide sequences of the rearranged genes from RF-producing hybridomas are compared with the sequence of the DP-10 germline gene to show nucleotide mutations. Bases similar to the germline gene are given as dashes, mutations that result in amino acid replacements are given in uppercase letters, and silent mutations are given in lowercase letters. Only codons that are different from the germline in the HID RF are given in the figure. RF established from the bone marrow (BM) B cells and peripheral blood (PBL) of RA patients are included in the figure to show that RF from RA patients, irrespective of their original anatomical compartment, have different patterns of mutations compared with HID RF. The data are based on references 45–48.

CLONAL EXPANSION AND AFFINITY MATURATION

It is now recognized that generation of mutations in the rearranged IgV genes alone would not be adequate to account for the phenomenon of affinity maturation in antibodies produced during the secondary phase of immune responses.[43] A process (or processes) capable of selectively activating and expanding B cells producing high-affinity antibodies is also essential. In T cell–dependent immune responses, the process of selective activation and expansion of higher affinity antibodies occurs initially in the T cell areas of the spleen and lymph nodes.[50] Subsequently, selected B cells migrate to B cell follicles where they expand and initiate a germinal center reaction, leading to clonal expansion of the higher affinity antibody–producing B cells. This feature of the immune response has been used to study the kinetics of immune responses to exogenous antigens.[51] Such studies have been achievable with small hapten antigens, such as oxazolone and nitrophenyl, but are thought to be difficult with complex antigens, which have numerous immunogenic epitopes. In our studies, however, two IgM RF (RF-SJ1 and RF-SJ2) isolated from the same RA patients were found to be clonally related.[52] The V_H of RF-SJ2 had only 2 nucleotide differences from its germline counterpart (GL-SJ), whereas RF-SJ1 had accumulated 18 nucleotide mutations. The light chain of RF-SJ1 also had acquired 18 nucleotide mutations compared with the RF-SJ2. Functional affinity studies showed that the extensively mutated antibody (RF-SJ1) had a 100-fold higher affinity for human IgG than the RF-SJ2. These observations provide further evidence that RF in RA do undergo maturation including clonal expansion.

The derivation of the clonally related RF from the normal immunized donor MR allowed a detailed examination of the relationship between somatic hypermutation and affinity (TABLE 4). Among this group of RF, there is very little increase in affinity with the accumulation of mutations in the FRs. On average, the RF had K_d values of 2×10^{-6} M (range, 0.6–5 $\times 10^{-6}$ M). When compared with the affinity of RF from RA patients, using the same gene segments, the mean K_d was approximately 10-fold lower, that is, 3×10^{-7} M (range, 8×10^{-8} M to 5×10^{-7} M) (TABLE 4). RF in RA thus do not appear to be subject to regulatory mechanisms that control their affinity.

REPERTOIRE SHIFT IN THE IgV GENES ENCODING RF

In addition to diversifying the antibody repertoire of an immune response by somatic mutation, maturation of the antibody response is frequently accompanied by a shift in the repertoire of the IgV genes used.[53] Studies of primary immune responses to defined hapten antigens, such as oxazolone, in mice revealed that, although the primary response was entirely dominated by a particular pair of V_H and V_L germline genes, only 20% of the antibodies utilized the same combination in the secondary and tertiary responses.[44] This modification in the repertoire is called "repertoire shift."

In humans, studies of immune responses to rabies vaccine have provided evidence for repertoire shift.[54] For RF, there are limited data to suggest that repertoire shift may contribute to the diversity of the RF repertoire in RA synovia (TABLE 5).

Repertoire shift signifies that IgV genes utilized by low-affinity antibodies in the

TABLE 4. Functional Affinities of IgM RF from Different Sources[a]

Source and Clone Examined	Nucleotide Mutations in FR1+2+3		Nucleotide Mutations in CDR1+2		
	R	S	R	S	K_d (M)
HID PBL					
RF-MR1	3	1	2	3	2×10^{-6}
RF-MR30	2	1	0	2	5×10^{-6}
RF-MR2	1	2	0	0	1×10^{-6}
RF-MR16	4	2	2	2	6×10^{-6}
RF-MR37	2	1	0	0	2×10^{-6}
RF-MR33	0	2	1	1	9×10^{-7}
RF-MR25	0	0	0	2	2×10^{-6}
RF-MR14	2	0	1	1	2×10^{-6}
RF-MR28	2	0	0	1	1×10^{-6}
RA SM					
RF-SJ1	7	1	2	6	2.4×10^{-8}
RF-SJ2	0	0	1	1	2.7×10^{-6}
RF-SJ3	1	2	1	0	4.6×10^{-8}
RF-SJ4	9	7	8	5	7.9×10^{-8}
RF-TS1	6	2	3	0	7.7×10^{-8}
RF-TS2	3	2	2	1	7.1×10^{-8}
RF-TS5	1	1	1	0	2.1×10^{-7}
RF-KL1	1	3	9	4	6.8×10^{-7}
EMC					
KAS	ND	ND	ND	ND	2.5×10^{-7}

[a]The data are based on references 45 and 52. Only IgM RF paraprotein KAS and IgM RF-producing lines/hybridomas that have been characterized for specificity and gene use are given. HID PBL and RA SM indicate the original RF-producing cells used to establish the lines/hybridomas. EMC indicates that the RF paraprotein KAS was from a patient with essential mixed cryoglobulinemia. All RF-producing hybridomas were sequenced at the mRNA level, whereas paraprotein KAS was sequenced at the amino acid level. ND = not determined. The dissociation constant, K_d, was deduced from the Scatchard plot using an ELISA assay for binding to native human IgG.

primary response may not be capable of, or adequate for, encoding high-affinity antibodies that dominate the secondary response. The reasons for this may lie in intrinsic properties of the sequence or may reflect regulatory influences of B cell selection in germinal centers.[55] In responses to exogenous antigens, the limiting factor in determining repertoire is Ag concentration. Levels of exogenous antigens decline gradually, reaching a minimum at the end of the acute response. This leads to competition for the limited concentration of Ag, thus allowing only B cells with the highest affinity to survive. In responses to self-antigens in normal individuals, however, the process of B cell recruitment in germinal centers is regulated by a number of mechanisms, including high levels of soluble self-antigens that block self-reactive B cells from reaching germinal centers and prevent maturation.[56] Some of these regulatory processes may be abnormal in the ectopic germinal

TABLE 5. IgV Gene Use in RF Paraproteins and Monoclonal RF-producing Clones Established by Hybridoma Technology from Peripheral Blood of Normal Immunized Donors and the Synovial Membrane of RA Patients[a]

RF	V_H Family	Closest Germline V_H Gene	V_L Family	Closest Germline V_L Gene	Source
RF-TT9	3	DP-54	κ3a	Kv328	HID PBL
RF-MR5/41	3	DP-54	κ3a	Kv328	HID PBL
RF-TT5	3	DP-54	κ3a	Kv328	HID PBL
RF-MRC	1	DP-10	κ3b	Kv325	HID PBL
RF-MR1	1	DP-10	κ3b	Kv325	HID PBL
RF-TT1	1	DP-10	κ3b	Kv325	HID PBL
M7	3	DP-54	κ3a	Kv328	EMC
BOR	1	DP-10	κ3b	Kv325	EMC
KAS	1	DP-10	κ3b	Kv325	EMC
HUL	1	DP-10	κ3b	Kv325	EMC
RF-TS1	1	DP-10	κ3b	Kv325	RA SM
RF-TS2	3	DP-49	κ3a	Kv328	RA SM
RF-TS3	1	4.16	κ2	A23	RA SM
RF-TS4	3	DP-49	ND	ND	RA SM
RF-TS5	3	DP-35	κ1	11L102	RA SM
RF-SJ1	3	DP-46	λ1	lv117	RA SM
RF-SJ2	3	DP-46	λ1	lv117	RA SM
RF-SJ3	3	DP-49	κ3b	Kv325	RA SM
RF-SJ4	4	DP-66	κ3b	Kv305	RA SM
RF-KL1	3	DP-47	κ1	Vd	JRA SM
B42	3	DP-47	λ1	lv1042	RA SM
C93	3	8-1B	λ3	ll150	RA SM
D53	4	4.41	λ3	ll150	RA SM
H4	3	DP-47	λ3	ll150	RA SM
H6	1	DP-75	κ4	k18	RA SM
HAF10	1	hvlf10	λ	lv801	RA SM
C6	3	ND	κ1	HK102	RA SM
G4	1	DP-46	κ3b	Vg	RA SM
D5	3	DP-46	κ3b	Vg	RA SM
G9	4	DP-79	λ3	lv318	RA SM
A2A2	3	DP-49	κ1	012/02	RA SM

[a]The data are based on references 4, 5, 45, and 57–63. Only IgM RF paraproteins or IgM RF-producing lines/hybridomas that have been well characterized are given. HID PBL and RA SM indicate the original RF-producing cells used to establish the lines/hybridomas. JRA refers to juvenile rheumatoid arthritis. M7, BOR, KAS, and HUL are RF paraproteins from patients with essential mixed cryoglobulinemia (EMC) or Waldenström's macroglobulinemia. These RF were sequenced at the protein level. ND = not determined.

centers in synovial membranes of patients with RA, leading to immune response maturation.

SUMMARY

Recent advances in molecular biological and human cell hybridization technology have significantly advanced the knowledge of mechanisms that underlie human rheumatoid factor (RF) production. These advances have provided insight into the etiopathogenesis of synovial inflammation and lymphocyte recruitment in rheumatoid arthritis (RA) joints.

We have examined the mechanisms that lead to RF production in RA patients and those that regulate RF production in normals. The studies revealed structural features that distinguish RF produced in normals from those produced in RA synovial tissue. There are significant differences in the use of V_L and V_H genes between the two RF populations. Furthermore, IgV genes encoding synovial RF in RA have extensive evidence for nucleotide changes, leading to amino acid replacement in the complementarity determining regions (CDRs). In addition, RF produced in RA synovia show evidence for affinity maturation, isotype switch to IgG RF, and repertoire shift indicative of a continued recruitment of B cells. Together with computer modeling and crystallographic studies, our data suggest that the mechanisms that operate on RF selection in RA synovia are similar to immune responses to exogenous antigens. In contrast, RF established from human immunized donors (HID) are characterized by a very low ratio of replacement to silent (R:S) nucleotide changes in the CDR1+2. In addition, there is little increase in affinity with increasing numbers of mutations. There is thus evidence for regulatory mechanisms that limit affinity maturation of RF in normals.

ACKNOWLEDGMENTS

We would like to thank D. G. Williams, of the Kennedy Institute of Rheumatology, for useful discussions and for the literature survey used in TABLE 5.

REFERENCES

1. KUNKEL, H. G., V. AGNELLO, F. G. JOSLIN, R. J. WINCHESTER & J. D. CAPRA. 1973. Cross-idiotypic specificity among monoclonal IgM proteins with anti-gamma-globulin activity. J. Exp. Med. **137:** 331–342.
2. KUNKEL, H. G., R. J. WINCHESTER, F. G. JOSLIN & J. D. CAPRA. 1974. Similarities in the light chains of anti-gamma-globulins showing cross-idiotypic specificities. J. Exp. Med. **139:** 128–136.
3. RANDEN, I., K. M. THOMPSON, V. PASCUAL, K. VICTOR, D. BEALE, J. COADWELL, Ø. FØRRE, J. D. CAPRA & J. B. NATVIG. 1992. Rheumatoid factor V genes from patients with rheumatoid arthritis are diverse and show evidence of an antigen-driven response. Immunol. Rev. **128:** 49–71.
4. BROWN, C. M., K. J. FITZGERALD, S. MOYES, R. A. MAGEED, D. G. WILLIAMS & R. N. MAINI. 1995. Sequence analysis of immunoglobulin heavy-chain variable region genes from the synovium of a rheumatoid arthritis patient shows little evidence of mutation, but diverse CDR3. Immunology **84:** 367–374.
5. THOMPSON, K. M., M. BØRRETZEN, I. RANDEN, Ø. FØRRE & J. B. NATVIG. 1995. V-gene repertoire and hypermutation of rheumatoid factors produced in rheumatoid synovial inflammation and immunized healthy donors. Ann. N.Y. Acad. Sci. **764:** 440–449.
6. NOSSAL, G. J. V. 1992. Cellular and molecular mechanisms of B-lymphocyte tolerance. Adv. Immunol. **52:** 283–331.
7. HARTLEY, S. B., J. CROSBIE, R. BRINK, A. B. KANTOR, A. BASTEN & C. C. GOODNOW. 1991. Elimination from peripheral lymphoid tissues of self-reactive B lymphocytes recognising membrane-bound antigens. Nature **353:** 765–769.

8. CARSON, D. A., P. P. CHEN & T. J. KIPPS. 1991. New roles for rheumatoid factor. J. Clin. Invest. **87:** 379–383.
9. BIKOFF, E. K. 1983. Tolerance for self Ig at the level of the Ly1+ T cell. J. Exp. Med. **158:** 1868–1880.
10. ROOSNEK, E. & A. LANZAVECCHIA. 1991. Efficient and selective presentation of antigen-antibody complexes by rheumatoid factor B cells. J. Exp. Med. **173:** 487–489.
11. TIGHE, H., P. P. CHEN, R. TUCKER, T. J. KIPPS, J. ROUDIER, F. R. JIRIK & D. A. CARSON. 1993. Function of B cells expressing a human immunoglobulin M rheumatoid factor autoantibody in transgenic mice. J. Exp. Med. **177:** 109–118.
12. THOMPSON, K. M., I. RANDEN, M. BØRRETZEN, Ø. FØRRE & J. B. NATVIG. 1994. Variable region gene usage of human monoclonal rheumatoid factors derived from healthy donors following immunisation. Eur. J. Immunol. **24:** 1771–1778.
13. RANDEN, I., O. J. MELLBYE, Ø. FØRRE & J. B. NATVIG. 1995. The identification of germinal centres and follicular dendritic cell networks in rheumatoid synovial tissue. Scand. J. Immunol. **41:** 481–486.
14. MUNTHE, E. & J. B. NATVIG. 1972. Immunoglobulin classes, subclasses, and complexes of IgG rheumatoid factor in rheumatoid plasma cells. Clin. Exp. Immunol. **12:** 55–70.
15. MOYNIER, M., M. ABDERRAZIK, C. DIDRY, J. SANY & J. BROCHIER. 1992. The B cell repertoire in rheumatoid arthritis. III. Preferential homing of rheumatoid factor–producing B cell precursors in the synovial fluid. Arthritis Rheum. **35:** 49–54.
16. POPE, R. M., D. C. TELLER & M. MANNIK. 1975. Intermediate complexes formed by self-association of IgG rheumatoid factors. Ann. N.Y. Acad. Sci. **256:** 82–87.
17. PANAYI, G. S., J. S. LANCHBURY & G. H. KINGSLEY. 1992. The importance of the T cell in initiating and maintaining the chronic synovitis of rheumatoid arthritis. Arthritis Rheum. **35:** 729–735.
18. ALARCON, G. S. 1995. Epidemiology of rheumatoid arthritis. Rheum. Dis. Clin. North Am. **21:** 589–604.
19. ZIFF, M. 1993. Role of endothelium in the pathogenesis of rheumatoid synovitis. Int. J. Tissue React. **15:** 135–137.
20. NATVIG, J. B. & A. J. QUAYLE. 1995. V-genes of T-cell receptors in rheumatoid arthritis. Ann. N.Y. Acad. Sci. **756:** 138–146.
21. MELCHERS, I., H. H. PETER & H. EIBEL. 1995. The T and B cell repertoire of patients with rheumatoid arthritis. Scand. J. Rheumatol. Suppl. **101:** 153–162.
22. SHMERLING, R. H. & T. L. DELBANCO. 1991. The rheumatoid factor: an analysis of clinical utility. Am. J. Med. **91:** 528–534.
23. GRIPENBERG, M., A. M. TEPPO, P. KURKI, G. GRIPENBERG & T. HELVE. 1988. Autoantibody activity of cryoglobulins and sera in systemic lupus erythematosus: association of IgM class rheumatoid factors with Raynaud's syndrome. Scand. J. Rheumatol. **17:** 249–254.
24. MULLER, K., P. OXHOLM, M. MIER-MADSEN & A. WIIK. 1989. IgA and IgM rheumatoid factors in patients with primary Sjögren's syndrome: correlation to extraglandular manifestations. Scand. J. Rheumatol. **18:** 29–31.
25. SASSO, E. H., C. V. BARBER, F. A. NARDELLA, W. J. YOUNT & M. MANNIK. 1988. Antigen specificities of human monoclonal and polyclonal IgM rheumatoid factors. J. Immunol. **140:** 3098–3107.
26. RANDEN, I., K. M. THOMPSON, J. B. NATVIG, Ø. FØRRE & K. WAALEN. 1989. Human monoclonal rheumatoid factors derived from the polyclonal repertoire of rheumatoid synovial tissue: production and characterization. Clin. Exp. Immunol. **78:** 13–18.
27. MAGEED, R. A., D. A. CARSON & R. JEFFERIS. 1988. Immunogenic and antigenic epitopes of immunoglobulins. XXIII. Idiotype and molecular specificity of human rheumatoid factors: analysis of cross-reactive idiotype of rheumatoid factor paraproteins from the Wa idiotype group in relation to their IgG subclass specificity. Scand. J. Immunol. **28:** 233–240.
28. NARDELLA, F. A., I. R. OPPLIGER, G. C. STONE, E. H. SASSO, M. MANNIK, J. SJÖQUIST, A. K. SCHRÖEDER, P. CHRISTENSEN, P. J. JOHANSSON & L. BJÖRCK. 1988. Fc epitopes for human rheumatoid factors and the relationships of rheumatoid factors to the Fc binding proteins of microorganisms. Scand. J. Rheumatol. Suppl. **75:** 190–198.

29. BONAGURA, V. R., N. AGOSTINO, T. KWONG, M. BØRRETZEN, K. M. THOMPSON, J. B. NATVIG & S. L. MORRISON. 1995. Healthy immunized donors (HIDs) and rheumatoid arthritis patients produce IgM rheumatoid factors (RF) that react differently with genetically engineered chimeric IgG antibodies (cIgG). Arthritis Rheum. **38**(suppl.): S166 (abstract).
30. JEFFERIS, R., M. I. NIK JAAFAR & M. STEINITZ. 1984. Immunogenic and antigenic epitopes of immunoglobulins. VIII. A human monoclonal rheumatoid factor having specificity for a discontinuous epitope determined by histidine/arginine interchange at residue 435 of immunoglobulin G. Immunol. Lett. **7:** 191–194.
31. HUNNEYBALL, I. M. & D. R. STANWORTH. 1976. The effect of chemical modification on the antigenicity of human and rabbit immunoglobulin G. Immunology **30:** 881–894.
32. AGNELLO, V., A. ARBETTER, G. I. DE KASEP, R. POWELL, E. M. TAN & F. JOSLIN. 1980. Evidence for a subset of rheumatoid factors that cross-react with DNA-histone and have a distinct cross-reactive idiotype. J. Exp. Med. **151:** 1514–1527.
33. MAGEED, R. A., M. DEARLOVE, D. M. GOODALL & R. JEFFERIS. 1986. Immunogenic and antigenic epitopes of immunoglobulins. XVII. Monoclonal antibodies reactive with common and restricted idiotopes to the heavy chain of human rheumatoid factors. Rheumatol. Int. **6:** 179–183.
34. SULEYMAN, S., K. M. THOMPSON, Ø. FØRRE, M. SIOUD, I. RANDEN, R. A. MAGEED & J. B. NATVIG. 1994. Three new cross-reacting idiotopes as markers for the products of two distinct human V_H3 genes expressed in the early repertoire. Scand. J. Immunol. **40:** 681–690.
35. MAGEED, R. A., D. M. GOODALL & R. JEFFERIS. 1990. A highly conserved conformational idiotope on human IgM rheumatoid factor paraproteins of the Wa cross-reactive idiotype family defined by a monoclonal antibody. Rheumatol. Int. **10:** 57–63.
36. CROWLEY, J. J., R. A. MAGEED, G. J. SILVERMAN, P. P. CHEN, F. KOZIN, R. A. ERGER, R. JEFFERIS & D. A. CARSON. 1990. The incidence of a new human cross-reactive idiotype linked to subgroup V_HIII heavy chains. Mol. Immunol. **27:** 87–94.
37. DEANE, M., L. E. MACKENZIE, F. K. STEVENSON, P. Y. YOUINOU, P. M. LYDYARD & R. A. MAGEED. 1993. The genetic basis of human V(H)4 gene family–associated cross-reactive idiotype expression in CD5+ and CD5− cord blood B-lymphocyte clones. Scand. J. Immunol. **38:** 348–358.
38. MAGEED, R. A., M. R. WALKER & R. JEFFERIS. 1986. Restricted light chain subgroup expression in human rheumatoid factor paraproteins determined by monoclonal antibodies. Immunology **59:** 473–478.
39. RADOUX, V., P. P. CHEN, J. A. SORGE & D. A. CARSON. 1986. A conserved human germline V kappa gene directly encodes rheumatoid factor light chains. J. Exp. Med. **164:** 2119–2124.
40. CROWLEY, J. J., R. D. GOLDFIEN, R. E. SCHROHENLOHER, H. L. SPIEGELBERG, R. A. MAGEED, R. JEFFERIS, W. J. KOOPMAN, D. A. CARSON & S. FONG. 1988. Incidence of two cross-reactive idiotypes defines two mutually exclusive kappa light chain variable region subgroups for human rheumatoid factor paraproteins. J. Immunol. **140:** 3411–3418.
41. SILVERMAN, G. J., R. E. SCHROHENLOHER, M. A. ACCAVITTI, W. J. KOOPMAN & D. A. CARSON. 1990. Structural characterization of the second major cross-reactive idiotype group of human rheumatoid factors: association with the V_H4 gene family. Arthritis Rheum. **33:** 1347–1360.
42. VENCOVSKY, J., R. A. MAGEED, W. E. OLLIER & R. N. MAINI. 1995. Monozygosity rheumatoid arthritis twin pairs express similar levels of conserved immunoglobulin V genes in polyclonal rheumatoid factors irrespective of disease status. Scand. J. Immunol. **42:** 147–157.
43. BEREK, C. & M. ZIEGNER. 1993. The maturation of the immune response. Immunol. Today **14:** 400–404.
44. BEREK, C., G. M. GRIFFITHS & C. MILSTEIN. 1985. Molecular events during the immune response to oxazolone. Nature **316:** 412–418.
45. BØRRETZEN, M., I. RANDEN, E. ZDARSKY, Ø. FØRRE, J. B. NATVIG & K. M. THOMPSON. 1994. Control of autoantibody affinity by selection against amino acid replacements in the complementarity determining regions. Proc. Natl. Acad. Sci. U.S.A. **91:** 12917–12921.
46. SHLOMCHIK, M. J., A. MARSHAK-ROTHSTEIN, C. B. WOLFOWICZ, T. L. ROTHSTEIN & M. G. WEIGERT. 1987. The role of clonal selection and somatic mutation in autoimmunity. Nature **328:** 805–810.

47. SHLOMCHIK, M., M. MASCELLI, H. SHAN, M. Z. RADIC, D. PISETSKY, A. MARSHAK-ROTHSTEIN & M. WEIGERT. 1990. Anti-DNA antibodies from autoimmune mice arise by clonal expansion and somatic mutation. J. Exp. Med. **171:** 265–292.
48. MAGEED, R. A., J. R. KIRWAN, P. W. THOMPSON, D. A. MCCARTHY & E. J. HOLBOROW. 1991. Characterization of the size and composition of circulating immune complexes in patients with rheumatoid arthritis. Ann. Rheum. Dis. **50:** 231–236.
49. RANDEN, I., V. PASCUAL, K. VICTOR, K. M. THOMPSON, Ø. FØRRE, J. D. CAPRA & J. B. NATVIG. 1993. Synovial IgG rheumatoid factors show evidence of an antigen-driven immune response and a shift in the V-gene repertoire compared to IgM rheumatoid factors. Eur. J. Immunol. **23:** 1220–1225.
50. LIU, Y-J., J. ZHANG, P. L. LANE, E. Y. CHAN & I. C. MACLENNAN. 1991. Sites of specific B cell activation in primary and secondary responses to T cell–dependent and T cell–independent antigens. Eur. J. Immunol. **21:** 2951–2962.
51. JACOB, J. & G. KELSOE. 1992. *In situ* studies of the primary immune response to (4-hydroxy-3-nitrophenyl)-acetyl. II. A common clonal origin for periarteriolar lymphoid sheath–associated foci and germinal centers. J. Exp. Med. **176:** 679–688.
52. RANDEN, I., D. BROWN, K. M. THOMPSON, N. C. HUGHES-JONES, V. PASCUAL, K. VICTOR, J. D. CAPRA, Ø. FØRRE & J. B. NATVIG. 1992. Clonally related IgM rheumatoid factors undergo affinity maturation in the rheumatoid synovial tissue. J. Immunol. **148:** 3296–3301.
53. BEREK, C., A. BERGER & M. APEL. 1991. Maturation of the immune response in germinal centers. Cell **67:** 1121–1129.
54. UEKI, Y., I. S. GOLDFARB, N. HARINDRANATH, M. GORE, H. KOPROWSKI, A. L. NOTKINS & P. CASALI. 1990. Clonal analysis of a human antibody response: quantitation of precursors of antibody-producing cells and generation and characterization of monoclonal IgM, IgG, and IgA to rabies virus. J. Exp. Med. **171:** 19–34.
55. LIU, Y-J., C. ARPIN, O. DE BOUTEILLER, C. GURET, J. BANCHEREAU, H. MARTINEZ-VALDEZ & S. LEBECQUE. 1996. Sequential triggering of apoptosis, somatic mutation, and isotype switch during germinal center development. Semin. Immunol. **8:** 169–177.
56. PULENDRAN, B., M. KARVELAS & G. J. V. NOSSAL. 1994. A form of immunologic tolerance through impairment of germinal center development. Proc. Natl. Acad. Sci. U.S.A. **91:** 2639–2643.
57. PASCUAL, V., I. RANDEN, K. M. THOMPSON, M. SIOUD, Ø. FØRRE, J. NATVIG & J. D. CAPRA. 1990. The complete nucleotide sequences of the heavy chain variable regions of six monospecific rheumatoid factors derived from Epstein-Barr virus–transformed B cells isolated from the synovial tissue of patients with rheumatoid arthritis: further evidence that some autoantibodies are unmutated copies of germline genes. J. Clin. Invest. **86:** 1320–1328.
58. YOUNGBLOOD, K., L. FRUCHTER, G. DING, J. LOPEZ, V. BONAGURA & A. DAVIDSON. 1994. Rheumatoid factors from the peripheral blood of two patients with rheumatoid arthritis are genetically heterogeneous and somatically mutated. J. Clin. Invest. **93:** 852–861.
59. EZAKI, I., H. KANDA, K. SAKAI, N. FUKUI, M. SHINGU, M. NOBUNAGA & T. WATANABE. 1991. Restricted diversity of the variable region nucleotide sequences of the heavy and light chains of a human rheumatoid factor. Arthritis Rheum. **34:** 343–350.
60. NEWKIRK, M. M., R. A. MAGEED, R. JEFFERIS, P. P. CHEN & J. D. CAPRA. 1987. Complete amino acid sequences of variable regions of two human IgM rheumatoid factors, BOR and KAS of the Wa idiotypic family, reveal restricted use of heavy and light chain variable and joining region gene segments. J. Exp. Med. **166:** 550–564.
61. ERMEL, R. W., T. P. KENNY, A. WONG, A. SOLOMON, P. P. CHEN & D. L. ROBBINS. 1994. Preferential utilization of a novel V lambda 3 gene in monoclonal rheumatoid factors derived from the synovial cells of rheumatoid arthritis patients. Arthritis Rheum. **37:** 860–868.
62. SOTO-GIL, R. W., T. OLEE, B. K. KLINK, T. P. KENNY, D. L. ROBBINS, D. A. CARSON & P. P. CHEN. 1992. A systematic approach to defining the germline gene counterparts of a mutated autoantibody from a patient with rheumatoid arthritis. Arthritis Rheum. **35:** 356–363.
63. ERMEL, R. W., T. P. KENNY, P. P. CHEN & D. L. ROBBINS. 1993. Molecular analysis of rheumatoid factors derived from rheumatoid synovium suggests an antigen-driven response in inflamed joints. Arthritis Rheum. **36:** 380–388.

Evidence for a Selected Humoral Immune Response Encoded by V_H4 Family Genes in the Synovial Membrane of a Patient with RA[a]

JAN VOSWINKEL, MICHAEL PFREUNDSCHUH, AND ANGELA GAUSE[b]

Internal Medicine I
Saarland Medical School
D-66421 Homburg/Saar, Germany

INTRODUCTION

Patients with rheumatoid arthritis (RA) often have abundant germinal center–like B cell infiltrates in their synovial membrane (SM). The analysis of rearranged V_L and V_H genes from B cell foci had characterized these cells as highly mutated memory B cells.[1,2] As we had found an overrepresentation of rearranged V_H4 genes in the B cell foci of two patients, we performed the following experiments in order to characterize the V_H4 response in one patient in more detail.

MATERIALS AND METHODS

SM was obtained from a 78-year-old woman with RA of 15-year duration undergoing total joint replacement of the knee. The SM was snap-frozen in liquid nitrogen and stored at $-70°C$. B cell–rich areas of the SM were identified by CD20 staining of frozen tissue sections, isolated by microdissection, and pooled. This method was chosen in order to enrich for B cells not preselected by cell culture procedures. An estimated amount of about 10^5 B cells was collected, DNA was extracted, and the DNA of a calculated number of about 5×10^3 B lymphocytes was submitted to 35 cycles of a PCR with V_H-family-specific oligonucleotides and a J_H oligonucleotide mix (one PCR for each V_H family 1 to 6). The V_H4 PCR product was cloned and sequenced by standard methods.

RESULTS AND DISCUSSION

Sequence analysis of 11 bacterial clones revealed that 7 of these 11 were potentially functional and all were mutated with 88% to 96% homology to known

[a]This work was supported by the DFG (Grant No. DFG-GA-320).

[b]To whom all correspondence should be addressed.

TABLE 1. List of Rearranged V_H4 Genes Analyzed[a]

Rearranged Gene	Germline Gene	Homology (%)	Mutations		R:S		CDR3 Length (bp)	D_H	J_H	Type of Rearrangement
			CDR	FR	CDR	FR				
$S8V_H44$	GL8 (99.6% $V_H4.34$)	91.0	7	5	5:2	3:2	44	DLR2	4	nf
$S8V_H45$	GL7 (100% DP71)	94.1	3	4	2:1	3:1	47	DA5	4	nf
$S8V_H46$	GL1 (100% DP66)	92.5	7	6	4:3	5:1	42	D21-10, DIR1	2	pf
$S8V_H47$	GL5 (100% DP68)	96.5	0	4	0:0	3:1	33	DN1	4	pf
$S8V_H48$	GL2 (99.6% $V_H4.34$)	94.7	3	8	3:0	5:3	33	DLR2	5	pf
$S8V_H49$	GL6 (100% DP65)	93.0	2	12	1:1	8:4	30	DK4	4	pf
$S8V_H410$	$V_H4.22$	90.1	8	11	7:1	5:6	35	DIR1	4	nf
$S8V_H411$	GL2 (99.6% $V_H4.34$)	93.8	4	8	4:0	5:3	33	DLR2	5	pf
$S8V_H412$	GL6 (100% DP64)	93.4	6	7	6:0	6:1	42	DXP′1	5	pf
$S8V_H414$	GL9 (99.1% DP67)	90.2	6	9	2:4	4:5	30	D21-9	1	pf
$S8V_H413$	GL4 (99.5% DP63)	93.8	5	9	4:1	5:4	41	DA1	1	nf

[a]The most homologous germline gene of the patient is given in the second column, with the percentage of nucleotide homology to published V_H4 germline genes in parentheses (according to Tomlinson[5] and Weng[6]). In the following columns, the percentage of homology, the absolute number of mutations and R:S ratios in CDR and FR, the nucleotide length of the CDR3, and D_H and J_H germline segments are given. The last column designates a potentially functional rearrangement (pf) and a nonfunctional rearrangement (nf). Homology is compared within the V_H segments from amino acid position 25 (FR1) up to 94 (end of FR3); the length of the CDR3 is measured between amino acid position 95 and 102 according to Kabat.[7]

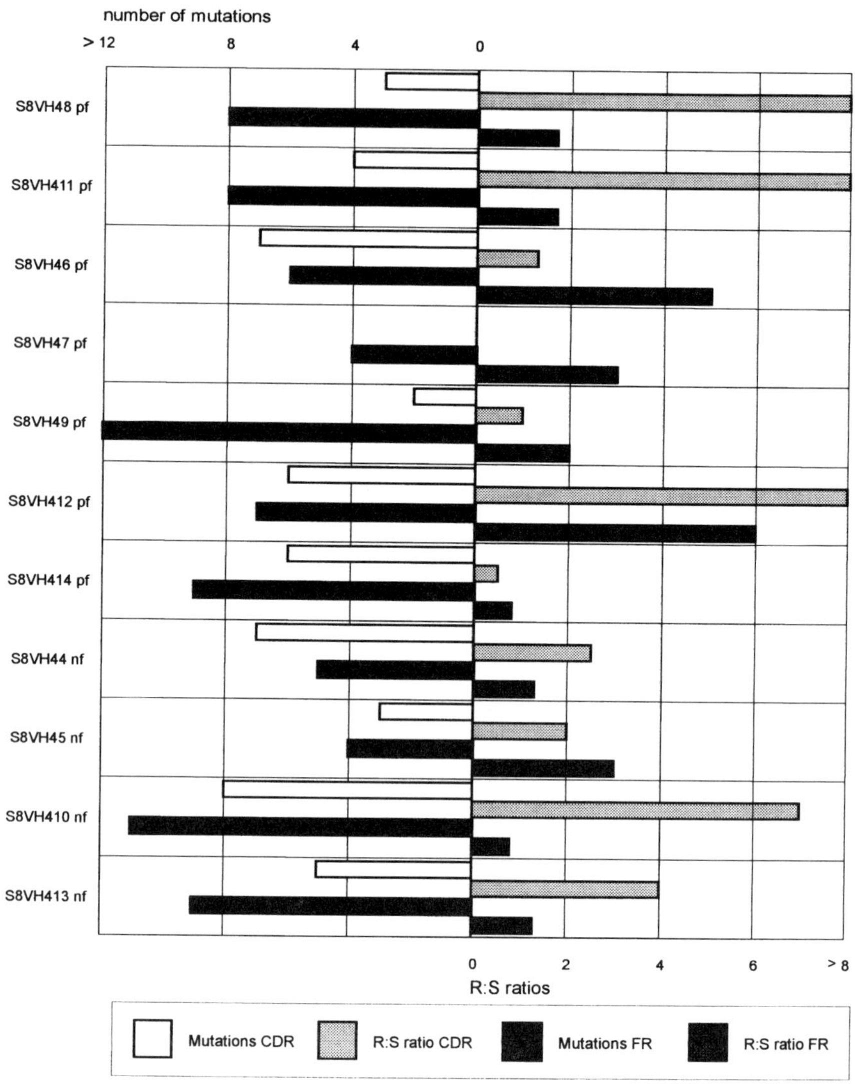

FIGURE 1. Number of mutations and R:S ratios of 11 SM-derived rearranged V_H4 genes in comparison, separated between CDR and FR. The R:S ratio is the quotient of replacement mutations and silent mutations. In all cases where R:S is >8, the denominator (S) is 0, so the quotient is infinity. $S8V_H48$ and $S8V_H411$ are the two members of one clone.

germline genes and to germline genes of the same patient (TABLE 1). Analysis of the complementarity determining region (CDR) 3 reveals that 9 products are clonally not related, whereas 2 represent members of 1 B cell clone that differ by five nucleotide exchanges. Three of the five mutations encode amino acid replacements in CDRs, indicating significant expansion of one specific clone. The most homologous germline gene of this clone is the $V_H4.34$ gene, which has so far rarely been identified.[3] The $V_H4.21$/DP63 germline gene, which has been found overrepresented in the autoimmune repertoire, was identified only in one nonfunctional rearrangement.[4] Overall, the pattern of mutations and the replacement-to-silent (R:S) ratios are diverse, with some products indicating antigen selection by their high R:S ratios in CDRs (FIGURE 1). Although we cannot prove antigen specificity, there is evidence for selection by antigen and expansion of specific clones in the SM on the background of a polyclonal stimulation.

REFERENCES

1. GAUSE, A., K. GUNDLACH, M. ZDICHAVSKY, G. JACOBS, B. KOCH, T. HOPF & M. PFREUNDSCHUH. 1995. Eur. J. Immunol. **25:** 2775–2782.
2. SCHRÖDER, A. E., A. GREINER, C. SEYFERT & C. BEREK. 1996. Proc. Natl. Acad. Sci. U.S.A. **93:** 221–225.
3. KLEIN, U., R. KÜPPERS & K. RAJEWSKY. 1994. J. Exp. Med. **180:** 1383–1393.
4. PASCUAL, V. & J. D. CAPRA. 1992. Arthritis Rheum. **35:** 11–18.
5. TOMLINSON, J. M. *et al.* 1992. J. Mol. Biol. **227:** 776–798.
6. WENG, N. P. *et al.* 1992. Eur. J. Immunol. **22:** 1075–1082.
7. KABAT, E. A. *et al.* 1991. NIH publication. Bethesda, Maryland.

Identification and Cloning of Genes Expressed by Human Tonsillar B Lymphocyte Subsets

J. KIMBLE FRAZER,[a] JANETTE LeGROS,[a]
ODETTE de BOUTEILLER,[b] YONG-JUN LIU,[b]
JACQUES BANCHEREAU,[b] VIRGINIA PASCUAL,[a]
AND J. DONALD CAPRA[a]

[a]*Molecular Immunology Center*
University of Texas Southwestern Medical Center
Dallas, Texas 75235

[b]*Schering-Plough Laboratory for Immunological Research*
69571 Dardilly, France

Mature B cells, as they pass through the germinal center reaction, may be distinguished and separated on the basis of a series of phenotypic cell surface markers.[1] These different B cell subsets, spanning from the naive to memory cell compartments (classified Bm1–5), not only reflect distinct anatomical locations within the secondary lymphoid organ, but also correlate with the onset of certain differentiation steps (FIGURE 1). For instance, both somatic hypermutation and isotype switch phenomena have been demonstrated to appear in the Bm3 (centroblast) and Bm4 (centrocyte) subsets, respectively.[2,3]

Representational Difference Analysis (RDA) is a technique that combines the advantages of subtractive hybridization methodologies with the power of PCR-based strategies to identify genes regulated differentially between two separate cDNA sources.[4,5] Using cDNAs prepared from 2×10^5 discrete twice-FACS-sorted cell populations, we have identified over 100 different candidate gene fragments that are either uniquely expressed or differentially regulated by mature tonsillar B cells as they move from the follicular mantle (FM; pooled Bm1/Bm2 subsets, CD38−) into the germinal center (GC; Bm3 subset, CD38+). Our preliminary findings are bolstered by the fact that a message known to be differentially regulated between subsets, CD38, has been independently isolated 11 times from the GC compartment (but not the FM), indicating that at least some of these candidates truly reflect messenger RNAs specific to centroblasts that have just entered germinal centers. In addition, five distinct novel sequence fragments have been isolated 8, 8, 12, 23, and 30 times, respectively, perhaps reflecting a similar level of upregulation of these mRNAs. In sum, these sequence fragments comprise genes of known identity, genes with similarity to known sequences, and genes with no significant homologies. Among those with known or notable homologies are sequences encoding cell surface molecules (including CD38), protein kinases, transport proteins, and hormone-binding proteins (TABLE 1). The

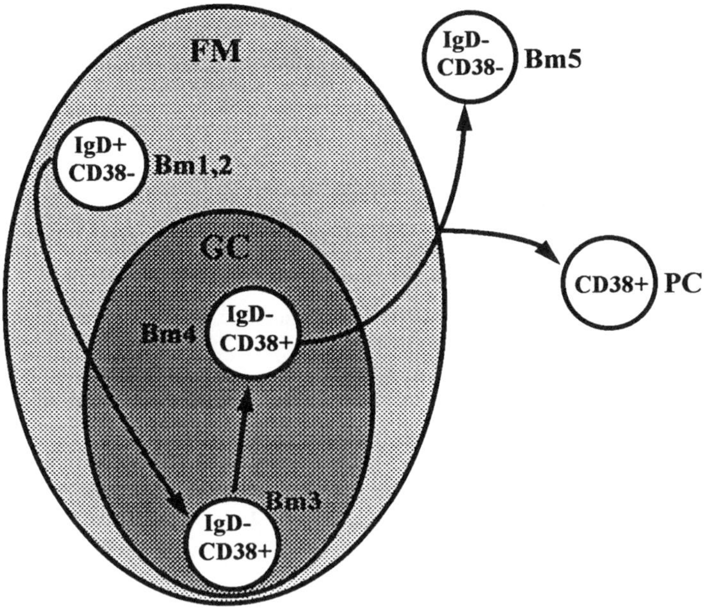

FIGURE 1. Schematic representation of B lymphocyte differentiation and subsetting through a germinal center reaction: FM, follicular mantle; GC, germinal center; Bm1/2, naive B cells; Bm3, centroblast in germinal center dark zone; Bm4, centrocyte in germinal center light zone; Bm5, memory B cell in intraepithelium or exiting the germinal center; PC, plasma cell.

TABLE 1. Germinal Center–specific Genes Identified by Representational Difference Analysis

- 217 total sequences processed; 103 unique sequences
- CD38 independently isolated 11 times (5%)
- 5 genes with no known homologies isolated 8 (4%), 8 (4%), 12 (6%), 23 (11%), and 30 (14%) times, respectively

Known Genes	Homologous Genes	Unknown Genes
2 cell surface proteins (including CD38)	1 cotransporter protein	91 sequences with no homology to known genes
2 protein kinases	1 guanylate kinase	
	1 hormone-binding protein	

verification, identification, and characterization of these messages, and subsequent experiments to ascertain their functional significance, should provide an exciting area of research for future studies.

REFERENCES

1. Liu, Y-J., O. de Bouteiller, C. Arpin, I. Durand & J. Banchereau. 1994. Adv. Exp. Med. Biol. **355:** 289–296.

2. Pascual, V., Y-J. Liu, A. Magalski, O. de Bouteiller, J. Banchereau & J. D. Capra. 1994. J. Exp. Med. **180:** 329–339.
3. Liu, Y-J., F. Malisan, O. de Bouteiller, C. Guret, S. Lebecque, J. Banchereau, F. Mills, E. Max & H. Martinez-Valdez. 1996. Immunity **4:** 241–250.
4. Lisitsyn, N., N. Lisitsyn & M. Wigler. 1993. Science **259:** 946–950.
5. Hubank, M. & D. G. Schatz. 1994. Nucleic Acids Res. **22:** 5640–5648.

Somatic Mutation and CDR3 Length of Immunoglobulin Lambda Variable Region Genes in the Synovium of Patients with Rheumatoid Arthritis

R. A. MAGEED,[a] S. P. MOYES,[a] J. VENCOVSKÝ,[b] AND R. N. MAINI[a]

[a]*Kennedy Institute of Rheumatology Hammersmith, London W6 7DW, United Kingdom*

[b]*Institute of Rheumatology Prague 2, the Czech Republic*

Our previous sequencing of immunoglobulin genes in B cell hybridomas established from rheumatoid arthritis (RA) synovial tissues has revealed evidence for both polyclonal activation and antigen-driven expansion of B cells. To further define the molecular and cellular basis for this observation, we have developed a novel approach that provides a more comprehensive representation of the B cell repertoire in RA synovia than hybridoma generation. The approach is based on antigen (Ag)–specific B cell separation, anchored RT-PCR, and identification of dominant and unique B cell clones by Ig gene fingerprinting (separated on the basis of CDR3 length). Dominant and unique clones separated on the basis of Vλ gene length within rheumatoid factor (RF)– and non-RF-producing B cells were identified and studied by DNA sequencing. The finding of dominant and unique clones in RA synovia compared with peripheral blood suggests that some synovial B cells are selectively expanded in the synovium. However, this expansion was not restricted to RF-producing B cells, suggesting that IgG is unlikely to be the only driving Ag in RA synovia. The data also provided evidence for frequent nontemplated (N) nucleotide additions at the V-J junctions of the Vλ light chains and extended CDR3 in synovial B cells.

DISCUSSION

The production of immunoglobulins (Ig), including RF, in the synovium of RA patients contributes to the pathogenesis of this disease.[1] The factors that lead to sustained synovial lymphocyte activation in RA, however, remain poorly defined. Although RF is a serological hallmark for RA and high levels are detected in the synovium, it is not clear if IgG is the only driving Ag for the synovial immune response. Furthermore, the immunological nature of the response in the synovium in terms of clonal expansion and maturation is not clear. To understand disease mechanisms, it is important to define how lymphocytes are continually recruited to the immune response in the synovium. One approach to achieve this is to study the

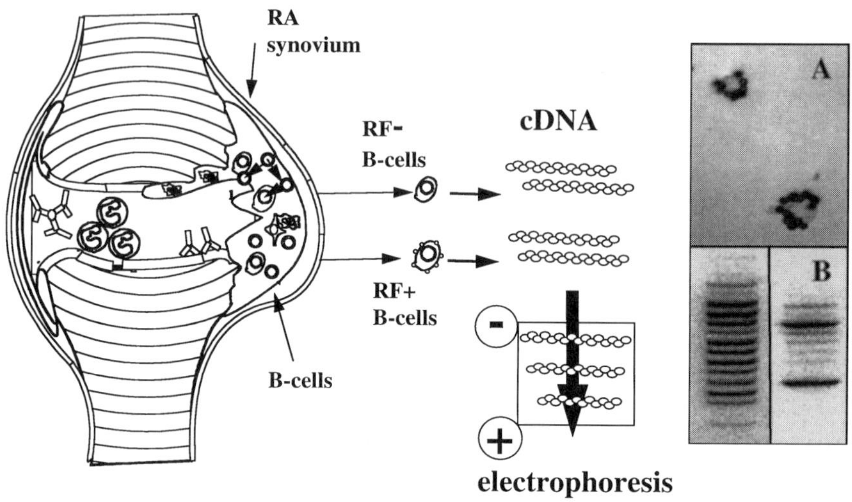

FIGURE 1. The strategy used to study the clonality and IgV sequences of synovial B cells. Synovial cells are isolated from synovial tissue or fluid after tissue dissection or treatment with hyaluronidase, and mononuclear cells are isolated using Ficoll-Hypaque fractionation. Cells of the monocyte/macrophage lineage and T cells are depleted with L-leucine methyl ester and by rosetting with nuraminidase-treated sheep red blood cells, respectively. RF-expressing cells are separated from non-RF-expressing B cells using magnetic beads coated with an IgG_4 paraprotein. Panel A shows the coated magnetic beads bound to RF B cells. mRNA from each cell population is then subjected to two sets of PCR. The first is an anchored-PCR using poly-G-tailed cDNA, whereas the second is an IgV gene family–specific PCR with a radiolabeled C-primer. The radiolabeled PCR products (panel B for V_H rearrangements) are then separated on a high-resolution gel and individual dominant or unique bands are cut, cloned, and sequenced.

specificity and the IgV genes expressed by synovial B cells because rearranged IgV genes harbor imprints characteristic of the way that B lymphocytes are selected, as well as the clonal relationship between different populations.[2] In this study, we use a new approach based on the separation of IgG-specific B cells from the synovial tissue of RA patients followed by identification of dominant/unique clones. The manner of immunological selection, the clonal maturation, and the relationship between different antigen-specific B cells are then studied by sequencing DNA isolated from high-resolution gels.

RESULTS AND CONCLUSIONS

The pattern of IgV gene rearrangement is a distinct feature of individual progenitor B cell clones. This feature is manifested in the pattern of V, D (for the heavy chain), and J gene recombination and in the size of the CDR3 of the heavy and light chains.[3] The length and nucleotide sequence of the CDR3 are determined not only by the random recombinatorial process and break/rearrangement, but also by nontemplated nucleotide addition (N-addition). Although the degree of diversity generated in the heavy-chain variable region is higher than that of the light chain, due to heavy-chain D_H genes, recent studies have shown that a significant degree of diversity is nevertheless generated in the light chain by the combinatorial process and N-additions.[4]

Using a new approach in which synovial B cells or RF-expressing B cells, separated with magnetic beads coated with IgG (FIGURE 1), are used for size fractionation of the rearranged IgV gene with the aid of PCR, cloning, and sequencing, we have observed dominant and unique Vλ rearrangements in synovial B cells (FIGURE 2). The data, however, reveal no restrictions in the use of individual Vλ genes from the larger families (Vλ1, 2, and 3) in any B cell population. The study of nucleotide sequences revealed that mutations were equally evident within RF and non-RF populations. This finding suggests that a significant proportion of the non-RF-expressing B cell population is also Ag-driven (FIGURES 3A and 3B). However, when the sequences were assessed for interclonal variations, it was evident that the RF B cells were more often clonally related than were non-RF-expressing B cells. These data may imply that the nature of clonal expansion is different between RF- and non-RF-expressing clones or that the non-RF-expressing clones have been selected by more than one Ag. Interestingly, when sequences from the smaller Vλ families were studied, there was a surprising similarity between the sequences obtained from the RF and non-RF B cells (FIGURE 3C). This may suggest the existence

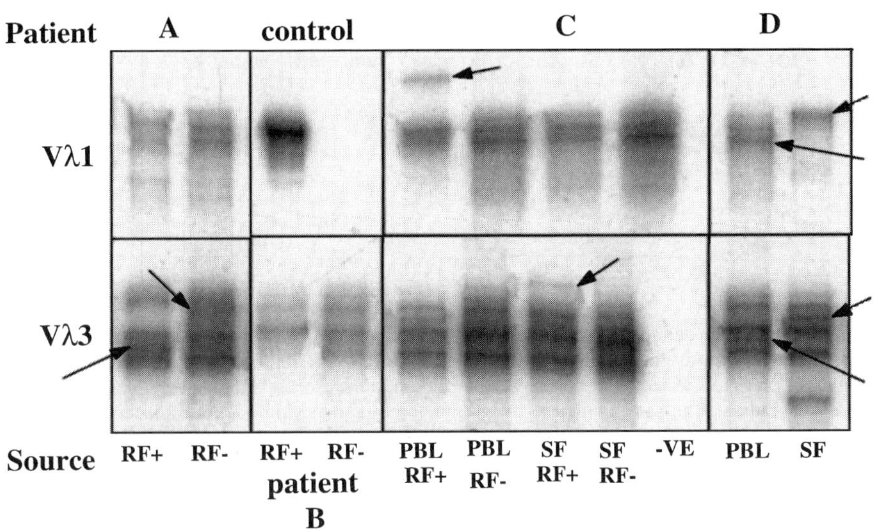

FIGURE 2. The fingerprinting profiles obtained for synovial fluid (SF), peripheral blood (PBL), and RF (RF+) and non-RF (RF−) B cells from synovial membrane (given as RF; synovial fluid RF, SF RF; and peripheral blood RF, PBL RF) expressing Vλ1 and 3 genes from four patients. The positive control was mRNA from a hybridoma expressing a Vλ1 gene. As a negative control, mRNA from a hybridoma not expressing the examined Vλ gene family was used. The arrows mark the bands detected in one population of B cells, but not in the corresponding population. Patients A, B, C, and D all had long-standing classical RA.

A -

Clone		CDR1	CDR2	CDR3			
DPL11	**(Vλ2)**	**TGTSSDVGGYNYVS**	**EVSNRPS**	**SSYTSSSTL**	**VV**	**FGGGTKLTVL**	Jλ2
RF-3		..I......SK...	D......	..H.AT..	.L	....	
					YV	**FGTGTKVTVL**	Jλ1
RF-4		S..T..I.PSD..A	D..R...	...S..GS	..	Y..A......	
RF+3		......I...D...	D......	I...I...	C.	....	
VL2.1	**(Vλ2)**	**TGTSSDVGSYNLVS**	**EGSKRPS**	**SSYTSSSTL**	**YV**	**FGTGTKVTVL**	Jλ1
RF+4		..SW..I..NKF..	DV.N...	.....AGI	V.	..S..T.S..	
RF+6		..SW..I..N.FI.	DV.N...	.....AGI	V.	..I..T.T..	

B -

Clone	CDR1	CDR2	CDR3	N- additions			
HUMLV413 (Vλ4)	**QGDSLRSYYAS**	**GKNNRPS**	**NSRDSSGNH**		**YV**	**FGTGTKVTV**	Jλ1
SF-3	......G....	.NS....	Q.Y...LTG	S	G.	.......I..	
SF-1	......G....	..D....	Q.Y...LIG	S	G.	....	
IGLV3S2 (Vλ3a)	**GGNNIGSKSVH**	**YDSDRPS**	**QVWDSSSDH**		**VV**	**FGGGTKLTV**	Jλ2/3
SF-4	......NEA.L	S.CY...	......C..	P	.L	....	
PBL-3	E......R.A.	..N....	....GI...		Q.	....	
Hsiggll295 (Vλ3b)	**SGDALPKKYAY**	**KDSKRPS**	**YSADYSGNE**		**YV**	**FGTGTKVTV**	Jλ2/3
PBL-6	....	E......	F.T.S..S.		G.	....	
Hsiggll150 (Vλ3b)	**SGDALPKQYAY**	**KDSERPS**	**QSADSSGNH**		**YV**	**FGTGTKVTV**	Jλ2/3
PBL-2	..E....K...	....	L......TD		..	....	

C -

Clone	**CDR1**	**CDR2**	**FR3**	**CDR3**	N-additions			
IGLV6S1 (Vλ6)	**TRSSGSIASNYVQ**	**EDNQRPS**	**SGSIDSS**	**QSYDSSN**	**GE**	**VV**	**FG**	Jλ2/3
RF-1	..........I...	....	F..V...	HT.NNT.	GK	E.	..	
RF-2	..........I...	....K..	F..V.G.	HT.NNT.	GE	E.	..	
RF-3	..........I...	....	F..V.P.	HT.NNT.	GE	E.	..	
RF+1	..........I...	....	F..V...	HT.NNT.	GE	E.	..	
RF+2	..........I...	....	F..V...	HT.NNT.	GE	E.	..	
RF+3	..........I...	....	F..V...	HT.NNT.	GE	E.	..	

FIGURE 3. The deduced amino acid sequences (given by single letters) of individual rearrangements representing single B cell clones. Only CDR regions (and FR3 in part C) are shown for clarity. The sequences are given in relation to the closest related germline gene (bold). Identity is indicated by a dot, whereas differences are given as single letter replacements. Part A shows the sequences of Vλ2 genes in RF (RF+3, +4, and +6) and non-RF B cells (RF−3 and −4) isolated from synovial membranes. This section reveals mutations in both populations of B cells and interclonal similarity in RF clones. Part B shows the sequences of expressed Vλ3a, 3b, and 4 in SF B cells (SF-1, 3, and 4) in comparison with PBL B cells. This section shows N-additions in SF B cells. Part C shows the sequences of the expressed Vλ6 gene in RF (RF+1, +2, and +3) and non-RF (RF−1, −2, and −3) B cells in synovial membranes. This section highlights the sequence and interclonal similarity between the two populations expressing this small Vλ6 gene family (one member).

of clonal relationships between RF- and non-RF-expressing B cells that express the smaller Vλ gene families or may reflect a singular manner in which genes from the smaller Vλ gene families are rearranged.

Collectively, our data attest to the fact that most RA synovial B cells are specifically selected for expansion and differentiation, perhaps by numerous antigens including self-IgG. Furthermore, the data may suggest that cells with N-additions are preferentially expanded in RA synovia and that some RF- and non-RF-expressing B cells may have arisen from the same ancestral B cell clones.

REFERENCES

1. HARRIS, E. D., JR. 1990. Rheumatoid arthritis: pathophysiology and implications for therapy. N. Engl. J. Med. **322:** 1277–1289.
2. BERMAN, J. E. & F. W. ALT. 1990. Human heavy chain variable region gene diversity, organization, and expression. Int. Rev. Immunol. **5:** 203–214.
3. TONEGAWA, S. 1983. Somatic generation of antibody diversity. Nature **302:** 575–581.
4. BRIDGES, S. L., S. K. LEE, M. L. JOHNSON, J. LAVELLE, P. FOWLER, W. J. KOOPMAN & H. W. SCHROEDER, JR. 1995. Somatic mutation and CDR3 lengths of immunoglobulin κ light chains expressed in patients with rheumatoid arthritis and normal individuals. J. Clin. Invest. **96:** 831–841.

Immunoglobulin Variable Region (IgV) Gene Expression in Rheumatoid Factors from Monozygotic Twins with Rheumatoid Arthritis

J. VENCOVSKÝ,[a] R. N. MAINI,[b] W. E. OLLIER,[c] AND R. A. MAGEED[b]

[a]*Institute of Rheumatology Prague 2, the Czech Republic*

[b]*Kennedy Institute of Rheumatology Hammersmith, London W6 7DW, United Kingdom*

[c]*Arthritis and Rheumatism Epidemiology Research Unit Manchester, United Kingdom*

INTRODUCTION

Patients with rheumatoid arthritis (RA) produce high levels of autoantibodies against IgG-Fc (rheumatoid factors, RF). The stimulus for the persistent production of RF, however, is not yet known. Knowledge of the pattern and level of IgV gene use within naturally occurring Ig and RF may help to answer the questions concerning RF cell clonality, mechanisms of cell selection, and persistent production.[1] The aim of this study was to examine the influence of RA disease mechanisms on determining the level of IgV gene use and mutation in RF. Monozygotic (MZ) twins were chosen for the study to compare the effect of genetic factors that regulate the level of IgV gene use with disease mechanisms on RF quantity and quality.

METHODS

Six MZ twin pairs were studied—three were concordant and three discordant for RA. The levels of RF and IgV gene use in the expressed repertoire of these RA twins were compared with those from four normal MZ twin pairs and ten randomly selected healthy controls. Individual immunoglobulin isotypes were purified using gel filtration and affinity chromatography. The RF content of each Ig fraction was then separated from the rest using affinity chromatography with an aggregated IgG column. The level of variable region gene use within the different Ig and RF fractions was determined by ELISA using specific mouse monoclonal antibodies. These antibodies have been shown to recognize protein products of IgV genes in germline, or minimally mutated germline, configurations on RF paraproteins as well as on RF produced by fetal or RA synovial B lymphocytes.

TABLE 1. Percent of IgV Gene Products in the Plasma of MZ Twins with RA (n = 12), Normal MZ Twin Pairs (n = 8), and Normal Controls (n = 10)[a]

Groups Examined	% Ig Reactive with G6	% Ig Reactive with G8	% Ig Reactive with B6	% Ig Reactive with D12	% Ig Reactive with Lc1	% Ig Reactive with 9G4	% Ig Reactive with C7
IgM							
RA twins	0.7 (0.9)	6.5 (4.2)	4.1 (2.0)	4.2 (2.5)	15.0 (6.0)	0.8 (0.8)	22.1 (4.7)
normal twins	0.01 (0.04)	0.9 (0.7)	1.5 (0.5)	1.7 (1.0)	4.1 (1.6)	0.2 (0.1)	7.4 (1.4)
normal controls	0	0.5 (0.6)	1.2 (0.6)	2.01 (1.6)	3.7 (2.5)	0.2 (0.1)	16.1 (20.4)
	$p < 0.01$	$p < 0.01$	$p < 0.01$	$p < 0.01$	$p < 0.01$	$p < 0.01$	$p < 0.01$
IgA							
RA twins	0.5 (0.7)	3.9 (1.4)	6.3 (2.3)	12.9 (5.3)	4.0 (2.6)	0.4 (0.5)	8.8 (8.2)
normal twins	0	1.2 (0.3)	5.3 (1.0)	7.6 (1.5)	0.5 (0.7)	0.3 (0.3)	3.9 (0.9)
normal controls	0	0.7 (0.5)	3.2 (1.8)	6.1 (3.1)	0.3 (0.5)	0.3 (0.1)	3.4 (1.5)
	$p < 0.01$	$p < 0.01$	$p < 0.05$	$p < 0.01$	$p < 0.01$	NS	$p < 0.05$
IgG							
RA twins	0.2 (0.2)	5.3 (4.2)	7.1 (2.7)	6.8 (2.3)	0.7 (0.5)	2.2 (1.0)	1.1 (0.6)
normal twins	0.05 (0.08)	2.1 (1.0)	5.4 (1.5)	16.7 (6.2)	0	2.8 (1.8)	1.0 (0.6)
normal controls	0.01 (0.04)	1.9 (0.7)	4.0 (1.4)	13.8 (6.5)	0	1.8 (1.5)	0.8 (0.2)
	$p < 0.01$	$p < 0.01$	$p < 0.05$	$p < 0.01$	$p < 0.01$	NS	NS

[a]The sum of the percentages of the IgV determinants in the RF and non-RF fractions in the RA twins was compared with the combined data of the IgV determinants in the normal twins and random controls. The results are given as the mean percentages (standard deviation). NS = not significant.

RESULTS

Levels of the examined IgV determinants were generally higher in the RA twins compared with the normal MZ twins and the random controls (TABLE 1). When levels of the IgV determinants were expressed as percentages of the total non-RF or RF in individual isotypes, a significant proportion of the RF in the RA twins expressed these determinants irrespective of disease status (TABLE 2). Correlation studies revealed that the level of the IgV determinants was significantly related to the levels of IgM RF and to total IgM levels. The level of the IgV determinants, on the other hand, did not

TABLE 2. Total IgV_H Determinant Levels in the RF and Non-RF Fractions in Six MZ RA Twin Pairs[a]

	IgV_H in:					
	IgM–non-RF (%)	IgM–RF (%)	IgA–non-RF (%)	IgA–RF (%)	IgG–non-RF (%)	IgG–RF (%)
mean	26.0	40.0	17.5	31.0	15.5	27.5
SD	6.5	22.1	7.0	10.9	4.2	10.3
significance	NS		$p = 0.005$		$p = 0.004$	

[a]Percentages of the IgV_H determinants detected by G8, B6 or D12, 9G4, and Lc1 monoclonal antibodies were added up for the purpose of this comparison. NS = not significant.

correlate to IgG and IgA isotype levels. The results of the correlation studies also demonstrated close interrelationships between levels of the different IgV determinants within IgM RF. Furthermore, the percentages of IgV determinants in each RF fraction were generally similar in related twins irrespective of disease concordance, but were different between unrelated twins. Similarities in the level of the IgV determinants were significant for the levels of Ig reactive with G6, G8, and Lc1 monoclonal antibodies. The levels of Vκ3 expression, as determined using the C7 monoclonal antibody, were 34% within IgM RF, 24% in IgA RF, 13% in IgG RF, and 19%, 2.3%, and 0.4% within non-RF IgM, non-RF IgA, and non-RF IgG, respectively. The higher level of Vκ3 expression in RF was highly significant (IgM, $p = 0.013$; IgA, $p = 0.06$; IgG, $p < 0.001$).

DISCUSSION

A significant proportion of the produced IgM, IgA, and IgG antibodies in RA twins is encoded by a limited set of germline, or minimally mutated germline, genes. IgV determinants encoded by these germline genes were strongly associated with RF activity. This finding suggests that the increased levels of IgV determinants in the RA twins are likely to be due to the overproduction of RF. This association also suggests that the increased levels may be due to some inherited defects in the molecular or cellular regulatory mechanisms of B lymphocytes expressing RF encoded by these genes. This argument is further substantiated by the observations that similar levels of IgV determinants were detected within twin pairs and different levels between unrelated twin pairs. These observations, however, were independent of disease status, suggesting that this abnormality is related to RF production rather than disease expression. Relatively high levels of IgV determinants were found also within IgA RF and IgG RF, which suggests that significant proportions of these Ig RF isotypes are not extensively mutated. These data also suggest that a significant proportion of RF in RA patients and their twins is not antigen-driven. Alternative mechanisms may include genetic abnormalities within B cells in these individuals or superantigen stimulation.

REFERENCE

1. Sasso, E. H. 1992. Immunoglobulin V genes in rheumatoid arthritis. Rheum. Dis. Clin. North Am. **18:** 809–836.

Comparison of Structural Characteristics of Antisubnucleosome and Anti-DNA Monoclonal Antibodies Derived from Lupus Mice[a]

S. KOUTOUZOV,[b] F. JOVELIN,[c] F. BRARD,[c] G. RAUX,[c]
F. TRON,[c] AND D. GILBERT[c]

[b]*INSERM U25*
Hôpital Necker
Paris, France

[c]*Groupe de Recherche en Immunopathologie*
(Institut Fédératif de Recherche Multidisciplinaire
sur les Peptides 23)
Faculté Mixte de Médecine et de Pharmacie
Hôpital Charles Nicolle
Rouen, France

Systemic lupus erythematosus (SLE) is an autoimmune disease characterized by the production of autoantibodies, in particular, those directed against nuclear antigens. Although the precise identification of the mechanisms involved in the breakdown of B cell tolerance is still lacking, several arguments suggest that the nucleosome might represent the prototype of immunogenic particles responsible for autoantibody production in both human and mouse lupus diseases: (i) besides antideoxyribonucleic acid (DNA) antibodies, IgG specific for nucleosome or subnucleosome structures like H2A-H2B or H2A-H2B/DNA are frequently observed in the course of SLE; (ii) in SLE sera, DNA circulates as DNA-protein complexes and has a size periodicity similar to a nucleosome ladder.[1] The determination of the relationships between antisubnucleosome and anti-DNA antibodies would help elucidate the mechanisms responsible for the breakdown of B cell tolerance to nuclear antigens in SLE. Herewith, we compared the structural characteristics of the variable heavy-chain (V_H) and light-chain (V_L) genes encoding anti–double-stranded DNA (dsDNA) and antisubnucleosome antibodies and showed that their variable regions shared similar structural characteristics and mutation patterns.

The mRNA sequences of the V_H and V_L regions of 6 antisubnucleosome monoclonal antibodies (mAb) obtained by our group and of 13 antisubnucleosome mAb obtained by others, which all derived from lupus mouse strains, were retained for alignment and statistical analysis. All mAb were specific for the H2A-H2B dimer or H2A-H2B/DNA, did not bind to ssDNA or dsDNA, and belonged to the IgG class.

[a]This work was supported by the Institut National de la Santé et de la Recherche Médicale (INSERM, CRI 950602) and the Direction de la Recherche et des Etudes Doctorales.

TABLE 1. Frequency[a] of Amino Acid (AA) Residues at Different Positions of the H-Chain Complementarity Determining Regions (CDR) of Antisubnucleosome mAb, Anti-DNA mAb, and Antibodies from Kabat *et al.*[2]

		mAb		
CDR	AA Position	Antisubnucleosome	Anti-dsDNA	Kabat
1	D/E 31	**63.2**	19.1	25.3
	N 33	0.0	**14.3**	2.5
2	K/R 50	**31.6**	23.8	12.9
	Y 52A	**15.8**	0.0	3.6
	K/R 52C	**25.0**	0.0	0.0
	K/R 53	0.0	**14.3**	2.5
	Y 54	0.0	**9.5**	0.7
	K/R 55	**5.3**	0.0	0.4
	D/E 55	**15.8**	0.0	4.3
	N 55	**10.5**	4.8	0.6
	D/E 56	5.3	**23.8**	3.4
	N 56	**31.6**	**28.6**	8.7
	D/E 58	**36.8**	28.6	14.8
	N 58	**0.0**	14.3	22.3
	D/E 61	**47.4**	33.3	26.8
	N 62	**15.8**	0.0	2.4
3	K/R 95	**42.1**	**23.8**	7.0
	K/R 96	**31.6**	**38.1**	9.7
	Y 96	**0.0**	**0.0**	19.9
	K/R 97	**26.3**	10.0	3.8
	Y 97	**10.5**	**10.0**	32.6
	K/R 98	**29.4**	**31.6**	4.6
	K/R 99	7.7	**27.8**	6.6
	K/R 100	**76.9**	**12.5**	6.0
	K/R 100A	**23.1**	**33.3**	5.5
	K/R 100B	**27.3**	**36.4**	5.8
	Y 100B	**0.0**	**0.0**	28.3
	K/R 100C	12.5	**25.0**	3.3
	Y 100D	50.0	**100.0**	14.9
	D/E 101	**94.7**	71.4	73.9
	N 102	0.0	**4.8**	0.3

[a]Numbers in bold type indicate that the frequency is significantly different from that observed in antibodies from Kabat. Underscored numbers indicate that the frequency is significantly different from that observed in anti-DNA mAb.

Twenty-one anti-DNA mAb were selected from the GenBank database, based on the following criteria: (i) they bound to dsDNA; (ii) the V_H family distribution was similar to that of selected antisubnucleosome mAb; and (iii) they belonged to the IgG isotype. The V_H and V_L mRNA sequences of the selected mAb were aligned according to the numbering of Kabat *et al.*[2] The chi-square and the corrected tests were used to compare, on the one hand, the V_H and V_L sequences of antisubnucleosome, anti-dsDNA, and the large compilation of antibodies reported in Kabat *et al.* and, on the other hand, the distribution of charged amino acids at different positions of the H- and L-chain complementarity determining regions (CDR) of the different antibody populations.

Analysis of the overall structure of the antisubnucleosome V_H regions indicated that they share several features with anti-DNA mAb: they frequently used inverted-D or D-D gene junctions; 14 utilized a J_H4 gene segment that has been demonstrated to be overused in lupus mouse strains; and their CDR3 often had a high content of arginine residues. We next examined, at each position of V_H and V_L CDR, the frequency of positively charged amino acids (aspartate and glutamate), potentially interacting with histones, and of amino acid residues (arginine, lysine, asparagine, and tyrosine) demonstrated to participate in DNA interaction. TABLE 1 shows the frequency of these amino acids in V_H CDR. The V_H CDR1 of antisubnucleosome mAb had two major significant characteristics: a higher frequency of D + E ($p < 0.001$) at position 31 and a lower frequency of asparagine ($p < 0.05$) at position 33 than in anti-dsDNA antibodies. In the V_H CDR2 of antisubnucleosome and anti-dsDNA antibody, the D + E content was similar, but significantly higher than in Kabat's compilation ($p < 0.01$). No significant difference in the V_H CDR3 was observed between the two autoantibody populations, which both exhibited a higher content of positively charged amino acids when compared to mAb contained in Kabat's compilation. The light chains of anti-DNA and antisubnucleosome did not exhibit particular features. However, anti-DNA mAb had a higher content of positively charged amino acids and asparagine residues at certain positions of CDR1 (TABLE 2).

These data show that antisubnucleosome and anti-dsDNA mAb structures differ

TABLE 2. Frequency[a] of Amino Acid (AA) Residues at Different Positions of the L-Chain Complementarity Determining Regions (CDR) of Antisubnucleosome mAb, Anti-DNA mAb, and Antibodies from Kabat *et al.*[2]

		mAb		
CDR	AA Position	Antisubnucleosome	Anti-dsDNA	Kabat
1	K/R 24	52.6	**95.2**	62.8
	D/E 28	**43.8**	14.3	20.7
	N 28	**0.0**	**47.6**	24.5
	N 29	**21.1**	0.0	1.2
	K/R 31	**31.6**	**38.1**	5.1
2	D/E 50	**0.0**	**0.0**	19.6
	N 52	**26.3**	4.8	7.9
	Y 52	**10.5**	0.0	0.6
	K/R 54	**10.5**	42.9	48.4
	N 55	0.0	**4.8**	0.1
	D/E 56	**21.1**	9.5	5.4
	N 56	**5.3**	0.0	0.6
	Y 56	**15.8**	0.0	0.3
3	Y 96	**55.6**	**42.9**	19.6

[a]See footnote to TABLE 1.

from those of antibodies compiled from Kabat's database. In addition, the two autoantibody populations have similar structural properties, in particular, in the V_H CDR2 and the V_H CDR3. Furthermore, study of the binding properties of clonally related antisubnucleosome mAb that differ by a few mutations in their CDR enabled us to show that antisubnucleosome mAb may share mutation patterns similar to those reported for anti-dsDNA antibodies.[3] Taken together, these data suggest that the nucleosome may constitute the common immunogenic structure that both selects and drives the anti-DNA and anti-H2A-H2B autoantibody response.

REFERENCES

1. TAX, W. *et al.* 1995. Apoptosis, nucleosomes, and nephritis in systemic lupus erythematosus. Kidney Int. **48:** 666–673.
2. KABAT, E. A., T. T. WU, H. M. PERRY, K. S. GOTTESMAN & C. FOELLER. 1991. Sequences of Proteins of Immunological Interest. Fifth edition. United States Department of Health and Human Services. Bethesda, Maryland.
3. BRARD, F., F. JOVELIN, S. PETIT, F. TRON & D. GILBERT. 1996. Structural properties and mutation patterns of anti-nucleosome monoclonal antibodies are similar to those of anti-DNA antibodies. Eur. J. Immunol. **26:** 1587–1594.

Site-directed Mutagenesis of Recombinant Human β_2-Glycoprotein I

Effect of Phospholipid Binding and Anticardiolipin Antibody Activity

YONG SHENG,[a] STEVEN A. KRILIS,[a] AND ANDREJ SALI[b]

[a]*Department of Immunology, Allergy, and Infectious Disease*
and
Department of Medicine
University of New South Wales
St. George Hospital
Kogarah NSW 2217, Australia

[b]*The Jane Coffin Child Memorial Fund for Medical Research*
The Rockefeller University
New York, New York 10021

β_2-Glycoprotein I (β_2GPI), a phospholipid-binding plasma protein, has been shown to be the target antigen for antiphospholipid (aPL) antibodies purified from patients with autoimmune disease.[1] Antiphospholipid antibodies that occur in association with infections are not associated with an increased risk of thromboembolic complications[2] and are directed against anionic phospholipids and not β_2GPI.[1]

These antibodies preferentially bind β_2GPI that has been immobilized on anionic phospholipid surfaces, whereas binding in the fluid phase is weak and nondetectable. A number of hypotheses have been put forward to explain this reactivity. It has been proposed that the binding of β_2GPI to PL induces a conformational change in β_2GPI, thus exposing a cryptic epitope for aPL antibodies to bind.[1] Alternatively, it has been suggested that binding of β_2GPI to phospholipid increases the local concentration of β_2GPI, thus promoting an increase in affinity of the aPL antibodies for β_2GPI.[3] β_2GPI is composed of five highly conserved domains of 60 repeating amino acids called complement control protein (CCP) repeats. In β_2GPI, the fifth domain is the most variable and contains a region that has been predicted to be critical for phospholipid binding. To study the interaction between native β_2GPI and anionic PL such as cardiolipin in more detail, we first calculated a 3D model of the fifth domain of β_2GPI (β_2GPI-5), relying on its similarity to the 15th module from human factor H, whose 3D structure has been determined by NMR. The electrostatic calculations confirm that the loop Lys282–Lys287 is likely to be part of the PL-binding site. To test this prediction, the cDNA for human β_2GPI was inserted into a baculovirus vector for expression in insect cells. Site-directed mutagenesis was then performed to assess the role of individual amino acids in the Lys282–Lys287 loop on the phospholipid binding and cofactor activity of β_2GPI. Expressed wild-type β_2GPI had activity equivalent to native β_2GPI. Four mutants were generated: mutants 1, Lys286 to Glu286; 2, Lys286,

287 to Glu286, 287; 3, Lys284, 287 to Glu284, 287; and 4, Lys284, 286, 287 to Glu284, 286, 287. Affinity-purified antibodies from patients with aPL syndrome exhibited binding in a CL-ELISA system only in the presence of recombinant wild-type β_2GPI in a dose-dependent manner similar to that obtained with native human β_2GPI (FIGURE 1). In contrast, no cofactor activity was obtained with mutants 2, 3, and 4 when these were tested up to a concentration of 64 μg/mL (FIGURE 1). However, mutant 1 exhibited a dose-dependent increase in binding that was only

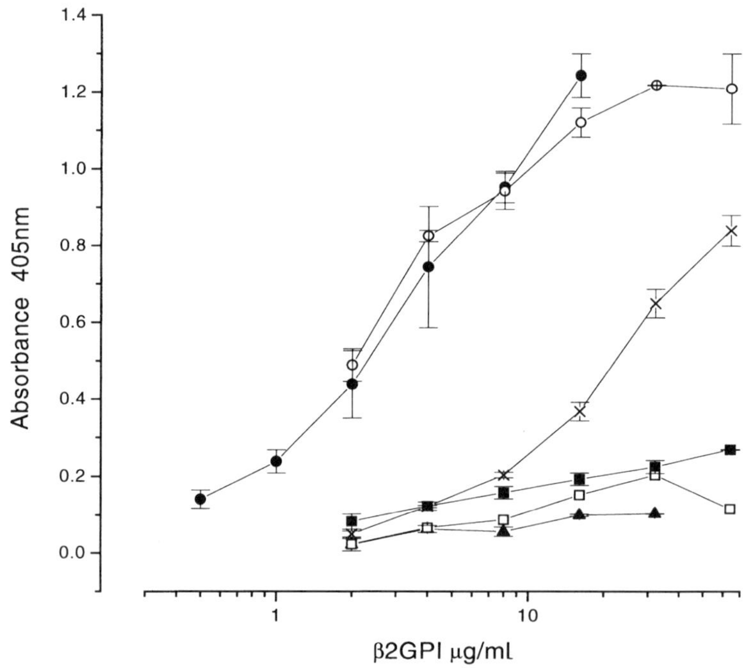

FIGURE 1. Dose response of binding activity of affinity-purified aPL antibody at 2 μg/mL from an autoimmune patient to CL in a modified CL-ELISA in the presence of different preparations of β_2GPI: native β_2GPI (●), recombinant wild-type β_2GPI (○), mutant 1 (×), mutant 2 (■), mutant 3 (▲), and mutant 4 (□). Results are expressed as the mean ± SE of duplicates.

demonstrated at high concentrations of β_2GPI and only reached approximately 50% of that obtained with wild-type β_2GPI (FIGURE 1).

In summary, comparative molecular modeling has predicted that a highly positive charged amino acid sequence, Lys282-Asn-Lys-Glu-Lys-Lys287, located in the fifth domain of β_2GPI is the major PL-binding site. We have tested this hypothesis and have shown that amino acid residues Lys284, 286, and 287 are critical for β_2GPI binding to PL and for cofactor activity for aPL antibodies.

REFERENCES

1. KRILIS, S. A. & J. E. HUNT. 1994. Immunology of antiphospholipid antibodies. *In* Immunology of Connective Tissue Disease. Volume 22. G. S. Panayi, Ed.: 279–304. Kluwer. Dordrecht.
2. MCNEIL, H. P., C. N. CHESTERMAN & S. A. KRILIS. 1991. Adv. Immunol. **49:** 193–279.
3. ROUBEY, R. A. S., R. A. EISENBERG, H. F. HARPER & J. B. WINFIELD. 1995. J. Immunol. **154**(2): 954–960.

Herpes Viruses in Multicase Families with Rheumatoid Arthritis and Systemic Lupus Erythematosus

C. DOSTÁL,[a] M. M. NEWKIRK,[b] K. N. WATANABE DUFFY,[b] A. PALEČKOVÁ,[a] V. BOŠÁK,[c] M. ČERNÁ,[a] E. ŽD'ÁRSKÝ,[a] AND J. ZVÁROVÁ[a]

[a]*Institute of Rheumatology Prague 2, the Czech Republic*

[b]*Division of Rheumatology McGill University Montreal, Canada*

[c]*Research Institute of Rheumatic Disease Piešt'any, Slovakia*

INTRODUCTION

The etiology of rheumatoid arthritis (RA) and systemic lupus erythematosus (SLE) is unknown, but likely involves a number of factors both genetic and environmental. The role of infection either as a trigger mechanism or as a contributor to the morbidity is receiving close attention. A number of viruses, among them the herpetic, have been suggested to have a role in the etiology of RA[1] and SLE.[2] The aim of this study was to investigate the presence of infection by Epstein-Barr virus (EBV), herpes-virus 6 (HHV-6), and cytomegalovirus (CMV), in cells from saliva and peripheral blood, of families (affected and nonaffected members) with multiple cases of RA or SLE, using polymerase chain reaction (PCR) techniques.

PATIENTS

Members of 13 families with RA, 5 families with SLE, and 1 family with no history of autoimmune disease, used as a control, were drawn from the Czech Republic and Slovakia. Altogether, there were 30 affected and 21 nonaffected members of RA families and 11 affected and 17 nonaffected members of SLE families. The diagnosis of definite RA and SLE disease was determined according to established diagnostic criteria. No family member had any evidence of clinical symptoms suggestive of EBV, HHV-6, or CMV infection and no patient had any symptoms of secondary Sjögren's syndrome.

METHODS

Isolation of DNA from Investigated Cells

Genomic DNA was isolated from saliva and peripheral blood leukocytes and lymphocytes using phenol-chloroform extraction.

TABLE 1. Presence of Viral DNA EBV, HHV-6, and CMV in Diseased and Healthy Members of 13 RA and 5 SLE Multicase Families and in 1 Control Healthy Family

Virus	Family Members	Saliva Cells (+/*n*)	%	PB Lymphocytes (+/*n*)	%	$PB_{polymorphonuclear}$ (+/*n*)	%
EBV	RA	19/27	70[a]	14/29	48[b]	8/30	27
	non-RA	11/20	55	2/20	10	2/20	10
	control	3/4	—	1/4	—	0/4	—
HHV-6	RA	8/27	30[a]	13/29	45[b]	5/30	17
	non-RA	7/19	37	2/18	11	7/19	37
	control	1/4	—	1/4	—	1/4	—
CMV	RA	4/27	15	2/30	7	1/30	3
	non-RA	3/19	16	3/20	15	3/20	15
	control	1/4	—	0/4	—	1/4	—
EBV	SLE	7/10	70	0/10	—	0/10	—
	non-SLE	11/16	69	0/10	—	0/10	—
	control	3/4	—	1/4	—	0/4	—
HHV-6	SLE	0/10	—	4/10	40[b]	0/10	—
	non-SLE	4/16	25	3/16	19	1/16	6
	control	1/4	—	1/4	—	1/4	—
CMV	SLE	0/10	—	0/10	—	0/10	—
	non-SLE	0/10	—	2/16	13	0/10	—
	control	1/4	—	0/4	—	1/4	—

[a]Fisher's test: not significant.
[b]Fisher's test: $p < 0.01$.

Viral DNA

For detection of viral DNA in the human genome, we used two techniques. In the first case, the amplified DNA products from the three different cells were resolved on the same agarose gel for each individual family and transferred to nitrocellulose to enable comparative analysis. After radioactive hybridization, the blots were exposed to X-ray film and the densities were quantitated by laser densitometry.[3] In the second case, an established semiquantitative PCR allowed the visualization in agarose gel after amplification, but with a higher quantity of input DNA.

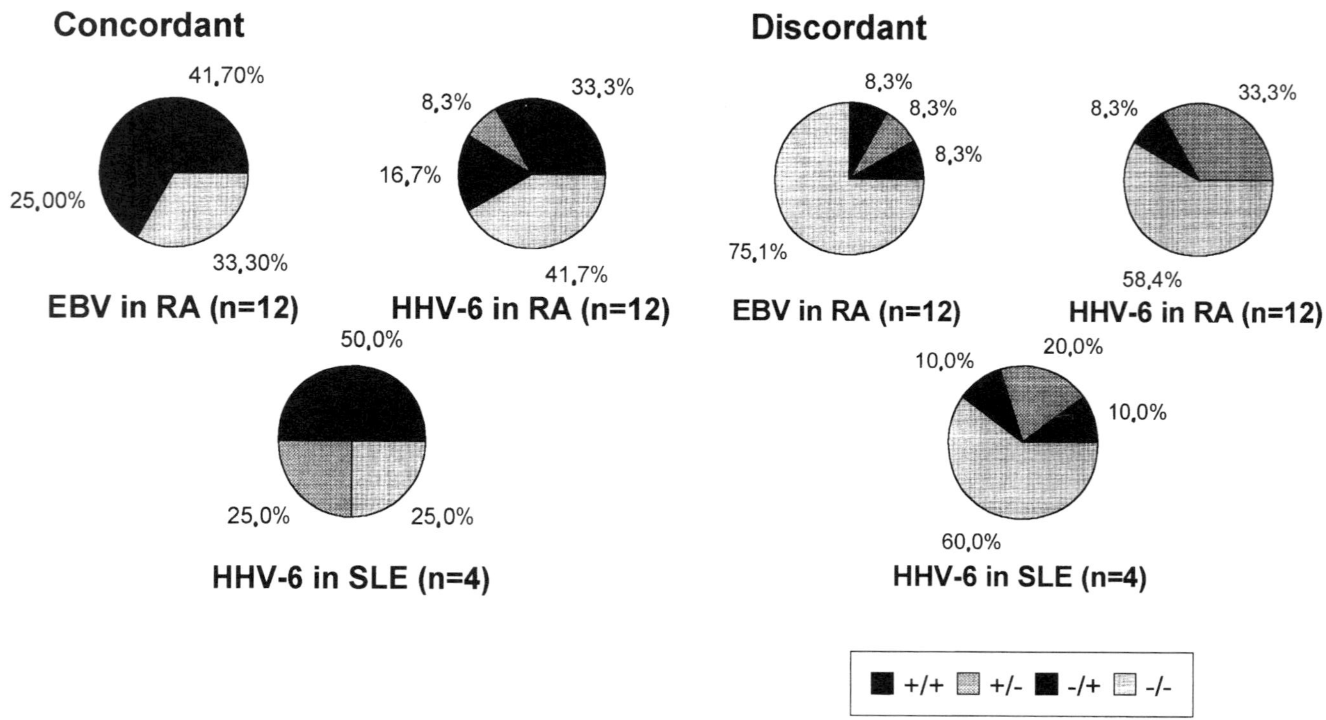

FIGURE 1. Presence of viral DNA in sibling pairs in peripheral blood lymphocytes according to RA and SLE concordance.

Tissue Typing

All individuals were tested for human leukocyte antigen class I and class II using the standard microlymphocytotoxicity assay and for HLA class II genes by sequence-specific primer PCR.

RESULTS

Of the three herpetic viruses investigated, the EBV DNA was found in the highest frequency in both the multicase RA and SLE families. Saliva appeared to be the most frequently colonized compartment, but without any difference between affected and nonaffected members (TABLE 1). Significantly increased EBV DNA accumulation was observed in lymphocytes from peripheral blood (PB) in the RA-affected members as compared to nonaffected members. For HHV-6 DNA, the same accumulation in members of RA families was seen, exhibiting a significantly increased difference in affected compared to nonaffected members in lymphocytes of peripheral blood. No significant differences in CMV DNA were observed. When comparing EBV and HHV-6 infection in peripheral blood lymphocytes of sibling pairs according to disease concordance, we found that there was a high frequency of discordant pairs who were completely negative for infection (approximately 65%). Disease-concordant sibling pairs were also concordant for infection, but only half were infected (FIGURE 1).

CONCLUSIONS

Our observation of elevated accumulation of selected herpetic viruses in lymphocytes from affected members of RA and SLE multicase families may reflect a possible role in the etiopathogenesis or in the process of the natural course of these diseases or that these individuals are more susceptible to such infections.

REFERENCES

1. ZHANG, L., S. NIKKARI, M. SKURNIK, T. ZIEGLER, R. LUNKKAINEN, T. MÖTTÖNEN & P. TOIVANEN. 1993. Detection of herpes viruses by polymerase chain reaction in lymphocytes from patients with rheumatoid arthritis. Arthritis Rheum. **36**(8): 1081–1086.
2. KALDEN, J. R. & S. GAY. 1994. Retroviruses and autoimmune rheumatic diseases. Clin. Exp. Immunol. **98:** 1–5.
3. NEWKIRK, M. M., K. N. WATANABE DUFFY, A. PALEČKOVÁ, E. IVAŠKOVÁ, A. GALIANOVÁ, K. SEEMAN, K. VOJTĚCHOVSKÝ & C. DOSTÁL. 1995. Herpes viruses in multicase families with rheumatoid arthritis. J. Rheumatol. **22:** 2055–2061.

Use of Phage Expression to Analyze Regions of a Human $V_{4\text{-}34}(V_H4\text{-}21)$-encoded IgG Autoantibody Required for Recognition of DNA

No Involvement of the 9G4 Idiotope[a]

IAN MOCKRIDGE, CAROLINE CHAPMAN, MYFANWY SPELLERBERG, DAVID ISENBERG, AND FREDA STEVENSON[b]

Molecular Immunology Group
Tenovus Laboratory
Southampton University Hospitals
Southampton SO16 6YD, United Kingdom

The $V_{4\text{-}34}$ gene encodes the majority of autoanti–red cell antibodies of I/i specificity[1] as well as a number of IgM and IgG anti-DNA antibodies from patients with systemic lupus erythematosus (SLE).[2] Nucleotide sequence analysis of a panel of monoclonal antibodies (MoAbs) that use this gene has indicated that discrimination between different autoantigens may arise from the CDR3 sequence of V_H. Specifically, anti-DNA activity may require basic amino acids, such as arginine, found in this region. To test this, we have expressed V_H and V_L sequences from a patient's IgG anti-DNA MoAb, as Fab molecules at the surface of phage. The influence of the basic CDR3, of somatic mutations in V_H, and of the V_L gene on recognition of DNA has been assessed. The 9G4 idiotope, located in FWR1 of V_H and known to be involved in red cell recognition, has been found to have no influence on DNA binding.

METHODS

V_H and V_L genes were amplified from D5, an IgG anti-DNA MoAb.[2] Control V_H was from FIF, a MoAb with anti–red cell activity, and unmutated sequence. Control V_L (17B) was an unmutated VκIIIb (A27) gene. Genes were amplified using specific primers[2] and ligated into pHEN expression system[3] in various combinations. The CDR3-J region of D5 V_H was PCR-amplified and used as a primer together with the 5′ V_H4-21 oligonucleotide to introduce this region into the control FIF V_H. pHEN1 Fab

[a]This study was supported by the Arthritis and Rheumatism Council, United Kingdom.
[b]To whom all correspondence should be addressed.

constructs were used to transform *E. coli* TG1 cells, and phage expression was induced by infection with helper phage and incubation overnight at 30 °C. Phage particles were purified as described.[3] Levels of expression of Fab, anti-DNA activity, and idiotope expression were measured by ELISA.

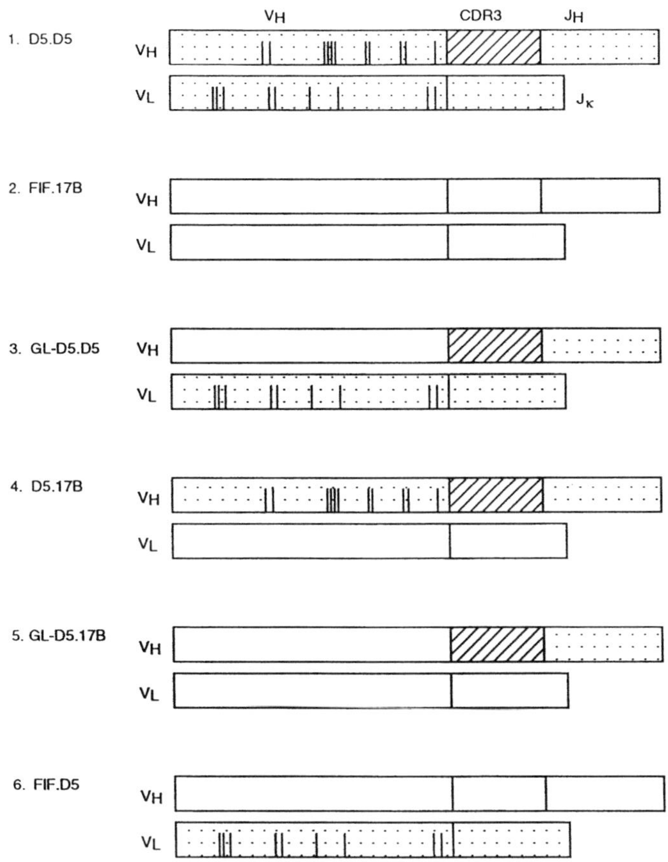

FIGURE 1. Constructs assembled as $V_{4\text{-}34}$/VκIIIb Fab on phage surfaces. Terms—1. D5.D5: homologous V_H-V_L pair from MoAb D5; 2. FIF.17B: control pair of unmutated V_H from an anti–red cell MoAb FIF, with unmutated VκIIIb 17B; 3. GL-D5.D5: homologous pair from D5 with somatic mutations removed from V_H; 4. D5.17B: heterologous pair; 5. GL-D5.17B: heterologous pair with somatic mutations removed from V_H; 6. FIF.D5: heterologous pair. Vertical lines indicate the positions of somatic mutations leading to replacement amino acids.

RESULTS

Recombinant Fab constructs were assembled (FIGURE 1) and tested. Specificity of homologous Fab (D5.D5) for ss/dsDNA reflected that of the original D5 MoAb (not shown), and control Fab gave insignificant binding. Comparison of binding of D5.D5 with a construct from which all somatic mutations in V_H had been removed (GL-D5.D5) revealed no loss of activity (FIGURE 2). In contrast, exchange of D5 V_L for unmutated 17B V_L (D5.17B) reduced binding by ~50%. However, D5 V_L could not confer anti-DNA activity on FIF V_H (FIF.D5). The construct with GL-D5 V_H paired with control V_L (GL-D5.17B) was inferior to D5.17B, suggesting that somatic mutations in V_H may play a minor role in this pairing.

All constructs expressed the 9G4 idiotope.[2] Change of Trp at position 7 of D5 V_H to Ser completely ablated idiotope expression, but there was no effect on binding of DNA.

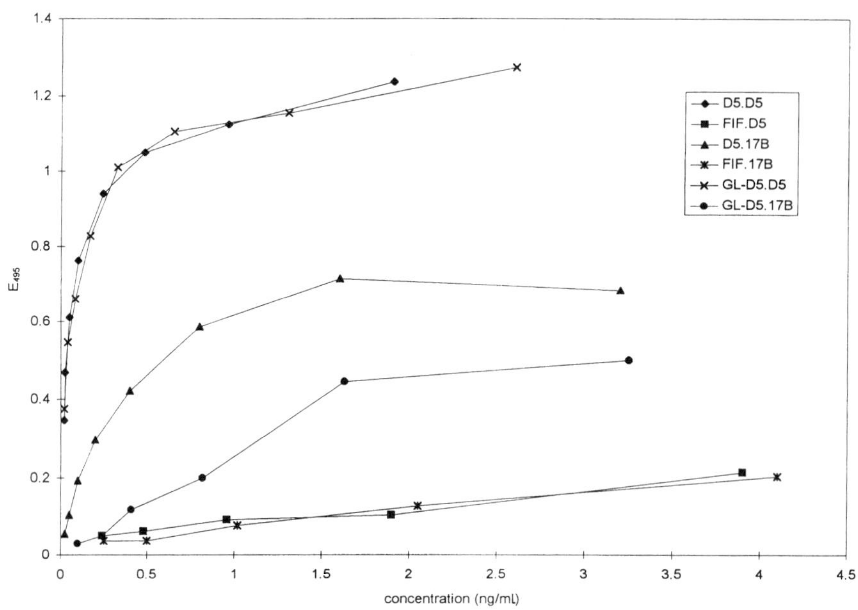

FIGURE 2. Binding of phage-expressed Fab molecules to ssDNA. Fab molecules derived from homologous, heterologous, or mutant V_H-V_L pairs were expressed at phage surfaces and tested for anti-ssDNA activity by ELISA. Bound phage was detected by sheep anti-phage antibody, followed by HRP-rabbit anti-sheep IgG.

DISCUSSION

Expression of recombinant Fab at the surface of phage has been used to assess the contribution of V region sequences to recognition of ssDNA, by a human IgG MoAb encoded by the $V_{4\text{-}34}$ V_H gene. A significant role for basic CDR3 has been confirmed, with a surprising lack of influence of somatic mutations in V_H. In contrast, mutations in V_L appear to have a role. The 9G4 idiotope lies in FWR1 and has a major influence on recognition of red cells by $V_{4\text{-}34}$-encoded IgM. The Trp at position 7 in FWR1 appears crucial for idiotope expression, but its removal has no effect on recognition of DNA. These findings indicate that DNA autoantigen, unlike red cell antigen, is acting as a conventional B cell antigen.

REFERENCES

1. PASCUAL, V., K. VICTOR, M. SPELLERBERG, T. J. HAMBLIN, F. K. STEVENSON & J. D. CAPRA. 1992. V_H restriction among human cold agglutinins: the V_H4-21 gene segment is required to encode anti-I and anti-i specificities. J. Immunol. **149:** 2337–2344.
2. STEVENSON, F. K., C. LONGHURST, C. J. CHAPMAN, M. EHRENSTEIN, M. B. SPELLERBERG, T. J. HAMBLIN, C. T. RAVIRAJAN, D. LATCHMAN & D. ISENBERG. 1993. Utilization of the V_H4-21 gene segment by anti-DNA antibodies from patients with systemic lupus erythematosus. J. Autoimmun. **16:** 809–825.
3. HOOGENBOOM, H. R., A. D. GRIFFITHS, K. S. JOHNSON, D. J. CHISWELL, P. HUDSON & G. WINTER. 1991. Multi-subunit proteins on the surface of filamentous phage: methodologies for displaying antibody (Fab) heavy and light chains. Nucleic Acids Res. **19:** 4133–4137.

Induction of Autoimmunity

A Role for the Idiotypic Network[a]

YEHUDA SHOENFELD AND JACOB GEORGE

Department of Medicine "B"
and
Research Unit of Autoimmune Diseases
Sheba Medical Center
Tel-Hashomer 52621, Israel
and
Sackler Faculty of Medicine
Tel Aviv University
Tel Aviv, Israel

INTRODUCTION

Autoimmune disorders are diverse and heterogeneous and their etiology remains enigmatic despite intensive and prolonged investigation. It has been suggested from cumulative data that the autoimmune state and disease "require" a triggering event (e.g., infectious episode) and a distinct milieu (e.g., HLA predisposition, distinct hormonal and immunologic status, and environmental conditions) to become clinically overt.[1]

The uncertainties spanning the definition and understanding of the nature of autoimmunity have been temporarily reduced following the establishment and subsequent revision of the Rose/Witebsky criteria[2] as means of characterizing the so-called "classic" autoimmune diseases. One of the principles set by these classic criteria requires the induction of autoimmune disease by immunization with the autoantigen (emulsified in adjuvant), towards which the immune system generates an attack (as has been shown, for example, in myasthenia gravis, autoimmune hemolytic anemia, and pemphigus vulgaris). Also addressed by these criteria is the issue of passive transfer of a pathogenic autoantibody with resultant clinical manifestations of the respective autoimmune disease, as a tool for defining a disease as autoimmune. In recent years, a significant number of studies performed by us[3–17] and others[18–21] have put forward the role of induction of autoimmune diseases by active immunization with the respective autoantibodies.[3] The roots of this concept lie in the initial hypothesis proposed by Jerne[22] in 1974, stating that the immune response may be modulated via unique antigenic determinants of the immunoglobulin variable regions (idiotypes). Accordingly, these determinants are complemented by other respective antibodies, thus establishing a functional network with alternating immunoglobulin expressions. The essentials of the idea are that an autoantigen may lead to the generation of

[a]This work was supported by the Felix and Ruta Zandman Grant for Research in Autoimmunity.

antibodies (Ab1), with the serologically unique structure of which (Ab1 idiotype) resulting in production of anti-idiotypic antibodies (Ab2). The latter antibodies recognize (similar to the antigen) the binding site of Ab1 and therefore may bear structural similarity and binding properties with the autoantigen. In the same manner, Ab2 are capable of eliciting the generation of anti-anti-idiotypic antibodies (Ab3) and so on. We may also view this intercalated network as arising following the introduction of an antibody acting much as the antigen in initiating this resultant cascade.

In the following lines, we will demonstrate the applications of the above-mentioned principles in clinical practice; namely, we will provide evidence supporting the role of idiotypic dysregulation (by immunization with a target autoantibody) in induction of experimental autoimmune diseases in murine models. Furthermore, circumstantial studies substantiating the importance of the idiotypic network in the emergence of the autoimmune state will be presented.

IDIOTYPIC INDUCTION OF AUTOIMMUNE DISEASE IN ANIMAL MODELS

Induction of Experimental SLE by Immunization with Anti-DNA Antibodies

It has been shown by us[4–6] and others[20,21] that immunization of different mice strains with monoclonal or polyclonal murine and human anti-DNA that carry a pathogenic idiotype results in the production of a wide array of lupus-associated antibodies (i.e., anti-DNA, anti-Sm, anti-Ro-SS-A, antihistones) by the mice, a phenomenon referred to by us as "autoantibody spread". In parallel, the mice were found to develop clinical findings consistent with human SLE, including increased erythrocyte sedimentation rate (ESR), leukopenia, thrombocytopenia, proteinuria, alopecia, and paralysis. Furthermore, the deposition of anti-DNA antibodies has been confirmed within the glomeruli, skin, and brain of the mice.

The studies were repeated successfully with a similar protocol containing monoclonal antibodies generated by the hybridoma technique with lymphocytes obtained from the mice with induced experimental SLE.[6]

The support for the role of idiotypes and T cells in this proposed model was validated by accomplishing induction of SLE with T cell lines specific for idiotypes[8] and by complete abolishment of the disease by transfusion of specific idiotype T suppressor cells following the disease induction.[9]

Experimental Antiphospholipid Syndrome (APS) Induced by Immunization with Anticardiolipin Antibodies (aCL)

The presence of anticardiolipin antibodies and/or lupus anticoagulant in the sera of patients with antiphospholipid syndrome is thought to predispose them to the occurrence of thrombocytopenia, thromboembolic phenomena, and fetal wastage. It was shown that immunization of naive mice with either human or mouse monoclonal or polyclonal aCL led to the production of murine aCL, 3–4 months following administration of the antibody.[10,11,18] Concomitant with the serological pattern generated by the immunized mice, they were also found to develop thrombocytopenia, prolonged activated thromboplastin time (aPTT), and a low fecundity rate with increased fetal resorptions upon mating. These clinical manifestations are consistent with human APS. *In vivo* evidence of a hypercoagulable state has been shown by the detection of significant thromboses in some of the fetuses.[10]

Idiotypic Manipulation with Antineutrophil Cytoplasmic Antibodies (ANCA)

Wegener's granulomatosis (WG) is a granulomatous vasculitis that involves the upper respiratory tract, lungs, and kidneys. Its clinical expression, however, is wider, encompassing fever, skin abnormalities, peripheral neuropathy, arthralgia/arthritis, and inflammatory changes in the eyes. WG is considered autoimmune, among other things, owing to its association with ANCA, which are predominantly directed against proteinase-3 (PR-3), a serine protease in the azurophil granules of polymorphonuclears. Immunization of naive mice with ANCA-enriched IgG[12,13] has led to the production of mouse ANCA. Starting from 6 months following immunization, the mice were shown to develop signs of vasculitis and focal mononuclear infiltrates in the lungs, and immunofluorescence studies of the renal section disclosed granular deposition of immunoglobulins in the glomeruli.[12] This histopathological picture may provide proof for the direct role of ANCA in the pathogenesis of Wegener's associated vasculitis.

Idiotypic Manipulation with Antithyroglobulin Antibodies (hTg)

Experimental autoimmune thyroiditis is an organ-specific autoimmune disease mediated by T cytotoxic cells. We have been able to show that immunization of naive mice with monoclonal mouse antihuman thyroglobulin antibodies has led to activation of the idiotypic cascade with resultant elaboration of mouse antihuman thyroglobulin antibodies (Ab3) and decreased levels of thyroid hormones.[14] Yet, it should be mentioned that we were not able to demonstrate histopathological changes in the immunized mice.

Idiotypic Manipulation with Antiglomerular Basement Membrane Antibodies (GBM)

Goodpasture's syndrome (GPS) is characterized by a triad of glomerulonephritis with hematuria, pulmonary hemorrhage, and anti-GBM antibodies. The syndrome is considered autoimmune in nature and anti-GBM antibodies that are incriminated as mediating the tissue damage are primarily directed to the $\alpha 3$ chain of type IV collagen. The epitope towards which the antibodies are aimed had been located to the globular noncollagenous domain (NC1) of the $\alpha 3$ (IV) chain. We have used mouse monoclonal anti-NC1 antibodies and IgG serum fractions from GPS patients to immunize naive mice in attempts to reproduce GPS-like findings.[15] The involvement of the idiotypic network could be observed by the emergence of murine anti-NC1 antibodies (Ab3) and either erythrocyturia or proteinuria in some of the mice.

Idiotypic Manipulation with Anti-U1-ribonucleoprotein (RNP) Antibodies

Mixed connective tissue disease (MCTD) is a hybrid autoimmune entity encompassing clinical findings of other well-defined autoimmune diseases. The serological hallmarks of MCTD are high titers of antibodies directed against various epitopes within the U1RNP complex. We have recently immunized several groups of naive mice with different epitope-specific anti-U1RNP preparations obtained from MCTD patients with different disease manifestations.[16] Although no histopathological findings were found in the mice, an intriguing pattern of autoantibody reactivity was produced: it was found by immunoblotting that, regardless of the epitope specificity of the antibody used for immunization, the mice developed antibodies against the 68–70-kDa protein in the RNP complex. This reaction, which has been termed "autoantibody dominance", provided additional support for the existence of idiotypic connectivities as engaged actively in the global immune response.

Idiotypic Manipulation with Antiendothelial Cell Antibodies (AECA)

Active immunization of BALB/c (naive) mice with affinity-purified AECA has also been recently contemplated.[17] Three months after a boost injection with human AECA, mice developed endogenous AECA (Ab3), but not antibodies to proteinase-3, cardiolipin, or DNA. Histological examination of lungs and kidneys revealed lymphoid cell infiltration surrounding arterioles and venules, as well as deposition of immunoglobulins at the outer part of blood vessel walls. This experimental animal model has provided the first direct proof for the pathogenicity of AECA.

CONCLUDING REMARKS

Apart from the comprehensive data furnished by the various experimental models (summarized in TABLE 1), it appears that the concept of idiotypic network is supported by indirect studies. Accordingly, because a complementary set of idiotypes are to be generated in response to an administered antibody, it has been assumed that the cascade of idiotypes to follow could be halted by various manipulations. Thus, it seems conceivable that the models of experimental SLE and APS could be suppressed by treatment with intravenous gamma globulin (IVGG)[23,24] preparations that possess specific anti-idiotypic properties. Moreover, it has been shown that successful modulation of experimental SLE has been accomplished by using specific monoclonal anti-idiotypic (anti-16/6 idiotype) antibodies conjugated to saporin,[25] thus further supporting the role of idiotypic dysregulation in the promotion of autoimmune disease induction.

TABLE 1. Representative Experimental Autoimmune Models Induced by Idiotypic Manipulation[a]

Autoantibody Used for Immunization	Characteristic Binding of Mice Autoantibodies	Clinical Findings	Reference
Anti-16/6 (H) mAb	DNA, histones, Sm, Ro/SSA	elevated ESR, leukopenia, thrombocytopenia, proteinuria, alopecia, paralysis	4
Anti-16/6 (H) polyclonal	DNA, nuclear antigen	proteinuria, alopecia	19
Anti-16/6 (M)	DNA, histones, Sm, Ro/SSA	elevated ESR, leukopenia, thrombocytopenia, alopecia, paralysis	6
Anti-16/6 (MIV 7) (H)	ssDNA, dsDNA, histones, CL, phosphatidylserine	elevated ESR, leukopenia, thrombocytopenia, alopecia, proteinuria, fetal wastage, prolonged aPTT	8
Anti-Sm, 4B4 idiotype (H) mAb	dsDNA, ssDNA, Sm, ribonucleoprotein	not evaluated	21
H-3 mAb aCL (H)	CL, dsDNA, lupus anticoagulant	thrombocytopenia, increased fetal resorption, prolonged aPTT, smaller size of fetuses and placenta	10
Purified aCL (H)	CL, lupus anticoagulant	thrombocytopenia, low fecundity rate, prolonged aPTT	11
Purified anti-cardiolipin (H)	CL, β_2GPI	not evaluated	18
Purified ANCA (H)	proteinase-3, endothelial cells	sterile microabscesses (lung), proteinuria	12
	MPO	perivascular lung infiltrates, induced respiratory burst in neutrophils	13
Purified AECA (H)	endothelial cells	lymphoid cell infiltration surrounding arterioles and venules, deposition of immunoglobulins at the outer part of blood vessel walls	17
hTg mAb (H)	thyroglobulin	low production of thyroid hormones	14
Anti-NC1 mAb (M)	NC1	erythrocyturia, proteinuria, beaded podocytes	15
Anti-U1RNP polyclonal (H)	restricted reactivity to 68–70-kDa epitope	not observed	16

[a]Abbreviations: H, human; M, mouse; mAb, monoclonal antibody; CL, cardiolipin; ESR, erythrocyte sedimentation rate; NC, noncollagenous; AECA, antiendothelial cell antibodies; hTg, human thyroglobulin; MPO, myeloperoxidase.

As can be viewed from most of the models presented above, active immunization of naive mice with various specific autoantibodies (Ab1) led to the production of mice Ab2, which resulted in the elaboration of anti-anti-antibodies (Ab3). Concomitant with the generation of Ab3 (mouse-respective antibodies), clinical findings of autoimmune character were exemplified in many of the mice, corresponding to the matching disease in humans. An additional intriguing phenomenon that we have observed following immunization with specific autoantibodies (found in sera of patients with the respective disease) is the production of mice autoantibodies with different antigenic specificities characteristic of the specific autoimmune disease. This diversification of the immune response seen in the sera of the mice has been designated by us as "autoantibody spread", which may explain the diverse panoply of autoantibodies detected in patients with autoimmune diseases.

The above animal models have led us to assume that, in humans, a similar phenomenon could be induced by a triggering event (e.g., an infectious agent resulting in the production of human antibodies carrying pathogenic idiotypes) in a "susceptible" individual (e.g., prone to autoimmune disease because of a certain genetic background or immunological or hormonal status). Circumstantial support for this hypothesis is based on studies in which high titers of pathogenic idiotypes have been detected in the sera of patients following infections with *Klebsiella*, *Mycobacterium tuberculosis*, and pneumococci.[3,26] This may provide an appealing theory to the emergence of autoimmune diseases.

Furthermore, the animal models by which idiotypic manipulations have been contemplated are well in accord with the concept of autoimmune diseases being multifactorial entities arising following an interplay of various immunological, genetic, hormonal, and environmental factors in the context of a pathogenic idiotype introduced to the immune system.

Future prospects regarding prevention and treatment of autoimmune disease in our opinion should take into account these assumptions and apply these principles when planning immunomodulatory regimens.

REFERENCES

1. SHOENFELD, Y. & D. A. ISENBERG. 1989. The mosaic of autoimmunity. Immunol. Today **10:** 123–126.
2. ROSE, N. R. & C. BONA. 1993. Defining criteria for autoimmune diseases: Witebsky's criteria revisited. Immunol. Today **14:** 426–430.
3. SHOENFELD, Y. 1994. Idiotypic induction of autoimmunity: a new aspect of the idiotypic network. FASEB J. **8:** 1296–1303.
4. MENDLOVIC, S., S. BROCKE, Y. SHOENFELD, *et al.* 1988. Induction of SLE-like disease in mice by a common anti-DNA idiotype. Proc. Natl. Acad. Sci. U.S.A. **85:** 2260–2264.
5. BLANK, M., S. MENDLOVIC, E. MOSES, *et al.* 1989. Induction of SLE-like disease in naive mice with monoclonal anti-DNA antibody derived from a patient with polymyositis carrying 16/6 Id. J. Autoimmun. **1:** 683–691.
6. BLANK, M., M. KRUP, S. MENDLOVIC, H. FRICK, E. MOSES, N. TALAL, A. R. M. COATES & Y. SHOENFELD. 1990. The importance of the pathogenic 16/6 idiotype in the induction of SLE in naive mice. Scand. J. Immunol. **31:** 45–52.

7. Blank, M., I. Krause, M. Ben-Bassat & Y. Shoenfeld. 1992. Induction of antiphospholipid associated with SLE following immunization with human monoclonal pathogenic anti-DNA idiotype. J. Autoimmun. **5:** 495–509.
8. Blank, M., S. Mendlovic, E. Moses, A. R. M. Coates & Y. Shoenfeld. 1991. Induction of SLE in naive mice with T cell lines specific for human anti-DNA antibody SA-1 (16/6+ Id) and for mouse tuberculous antibody (16/6+ Id). Clin. Immunol. Immunopathol. **60:** 471–483.
9. Blank, M., M. Ben-Bassat & Y. Shoenfeld. 1991. Modulation of SLE induction in naive mice by specific T cells with suppressor activity to pathogenic anti-DNA idiotype. Cell. Immunol. **137:** 474–486.
10. Bakimer, R., P. Fishman, M. Blank, B. Srendi, M. Djaldetti & Y. Shoenfeld. 1992. Induction of primary anti-phospholipid syndrome in naive mice by immunization with a human monoclonal anti-cardiolipin antibody. J. Clin. Invest. **89:** 1558–1563.
11. Cohen, J., R. Bakimer, M. Blank, G. Valesini & Y. Shoenfeld. 1994. Pathogenic anticardiolipin antibodies: the experience from monoclonal gammopathy. Clin. Exp. Immunol. **97:** 181–186.
12. Blank, M., Y. Tomer, M. Stein, J. Kopolovic, A. Wiik, P. L. Meroni, G. Conforti & Y. Shoenfeld. 1995. Immunization with anti-neutrophil cytoplasmic antibody (ANCA) induces the production of mouse ANCA and perivascular lymphocyte infiltration. Clin. Exp. Immunol. **102:** 120–130.
13. Tomer, Y., B. Gilburd, M. Blank, O. Lider, R. Hershkoviz, P. Fishman, R. Zigelman, P. L. Meroni, A. Wiik & Y. Shoenfeld. 1995. Characterization of biologically active antineutrophil cytoplasmic antibodies induced in mice. Arthritis Rheum. **38:** 1375–1381.
14. Tomer, Y., B. Gilburd, J. Sack, T. F. Davies, A. Meshorer, C. L. Burek, N. R. Rose & Y. Shoenfeld. 1996. Induction of thyroid autoantibodies in naive mice by idiotypic manipulation. Clin. Immunol. Immunopathol. In press.
15. Shoenfeld, Y., B. Gilburd, M. Hojnic, M. Damianovich, S. Hacham, Y. Kopolovic, S. Polak-Charcon, I. Goldberg, A. Afec, L. Hun-Chi & J. B. Peter. 1996. Induction of Goodpasture antibodies to noncollagenous domain (NC1) of type IV collagen in mice by idiotypic manipulation. Hum. Antib. Hybrid. **6:** 122–128.
16. Gilburd, B., J. George, A. Afec, M. Damianovich, A. Doria, S. Todesco & Y. Shoenfeld. 1996. "Autoantibody dominance" pattern following idiotypic manipulation of naive mice with different epitope-specific anti-U1RNP antibodies. Submitted.
17. Damianovich, M., B. Gilburd, J. George, N. Del Papa, A. Afec, I. Goldberg, Y. Kopolovic, D. Roth, G. Barkai, P. L. Meroni & Y. Shoenfeld. 1996. Pathogenic role of antiendothelial cell antibodies (AECA) in vasculitis: an idiotypic experimental model. J. Immunol. **156:** 4946–4951.
18. Pierangeli, S. S. & E. N. Harris. 1993. Induction of phospholipid antibodies in mice and rabbits by immunization with human beta-2 glycoprotein-1 or anticardiolipin antibodies alone. Clin. Exp. Immunol. **93:** 269.
19. Tincani, A., G. Balestrieri, F. Allegri, R. Cattaneo, A. Fornasieri, M. Li, A. Sinico & G. D'Amico. 1993. Induction of experimental SLE in naive mice by immunization with human polyclonal anti-DNA antibody carrying the 16/6 idiotype. Clin. Exp. Rheumatol. **11:** 129–134.
20. Rombach, E., D. A. Stetler & J. C. Brown. 1992. Rabbits produce SLE-like anti-RNA polymerase I and anti-DNA autoantibodies in response to immunization with either human or murine SLE anti-DNA antibodies. Autoimmunity **13:** 291–302.
21. Dang, H., N. Ogawa, M. Takei, K. Lazaridis & N. Talal. 1993. Induction of lupus-associated autoantibodies by immunization with native and recombinant Ig polypeptides expressing a cross-reactive idiotype 4B4. J. Immunol. **151:** 7260.
22. Jerne, N. K. 1974. Towards a network theory of the immune system. Ann. Immunol. (Paris) **125c:** 373–389.
23. Bakimer, R., B. Gilburd, N. Zurgil & Y. Shoenfeld. 1993. The effect of intravenous γ-globulin on the induction of experimental antiphospholipid syndrome. Clin. Immunol. Immunopathol. **69:** 97–102.

24. KRAUSE, I., M. BLANK, J. KOPOLOVIC, A. AFEC, I. GOLDBERG, Y. TOMER & Y. SHOENFELD. 1995. Abrogation of experimental systemic lupus erythematosus and primary antiphospholipid syndrome with intravenous gamma globulin. J. Rheumatol. **22:** 1068–1074.
25. BLANK, M., J. MANSROI, Y. TOMER, A. MANSROI, J. KOPOLOVIC, S. POLAK-CHARCON & Y. SHOENFELD. 1994. Suppression of experimental SLE with specific anti-idiotypic antibody-saporin conjugate. Clin. Exp. Immunol. **98:** 434–441.
26. SHOENFELD, Y. & E. MOSES. 1990. Pathogenic idiotypes of antibodies and autoimmunity: lessons from new experimental models of SLE. FASEB J. **4:** 2646–2651.

B Cell Presentation of Cartilage Type II Collagen to T Cells

RIKARD HOLMDAHL, ERIK MICHAËLSSON, AND MIKAEL VESTBERG

Department of Cell and Molecular Biology
Section for Medical Inflammation Research
Lund University
S-22100 Lund, Sweden

Arthritis can be induced in mice after a single immunization with the cartilage-specific type II collagen (CII)—the collagen-induced arthritis (CIA) model for rheumatoid arthritis. The complexities of structures on CII recognized by lymphocytes are beginning to be unraveled in this model. Immune response to these will be used to investigate how tolerance is maintained and how disease may develop after CII immunization.

Immunization of H-2^q haplotype mice with rat CII leads to activation and expansion of A^q-restricted T cells directed towards an immunodominant peptide in rat CII, located at position 256–270.[1] The peptide is naturally, and variably, glycosylated and T cells can discriminate between the different modifications.[2,3] Expression of this peptide in transgenic type I collagen, that is, in a systemically occurring collagen, will impair the T cell response.[4] These mice are not susceptible to CIA. Expression of the peptide in mouse CII, that is, in cartilage only, leads to an impaired, but not deleted, T cell response. A CII-specific B cell response is maintained and, in similarity with wild-type mice, does not cross-react with type I collagen.[5] These mice develop CIA, although with a lower incidence than wild-type controls. Taken together, this shows that T cells recognize CII-derived peptides in the physiologic situation and thereby become tolerized, whereas B cells are tolerized only by systemic expression of collagen. Immunization with rat CII leads to a strong B cell response towards mouse CII. These B cells are isotype-switched, but not somatically mutated, possibly reflecting antigen-specific interactions between T and B cells outside germinal centers.[6] After immunization, they will develop into plasma cells, producing antibodies able to bind to cartilage, thereby playing a major role in the disease course.[7]

To understand how CII-reactive T cells are activated *in vivo* and how they trigger antigen-specific activation of B cells, we need to know the nature of the antigen-presenting cells. The most-efficient antigen-presenting cells (APC) are dendritic cells, macrophages, and B cells. Both MHC class II–expressing dendritic cells and B cells have been suggested to be the crucial cell type for antigen priming and the most efficient for antigen presentation. We first investigated the ability of dendritic cells to present CII to antigen-specific A^q-restricted T hybridomas.[8] The data summarized in TABLE 1 show that the dendritic cells are unable to present the CII256–270 peptide when located in a collagen α-chain. The failure to present is not dependent on the

TABLE 1. Dendritic Cells Cannot Present Collagen[a]

APC	Antigen		
	CII	CII256–270	OVA
Langerhans' cells *in vivo*	−	nd	+++
Langerhans' cells *in vitro*	−	+++	+++
blood dendritic cells	−	+++	+++
peritoneal macrophages	+++	+++	+++
spleen cells	+++	+++	+++
spleen cells lacking B cells	+++	+++	+++

[a]Different antigen-presenting cells (APC) tested for capacity to stimulate antigen-specific IL-2-secreting T cell hybridomas. All cells are from H-2[q] haplotype mice. Langerhans' cells *in vivo* are derived from mouse ears injected with respective antigens. Blood dendritic cells are isolated after GM-CSF expansion. Spleen cells lacking B cells are from IgM gene–deleted mice. nd = not determined.

triple-helical structure, posttranslational modifications, type II–specific sequences, or the maturity state of the dendritic cell. Thus, it raises the question of which antigen-presenting cell primes a collagen response and which is the most potent cell for presentation of CII to already primed T cells. An obvious candidate is the B cell and, to address this, we used C3H.Q mice lacking B cells, due to a deletion of the gene coding for the IgM heavy chain. However, spleen cells from these mice and spleen cells from wild-type littermates presented CII to T cells equally well, indicating an important role for macrophages. However, it does not exclude a role for B cells. To directly investigate if B cells are able to present CII, we purified spleen cells from

TABLE 2. Antigen Presentation by B Cells[a]

APC	Antigen		
	CII	CII256–270	OVA
From Naive Mice			
bulk SpC	+++	+++	++
μMT SpC	+++	+++	+++
B220[+] SpC	+	++	−
LPS blasts	−	+++	−
anti-kappa blasts	+	++++	−
anti-CD40 (FGK)	+++	++++	(+)
anti-kappa + FGK	(+)	++++	−
From Ag-primed Mice			
B220[+] OVA-primed	(+)	+++	++++
B220[+] CII-primed	(+)	+++	−
B220[+] OVA-primed + FGK	(+)	+++	++++
B220[+] CII-primed + FGK	(+)	+++	(+)

[a]Different antigen-presenting cells (APC) tested for capacity to stimulate antigen-specific IL-2-secreting T cell hybridomas. All cells are from H-2[q] haplotype mice. Spleen cells (SpC) lacking B cells are from mice lacking B cells (μMT mice). B220[+] B cells are purified from spleens with positive magnetic bead selection.

naive H-2^q mice (B10.Q × DBA/1) with magnetic bead–coupled B220-specific antibody (TABLE 2). This population could present CII, but not as well as bulk spleen cells. Incubation with anti-CD40 antibodies augmented the response, whereas LPS treatment or cross-linking of surface immunoglobulin did not enhance presentation. In contrast, when the mouse had been immunized prior to B cell purification, the purified B cell population was not able to present CII. Ovalbumin-primed B cells presented ovalbumin well to T cell hybridomas. We suggest the following: (1) in contrast to dendritic cells, B cells are able to present CII; (2) CII-primed B cells derived from the primary response are not capable of antigen presentation *in vitro*; and (3) such B cells, which are isotype-switched, but not somatically mutated, may play a regulatory role for the activation of CII-specific T cells.

REFERENCES

1. MICHAËLSSON, E., M. ANDERSSON, Å. ENGSTRÖM & R. HOLMDAHL. 1992. Eur. J. Immunol. **22:** 1819–1825.
2. MICHAËLSSON, E., *et al.* 1994. J. Exp. Med. **30:** 745–749.
3. MICHAËLSSON, E., J. BRODDEFALK, J. KIHLBERG, Å. ENGSTRÖM & R. HOLMDAHL. 1996. Eur. J. Immunol. **26:** 1906–1910.
4. MALMSTRÖM, V., *et al.* 1996. Proc. Natl. Acad. Sci. U.S.A. **93:** 4480–4485.
5. HOLMDAHL, R., K. RUBIN, L. KLARESKOG, E. LARSSON & H. WIGZELL. 1986. Arthritis Rheum. **29:** 400–410.
6. MO, J. A., C. A. BONA & R. HOLMDAHL. 1993. Eur. J. Immunol. **23:** 2503–2510.
7. TERATO, K., *et al.* 1992. J. Immunol. **148:** 2103–2108.
8. MICHAËLSSON, E., *et al.* 1995. Eur. J. Immunol. **25:** 2234–2241.

Correlation between HLA-DR Sequence Polymorphisms and Rheumatoid Factor Production

CORNELIA M. WEYAND AND JÖRG J. GORONZY

Department of Internal Medicine
Mayo Foundation
Rochester, Minnesota 55905

Rheumatoid arthritis (RA) is a heterogeneous disease with a wide spectrum of destructive polyarthritis. The production of autoantibodies with specificity for the Fc portion of IgG may or may not be a component of the disease process. The distinction of patients with (seropositive) and without (seronegative) rheumatoid factor (RF) has significant clinical impact. Seronegative RA patients have a more-benign disease course, respond to less-aggressive therapeutic management, and very rarely develop the most-feared complication of RA, namely, extra-articular progression of the disease manifesting with either nodulosis or rheumatoid organ disease.

Why some patients produce RF, whereas others lack that autoantibody, remains an unresolved issue. One possible explanation holds that seronegative RA and seropositive RA represent two entirely distinct disease entities. In that scenario, pathomechanisms in seronegative and seropositive RA would be disease-specific and would be different for the two types of inflammatory polyarthritis. It is also possible that seronegative and seropositive RA patients principally have the same condition, but RF− patients lack appropriate B cell precursor cells necessary to synthesize IgG Fc autoantibodies. Alternatively, T cell help required for RF production is more abundant in RF+ patients compared to RF− patients.

To examine these hypotheses, the frequencies of B cells able to produce RF as determined by limiting dilution analysis were compared in seropositive and seronegative RA patients and normal controls. Limiting numbers of peripheral blood B cells were expanded in the presence of anti-CD3-activated cloned CD4+ T cells, and microcultures with evidence for IgM and RF production were identified.[1] In healthy individuals, 0.3% of IgM-secreting B cells released immunoglobulins with RF activity (TABLE 1). This frequency was expanded about 30-fold in patients with seropositive RA. Seronegative patients could be distinguished from the normal controls as well as the seropositive patients. The subset of RF+ B cell precursors was approximately 3% in seronegative patients. In summary, individuals with seronegative RA have a 10-fold increased frequency of B cells in the circulation that can synthesize RF when compared to healthy controls. RF-positivity appears to be a matter of threshold because the RF+ B cell subset in seropositive patients is yet 3 times larger.

The presence of B cell precursors able to secrete RF in RA patients lacking RF antibodies in the serum was confirmed in experiments using the bacterial superantigen, staphylococcal enterotoxin D (SE D), as a stimulator.[2] In T-B cell cocultures

TABLE 1. Frequencies of RF+ B Cell Precursor Cells in Seropositive and Seronegative Patients with RA[a]

Stimulation	Controls (n = 7)	Seropositive RA (n = 6)	Seronegative RA (n = 8)
anti-CD3	1:360	1:9.5	1:34
SE D	1:3.6	1:3.7	1:4.4

[a]Replicate cultures of limiting numbers of B cells obtained from peripheral blood of normal controls and RA patients with RF+ or RF− disease were established by coculture with activated T cell clones. T cells were activated either by immobilized anti-CD3 or by 1 μg/mL SE D. Supernatants were harvested after 15 days and microcultures containing IgM and/or RF were identified. Frequencies of IgM-producing and of RF-producing B cells were determined. Results are given as the ratio of RF-producing per IgM-producing cells.

driven by SE D, RF+ B cells are preferentially activated and up to 30% of B cells producing IgM upon SE D stimulation can be found to be RF+. The proportion of B cells releasing RF upon SE D stimulation was similar in normals, seronegative, and seropositive patients, documenting that the seronegativity of RF− patients is not the result of a lack in the B cell repertoire. These data are compatible with the existence of a more-pronounced T cell help for RF+ B cells in seropositive patients. Because T cell help is an HLA-restricted phenomenon, evidence was sought for differences in the HLA association of seronegative and seropositive RA.

Our previous studies have demonstrated that 80–95% of patients with severe seropositive RA carry an RA-associated HLA-DRB1 allele. Disease association for RA has been established for a set of alleles, all of which share a sequence motif spanning amino acid position 70–74 of the HLA-DRB1 gene.[3] The set of disease-associated HLA-DRB1 variants includes HLA-DRB1*01, 04, 10, and 1402. Within the HLA-DRB1*04 family, several allelic subtypes have been found enriched in RA patients, including DRB1*0401, 0404, 0405, and 0408. A larger-than-expected fraction of these patients have inherited two disease-associated alleles. Correlation of allelic combinations and clinical presentation leads to the observation that patients with two disease-associated alleles have more severe disease and frequently extra-articular disease.[4,5] Thus, HLA-DR molecules function to affect severity in RA. Among patients with seropositive RA, more than 90% of patients express at least one disease-relevant HLA-DR allele. Most patients type HLA-DRB1*04 and the DRB1*0401 allelic variant is dominant in RF-producing RA patients (FIGURE 1A). A different picture emerged for RF− patients. Only about one-third of those patients were HLA-DRB1*04; one-third carried an HLA-DRB1*01 allele and one-third of the patients lacked an RA-associated haplotype. Of the HLA-DRB1*04 alleles, they preferred the DRB1*0404 and 0408 allelic variants and rarely expressed B1*0401 (FIGURE 1A). A sequence comparison of B1 alleles associated with the seropositive and seronegative variants of the disease identifies the dimorphism expressed in position 71 as the distinguishing factor (FIGURE 1B). A lysine substitution in B71 is a characteristic feature of seropositive patients, whereas seronegative patients typically have an arginine substitution in this position. A double-dose of disease-associated DRB1 alleles, either as a combination of two lysine-containing HLA-DRB1 alleles or

A

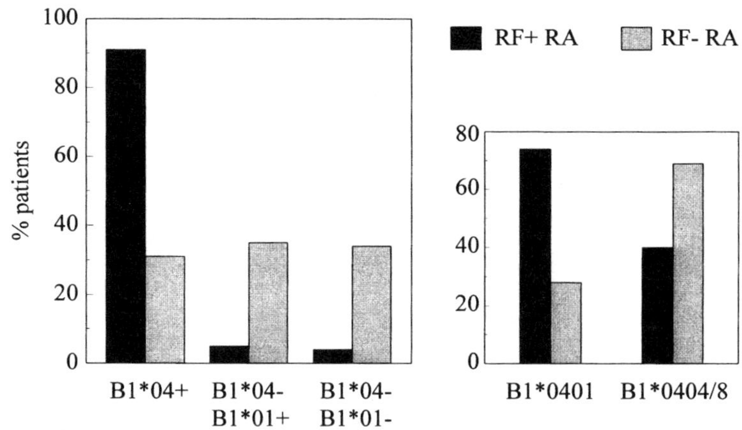

B

	Amino acid polymorphism position 70	71	72	73	74
RA associated alleles dominant in seropositive disease					
B1*0401	Q	K	R	A	A
RA associated alleles dominant in seronegative disease					
B1*0404	Q	R	R	A	A
B1*0408	Q	R	R	A	A
B1*01	Q	R	R	A	A

FIGURE 1. HLA-DRB1 association of RF+ and RF− RA. One hundred forty-two patients with seropositive RA and 60 patients with seronegative RA were characterized for their HLA-DRB1 alleles. The majority of seropositive RA patients expressed an HLA-DRB1*0401 allele, whereas seronegative RA was associated with HLA-DRB1*01 and 0404(8) (A). All disease-associated alleles expressed the RA-linked sequence motif in the third hypervariable region of the DRB1 gene; however, they differed in a sequence polymorphism in position 71 (B). Our data suggest that a lysine versus arginine substitution in the rheumatoid epitope is important for rheumatoid factor production.

as a combination of an arginine and a lysine amino acid in position 71, is almost exclusively found in patients with RF production.[6] The lysine-arginine exchange has been considered conservative, which is the case for charge. Position 71 is a critical component of binding pocket 4 that accommodates peptide side chains of antigenic peptides bound to HLA-DR molecules.[7] Because lysine and arginine differ in size, differences in the binding affinities can be anticipated.

In summary, RF production appears to result from an HLA-DR-restricted immune response. The data are best compatible with an antigen-driven immune response in which the HLA-DR-antigen complex is recognized by T helper cells promoting the differentiation of B cells, producing immunoglobulins with RF activity. It can be predicted that antigens of interest bind with high affinity to RA-associated alleles with a B71 lysine substitution and with lower affinity to HLA-DR molecules expressing arginine at the entrance to binding pocket 4. Testing candidate antigens for their interaction with HLA-DR molecules might provide an approach to identify agents eliciting the formation of RF.

REFERENCES

1. HE, X., W. ZHONG, T. G. MCCARTHY, C. M. WEYAND & J. J. GORONZY. 1996. Increased responsiveness of rheumatoid factor–producing B cells in seronegative rheumatoid arthritis. Arthritis Rheum. **39:** 1499–1506.
2. HE, X., J. J. GORONZY & C. M. WEYAND. 1992. Selective induction of rheumatoid factors by superantigens and human helper T cells. J. Clin Invest. **89:** 673–680.
3. WINCHESTER, R. 1994. The molecular basis of susceptibility to rheumatoid arthritis. Adv. Immunol. **56:** 389–466.
4. WEYAND, C. M., C. XIE & J. J. GORONZY. 1992. Homozygosity for the HLA-DRB1 allele selects for extra-articular manifestations in rheumatoid arthritis. J. Clin. Invest. **89:** 2033–2039.
5. WEYAND, C. M., K. C. HICOK, D. L. CONN & J. J. GORONZY. 1992. The influence of HLA-DRB1 genes on disease severity in rheumatoid arthritis. Ann. Intern. Med. **117:** 801–806.
6. WEYAND, C. M., T. G. MCCARTHY & J. J. GORONZY. 1995. Correlation between disease phenotype and genetic heterogeneity in rheumatoid arthritis. J. Clin. Invest. **95:** 2120–2126.
7. STERN, L. J., J. H. BROWN, T. S. JARDETZKY, *et al.* 1994. Crystal structure of the human class II MHC protein HLA-DR1 complexed with an influenza virus peptide. Nature **368:** 215–221.

Superantigens, V_H Gene Polymorphism, and Rheumatoid Factor (RF) Production

JÖRG J. GORONZY, XIAOWEN HE, AND CORNELIA M. WEYAND

Department of Internal Medicine
Mayo Foundation
Rochester, Minnesota 55905

In an attempt to study T-B cell interaction leading to RF synthesis, we began in the early 1990s to explore the action of bacterial superantigens to cross-link T cell receptors (TCR) with MHC complexes expressed on B cells. This led us to the serendipitous finding that staphylococcal enterotoxin D (SE D) preferentially induced the production of anti-IgG Fc antibodies in normal peripheral B cells.[1] In limiting dilution analyses, RF production was an infrequent event among normal B cells activated in the presence of anti-CD3-stimulated T cells. Approximately 1 out of 500 B cells released RF. Stimulation of T-B cell cultures with SE D led to a preferential activation of RF+ B cells.[2] One out of 3–4 IgM+ B cells was positive for RF. Interestingly, the bias of SE D–stimulated B cells toward RF specificity was indistinguishable in normal individuals and patients with rheumatoid arthritis (RA). The fraction of B cells secreting RF when help was provided by anti-CD3-stimulated T cells, however, was expanded in RA patients. These data were best compatible with SE D targeting a B cell subset highly enriched for RF+ B cell precursors that in normals is not responsive to anti-CD3-activated T cells.

To address the mechanism of SE D–induced RF production, we proceeded with a molecular analysis of stimulated B cells. B cell clones were established from normal donors by expanding individual B cells in the presence of clonal T helper cells. Cultures were stimulated either by cross-linked anti-CD3 or by SE D. B cell clones were characterized for RF production and the V_H gene family usage was determined by RT-PCR. As given in FIGURE 1, V_H3 gene segments were particularly enriched among RF+ B cell clones induced by SE D. Sequence analysis of RF+ V_H3+ immunoglobulins revealed that they were frequently in germline configuration with a low replacement-to-silent ratio and no clustering of mutations in the complementarity determining regions (CDR).[3] SE D–mediated activation was correlated with an unusual pattern of V_H3 gene segment usage. In particular, transcription of V3-21 was exclusively found in SE D–responsive B cell clones (28% of all RF+ B cell clones) and was not encountered in B cell clones derived by anti-CD3 activation. B cell clones established in the presence of anti-CD3-triggered T cells frequently utilized the V3-23 gene segment. Sequence polymorphisms distinguishing V3-21 (preferred by SE D) and V3-23 (disfavored by SE D) can be localized to the CDR1 and CDR2. The most-intriguing difference is a stretch of five serines in the CDR2. Based upon these

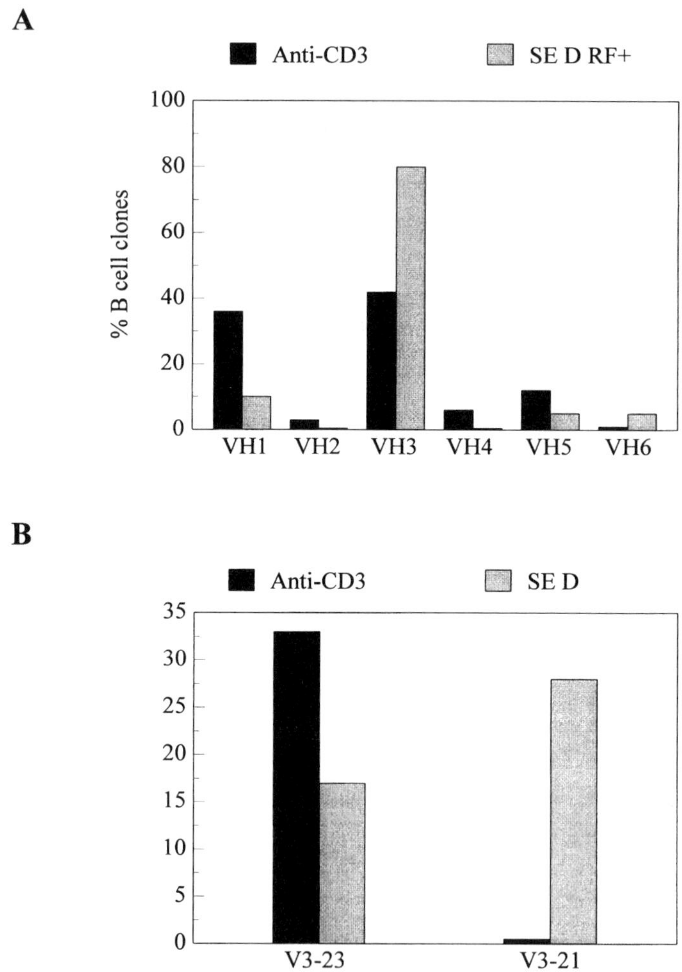

FIGURE 1. V_H gene repertoire of RF-producing B cells stimulated by SE D–activated T cells. Clonal B cell cultures were established by coculturing a limiting number of B cells from peripheral blood of normal individuals either with cloned cells stimulated with immobilized anti-CD3 or with T cells and 1 μg/mL SE D. Culture supernatants were harvested after 15 days and analyzed for the presence of IgM and RF. Total RNA was obtained from the microcultures and V_H gene family usage was determined in a nested RT-PCR using family-specific primer sets (A). Amplified products were sequenced and the V_H germline gene segment was identified (B).

data, we have proposed that SE D interacts with selected B cells through binding CDR2-encoded determinants. The selective activation of RF+ B cells by SE D raised the question of how SE D–induced RF from normals is related to RF from patients. To address this question, clones from patients with seropositive RA and primary Sjögren's syndrome (pSS) were generated by coculture with anti-CD3-stimulated T helper cells. A total of 127 B cell clones from normal donors were established. As expected, all were negative for Ig Fc binding. From RA patients, 113 RF− and 60 RF+ B cell clones were obtained. Eighty-two RF− and 47 RF+ B cell clones were derived from pSS patients. The cross-reactivity of the RF antibodies was determined by ELISA on Ig Fc, actin, keratin, ssDNA, thyroglobulin, and tetanus toxoid. Only 10% of the RF+ B cell clones released were truly polyreactive. Forty-five of 68 anti-Fc antibodies tested were monospecific for Ig Fc on the panel of antigens tested.[4]

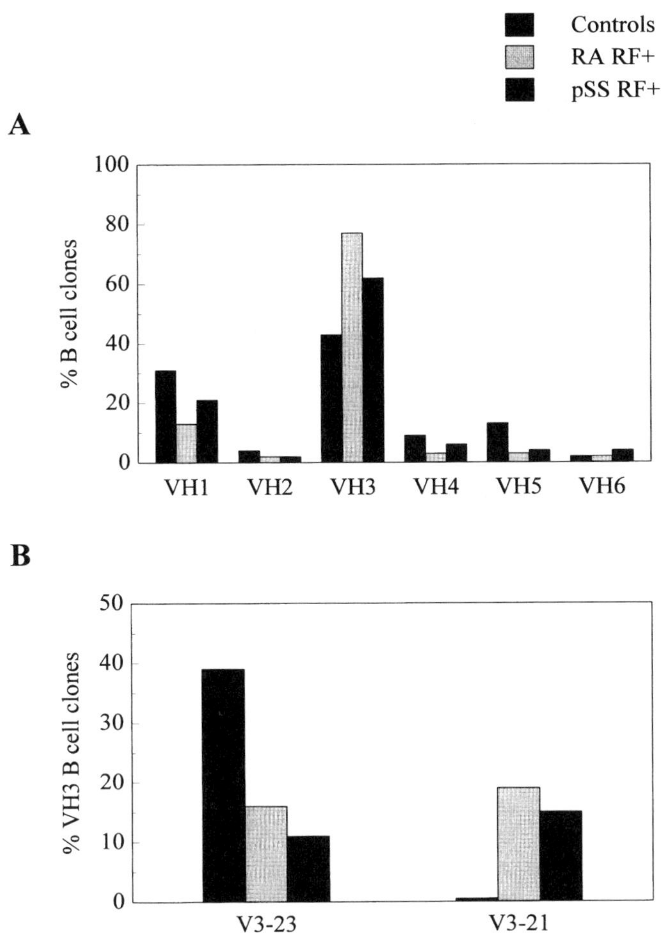

FIGURE 2. V_H gene repertoire of RF-producing B cells derived from patients with RA and Sjögren's syndrome. Clonal B cell cultures were established from PBMC of normal controls and patients with seropositive RA and pSS by coculture with anti-CD3-activated cloned T cells. Supernatants were assessed for IgM secretion and RF activity by ELISA. Under these culture conditions, all B cell clones from normals did not produce RF. V_H gene family usage (A) and V_H3 germline gene segment usage (B) were determined as described in FIGURE 1.

Immunoglobulin genes transcribed by the B cell clones were sequenced following V_H family–specific amplification (FIGURE 2). Compared to RF− B cell clones from normals, RF+ B cell clones preferentially used V_H3 gene elements. V_H3 was detected in 42% of the RF− B cell clones from normals compared to 77% in RF+ B cell clones isolated from RA patients. Results for V_H3 family subtypes are shown in FIGURE 2. V3-23 and V3-30 accounted for two-thirds of the V_H3+ B cell clones. In RA patients and pSS patients, the frequency of V3-23, however, was decreased with a compensatory increase in V3-21. V3-21 was exclusively found in patient-derived B cells and was not encountered in the 127 control clones. Transcription of V3-21 was correlated with RF specificity in both patient subsets. From these results, the hypothesis emerged that secretion of anti-Fc autoantibodies is a feature of a specialized B cell subset that is exquisitely responsive to the bacterial superantigen SE D. In two different RF-producing diseases, RA and pSS, RF+ B cells derived from the peripheral blood frequently expressed the V3-21 gene fragment that we have correlated with SE D responsiveness. By random B cell cloning, V3-21+ RF+ B cells were unique for patients and were not detected in normals. However, V3-21 transcripts are present in nonstimulated B cells from normals. We therefore hypothesize that V3-21+ B cells are in a state of tolerance from which they escape in RA or pSS. This state of tolerance can be broken by SE D, resulting in RF production in normal donors. Experimental evidence for this model was provided by semiquantifying V3-23 and V3-21 transcripts in anti-CD3– and SE D–driven B cells from control individuals.[4]

This series of studies provides insight into the regulation of RF+ B cells. These B cells are characterized by a molecular fingerprint with preferential usage of V_H3. Within the V_H3 family, V3-21 has a unique position. This gene segment is detected among RF+ B cells isolated from RA patients and pSS patients. V3-21+ B cells have an additional feature that distinguishes them from other V_H3+ B cells, namely, their selective responsiveness to the bacterial superantigen SE D. V3-21+ B cells in normals remain silent and are anergic to conventional T cell–dependent stimuli. Breaking this tolerant state appears to be a mechanism associated with disease. It is conceivable that bacterial superantigens could be involved in releasing V3-21+ B cells from their anergic state. As suggested by the germline configuration of V3-21+ sequences, antigen selection and affinity maturation may be a secondary process occurring in patients synthesizing pathogenic RF molecules.

REFERENCES

1. HE, X., J. J. GORONZY & C. M. WEYAND. 1992. Selective induction of rheumatoid factors by superantigens and human helper T cells. J. Clin. Invest. **89:** 673–680.
2. HE, X., J. J. GORONZY & C. M. WEYAND. 1993. The repertoire of rheumatoid factor–producing B cells responsive to bacterial superantigen and bystander help in normals and patients with rheumatoid arthritis. Arthritis Rheum. **36:** 1061–1069.
3. XIE, C., H. BRÜHL, X. HE, C. M. WEYAND & J. J. GORONZY. 1995. Selective activation of L3A10^{+} rheumatoid factor–producing B cells by the staphylococcal enterotoxin D. Int. Immunol. **7:** 425–434.
4. HE, X., J. J. GORONZY, W. ZHONG, C. XIE & C. M. WEYAND. 1995. V_H3-21 B cells escape from a state of tolerance in rheumatoid arthritis and secrete rheumatoid factor. Mol. Med. **1:** 768–780.

Regulation of Rheumatoid Factor Production by B Cells from Healthy Individuals and Patients with Rheumatoid Arthritis

W. J. E. VAN ESCH,[a] C. C. REPARON-SCHUIJT,[a]
C. VAN KOOTEN,[b] F. C. BREEDVELD,[a] AND C. L. VERWEIJ[a]

[a]*Department of Rheumatology*
[b]*Department of Nephrology*
University Hospital
Leiden, the Netherlands

The presence of rheumatoid factor (RF) in the circulation is a characteristic phenomenon in patients with rheumatoid arthritis (RA). However, RF is not specific for RA. Healthy individuals carry RF$^+$ B lymphocytes and immunization regularly induces synthesis of RF.[1–3] Evidence exists demonstrating that RF that circulates in patients with RA is structurally different from that present in healthy individuals. Furthermore, in contrast to RA patients, RF production in normals is a transient phenomenon with clear correlation to an initiating stimulus.[4]

To compare the regulation of RF production by peripheral B cells derived from RF-seropositive RA patients and RF-seronegative healthy individuals, we have studied RF production in a T-B cell coculture system. Antibody production by B cells was induced by either anti-CD3-stimulated T helper cell activity or staphylococcal enterotoxin D (SED)–induced T-B cell interaction.[5] For this purpose, we have selected a T cell clone, K15, that exhibited helper capacities in the presence of anti-CD3 and SED. Clone K15 is a synovial fluid autoreactive Vβ19$^+$ CD4$^+$ T cell clone isolated from the inflamed joint of an RA patient.[6]

As shown in FIGURE 1, in the anti-CD3-driven system, a significant ($n = 8$, $p = 0.012$) increase in IgM-RF production per μg IgM by RA B cells compared to B cells from normals was observed. In contrast to the anti-CD3-driven system, the SED system revealed a distinction between responders and nonresponders with respect to IgM-RF production in both RA and healthy individuals. The SED-responder phenotype was irrespective of total IgM production (TABLE 1). The SED-responsive RA B cells produced more IgM-RF per μg IgM than SED-responsive B cells from healthy individuals (FIGURE 1). From these findings, we conclude the following:

(1) usage of the anti-CD3- and SED-driven T-B cell coculture systems did not provide evidence for differential regulation of RF production between RA patients and healthy controls;
(2) a dichotomy in SED responsiveness exists with respect to IgM-RF production.

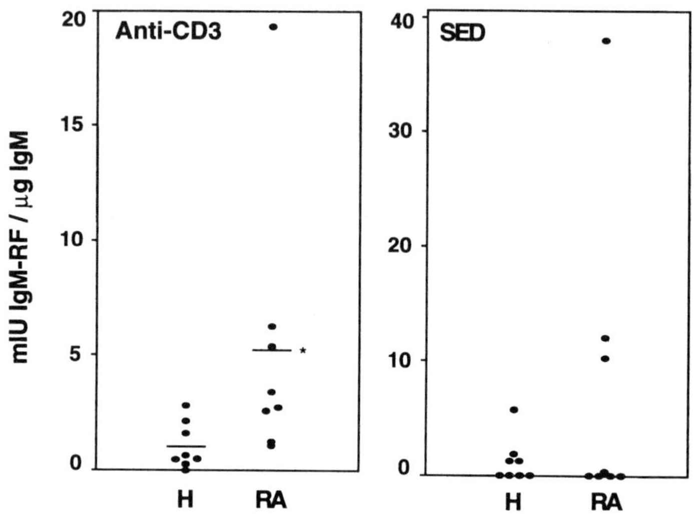

FIGURE 1. Individual production of IgM-RF per µg IgM as determined in culture supernatants of the anti-CD3- and SED-driven T-B cell coculture system. Peripheral B lymphocytes (10^4/well) were cocultured in duplicate with T cells (clone K15; 10^5/well) in the presence of SED (0.5 µg/mL) or immobilized anti-CD3 mAb (50 µg/mL). Culture supernatants were harvested after 13 days and analyzed for their concentrations of IgM and IgM-RF. Data were pooled from three independent experiments using B cells from different donors (H, healthy individuals; RA, RA patients). *: $p = 0.012$ compared to healthy controls (Mann-Whitney *U*-test).

TABLE 1. IgM and IgM-RF Production in Culture Supernatants of the SED-driven T-B Cell Coculture System[a]

Donor of Purified B Cells	IgM [µg/mL]	IgM-RF [mIU/mL]	Donor of Purified B Cells	IgM [µg/mL]	IgM-RF [mIU/mL]
H2	0.3	0	RA1	0.6	0
H3	11.6	0	RA2	0.5	0
H6	1.4	0	RA3	2.4	0
H7	3.3	0	RA5	5.8	2.0
H1	3.6	6.6	RA7	1.6	0
H4	83.0	104.0	RA4	1.6	60.0
H5	1.5	1.9	RA6	1.1	11.2
H8	1.6	9.2	RA8	1.6	19.8

[a]H, healthy individual; RA, RA patient.

REFERENCES

1. Slaughter, L., D. A. Carson, F. C. Jensen, T. L. Holbrook & J. H. Vaughan. 1978. *In vitro* effects of Epstein-Barr virus on peripheral blood mononuclear cells from patients with rheumatoid arthritis and normal subjects. J. Exp. Med. **148:** 1429–1434.

2. TARKOWSKI, A., C. CZERKINSKY & L.-Å. NILSSON. 1985. Simultaneous induction of rheumatoid factor– and antigen-specific antibody-secreting cells during the secondary immune response in man. Clin. Exp. Immunol. **61:** 379–387.
3. WELCH, M. J., S. FONG, J. VAUGHAN & D. CARSON. 1983. Increased frequency of rheumatoid factor precursor B lymphocytes after immunization of normal adults with tetanus toxoid. Clin. Exp. Immunol. **51:** 299–304.
4. CARSON, D. A., P. P. CHEN & T. J. KIPPS. 1991. New roles for rheumatoid factor. J. Clin. Invest. **87:** 379–383.
5. HE, X., J. GORONZY & C. WEYAND. 1992. Selective induction of rheumatoid factors by superantigens and human helper T cells. J. Clin. Invest. **89:** 673–680.
6. MAURICE, M. M., P. C. M. RES, A. LEOW, T. VAN HALL, M. R. DAHA, L. STRUYK, P. E. VAN DEN EBREN, F. C. BREEDVELD & C. L. VERWEIJ. 1994. Joint-derived T cells in rheumatoid arthritis proliferate to antigens present in autologous synovial fluid. Scand. J. Rheumatol. **23:** 157–165.

Tumor Necrosis Factor (TNF) Enhances the Locomotion of Low-Density Human Tonsillar B Lymphocytes through the Selective Triggering of Type II Receptor

A. CORCIONE,[a] L. OTTONELLO,[b] G. TORTOLINA,[b]
P. TASSO,[a] F. GHIOTTO,[a] I. AIROLDI,[a] R. D'AGOSTINO,[c]
F. DALLEGRI,[b] AND V. PISTOIA[a]

[a]*Laboratory of Oncology*
Scientific Institute G. Gaslini
16147 Genova, Italy

[b]*Department of Internal Medicine*
University of Genova
16132 Genova, Italy

[c]*Division of Otolaryngology*
Scientific Institute G. Gaslini
16147 Genova, Italy

TNF accomplishes various biological activities in different cell types including B lymphocytes.[1] Here, the chemotactic activity of recombinant (r) TNF versus human tonsillar B cells has been investigated.

Tonsillar B lymphocytes were purified (>95%) by sequential depletion of T cells, NK cells, and macrophages and were fractionated into low-density (LD) and high-density (HD) cells on a Percoll gradient.[2] Low-density B lymphocytes were further separated into CD39−, IgD− and CD39+, IgD+ cells by immune-rosetting. The aforementioned B cell fractions were tested for their ability to undergo polarization and migration in the presence or absence of rTNF. Migration studies were performed using the leading front method and the checkerboard analysis.[3]

LD B cells displayed a higher spontaneous migration than HD cells; furthermore, rTNF enhanced the locomotion of LD, but not HD, cells in a dose-dependent manner (FIGURE 1A). On the grounds of these experiments, 1 ng/mL rTNF was used in all subsequent experiments.

LD B lymphocytes are enriched for germinal center (GC) cells that can be purified as CD39−, IgD− cells. The CD39+, IgD+ LD B cell fraction contains a majority of follicular mantle (FM) lymphocytes (60–70%) admixed with memory cells (30–40%). FIGURE 1B shows the results of the chemotactic assays carried out with CD39−, IgD− and CD39+, IgD+ B lymphocytes in comparison with unfractionated LD B cells. CD39−, IgD− GC B cells did not enhance their locomotory capability upon exposure to rTNF, whereas CD39+, IgD+ cells did (FIGURE 1B). The locomotion of CD39+, IgD+ B lymphocytes was superimposable to that of unfractionated LD cells (FIGURE

1B). Checkerboard experiments (where different concentrations of rTNF above and below the filters were tested) demonstrated that B cell migration was attributable to both a chemotactic and a chemokinetic activity of the cytokine.

FACS analysis of CD39−, IgD− and CD39+, IgD+ LD B lymphocytes showed that the latter, but not the former, cells expressed surface type I and II TNF receptors (TNFRs), thus accounting for the failure of CD39−, IgD− GC B cells to migrate in response to rTNF. Notably, however, the transcripts of both TNFR genes were detected by RT-PCR in GC B lymphocytes.

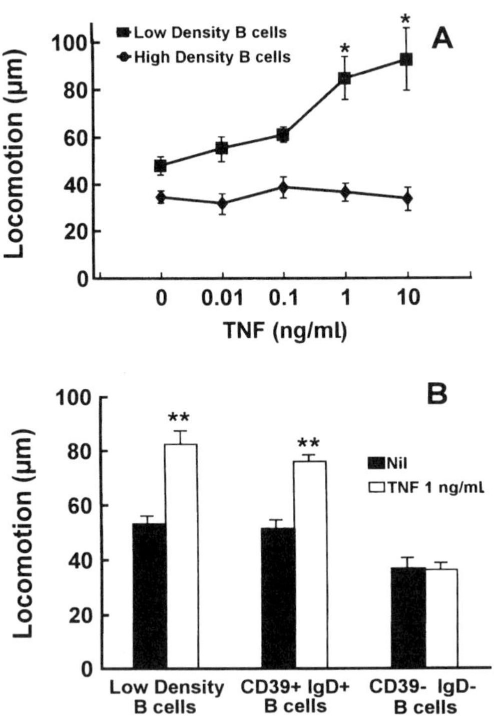

FIGURE 1. Locomotion of freshly isolated tonsillar B cell subsets. (A) Response of HD and LD B cells to different concentrations of rTNF. (B) Migration of unfractionated, CD39+, IgD+, and CD39−, IgD− LD B cells in the presence or absence of 1 ng/mL rTNF. Data are means ± SE from ten experiments: (*) $p < 0.01$; (**) $p < 0.005$.

In subsequent experiments, we investigated the involvement of TNFRs in the TNF-mediated enhancement of CD39+, IgD+ B cell locomotion by incubating the latter cells with blocking monoclonal antibodies (mab) to TNFRs or with an irrelevant, isotype-matched mab before running the chemotactic assays (FIGURE 2). The anti-TNFR-II mab abrogated the TNF-induced locomotion of CD39+, IgD+ cells (FIGURE 2). In contrast, the anti-TNFR-I mab had no effect (FIGURE 2), demonstrating that TNFR-II was selectively involved in the phenomenon.

Next, we investigated the ability of CD39−, IgD− and CD39+, IgD+ B cells to release TNF *in vitro*. TNF was assayed by ELISA in the supernatants from 48-h

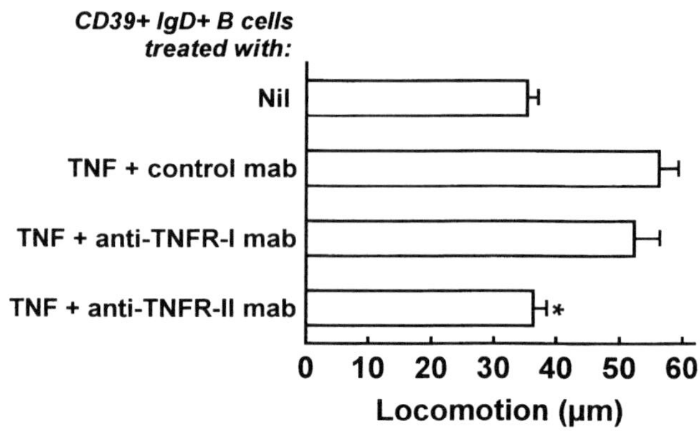

FIGURE 2. Involvement of TNFRs in the TNF-induced CD39+, IgD+ LD B cell locomotion. Freshly purified CD39+, IgD+ LD B cells were treated with anti-TNFR-I, anti-TNFR-II, or an isotype-matched mab of irrelevant specificity (control mab). Cells were subsequently washed and tested in locomotor assays in the absence (nil) or presence of 1 ng/mL rTNF. Results are means ± SE from four different experiments: (∗) $p < 0.05$.

unstimulated cultures. Both cell fractions released TNF (range: 800–1200 pg/mL), suggesting the possible autocrine and/or paracrine utilization of the cytokine.

Because, as mentioned, CD39+, IgD+ LD B cells are heterogeneous, we are investigating the TNF-mediated locomotor capabilities of FM (IgD+) and memory (IgD−, CD38−) tonsillar lymphocytes. Although both cell fractions migrate, these preliminary studies suggest that memory B cells display a stronger response to rTNF than FM B cells.

REFERENCES

1. Vassalli, P. 1992. Annu. Rev. Immunol. **10:** 411–452.
2. Corcione, A., L. Baldi, S. Zupo, M. Dono, G. Biolcati Rinaldi, S. Roncella, G. Taborelli, M. Truini, M. Ferrarini & V. Pistoia. 1994. J. Immunol. **153:** 2868–2877.
3. Wilkinson, P. C. 1986. Immunology **57:** 281–289.

Treatments with Tamoxifen and an Antiestradiol Antibody Have Beneficial Effects on Experimental SLE via Cytokine Modulation

Z. STHOEGER,[a] M. DAYAN,[a] H. ZINGER,[a] F. KALUSH,[a]
G. MOR,[b] Y. AMIR ZALTMAN,[b] F. KOHEN,[b] AND E. MOZES[a]

[a]*Department of Immunology*
[b]*Department of Hormone Research*
Weizmann Institute of Science
Rehovot 76100, Israel

Various studies demonstrated that estrogens accelerate and androgens ameliorate the course of human and murine systemic lupus erythematosus (SLE).[1] Recently, we reported that tamoxifen (antiestrogen with relatively minor side effects) has beneficial effects on the clinical manifestations of experimental SLE induced in BALB/c mice by immunization with the human monoclonal anti-DNA antibody that bears a common idiotype, 16/6 Id.[2] To elucidate the mechanism(s) involved in the therapeutic effects of tamoxifen, we further investigated the influence of an antiestrogen (E_2) monoclonal antibody (mAb) on 16/6 Id–immunized mice and the effects of both treatments on cytokine secretion.

MATERIALS AND METHODS

The human 16/6 Id is an anti-DNA monoclonal antibody.[3] This antibody was used to immunize female BALB/c mice (1 μg in complete Freund's adjuvant at the footpads and a boost of 1 μg in PBS three weeks later).[2,3] Tamoxifen was given subcutaneously, twice a week at 800 μg/mouse. The anti-E_2 mAb (IgG) was injected weekly, intraperitoneally at 50 μg/mouse. Clinical manifestations of experimental SLE were determined by leukocyte counts of heparinized blood, proteinuria by Combistix Kit, and immunohistology of frozen kidney sections by staining with FITC-rabbit anti-mouse IgG (γ-chain-specific). Levels of autoantibodies were measured by ELISA.[2,3] Cytokine levels were determined in supernatants of LPS-stimulated and unstimulated peritoneal macrophages (IL-1) or in supernatants of ConA-stimulated and unstimulated splenocytes (IL-2, IL-4, IFNγ, IL-10, and TNFα) by ELISA (IL-10 and IFNγ) or by bioassays (IL-1, IL-2, IL-4, and TNFα).

RESULTS AND DISCUSSION

Three weeks following the 16/6 Id immunization, when autoantibody titers started to raise, the mice were divided into untreated (PBS) and treated (either tamoxifen or anti-E_2 mAb) groups. Three additional nonimmunized groups of mice were treated with PBS, tamoxifen, or anti-E_2 mAb and served as controls. All mice were bled monthly and sacrificed seven months following booster injections. The autoantibody titers (against DNA, NE, 16/6, and anti-16/6 Id) in all immunized mice were significantly higher than those of the control groups. No differences could be observed in the total IgG autoantibody levels between the immunized treated or untreated groups; however, the levels of pathogenic IgG_{2a} autoantibodies were significantly lower in the treated mice. Treatment with tamoxifen and the anti-E_2 mAb had remarkable beneficial effects on the SLE-related clinical manifestations. Thus, 16/6 Id–immunized and either tamoxifen- or anti-E_2-treated mice had normal white blood cell counts, no proteinuria, and no immune complex glomerulonephritis. We have previously shown dysregulation of the cytokine network in mice with 16/6 Id–induced experimental SLE.[4] It therefore has been of interest to find out whether the treatment protocols act via modulation of the cytokine network. Immunocytes of the 16/6 Id–immunized mice secreted, *in vitro*, higher levels of the inflammatory cytokines IL-1 and TNFα and of IL-10 (about five times greater than control) and lower levels of IL-2, IFNγ, and IL-4 (about one-third of control) as compared to all control groups. Treatment with either tamoxifen or anti-E_2 restored the cytokine production to normal levels. Thus, cytokine modulation may be the basis for the therapeutic effects of both antiestrogens in experimental SLE.

REFERENCES

1. LAHITA, R. G. 1985. Sex steroids and the rheumatic diseases. Arthritis Rheum. **28:** 126.
2. STHOEGER, Z. M., Z. BENTWICH, H. ZINGER & E. MOZES. 1994. The beneficial effect of the estrogen antagonist tamoxifen on experimental SLE. J. Rheumatol. **21:** 2231–2238.
3. MENDELOVIC, S., S. BROCKE, Y. SHOENFELD, M. BEN-BASSAT, A. MESHORER, R. BAKIMER & E. MOZES. 1988. Induction of SLE-like disease by a common human anti-DNA idiotype. Proc. Natl. Acad. Sci. U.S.A. **85:** 2260–2264.
4. MOZES, E., F. KALUSH & B. TARTAKOVSKY. 1990. The physiological and pathological effects of cytokines. *In* Progress in Leukocyte Biology, p. 111–116. Wiley–Liss. New York.

Screening of Immunological Properties of Vermiculine in Selected Model Situations[a]

J. ROVENSKÝ,[b] M. BUC,[c] S. BLAŽÍČKOVÁ,[b]
M. FERENČÍK,[c] Ľ. RAUOVÁ,[b] J. FUSKA,[d]
AND M. STANČÍKOVÁ[b]

[b]*Research Institute of Rheumatic Diseases
Piešťany, Slovakia*

[c]*Department of Immunology
Faculty of Medicine
Comenius University
Bratislava, Slovakia*

[d]*Faculty of Chemistry and Technology
Slovak Technical University
Bratislava, Slovakia*

Vermiculine is a macrocyclic aglycosidic dilactone isolated from *Penicillium vermiculatum* with antibacterial, antiprotozoal, and cancerolytic properties.[1,2] Recent experimental results show that vermiculine has an immunosuppressive effect. However, immunosuppressive properties of vermiculine were demonstrated from the point of view of T cell immunity only. We thus attempted to determine the effect of vermiculine on the metabolic and functional activities of human peripheral neutrophils, which represent the basic component of the first line of defense of the immune system and are an essential part of the mechanisms of natural immunity. Furthermore, we investigated the immunomodulatory activities of vermiculine in the test of blastic transformation of lymphocytes using monoclonal anti-CD2/CD2R antibody and stimulation of lymphocytes by mitogens.

THE EFFECT OF VERMICULINE ON THE METABOLIC AND FUNCTIONAL ACTIVITIES OF HUMAN PERIPHERAL NEUTROPHILS

We investigated the effect of vermiculine on INT-reductase activity, superoxide production, phagocytic activity (PA), and candidacidal activity (CA) of neutrophils isolated from peripheral blood. Vermiculine in the highest concentration tested (100 μg/mL or 100 pg/neutrophil) significantly inhibited the INT activity and superoxide production of unstimulated neutrophils, as well as of neutrophils stimulated with opsonized zymosan (phagocytable stimulus) or with phorbol myristate acetate (activa-

[a]This work was supported by PECO Project No. BMHICT 9210.8 entitled "Immunotherapy of Chronic Arthritis: Experimental Basis".

tor of the protein kinase C). At this concentration, vermiculine significantly decreased the phagocytic activity, the phagocytic index (PI), and the candidacidal activity of neutrophils. The phagocytic index and candidacidal activity were also significantly decreased in the presence of 10 pg/neutrophil. These results show that vermiculine in the concentration of 100 pg of vermiculine per single neutrophil is able to inhibit metabolic activation as well as functional activity of human peripheral neutrophils *in vitro* (FIGURE 1).

INVESTIGATION OF IMMUNOMODULATORY PROPERTIES OF VERMICULINE BY THE TEST OF BLASTIC TRANSFORMATION OF LYMPHOCYTES

The stimulations of lymphocytes by monoclonal antibody anti-CD3, anti-CD2/CD2R, and polyclonal activators [phytohemagglutinin (PHA), concanavalin A (ConA), and pokeweed mitogen (PWM)] represent different models of lymphocyte activation. The aim of our work was to investigate if vermiculine would stimulate or inhibit the mitotic activity of lymphocytes induced by the polyclonal mitogens, that is, PHA, ConA, and PWM. The obtained results indicate the following:

(a) vermiculine inhibits especially the stimulation of lymphocytes by ConA and PWM, whereas its effect on stimulation of lymphocytes by PHA is negligible;
(b) vermiculine has neither stimulating nor inhibitory effect on unstimulated lymphocytes;
(c) the effect of vermiculine depends on the concentration used (FIGURE 2).

Analysis of stimulated lymphocytes by means of flow cytometry offers a more-

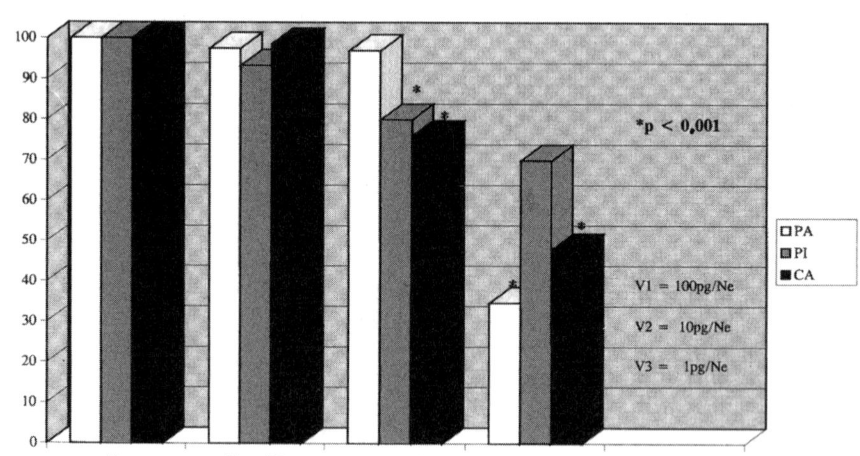

FIGURE 1. Effect of vermiculine on the phagocytic activity and candidacidal activity of human peripheral neutrophils (Ne).

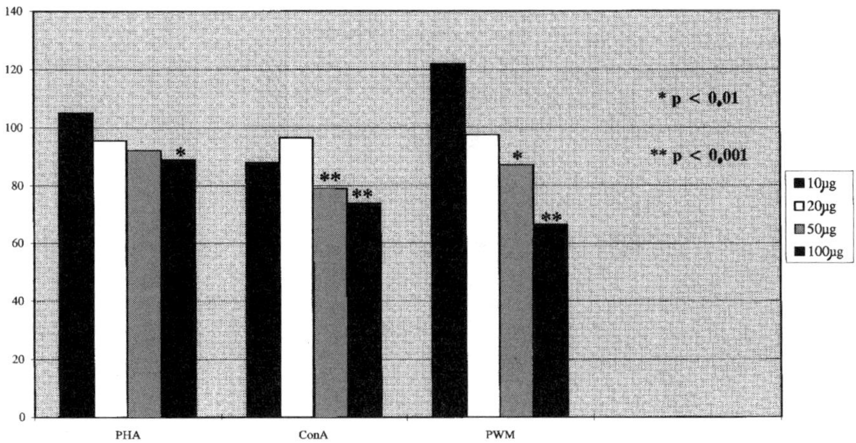

FIGURE 2. Effect of vermiculine on the mitotic activity of lymphocytes induced by the polyclonal mitogens: PHA, ConA, and PWM.

precise analysis of stimulated lymphocyte subpopulations. On using three-color analysis, we studied the expressivity of activation antigens CD69, CD25, and CD71. Vermiculine was found to diminish particularly the activation of $CD8^+$ lymphocytes (significantly reduced expressivity of CD69 was observed already after 4 hours of cultivation and that of CD25 after 48 hours). The intensity of inhibition was more pronounced in the concentration of 0.01 µg/mL.

Our results suggest that vermiculine might be a new immunosuppressive drug with possible use in the therapy of autoimmune diseases.[3,4]

REFERENCES

1. Fuska, J., L. P. Ivanickaja, L. V. Makucho & L. J. Volkova. 1974. Antibiotiki **19:** 890.
2. Fusková, A., J. Fuska & M. Kettner. 1978. Neoplasma **24:** 239.
3. Rovenský, J., J. Fuska, J. Jakubovský, L. Korčáková, E. Rovenská, D. Žitňan & Š. Kopecký. 1984. *In* Abstracts: New Trends in Antimicrobial and Anticancer Chemotherapy, p. 171. Prague.
4. Rovenský, J., J. Grimová, J. Fuska, J. Lastovička, J. Pekárek & D. Pokorná. 1990. Int. J. Immunopathol. Pharmacol. **3:** 35–40.

Analysis of CD40–CD40 Ligand Interactions in the Regulation of Human B Cell Function[a]

PETER E. LIPSKY, JEANNE F. ATTREP,
AMRIE C. GRAMMER, MELISSA J. McILRAITH,
AND YUICHI NISHIOKA

Harold C. Simmons Arthritis Research Center
University of Texas Southwestern
Medical Center at Dallas
Dallas, Texas 75235

During T cell–dependent B cell activation, interactions between a variety of cell surface molecules expressed by B cells and their ligands expressed by activated T cells play a role in facilitating B cell activation, proliferation, and differentiation. Prominent among these is an interaction between CD40 expressed by B cells and CD40 ligand expressed by activated T cells.[1,2] CD40 is a 45- to 50-kDa member of the TNFαR family of molecules expressed by B cells, myeloid cells, dendritic cells, follicular dendritic cells, endothelial cells, fibroblasts, epithelial cells, and keratinocytes.[2–7] The ligand for CD40 is a 33-kDa molecule expressed by activated T cells, as well as by mast cells.[8–13] Interactions between CD40 and CD40 ligand play a critical role in a variety of phases of B cell activation.[1,2,14] The essential role of this interaction is underscored by the finding that children with X-linked hyper-IgM syndrome express a defective CD40 ligand and produce little IgG, IgA, or IgE and have no germinal centers in their lymph nodes.[15–20] Similarly, CD40 ligand–deficient[21,22] and CD40-deficient[23] mice exhibit marked defects in the ability of B cells to switch to downstream immunoglobulin isotypes and do not generate germinal centers in response to immunization, reminiscent of the defects manifested by children with X-linked hyper-IgM syndrome.

A number of studies have focused on the impact of ligation of CD40 on B cell function. These studies have included the use of monoclonal antibodies to CD40 to stimulate B cells directly, the use of monoclonal antibodies to CD40 ligand to interfere with T cell/B cell collaboration *in vivo* and *in vitro*, and investigations of the impact of variety of recombinant CD40 ligand constructs, as well as the use of mice rendered deficient in CD40 ligand or CD40 by targeted gene disruption.[1,2,14,21–23] All have come to the conclusion that CD40–CD40 ligand interactions play a central role in facilitating T cell/B cell collaboration and stimulating quiescent B cells to enter the cell cycle, undergo clonal expansion, produce immunoglobulin, and undergo immunoglobulin isotype switching to produce downstream immunoglobulin isotypes.

[a]This work was supported by Grant No. AI-31229 from the National Institutes of Health.

IMPACT OF LIGATION OF B CELL CD40 WITH BACULOVIRUS-EXPRESSED CD40 LIGAND

One means to study the impact of CD40 ligation on B cell function *in vitro* involves an analysis of the capacity of recombinant CD40 ligand to stimulate purified B lymphocytes. Although a number of CD40 ligand constructs have been employed for this purpose, it is not certain that they accurately reflect the physiologic impact of CD40 ligation. In an attempt to develop a physiologically relevant means to simulate CD40 ligation, recombinant CD40 ligand was expressed in baculovirus-infected Sf9 cells.[24] It was reasoned that these cells were sufficiently phylogenetically distant from

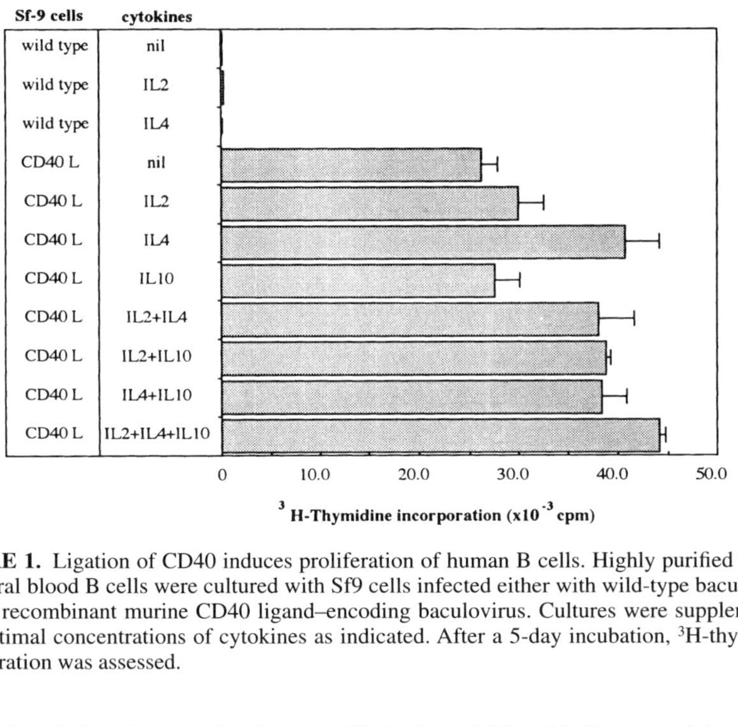

FIGURE 1. Ligation of CD40 induces proliferation of human B cells. Highly purified human peripheral blood B cells were cultured with Sf9 cells infected either with wild-type baculovirus or with recombinant murine CD40 ligand–encoding baculovirus. Cultures were supplemented with optimal concentrations of cytokines as indicated. After a 5-day incubation, ^{3}H-thymidine incorporation was assessed.

mammalian B lymphocytes that it was unlikely that additional influences of these cells conveyed by surface molecules or secreted proteins would influence the stimulatory impact of the expressed recombinant CD40 ligand. Moreover, analyzing the impact of baculovirus-expressed CD40 ligand allowed for an assessment of the effect of a membrane-bound molecule that might be more relevant than that of a variety of soluble constructs because the membrane association could allow the ligand to assume its physiologic conformation.

Culture of highly purified human peripheral B cells with baculovirus-expressed CD40 ligand led to initial aggregation of B cells around the Sf9 cells.[24] Subsequently, as shown in FIGURE 1, B cells entered the cell cycle and underwent proliferation as

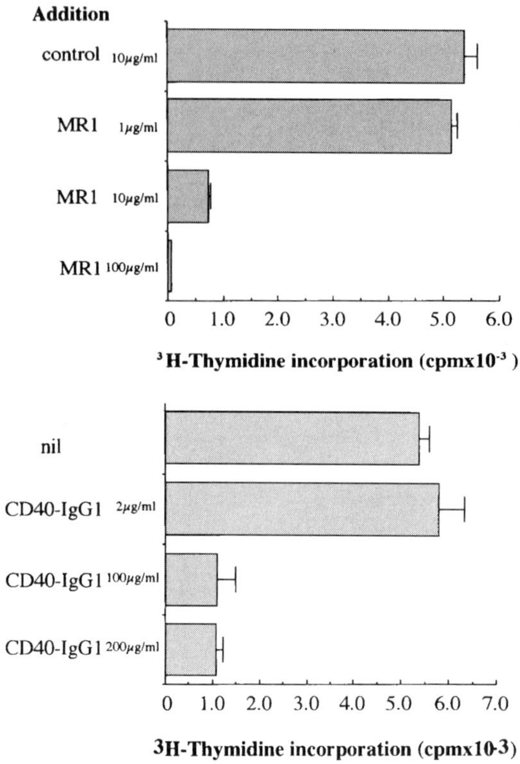

FIGURE 2. Specificity of the impact of Sf9-expressed CD40 ligand on human B cell responses. Highly purified human peripheral blood B cells were cultured with Sf9 cells infected with recombinant murine CD40 ligand–encoding baculovirus. Cultures were supplemented with various concentrations of a monoclonal antibody to murine CD40 ligand (MRI) or a CD40 IgG1 construct. After a 5-day incubation, ^{3}H-thymidine incorporation was assessed.

TABLE 1. Baculovirus-expressed CD40 Ligand–induced Immunoglobulin Production: Effect of Cytokines[a]

Addition to Culture		Secreted Ig (ng/mL)			
Sf9 Cells	Cytokines	IgM	IgG	IgA	IgE
WT	nil	0	0	0	0.00
WT	IL2 + IL4	<24	12	16	0.00
CD40L	nil	152	963	67	0.14
CD40L	IL2	1451	7766	573	0.14
CD40L	IL4	101	2703	115	1.95
CD40L	IL6	276	1101	90	0.00
CD40L	IL2 + IL4	556	13,606	1084	2.40
CD40L	IL2 + IL6	775	10,124	1122	0.00
CD40L	IL4 + IL6	126	1356	119	2.10
CD40L	IL2 + IL4 + IL6	599	11,377	575	7.38

[a]Purified human B cells were cultured with Sf9 cells infected with wild-type (WT) baculovirus or with recombinant murine CD40 ligand (CD40L)–encoding baculovirus. Cultures were supplemented with optimal concentrations of cytokines. After a 14-day incubation, the amount of immunoglobulin in the supernatants was detected by isotype-specific ELISA.

assessed by tritiated thymidine incorporation. This occurred without supplementation of cultures with cytokines, although additional cytokines, including IL2 or IL4, but not IL10, enhanced proliferation modestly. The effect of baculovirus-expressed CD40 ligand was specific in that it was blocked by a monoclonal antibody to CD40 ligand as well as by a soluble CD40 IgG construct (FIGURE 2). Culture of purified B cells with recombinant CD40 ligand also led to the production of small amounts of immunoglobulin without supplemental cytokines (TABLE 1). This resulted largely from stimulation of postswitch memory B cells, with IgG being the predominant Ig isotype produced. Immunoglobulin production could be enhanced by costimulation with a variety of cytokines. The isotype of Ig produced could be biased depending upon the specific cytokine employed. IL2 enhanced IgM, IgG, and IgA comparably, whereas IL4 increased production of IgG and IgE. IL6 enhanced the production of IgG and IgA

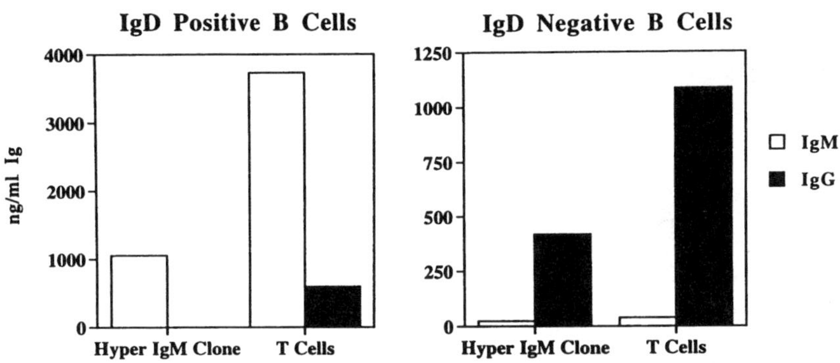

FIGURE 3. CD40 ligand-deficient T cells promote immunoglobulin production by both naive and memory B cells, but not heavy-chain isotype switching. Human peripheral blood B cells were separated into IgD(+) naive and IgD(−) postswitch memory subpopulations with the fluorescence-activated cell sorter. Each was cultured with a T cell clone derived from a child with hyper-IgM syndrome that lacked expression of a functional CD40 ligand or with normal T cells and stimulated with immobilized monoclonal antibody to CD3. After a 14-day incubation, the amount of immunoglobulin in the supernatants was determined.

supported by IL2, but not Ig promoted by IL4. Of note, IL6 had little effect in cultures that were not also stimulated by IL2. Thus, stimulation with recombinant CD40 ligand in combination with IL4 and IL6 led to production of no additional immunoglobulin above that produced by CD40 ligand and IL4 alone.

Although CD40 ligand could stimulate B cells to proliferate and produce immunoglobulin, it was not essential, as clones obtained from a child with hyper-IgM syndrome that failed to express a functional CD40 ligand could induce immunoglobulin production by both naive and postswitch memory B cells (FIGURE 3) as has previously been shown.[1,25] However, naive B cells could not undergo isotype switching to produce downstream immunoglobulin isotypes in the absence of CD40 ligand. Thus, anti-CD3-stimulated CD40 ligand–deficient T cells alone induced IgM production, but minimal IgG, from naive B cells, whereas normal T cells stimulated in

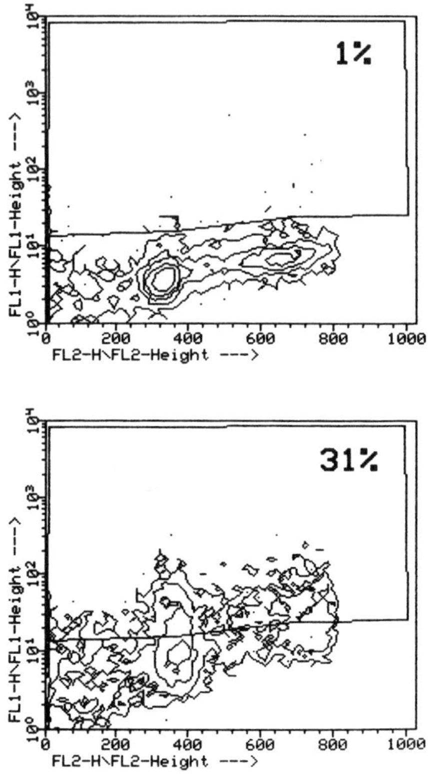

FIGURE 4. Ligation of CD40 induces apoptosis. IgG-secreting hybridoma 39 was incubated alone (upper panel) or with a large concentration of a murine CD40 ligand–CD8 construct (lower panel). After 40 hours of incubation, the cells were analyzed by FACS for the number of apoptotic cells following staining with propidium iodide and FITC-labeled ATP with terminal deoxynucleotide transferase. The x-axis is propidium iodide fluorescence and indicates the position of cells in the cell cycle, whereas the y-axis is FITC-ATP fluorescence and indicates the extent of DNA-strand breaks. The figures in each panel indicate the percentage of apoptotic cells.

a similar manner caused Ig isotype switching with production of IgG. This is consistent with the finding that children with hyper-IgM syndrome produce IgM antibodies, but do not switch to secrete downstream immunoglobulin isotypes. Of note, however, the requirement for B cells to undergo isotype switching does not appear to be absolute, as CD40-deficient mice can produce downstream immunoglobulin isotypes in response to *Borrelia burgdorferi.*[26] Moreover, CD40 ligand–deficient mice bred to express the *lpr* defect in Fas expression can produce IgG autoantibodies.[27] Although CD40 ligand can facilitate switching to downstream immunoglobulin isotypes, these results indicate that it may not be absolutely required in all circumstances.

One impact of CD40 ligand in the process of immunoglobulin isotype switching appears to involve the direct induction of transcription of downstream isotype genes before switch recombination.[24] The process of switch recombination is a multistep one in which one of the initial steps is transcription of the downstream isotype gene before deletional recombination occurs.[28] It has become clear that recombinant CD40 ligand in the absence of cytokines is capable of inducing transcription of downstream isotype genes, especially the ϵ gene.[24] This appears to result from activity of a unique promoter element in the 5′ region of the germline ε promoter.[29] Of note, however, engagement of CD40 ligand alone does not appear to be sufficient to induce subsequent steps in switch recombination and secretion of downstream immunoglobulin isotypes. Rather, this appears to require costimulation, usually with specific cytokines, although engagement of other surface receptors may also play a role.

Although most of the influences of CD40 engagement on B cell function appear to be positive, recent data suggest that CD40 engagement can also limit B cell responses and even induce apoptosis.[30] Thus, ligation of CD40 on human B cell hybridomas suppressed growth and immunoglobulin production. Moreover, such ligation of CD40 could induce apoptosis by a TNFα and Fas–independent mechanism (FIGURE 4). The induction of apoptosis by B cell hybridomas usually required a high level of CD40 engagement, although with some hybridomas engaging approximately 30% of surface CD40 induced programmed cell death. These results suggest the possibility that CD40 not only can induce activation of B cells, but also may limit their ongoing responses and even induce apoptosis. Of note, additional preliminary experiments using normal peripheral B cells have found that these differ in their sensitivity to inhibition by ligation of CD40. Memory B cells are more sensitive than naive B cells, and activated B cells are more susceptible to inhibition than resting B cells. These results are consistent with the idea that engagement of CD40 after initial activation may serve to limit the scope of the antibody response and thereby play a more complex regulatory function in the control of antibody production than previously appreciated.

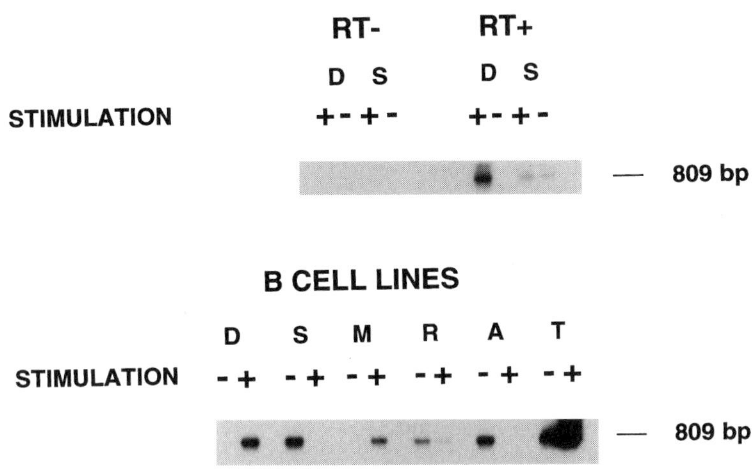

FIGURE 5. Human B cell lines express mRNA for the CD40 ligand. A variety of human EBV-transformed B lymphoblastoid cell lines [including SDL-Ml (S), Mar.B27 (M), and AO.EBV (A)], Burkitt lymphoma cell lines [Daudi (D) and Ramos (R)], and human peripheral blood T cells (T) were cultured alone (−) or stimulated with phorbol myristate acetate and ionomycin (+) and analyzed for CD40 ligand by RT-PCR using specific primers that would amplify the entire CD40 ligand cDNA. Amplifications were carried out with and without production of cDNA with reverse transcriptase (RT) as a control for DNA carryover.

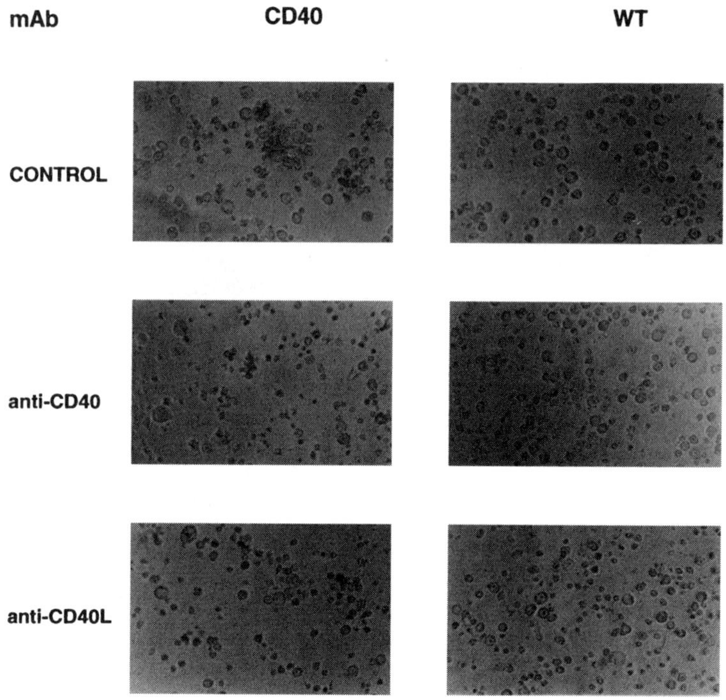

FIGURE 6. Human B cells express a functional CD40 ligand. The EBV-transformed B lymphoblastoid cell line, SDL-Ml, that constitutively expressed CD40 ligand mRNA was cultured with Sf9 cells infected with wild-type (WT) baculovirus or recombinant human CD40-encoding baculovirus. Cultures were supplemented with a control monoclonal antibody, an anti-CD40 (G28.5) monoclonal antibody, or an anti-human CD40 ligand (24-43) monoclonal antibody. Cultures were observed microscopically for the development of aggregates.

EXPRESSION OF CD40 LIGAND BY ACTIVATED B CELLS

Most experiments have examined the impact of CD40 ligand expressed on activated T cells. It has become apparent, however, that CD40 ligand expression is not limited to cells of T lymphocyte lineage. Of importance, activated B cells can also express CD40 ligand.[31] Thus, as shown in FIGURE 5, a variety of B cell lines express mRNA for CD40 ligand either constitutively or after activation. CD40 ligand mRNA was detected in B cells using primers that were derived from the known sequence of the T cell–expressed molecule. Moreover, the nucleotide sequence of the CD40 ligand cDNA obtained from human B cells was found to be identical to that expressed by activated T cells.[31] These results clearly show that the gene for the CD40 ligand is transcribed in human B cells.

Additional studies were carried out to document that the protein was expressed and functionally active. Initially, a 33-kDa protein was precipitated specifically from activated B cell lines with a CD40 IgG construct,[31] consistent with the conclusion that

CD40 ligand protein is expressed by activated B cells. It was difficult to identify CD40 ligand expression on activated B cells with monoclonal antibodies, however, because of its low abundance. Alternative means were therefore employed to detect expression of CD40 ligand protein on B cells. As shown in FIGURE 6, a B cell line that constitutively expressed CD40 ligand mRNA bound to Sf9 cells expressing recombinant CD40. This interaction was specifically blocked by monoclonal antibodies to either CD40 or CD40 ligand. These findings document that functional CD40 ligand is expressed by human B cells. Moreover, the results are consistent with the conclusion that under certain conditions CD40 ligand may function to facilitate homotypic aggregation by activated B cells.

The functional importance of CD40 ligand expressed by B cells was documented in a number of ways. First, B cell lines that express both CD40 and CD40 ligand were noted to undergo spontaneous homotypic aggregation that was inhibited with a CD40 IgG construct.[30,31] Second, ongoing proliferation of B cell lines or polyclonally activated normal human B cells could be blocked by a CD40 Ig construct or a monoclonal antibody to the CD40 ligand (FIGURES 7 and 8). Finally, immunoglobulin production by stimulated B cell lines or highly purified peripheral B cells was also

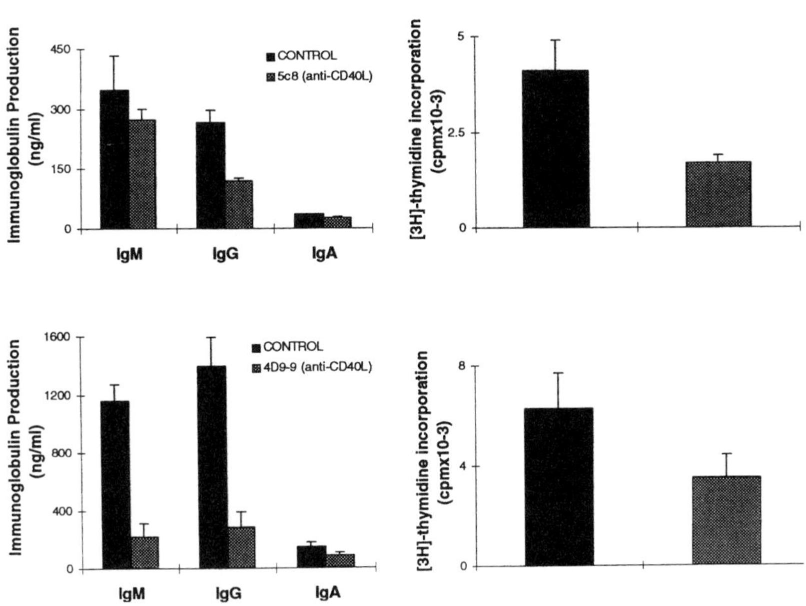

FIGURE 7. The CD40 ligand expressed by B cells is functionally active. Highly purified human peripheral blood B cells were stimulated with *S. aureus* Cowan I strain and IL2. In addition, cultures were supplemented with a control monoclonal antibody (black bars) or a monoclonal antibody to human CD40 ligand (gray bars) (5c8, upper panels; 4D9-9, lower panels). After a 5-day incubation, ^{3}H-thymidine incorporation was determined (right panels); after a 10-day incubation, supernatants were harvested and the content of immunoglobulin was assayed (left panels).

blocked by interfering with CD40–CD40 ligand interactions (FIGURES 7 and 8). All of these results are consistent with the conclusion that activated B cells express CD40 ligand and that homotypic B cell interactions mediated by CD40 ligand binding of CD40 play an essential role in facilitating ongoing B cell responses. It is therefore likely that during immune responses *in vivo,* following initial B cell activation mediated by interaction of resting B cells with CD40 ligand–expressing activated T cells, subsequent propagation of B cell responses within germinal centers of secondary lymphoid organs may well involve homotypic aggregation between CD40 ligand expressed by B cells and CD40 expressed by either the same or other B cells.

T CELL EXPRESSION OF CD40

Although initially thought to be a B cell lineage marker, recent evidence indicates that CD40 is more widely expressed. As has been shown,[32,33] CD40 is also expressed by activated T cells (FIGURE 9). Moreover, CD40 expressed by activated T cells is functionally active, in that it has the capacity to costimulate cytokine production by T cells and also to rescue T cells activated by signaling through the T cell receptor from apoptosis.[34] Thus, CD40 appears to play a similar role on T cells that it does on B cells. These findings suggest that the involvement of CD40–CD40 ligand interactions in ongoing T cell–dependent B cell responses is likely to be bidirectional and to involve a finely tuned regulatory mechanism that controls ongoing responses of both T and B cells.

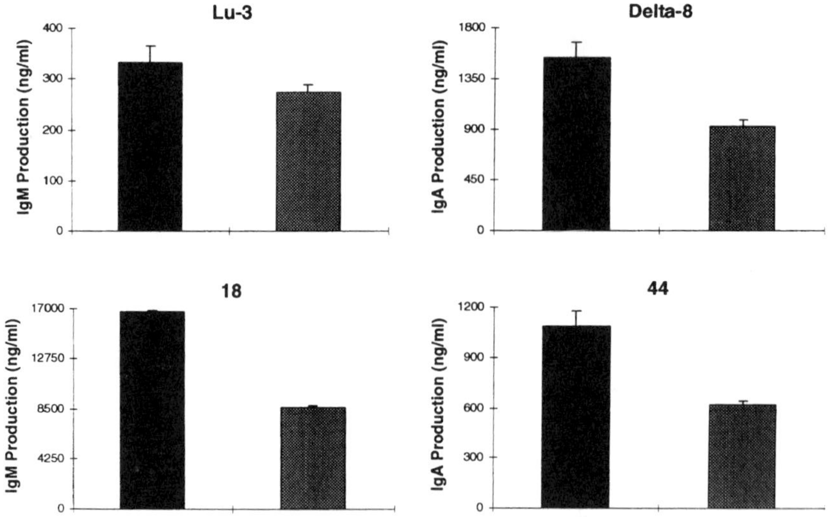

FIGURE 8. The CD40 ligand expressed by B cells is functionally active. Two IgM-secreting (Lu-3, 18) and two IgA-secreting (Delta-8, 44) hybridomas were cultured with a CD40 Ig construct (gray bars) or with a comparable concentration of control IgG (black bars). After a 10-day incubation, the amount of immunoglobulin in the supernatant was assessed.

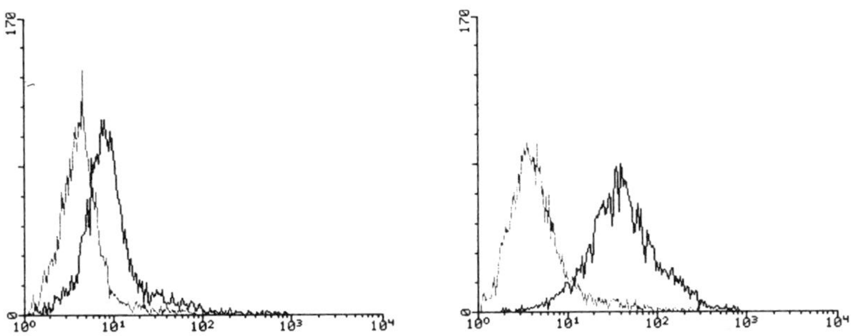

FIGURE 9. Activated human T cells express CD40. Highly purified human peripheral blood CD4(+) T cells were obtained by panning (purity, >96%) and were immediately stained with a control monoclonal antibody (gray histogram) or an anti-CD40 monoclonal antibody (G28.5, black histogram) and analyzed with the fluorescence-activated cell sorter (left panel). The same cells were stimulated with an immobilized monoclonal antibody to CD3 (64.1) for 24 hours and analyzed in the same manner (right panel).

SUMMARY

CD40–CD40 ligand interactions play an essential role in T cell/B cell collaboration. The data presented in this review have served to widen the scope of CD40–CD40 ligand interactions to include initial activation, proliferation, differentiation, and isotype switching of B cells, as well as subsequent downregulation of B cell function. Moreover, CD40 ligand expression by activated B cells is likely to play an essential role in facilitating ongoing responses of stimulated B cells maturing in germinal centers. Finally, CD40 expression by activated T cells may also play an important role in regulating the function of helper T cells within germinal centers. In summary, emerging data have expanded the role of CD40–CD40 ligand interaction during T cell/B cell collaboration and have emphasized its potential to regulate many of the functions of both partners in this essential interaction involved in antibody production.

REFERENCES

1. NISHIOKA, Y. & P. E. LIPSKY. 1994. The role of CD40–CD40 ligand interaction in human T cell–B cell collaboration. J. Immunol. **153:** 1027–1036.
2. VAN KOOTEN, C. & J. BANCHEREAU. 1996. CD40–CD40 ligand: a multifunctional receptor-ligand pair. Adv. Immunol. **61:** 1–77.
3. STAMENKOVIC, I., E. A. CLARK & B. SEED. 1989. A B-lymphocyte activation molecule related to the nerve growth factor receptor and induced by cytokines in carcinomas. EMBO J. **8:** 1403–1410.
4. SMITH, C. A., T. FARRAH & R. G. GOODWIN. 1994. The TNF receptor super-family of cellular and viral proteins: activation, co-stimulation, and death. Cell **76:** 959–962.
5. FREUDENTHAL, P. S. & R. M. STEINMAN. 1990. The distinct surface of human blood dendritic cells, as observed after an improved isolation method. Proc. Natl. Acad. Sci. U.S.A. **87:** 7698–7702.

6. SCHREIVER, F., A. S. FREEDMAN, G. FREEMAN, E. MESSNER, G. LEE, J. DALEY & L. M. NADLER. 1989. Isolated follicular dendritic cells display a unique antigenic phenotype. J. Exp. Med. **169:** 2043–2058.
7. GASPARI, A. A., G. D. SEMPOWSKI, P. CHESS, J. GISH & R. P. PHIPPS. 1996. Human epidermal keratinocytes are induced to secrete interleukin-6 and co-stimulate T lymphocyte proliferation by a CD40-dependent mechanism. Eur. J. Immunol. **26:** 1371–1377.
8. SPRIGGS, M. K., R. J. ARMITAGE, L. STROCKBINE, K. N. CLIFFORD, B. M. MACDUFF, T. A. SATO, C. R. MALISZEWSKI & W. C. FANSLOW. 1992. Recombinant human CD40 ligand stimulates B cell proliferation and immunoglobulin E secretion. J. Exp. Med. **176:** 1543–1550.
9. HOLLENBAUGH, D., L. S. GROSMAIRE, C. D. KULLAS, N. J. CHALUPNY, S. BRAESCH-ANDERSON, R. J. NOELLE, I. STAMENKOVIC, J. A. LEDBETTER & A. ARUFFO. 1992. The human T cell antigen gp39, a member of the TNF gene family, is a ligand for the CD40 receptor: expression of a soluble form of gp39 with B cell co-stimulatory activity. EMBO J. **11:** 4313–4321.
10. GAUCHET, J-F., J-P. AUBRY, G. MAZZEI, P. LIFE, T. JOMOTTE, G. ELSON & J-Y. BONNEFOY. 1993. Human CD40-ligand: molecular cloning, cellular distribution, and regulation of expression by factors controlling IgE production. FEBS Lett. **315:** 259–266.
11. GRAF, D., U. KORTHAUER, H. W. MAGES, G. SENGER & R. A. KROCZEK. 1992. Cloning of TRAP, a ligand for CD40 on human T cells. Eur. J. Immunol. **22:** 3191–3194.
12. VILLA, A., L. D. NOTARANGELO, J. P. DI SANTO, P. P. MACCHI, D. STRINA, A. FRATTINI, F. LUCCHINI, C. M. PATROSSO, S. GILIANI, E. MANTUANO, S. AGOSTI, G. NOCERA, R. A. KROCZEK, A. FISCHER, A. G. UGAZIO, G. DE SAINT BASILE & P. VEZZONI. 1994. Organization of human CD40L gene: implications for molecular defects in X chromosome–linked hyper-IgM syndrome and prenatal diagnosis. Proc. Natl. Acad. Sci. U.S.A. **91:** 2110–2114.
13. GAUCHET, J-F., S. HENCHOZ, G. MAZZEI, J-P. AUBRY, T. BRUNNER, H. BLASEY, P. LIFE, D. TALABOT, L. FLORES-REMO, J. THOMPSON, K. KISHI, J. BUTTERFIELD, C. DAHINDEN & J-Y. BONNEFOY. 1993. Induction of human IgE synthesis in B cells by mast cells and basophils. Nature **365:** 340–343.
14. SPRIGGS, M. K., W. C. FANSLOW, R. J. ARMITAGE & J. BELMONT. 1993. The biology of the human ligand for CD40. J. Clin. Immunol. **13:** 373–380.
15. ALLEN, R. C., R. J. ARMITAGE, M. E. CONLEY, H. ROSENBLATT, N. A. JENKINS, N. G. COPELAND, M. A. BEDELL, S. EDELHOFF, C. M. DISTECHE, D. K. SIMONEAUX, W. C. FANSLOW, J. BELMONT & M. K. SPRIGGS. 1993. CD40 ligand gene defects responsible for X-linked hyper-IgM syndrome. Science **259:** 990–993.
16. KORTHAUER, U., D. GRAF, H. W. MAGES, F. BRIÈRE, M. PADAYACHEE, S. MALCOLM, A. G. UGAZIO, L. D. NOTARANGELO, R. J. LEVINSKY & R. A. KROCZEK. 1993. Defective expression of T-cell CD40 ligand causes X-linked immunodeficiency with hyper-IgM. Nature **361:** 539–541.
17. FULEIHAN, R., N. RAMESH, R. LOH, H. JABARA, F. S. ROSEN, T. CHATILA, S. M. FU, I. STAMENKOVIC & R. S. GEHA. 1993. Defective expression of the CD40 ligand in X chromosome–linked immunoglobulin deficiency with normal or elevated IgM. Proc. Natl. Acad. Sci. U.S.A. **90:** 2170–2173.
18. DI SANTO, J. P., J-Y. BONNEFOY, J-F. GAUCHET, A. FISCHER & G. DE SAINT BASILE. 1993. CD40 ligand mutations in X-linked immunodeficiency with hyper-IgM. Nature **361:** 541–543.
19. ARUFFO, A., M. FARRINGTON, D. HOLLENBAUGH, X. LI, A. MILATOVICH, S. NONOYAMA, J. BAJORATH, L. S. GROSMAIRE, R. STENKAMP, M. NEUBAUER, R. L. ROBERTS, R. J. NOELLE, J. A. LEDBETTER, U. FRANCKE & H. D. OCHS. 1993. The CD40 ligand, gp39, is defective in activated T cells from patients with X-linked hyper-IgM syndrome. Cell **72:** 291–300.
20. CALLARD, R. E., R. J. ARMITAGE, W. C. FANSLOW & M. K. SPRIGGS. 1993. CD40 ligand and its role in X-linked hyper-IgM syndrome. Immunol. Today **14:** 559–564.
21. XU, J., T. M. FOY, J. D. LAMAN, E. A. ELLIOTT, J. J. DUNN, T. J. WALDSCHMIDT, J. ELSMORE, R. J. NOELLE & R. A. FLAVELL. 1994. Mice deficient for the CD40 ligand. Immunity **1:** 423–431.

22. RENSHAW, B. R., W. C. FANSLOW III, R. J. ARMITAGE, K. A. CAMPBELL, D. LIGGITT, B. WRIGHT, B. L. DAVIDSON & C. R. MALISZEWSKI. 1994. Humoral immune responses in CD40 ligand–deficient mice. J. Exp. Med. **180:** 1889–1900.
23. KAWABE, T., T. NAKA, K. YOSHIDA, T. TANAKA, H. FUJIWARA, S. SUEMATSU, N. YOSHIDA, T. KISHIMOTO & H. KIKUTANI. 1994. The immune responses in CD40-deficient mice: impaired immunoglobulin class switching and germinal center formation. Immunity **1:** 167–178.
24. JUMPER, M. D., Y. NISHIOKA, L. S. DAVIS, P. E. LIPSKY & K. MEEK. 1995. Regulation of human B cell function by recombinant CD40 ligand and other TNF-related ligands. J. Immunol. **155:** 2369–2378.
25. SPLAWSKI, J. B., J. NISHIOKA, Y. NISHIOKA & P. E. LIPSKY. 1996. CD40 ligand is expressed and functional on activated neonatal T cells. J. Immunol. **156:** 119–127.
26. FIKRIG, E., S. W. BARTHOLD, M. CHEN, I. S. GREWAL, J. CRAFT & R. A. FLAVELL. 1996. Protective antibodies in murine lyme disease arise independently of CD40 ligand. J. Immunol. **157:** 1–3.
27. MA, J., J. XU, M. P. MADAIO, Q. PENG, J. ZHANG, I. S. GREWAL, R. A. FLAVELL & J. CRAFT. 1996. Autoimmune lpr/lpr mice deficient in CD40 ligand: spontaneous Ig class switching with dichotomy of autoantibody responses. J. Immunol. **157:** 417–426.
28. STAVNEZER, J. 1996. Antibody class switching. Adv. Immunol. **61:** 79–146.
29. FUJITA, K., M. D. JUMPER, K. MEEK & P. E. LIPSKY. 1995. Evidence for a CD40 response element, distinct from the IL-4 response element in the germline ϵ promoter. Int. Immunol. **7:** 1529–1533.
30. BERGMAN, M. C., J. F. ATTREP, A. C. GRAMMER & P. E. LIPSKY. 1996. Ligation of CD40 influences the function of human Ig-secreting B cell hybridomas both positively and negatively. J. Immunol. **156:** 3118–3132.
31. GRAMMER, A. C., M. C. BERGMAN, Y. MIURA, K. FUJITA, L. S. DAVIS & P. E. LIPSKY. 1995. The CD40 ligand expressed by human B cells co-stimulates B cell responses. J. Immunol. **154:** 4996–5010.
32. ARMITAGE, R., T. TOUGH, B. MACDUFF, W. FANSLOW, M. SPRIGGS, F. RAMSDELL & M. ALDERSON. 1993. CD40 ligand is a T cell growth factor. Eur. J. Immunol. **23:** 2326–2331.
33. INDZHIIA, L., L. YAKOVLEVA, J. OVERBAUGH, K. LICCIARDI, M. CHIKOBAVA, I. KLOTZ, R. TORRES, V. INDZHIIA, B. LAPIN, E. CLARK & M. VALENTINE. 1992. Baboon T cell lymphomas expressing the B cell–associated surface proteins CD40 and Bgp95. J. Clin. Immunol. **12:** 225–236.
34. ATTREP, J., H-P. BREZINSCHEK, R. BREZINSCHEK & P. E. LIPSKY. 1996. Regulatory influences of CD40 on T lymphocytes. FASEB J. **10:** A1454.

CD40 and Its Ligand in Autoimmunity

RANDOLPH J. NOELLE,[a] MATTHEW MACKEY,[a]
TERESA FOY,[a] JANET BUHLMANN,[a]
AND CHRISTOPHER BURNS[b]

[a]*Department of Microbiology*
[b]*Department of Medicine*
Dartmouth Medical School
Lebanon, New Hampshire 03756

INTRODUCTION

CD40, a mitogenic receptor expressed on all mature B lymphocytes,[1,2] is a member of the nerve growth factor receptor (NGFR) family of receptors.[3] The ligand for CD40, gp39, is a type II membrane protein that is homologous to TNF-α and -β,[4,5] other NGFR family ligands. Evidence that CD40 is an important mitogenic receptor on B cells is derived from studies that show highly efficient triggering of human B cells by anti-CD40 and cofactors such as anti-CD20, anti-Ig, and lymphokines.[4–9] In the presence of these cofactors, anti-CD40 has been shown to initiate both B cell growth and differentiation. Similar to anti-CD40, gp39, expressed as a recombinant membrane protein or a soluble protein, also activates B cells in the presence of costimulators.[4,10] gp39 is transiently expressed on activated $CD4^+$ T_h *in vitro* and is induced *in vivo* on $CD4^+$ T cells as a result of antigen administration.[11] The $CD4^+$ T cell population expressing gp39 *in vivo* has been localized *in situ* juxtaposed to B cells producing antibodies to the immunizing antigen. *In vitro* and *in vivo* data suggest that, during the course of cognate T_h-B interaction, transient expression of gp39 by $CD4^+$ T cells is the result of antigen presentation.[12] Once expressed, gp39 binds to CD40 and reciprocally triggers B cell activation. The ability of a monoclonal antibody (mAb) specific for gp39, MR1, to block the capacity of gp39-bearing T_h to activate B cells *in vitro* has implicated gp39 as an important molecule in T cell–dependent B cell activation, as reviewed in reference 13.

Further evidence implicating gp39-CD40 involvement in humoral immune responses has recently been provided by several groups demonstrating that mutations in the gene encoding gp39 result in the inability of humans to respond to TD antigens, as reviewed in reference 13. An immunodeficiency characterized by failure to mount TD humoral immune responses, hyper-IgM syndrome (HIM), results in the expression of a defective gp39 molecule that lacks CD40 binding capacity. Although the B lymphocytes from these patients are reported to be normal, mutations in the gp39 molecule interrupt B cell triggering through CD40 and subsequent B cell activation and immunoglobulin production. Over the past few years, insights into the function of gp39 and CD40 in the regulation of humoral immunity have been provided by studies in gp39-deficient[14,15] and CD40-deficient[16] mice and in mice treated with anti-gp39.[11,17,18] For the most part, all of these systems agree that gp39 interactions are essential for secondary immune responses to TD antigens and in the formation of GC.

Studies using anti-gp39[18] or a soluble form of CD40[19] to inhibit the *in vivo* function of gp39 showed that the generation of memory B cells is also dependent on this ligand-receptor pair.

CD40 PLAYS A CENTRAL ROLE IN THE REGULATION OF ANTIGEN PRESENTATION

CD40 signaling has been shown to regulate the expression of B7.1 and B7.2 on B cells. We have proposed the following scheme for the regulation of B7 on B cells. Antigen recognition by the T cell antigen receptor (TCR) triggers the upregulation of gp39 on the T cells (FIGURE 1; signal 1). The expression of gp39 reciprocally triggers

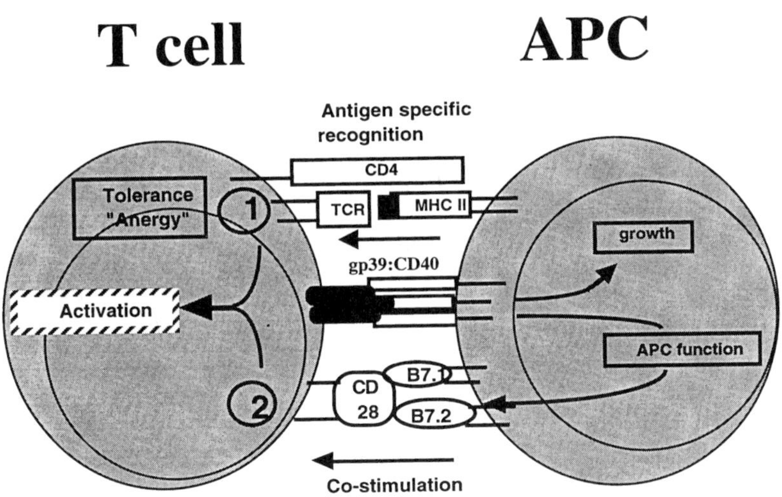

FIGURE 1. A model of CD40-regulated expression of B7.1 and B7.2.

the upregulation of B7.1 and B7.2 via CD40 on the cognate B cells. Having upregulated B7.1 and B7.2, the B cell costimulates the T cells to proliferate and to produce lymphokines (signal 2). Therefore, if the reciprocal signal via gp39 is blocked, the T cells will only receive signal 1 and are rendered anergic.

To test the hypothesis that antigen-bearing B cells could induce tolerance in the presence of anti-gp39, B cells were prepared from C57BL/6 (H-2[b]) mice by T cell depletion using Thy 1.2 and complement treatment and were injected into Balb/c (H-2[d]) mice. Some groups received anti-gp39 (250 μg/mouse/2 days) for 6 days, at which point the spleens from these recipient animals were removed and a single cell suspension was prepared and used as effector cells in a standard 4-hour chromium release assay. Targets in the assay were H-2[b]-bearing tumor cells. FIGURE 2 represents the allo-CTL response and MLR obtained for such an experiment. FIGURE 2 demonstrates that *in vivo* administration of allogeneic splenic B cells and anti-gp39 results in hyporesponsiveness of alloantigen-specific CTL activity (FIGURE 2A) and in $CD4^+$ proliferative responses (FIGURE 2B) to alloantigen. Assessment of third-party responses in the CTL and MLR assays confirms that the tolerogenic effect is allospecific (data not shown). These data have been published elsewhere.[20]

In lieu of using anti-gp39 to block the function of gp39, one would predict that the administration of allogeneic B cells into gp39−/− mice[14] would induce allospecific tolerance. The administration of allogeneic B cells into gp39−/− mice induces allospecific hyporesponsiveness of CD4 and CD8 T cells. These observations confirm the results observed with anti-gp39 administration and show that, in the absence of a CD40 signal, B cells are tolerogenic.

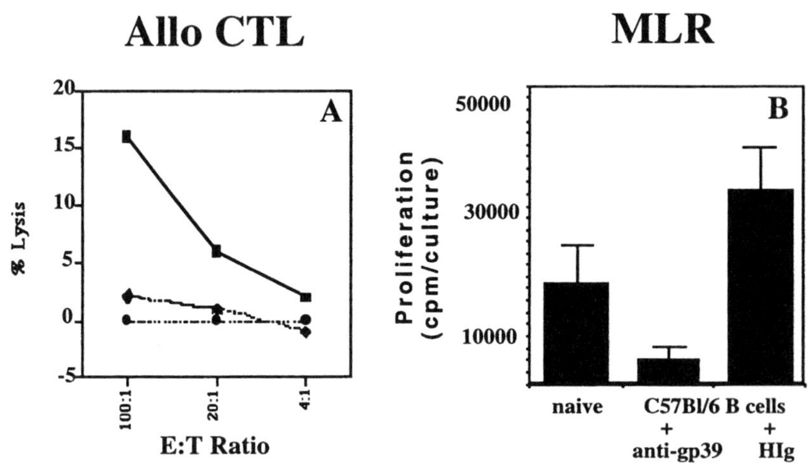

FIGURE 2. Anti-gp39 and allogeneic B cells prevent the generation of allospecific CTL and MLR. Balb/c mice (H-2^d) were administered T-depleted C57BL/6 (H-2^b)–derived splenic B cells. Recipient mice were either untreated or administered anti-gp39 (250 μg/mouse/2 days) for 6 days. A 4-hour chromium release assay was then performed using LB27.4 (H-2^{bd}) cells as the targets (A) or MLR against C57BL/6-irradiated spleen cells (B). Symbols in panel A: (■) C57BL/6 only; (◆) C57BL/6 + anti-gp39; (●) naive Balb/c + anti-gp39.

INDUCTION OF TRANSPLANTATION TOLERANCE USING ALLOGENEIC B CELLS AND ANTI-gp39

In collaboration with David Parker, Aldo Rossini, Dale Greiner, and coworkers at the University of Massachusetts, the tolerization regime of using allogeneic B cells and anti-gp39 was applied to a system of transplantation tolerance, as published.[21] Mice were induced to become diabetic by the chemical destruction of the endogenous islet cells, were given allogeneic B cells and/or anti-gp39, and were then transplanted with allogeneic islets. Without any prior tolerization or simply by the administration of allogeneic B cells, the mice rapidly rejected the allogeneic islet cells. The administration of anti-gp39 prolonged graft survival indefinitely in 40–50% of the mice. This observation will be discussed later in the context of the anti-inflammatory effect of anti-gp39. Virtually all of the transplanted mice pretreated with allogeneic B cells and anti-gp39 retained the allogeneic grafts indefinitely. If the allogeneic B cells and the allogeneic islet grafts were mismatched for the alloantigen, the success rate of graft survival dropped to that observed with anti-gp39 alone. These data, together with the data presented above, confirm that allogeneic B cells, if deprived of the CD40 signal, will induce T cell unresponsiveness.

IS CD40 SIGNALING CRITICAL FOR THE COSTIMULATION BY ALL APC?

To gain a more comprehensive view of the role of CD40 signaling in APC function, the role of CD40 in graft-versus-host disease (GVHD) was evaluated. Because studies clearly show that some dendritic cells constitutively express costimulatory molecules, it was not necessarily anticipated that anti-gp39 administration would impede their ability to present alloantigen. These questions were addressed indirectly by asking whether GVHD was blocked by anti-gp39 administration. The hallmark feature of a GVHD is that the donor T cells mount a CTL response against the F1 host alloantigens. Published studies have shown that anti-gp39 can block the generation of a GVHD in mice.[22] A brief treatment with anti-gp39 produced long-lived protection from a GVHD, suggesting that even after the antibody disappeared from the periphery no disease developed. In order to evaluate if T cell unresponsiveness was induced as a consequence of anti-gp39 treatment, T cells from GVHD mice that were treated with anti-gp39 were asked to transfer disease. No transfer of GVHD could be obtained from mice treated with anti-gp39, suggesting that the anti-gp39 resulted in T cell tolerance. Alternative to using anti-gp39 to interfere with the development of GVHD, we have also shown that no indication of GVHD was noted if T cells from gp39−/− mice were transferred into an F1 host. When WT parental T cells were transferred into an F1, a profound reduction in splenic cellularity was obvious; however, when gp39−/− T cells were transferred, no reduction in cellularity was noted. A GVHD typically is lethal to >95% of the mice within 21 days. Indeed, the transfer of WT T cells caused death in >95% of the recipients. In those recipients receiving WT T cells and anti-gp39 or gp39−/− T cells, >90% were alive with no signs of disease at >50 days. Upon more extensive analysis of mice receiving gp39−/− T cells, minimal (if any) features of GVHD were observed. These data suggest that the host is inducing tolerance to host MHC molecules in the donor T cell population. This implies that, in the absence of the CD40 signal, host APC are tolerogenic and therefore would include host dendritic cells and macrophages (see FIGURE 3). This observation raises the issue of whether professional APC (like dendritic cells and macrophages) need a CD40 signal to prime T cells.

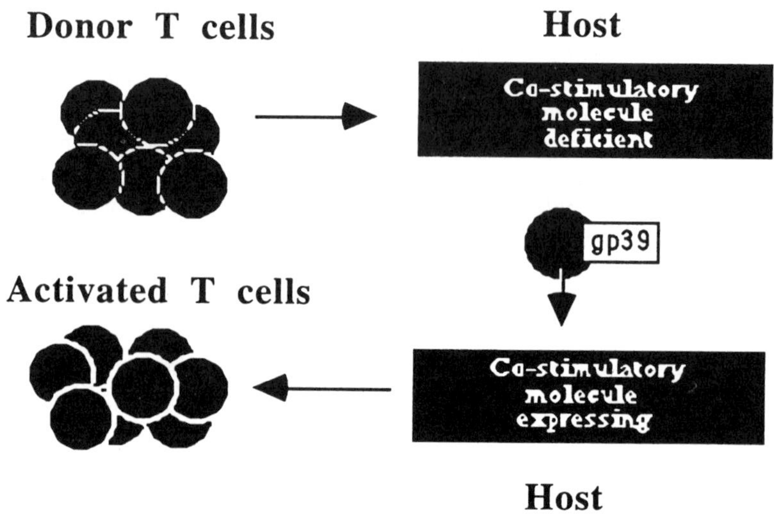

FIGURE 3. Do even dendritic cells need a CD40 signal? Alloreactive donor T cells, once administered, activate the host to upregulate costimulatory molecules. Once upregulated, the host can then reciprocally activate the donor T cells to mount a GVHD response.

ROLE OF CD40-gp39 INTERACTIONS IN AUTOIMMUNE DISEASE

Given the broad impact of anti-gp39 on the regulation of humoral immunity and on antigen presentation, the effect of anti-gp39 was assessed on different models of antibody- and T cell–mediated autoimmune disease. We have already demonstrated that anti-gp39 can prevent the onset of collagen-induced arthritis.[23] To address whether anti-gp39 can interfere with a spontaneous, antibody-mediated autoimmune disease, Christopher Burns and colleagues (Dartmouth Medical School) treated NZB/NZW F1 mice at an early age, weekly with anti-gp39. Treatment of mice prior to significant disease onset completely protected the mice from disease. This is consistent with the report from Datta and coworkers[24] that showed that brief treatment caused delayed onset of disease. After mice were treated with anti-gp39 and allowed to clear the anti-gp39, the humoral immune response to test antigens appeared normal, suggesting that there was no long-term immune suppression imposed by the treatment. Experiments currently in progress are investigating if anti-gp39 therapy can reverse established disease.

Recent work in collaboration with Eric Claassen and his colleagues has evaluated the role of CD40 and gp39 in the development and progression of experimental allergic encephalomyelitis (EAE). These studies have been published[25] and show that treatment of mice prior to disease onset with anti-gp39 can completely block the development of EAE. Furthermore, even late treatment with anti-gp39 can partially reverse disease. These data provide compelling evidence that anti-gp39 may have an impact on the priming and/or differentiation of effector T cells that mediate this disease. Histological studies by this group show the presence of gp39-bearing T cells in the brains of mice with EAE and in human brains from patients with multiple sclerosis. Moreover, CD40-bearing macrophages or microglia were also prominent in the perivascular infiltrates.

How does anti-gp39 interfere with the development and progression of a T cell–mediated autoimmune disease? Studies from a number of sources have now documented that the lack of CD40L (or the administration of anti-CD40L) blocks multiple mechanisms that are responsible for the development of inflammation (FIGURE 4). First, lack of CD40L function either alters or diminishes the priming and expansion of T cells in response to antigen, and likely polarizes the course of T cell differentiation toward a Th2 response.[26,27] This effect is due to the role of CD40L in the regulation of costimulatory molecules on APC and/or the regulation of IL12 production. Second, even though some effector T cells may be generated in the absence of CD40L, their ability to traffic to the appropriate target organ may be diminished. One would anticipate that the lack of CD40L will interfere with the localization of the effector cells in the target organ by prohibiting the upregulation of adhesion molecules required for effector T cell diapedesis and accumulation.[28,29] Third, even though some effector T cells may be identified within the target organ, the lack of CD40L would seriously compromise their ability to optimally trigger macrophage functions—like the production of proinflammatory cytokines and inflammatory cytokines, as well as the upregulation of costimulatory molecules and other mediators of inflammatory pathology.[30–32] In sum, the role of CD40L at all of these levels of cell-mediated immunity helps to explain why one can so effectively interfere with the development of autoimmune disease by the administration of anti-CD40L.

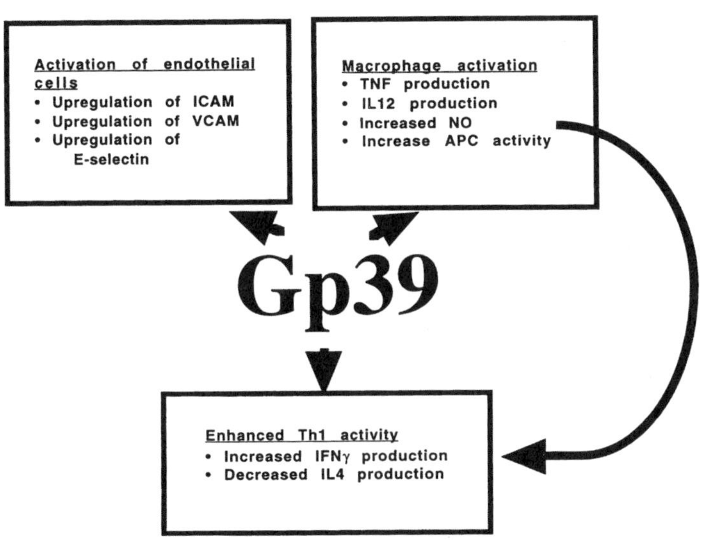

FIGURE 4. The multiple effects of gp39 on the inflammatory response.

CONCLUSIONS

gp39 is not just for humoral immune responses anymore. Recent studies from a number of laboratories have shown that gp39-CD40 interactions play a significant role in the regulation of APC activities, in the expression of adhesion molecules, and in the activation of macrophages. Because of these roles, gp39-CD40 interactions play a central role in the development of inflammatory responses. Coupled with its role as a critical regulator of humoral immunity, gp39 is a prime target for immune intervention in the treatment of both T cell–mediated and antibody-mediated autoimmune disease.

REFERENCES

1. GORDON, J., M. J. MILLSUM, G. R. GUY & J. A. LEDBETTER. 1987. Synergistic interaction between interleukin 4 and anti-Bp50 (CDw40) revealed in a novel B cell restimulation assay. Eur. J. Immunol. **17:** 1535–1538.
2. CLARK, E. A. & J. A. LEDBETTER. 1986. Activation of human B cells mediated through two distinct cell surface differentiation antigens, Bp35 and Bp50. Proc. Natl. Acad. Sci. U.S.A. **83:** 4494.
3. STAMENKOVIC, I., E. A. CLARK & B. SEED. 1989. A B-lymphocyte activation molecule related to the nerve growth factor receptor and induced by cytokines in carcinomas. EMBO J. **8:** 1403–1410.
4. HOLLENBAUGH, D., L. GROSMAIRE, C. D. KULLAS, N. J. CHALUPNY, R. J. NOELLE, I. STAMENKOVIC, J. A. LEDBETTER & A. ARUFFO. 1992. The human T cell antigen gp39, a member of the TNF gene family, is a ligand for the CD40 receptor: expression of a soluble form of gp39 with B cell co-stimulatory activity. EMBO J. **11:** 4313–4321.
5. ARMITAGE, R. J., W. C. FANSLOW, L. STROCKBINE, T. A. SATO, K. N. CLIFFORD, B. M. MACDUFF, D. M. ANDERSON, S. D. GIMPEL, T. DAVIS-SMITH, C. R. MALISZEWSKI, E. A. CLARK, C. A. SMITH, K. H. GRABSTEIN, D. COSMAN & M. K. SPRIGGS. 1992. Molecular and biological characterization of a murine ligand for CD40. Nature **357:** 80–82.
6. VALLE, A., C. E. ZUBER, T. DEFRANCE, O. DJOSSOU, R. M. DE & J. BANCHEREAU. 1989. Activation of human B lymphocytes through CD40 and interleukin 4. Eur. J. Immunol. **19:** 1463–1467.
7. GORDON, J., M. J. MILLSUM, R. L. FLORES & S. GILLIS. 1989. Regulation of resting and cycling human B lymphocytes via the surface accessory molecules interleukin-4, CD23, and CD40. Immunology **68:** 526–531.
8. JABARA, H. H., S. M. FU, R. S. GEHA & D. VERCELLI. 1990. CD40 and IgE: synergism between anti-CD40 monoclonal antibody and interleukin 4 in the induction of IgE synthesis by highly purified human B cells. J. Exp. Med. **172:** 1861–1864.
9. BANCHEREAU, J. & F. ROUSSET. 1991. Growing human B lymphocytes in the CD40 system. Nature **353:** 678–679.
10. ARMITAGE, R. J., T. A. SATO, B. M. MACDUFF, K. N. CLIFFORD, A. R. ALPERT, C. A. SMITH & W. C. FANSLOW. 1992. Identification of a source of biologically active CD40 ligand. Eur. J. Immunol. **22:** 2071–2076.
11. VAN DEN EERTWEGH, A. J. M., R. J. NOELLE, M. ROY, D. M. SHEPHERD, A. ARUFFO, J. A. LEDBETTER, W. J. A. BOERSMA & E. CLAASSEN. 1993. *In vivo* CD40-gp39 interactions are essential for thymus-dependent immunity: I. CD40-gp39 interactions are essential for thymus-dependent humoral immunity and identify sites of cognate interactions *in vivo*. J. Exp. Med. **178:** 1555–1565.
12. NOELLE, R. J., J. A. LEDBETTER & A. ARUFFO. 1992. CD40 and its ligand, an essential ligand-receptor pair for thymus-dependent B cell activation. Immunol. Today **13:** 431–434.
13. FOY, T., A. ARUFFO, J. BAJORATH, J. E. BUHLMANN & R. J. NOELLE. 1996. Immune regulation by CD40 and its ligand gp39. Annu. Rev. Immunol. **14:** 591–617.

14. XU, J., T. M. FOY, J. D. LAMAN, J. J. DUNN, T. J. WALDSCHMIDT, J. ELSEMORE, R. J. NOELLE & R. A. FLAVELL. 1994. Mice deficient for the CD40 ligand. Immunity **1:** 423–431.
15. RENSHAW, B. R., W. FANSLOW, R. J. ARMITAGE, K. A. CAMPBELL, D. LIGGITT, B. WRIGHT, B. L. DAVISON & C. R. MALISZEWSKI. 1994. Humoral immune responses in CD40 ligand–deficient mice. J. Exp. Med. **180:** 1889–1900.
16. KAWABE, T., T. NAKA, K. YOSHIDA, T. TANAKA, H. FUJIWARA, S. SUEMATSU, N. YOSHIDA, T. KISHIMOTO & H. KIKUTANI. 1994. The immune responses in CD40-deficient mice: impaired immunoglobulin class switching and germinal center formation. Immunity **1:** 167–178.
17. FOY, T. M., A. ARUFFO, J. A. LEDBETTER & R. J. NOELLE. 1993. *In vivo* CD40-gp39 interactions are essential for thymus-dependent immunity: II. Prolonged *in vivo* suppression of primary and secondary humoral immune responses by an antibody targeted to the CD40 ligand, gp39. J. Exp. Med. **178:** 1567–1575.
18. FOY, T. M., J. D. LAMAN, J. A. LEDBETTER, A. ARUFFO, E. CLAASSEN & R. J. NOELLE. 1994. gp39-CD40 interactions are essential for germinal center formation and the development of B cell memory. J. Exp. Med. **180:** 157–164.
19. GRAY, D., P. DULLFORCE & S. JAINANDUNSING. 1994. Memory B cell development, but not germinal center formation, is impaired by *in vivo* blockade of CD40–CD40-ligand interaction. J. Exp. Med. In press.
20. BUHLMANN, J. E., T. M. FOY, A. ARUFFO, K. M. CRASSI, J. A. LEDBETTER, W. R. GREEN, J. XU, L. D. SHULTZ, D. ROOPESIAN, R. A. FLAVELL, L. FAST, R. J. NOELLE & F. H. DURIE. 1995. In the absence of a CD40 signal, B cells are tolerogenic. Immunity **2:** 645–653.
21. PARKER, D. C., D. L. GREINER, N. E. PHILLIPS, M. C. APPEL, A. W. STEELE, F. H. DURIE, R. J. NOELLE, J. P. MORDES & A. A. ROSSINI. 1995. Survival of mouse pancreatic islet allografts in recipients treated with allogeneic small lymphocytes and antibody to CD40 ligand. Proc. Natl. Acad. Sci. U.S.A. **92:** 9560–9564.
22. DURIE, F. H., A. ARUFFO, J. A. LEDBETTER, K. M. CRASSI, W. R. GREEN & R. J. NOELLE. 1994. Antibody to the ligand of CD40, gp39, blocks the occurrence of the acute and chronic forms of graft-versus-host disease. J. Clin. Invest. **94:** 1333–1338.
23. DURIE, F. H., R. A. FAVA, T. M. FOY, A. ARUFFO, J. A. LEDBETTER & R. J. NOELLE. 1993. Prevention of collagen-induced arthritis with an antibody to gp39, the ligand for CD40. Science **261:** 1328–1330.
24. MOHAN, C., Y. SHI, J. D. LAMAN & S. K. DATTA. 1995. Interaction between CD40 and its ligand gp39 in the development of murine lupus nephritis. J. Immunol. **154:** 1470–1480.
25. GERRITSE, K., R. J. NOELLE, A. ARUFFO, J. A. LEDBETTER, J. D. LAMAN, W. J. A. BOERSMA & E. CLAASSEN. 1995. Functional and histological evidence for the involvement of gp39 (CD40 ligand) in multiple sclerosis. Proc. Natl. Acad. Sci. U.S.A. In press.
26. GREWAL, I. S., J. XU & R. A. FLAVELL. 1995. Impairment of antigen-specific T-cell priming in mice lacking CD40 ligand. Nature **378:** 617–620.
27. STUBER, E., W. STROBER & M. NEURATH. 1996. Blocking of CD40-CD40L interaction *in vivo* specifically prevents the priming of T helper 1 cells through the inhibition of interleukin 12 secretion. J. Exp. Med. **183:** 693–698.
28. HOLLENBAUGH, D., N. MISCHEL-PETTY, C. P. EDWARDS, J. C. SIMON, R. W. DENFIELD, P. A. KIENER & A. ARUFFO. 1995. Expression of functional CD40 by vascular endothelial cells. J. Exp. Med. **182:** 33–40.
29. KARMANN, K., C. W. HUGHES, J. SCHECHNER, W. C. FANSLOW & J. S. POBER. 1995. CD40 on human endothelial cells: inducibility by cytokines and functional regulation of adhesion molecule expression. Proc. Natl. Acad. Sci. U.S.A. **92:** 4342–4346.
30. KIENER, P. A., D. P. MORAN, B. M. RANKIN, A. F. WAHL, A. ARUFFO & D. HOLLENBAUGH. 1995. Stimulation of CD40 with purified soluble gp39 induces proinflammatory responses in human monocytes. J. Immunol. **155:** 4917–4925.
31. TIAN, L., R. J. NOELLE & D. A. LAWRENCE. 1995. Activated T cells enhance nitric oxide production by murine splenic macrophages through gp39 and LFA-1. Eur. J. Immunol. **25:** 306–309.
32. STOUT, R. D., J. SUTTLES, J. XU, I. S. GREWAL & R. A. FLAVELL. 1996. Impaired T cell–mediated macrophage activation in CD40 ligand–deficient mice. J. Immunol. **156:** 8–11.

Regulation of T and B Cell Responses by Modulating Interactions between CD28/CTLA4 and Their Ligands, CD80 and CD86[a]

PETER LANE[b]

Basel Institute for Immunology
Basel CH-4005, Switzerland

INTRODUCTION

The initiation of appropriate immune responses requires cooperation between both B and T lymphocytes and accessory cells. Whether these interactions lead to activation, differentiation, or death is determined by the state of maturity of the interacting cells and is a consequence of interactions between pairs of accessory molecules that direct immune responses down different pathways. It is now clear that both B and T cell responses are regulated by both positive and negative signals, which direct immune responses against foreign antigens while imposing a degree of control preventing the overexpansion of self-reactive clones that leads to autoimmune disease. Understanding the molecular mechanisms that mediate these positive and negative signals provides opportunities for the manipulation of inappropriate immune responses and thus generates new therapeutic approaches to tackling autoimmune disease.

In this regard, the interactions between the coreceptors, CD28/CTLA4, and their ligands, B7.1 (CD80) and B7.2 (CD86), seem to play a crucial role in both the positive and negative regulation of B and T cell responses. To address the role of these molecules in regulating lymphocyte responses, we have generated transgenic mice where CD28 is blocked by the soluble competitor CTLA4-Ig and, more recently, mice that express CD80-Ig, a potential soluble agonist for CTLA4. Immunological function in these mice is discussed in the light of recent knowledge of the function of CD28, CTLA4, and CD80 and CD86.

ROLE OF CD28 IN T CELL ACTIVATION

A two-signal model of T cell activation has been central to immunological thinking for 25 years[1] and, in recent times, the focus of attention for the molecular

[a]This work was supported by F. Hoffmann–La Roche Limited, Basel, Switzerland, which founded and supports the Basel Institute.

[b]Present address: Department of Immunology, Medical School, University of Birmingham, Birmingham B15 2TT, United Kingdom.

basis of that second signal has been on CD28, a homodimeric molecule expressed by the majority of CD4+ T cells.[2] A second ligand for CD80 and CD86 is CTLA4, which is expressed on activated T cells.[3] CTLA4 binds these molecules with a 100-fold higher affinity than does CD28.

There is overwhelming evidence from *in vitro* and *in vivo* studies that costimulation through CD28 either with mAb or with the natural ligands amplifies T cell immune responses.[1] What is more controversial is whether costimulation through CD28 is absolutely required for CD4+ T cell priming.

THE LIGANDS FOR CD28 AND CTLA4, CD80 AND CD86, ARE EXPRESSED DIFFERENTLY

There are currently two published ligands for CD28 and CTLA4, CD80[4] and CD86,[2] which bind to CD28 with micromolar affinity and are expressed on professional antigen-presenting cells like dendritic cells, but also on activated macrophages, B cells, T cells, and epithelium. The temporal expression of CD80 and of CD86 are different: CD86 is expressed earlier and more rapidly than CD80, which appears later on dendritic cells,[3] T cells,[5] and B cells.[4] CD80 and CD86 bind CD28 and CTLA4 with comparable overall affinities, but the kinetics of dissociation are faster for CD86.[6] Thus, although CD80 binds more slowly to CTLA4, it remains bound longer. This may be important for signaling differences through CTLA4 by CD80 and CD86. Furthermore, mutagenesis studies show that CD80 and CD86 bind differently to CTLA4. These potential signaling differences may be important in explaining the sometimes contradictory data on the function of CD28 and CTLA4.

IMMUNE FUNCTION IN MICE WHERE CD80 AND CD86 ARE BLOCKED BY SOLUBLE FORMS OF CTLA4-Ig

To address the role of CD28 *in vivo,* we generated transgenic (tg) mice that expressed 10–20 μg/mL of CTLA4-Ig in their serum. As CTLA4-Ig binds with nanomolar affinity to CD80 and CD86, virtually all endogenous CD80 and CD86 molecules should be bound *in vivo* to the soluble competitor, abrogating the normal signaling pathway through CD28. The close similarities in immune function between these mice and CD28-deficient mice suggest that this is the case.[7,8]

PRIMING OF CD4 CELLS

The CTLA4-Ig tg mice are clearly immunodeficient, but not in the way that we expected initially. There is abundant evidence from *in vitro* studies that CTLA4-Ig will block CD4+ T cell proliferation—not completely, but 80–90%—so we anticipated that priming of CD4+ cells would be compromised, in line with the conventional wisdom that T cells are anergized in the absence of the second signal.[9]

We immunized tg mice and control littermates with the soluble protein antigen, KLH, and enumerated the frequency of antigen-specific T cells in transgenic and control animals. To our surprise, there was little difference in the frequency of primed T cells assessed *ex vivo*; in fact, when the animals were subsequently boosted, augmented frequencies were observed in tg mice.[10] Furthermore, there was no obvious bias in the class of lymphokines secreted by the primed T cells, and these T cells were functionally competent to help B cells make T-dependent antibody responses when adoptively transferred into nude mice.

It could be argued that CD80 and CD86 are incompletely blocked in these experiments, but compatible results have recently been reported in the CD28-deficient mice. In these experiments, T cells from CD28−/− mice clearly proliferated *in vitro*, indicating the mice had been primed.[8] Because T cells from CD28−/− mice proliferated less well *in vitro* than CD28+/− mice, the investigators concluded that priming was less efficient in CD28−/− mice. However, this decreased proliferation *in vitro* is at least partly due to the absence of costimulation through CD80 and CD86.

DEPENDENCY ON CD28 COSTIMULATION DIFFERS AMONG T CELL CLONES

Our data suggest that costimulation through CD28 is not absolutely required for $CD4^+$ T cell priming *in vivo*. In accord with this, we have seen that the proliferation of T cell clones is variably sensitive to inhibition by CTLA4-Ig,[11] which implies that a strong signal through the TCR compensates. We have also found that naive T cells from TCR transgenic mice that express a $CD4^+$ TCR specific for the hemagglutinin of influenza virus are relatively resistant to the blocking effects of CTLA4-Ig (personal observation). An important prediction from this is that pathogenic organisms would not induce T cell tolerance if presented initially to the immune system on non-B7-ligand-expressing antigen-presenting cells.

Antigens closely related to self, where the repertoire of potentially responsive T cells is small, are the most likely antigens in my view to be B7-dependent. An example of this is tumor antigens. Transfection of tumor cells with CD80 and CD86 renders them immunogenic to the immune system.[12,13]

B CELL FUNCTION

In contrast to the question of T cell priming, there is good evidence that effector immune functions mediated by helper T cells are grossly impaired. T-dependent antibody responses are reduced in CD28−/−[7] or CTLA4-Ig tg mice[14] and also when CTLA4-Ig is injected.[15] This is reflected in the decreased levels of T-dependent IgG isotypes in CTLA4-Ig tg and CD28−/− mice and, in CTLA4-Ig tg mice, germinal centers are absent in spleen and lymph nodes of immunized animals; they also exhibit clonal selection and somatic mutation deficiency. T-independent responses are normal.

The absence of germinal centers is reminiscent of the B cell phenotype of CD40-ligand-deficient[16] and CD40-deficient mice.[17] The most direct explanation for the results is that, in addition to decreased lymphokine production, upregulation of surface molecules involved in contact-dependent T cell help on primed T cells, such as CD40-ligand, is also impaired. This would fit the considerable evidence suggesting that there is a positive feedback loop where costimulation through CD28 upregulates CD40-ligand,[18,19] which then acts through CD40 to upregulate CD80 and CD86.[20]

Alternatively, CTLA4-Ig may exert its effect by altering the type of T cells that develop. It has been reported that CTLA4-Ig can switch T cells to a Th1 phenotype[21] and, although we did not observe a biased cytokine profile on T cells analyzed *ex vivo,*[10] this may not reflect the *in vivo* function of primed T cells.

ESTABLISHED MEMORY ANTIBODY RESPONSES

Initial data suggested that it was difficult to suppress secondary antibody responses with CTLA4-Ig.[15] We have adoptively transferred primed lymphocytes into CTLA4-Ig tg or control recipients and found that tg mice can make secondary antibody responses, but the responses are poorly sustained and become exhausted (unpublished observations). This suggests that differentiation of memory B cells is unimpaired in the CTLA4-Ig environment, but self-renewal of memory B cells is compromised. Recent data suggest that treatment of lupus-prone mice with mCTLA4-Ig reduced established autoantibody production, which is consistent with the idea that memory B cell function is inhibited by CTLA4-Ig.[22]

EFFECTOR T CELL RESPONSES

Analogous to B lymphocyte activation, CD4-dependent CD8 responses are grossly reduced in CTLA4-Ig tg mice. This includes cytotoxic responses to male and other minor antigens in C57Bl/6 mice (Livingstone and Lane, unpublished observations) and also cytotoxic responses to vesicular stomatitis virus (VSV) (Zingernagel *et al.,* unpublished observations). In contrast, cytotoxic responses to major MHC determinants and cytotoxic responses to lymphocytic choriomeningitis virus (LCMV), which elicits a CD4-independent CD8 response, are normal. LCMV responses are also normal in CD28−/− mice.[7]

TRANSPLANTATION

It is understandable that CTLA4-Ig prevents the rejection of nonvascular xenografts,[23] which are predominantly mediated by effector functions such as specific antibody.

The data on allograft rejection are more controversial. We found that MHC-mismatched heart grafts into CTLA4-Ig tg mice (Balb/c into C57Bl/6) were rejected in a comparable period to control mice (Lane and Schultz, unpublished observations), but others have reported prolonged allograft survival.[24,25] However, Turka *et al.* found no evidence of tolerance induction, whereas Pearson *et al.* found that animals that had accepted heart grafts were now tolerant to skin grafts. In the latter case, it seemed likely that tolerance had been induced by the heart allograft, as CTLA4-Ig alone failed to induce skin engraftment. Similarly, in graft-versus-host disease, whereas CTLA4-Ig ameliorates symptoms, there is little evidence of CD4 tolerance induction.[26] Overall, the data seem to be consistent with the idea that it is difficult to tolerize $CD4^+$ T cells and it is likely that CTLA4 fusion proteins will be used in combination with other immunosuppressive agents. Recently, it has been reported that induction of tolerance is much more effective if CTLA4-Ig is delayed until after the transplantation, suggesting that the timing of the signal is critical.[27]

DIFFERENTIAL EFFECTS OF BLOCKING CD80 AND CD86 *IN VIVO*

Several studies have shown that immune responses are differentially affected by blocking of CD80 and CD86.[28–32] In general, blocking CD86 inhibits antibody responses and favors the development of T cells with a Th1 phenotype, exacerbating autoimmune diseases mediated by Th1 cells. In contrast, blocking CD80 ameliorates diseases mediated by Th1 cells such as autoimmune encephalitis.

The timing of the blocking of CD80 and CD86 during immune responses may also critically affect the immune response outcome.[21,27] Transplants are more readily accepted if CTLA4-Ig treatment is delayed and, paradoxically, CTLA4-Ig protects susceptible mice from experimental leishmaniasis.

NEGATIVE REGULATION OF T CELL CLONES

The most difficult observation to explain in CTLA4-Ig tg mice was the apparent increased frequency of primed T cells following immunization with protein antigens.[10] However, the recent findings that CTLA4-deficient mice die from an aggressive lymphoproliferative disorder much more severe than that associated with Fas-ligand-deficient T cell regulation[33,34] may explain this paradox. These studies clearly show that signaling to T cells can deliver a negative signal to T cells and, just as positive signals through CD28 are blocked in CTLA4-Ig tg mice, it is probable that signaling through endogenous CTLA4 is also impaired, accounting for the excessive priming of CD4 cells that was seen in mice that overexpressed a soluble form of CTLA4.[10]

DISTINCT MECHANISMS INDUCING T CELL SUICIDE AND ANERGY

There now appear to be at least two mechanisms for regulating T cells, through Fas[35] and through CTLA4. It appears that CTLA4 and Fas represent distinct mechanisms for regulating T cells as Fas killing is intact in CTLA4-deficient mice.[33] Second, induction of T cell anergy is present in mice with deficient Fas signaling where deletion of T cells fails to occur.[36] It has generally been thought that T cell anergy is due to deficient costimulation. However, we have found that the induction of "anergy," but not the Fas-ligand-dependent deletion, seen following immunization with the superantigen, staphylococcal enterotoxin B, is blocked in CTLA4-Ig transgenic mice.[37] This is consistent with the idea that signaling through CTLA4 may actively induce anergy (proliferative unresponsiveness) in T cells. This need not mean that T cell capacity to deliver help for other effector cells is prejudiced. CTLA4 is expressed by activated T cells within germinal centers[38] where T cells help antigen-selected B cells, but do not usually proliferate themselves. The overproduction of autoantibody in Fas-signaling-deficient mice is associated with plasma cell proliferation in the T zones,[39] but there is little evidence for Fas being involved in germinal centers despite the fact that Fas is strongly expressed by germinal center B cells.[40] This emphasizes the possibility that these mechanisms may operate in distinct microenvironments.

USE OF SOLUBLE COMPETITORS AND AGONISTS TO REGULATE IMMUNE FUNCTION

The criteria for a competitive antagonist are that it should be present in saturating quantities for a readily accessible ligand(s) to which it binds with high affinity, greater than the molecule for which it competes. CTLA4-Ig can effectively fulfill these criteria as a competitive antagonist for CD28. Unfortunately for many other potential soluble competitors, even though they bind with high affinity to their ligands (e.g., CD40 family members), accessibility and lack of a competitive advantage over the endogenous molecule make them poor competitive antagonists, which limits their usefulness. The second limitation of competitors is that their efficacy depends on their expression in saturating amounts.

An alternative strategy is to use soluble molecules as molecular agonists. As signal transduction through surface molecules usually involves dimerization of receptors, this effectively precludes small chemical agonists. However, Ig fusion proteins have the potential to dimerize and activate receptors. We have recently explored this possibility by generating CD80-Ig transgenic mice in the hope that this molecule will selectively bind and inhibit CTLA4-expressing T cells.

SUMMARY

In recent years, it has become clear that the fate of lymphocyte interactions with antigen is determined not only by signals through antigen-specific receptors, but by interactions between pairs of accessory molecules. One such crucial pair of ligands is that between CD80/CD86, expressed by professional APCs and activated T and B cells, and CD28 (resting and activated T cells primarily) and CTLA4 (activated T cells). Signals in this system can amplify (CD28) or inhibit (CTLA4) T cell responses. The uses of soluble competitors for CD28 (CTLA4-Ig) and agonists for the inhibitory receptor CTLA4 (CD80-Ig) offer therapeutic possibilities to tailor autoimmune responses in nonpathogenic directions.

REFERENCES

1. LINSLEY, P. S. & J. A. LEDBETTER. 1993. The role of the CD28 receptor during T cell responses to antigen. Annu. Rev. Immunol. **11:** 191–212.
2. FREEMAN, G. J., J. G. GRIBBEN, V. A. BOUSSIOTIS, J. W. NG, V. A. RESTIVO, L. A. LOMBARD, G. S. GRAY & L. M. NADLER. 1993. Cloning of B7-2: a CTLA-4 counter-receptor that co-stimulates human T cell proliferation. Science **262:** 909–911.
3. MCLELLAN, A. D., G. C. STARLING, L. A. WILLIAMS, B. D. HOCK & D. N. HART. 1995. Activation of human peripheral blood dendritic cells induces the CD86 co-stimulatory molecule. Eur. J. Immunol. **25:** 2064–2068.
4. LENSCHOW, D. J., G. H. SU, L. A. ZUCKERMAN, N. NABAVI, C. L. JELLIS, G. S. GRAY, J. MILLER & J. A. BLUESTONE. 1993. Expression and functional significance of an additional ligand for CTLA-4. Proc. Natl. Acad. Sci. U.S.A. **90:** 11054–11058.
5. PRABHU DAS, M. R., S. S. ZAMVIL, F. BORRIELLO, H. L. WEINER, A. H. SHARPE & V. K. KUCHROO. 1995. Reciprocal expression of co-stimulatory molecules, B7-1 and B7-2, on murine T cells following activation. Eur. J. Immunol. **25:** 207–211.
6. LINSLEY, P. S., J. L. GREENE, W. BRADY, J. BAJORATH, J. A. LEDBETTER & R. PEACH. 1994. Human B7-1 (CD80) and B7-2 (CD86) bind with similar avidities but distinct kinetics to CD28 and CTLA-4 receptors. Immunity **1:** 793–801.
7. SHAHINIAN, A., K. PFEFFER, K. P. LEE, T. M. KUNDIG, K. KISHIHARA, A. WAKEHAM, K. KAWAI, P. S. OHASHI, C. B. THOMPSON & T. W. MAK. 1993. Differential T cell costimulatory requirements in CD28-deficient mice. Science **261:** 609–612.
8. GREEN, J. M., P. J. NOEL, A. I. SPERLING, T. L. WALUNAS, G. S. GRAY, J. A. BLUESTONE & C. B. THOMPSON. 1994. Absence of B7-dependent responses in CD28-deficient mice. Immunity **1:** 501–508.
9. SCHWARTZ, R. H. 1992. Costimulation of T lymphocytes: the role of CD28, CTLA-4, and B7/BB1 in interleukin-2 production and immunotherapy. Cell **71:** 1065–1068.
10. RONCHESE, F., B. HAUSMANN, S. HUBELE & P. LANE. 1994. Normal T cell priming to a protein antigen in mice transgenic for soluble CTLA-4. J. Exp. Med. **179:** 809–817.
11. LANE, P., W. GERHARD, S. HUBELE, A. LANZAVECCHIA & F. MCCONNELL. 1993. Expression and functional properties of mouse B7/BB1 using a fusion protein between mouse CTLA4 and human γ1. Immunology **80:** 56–61.
12. TOWNSEND, S. E. & J. P. ALLISON. 1993. Tumor rejection after direct costimulation of CD8+ T cells by B7-transfected melanoma cells. Science **259:** 368–370.
13. HARDING, F. A. & J. P. ALLISON. 1993. CD28-B7 interactions allow the induction of CD8+ cytotoxic T lymphocytes in the absence of exogenous help. J. Exp. Med. **177:** 1791–1796.
14. LANE, P., C. BURDET, S. HUBELE, D. SCHEIDEGGER, U. MÜLLER, F. MCCONNELL & M. KOSCO-VILLBOIS. 1994. B cell function in mice transgenic for mCTLA4-H gamma-1: lack of germinal centers correlated with poor affinity maturation and class switching despite normal priming of CD4+ T cells. J. Exp. Med. **179:** 819–830.
15. LINSLEY, P. S., P. M. WALLACE, J. JOHNSON, M. G. GIBSON, J. L. GREENE, J. A. LEDBETTER, C. SINGH & M. A. TEPPER. 1992. Immunosuppression *in vivo* by a soluble form of the CTLA-4 T cell activation molecule. Science **257:** 792–795.
16. XU, J., T. M. FOY, J. D. LAMAN, T. J. WALDSCHMIDT, J. ELSEMORE, R. J. NOELLE & R. A. FLAVELL. 1994. Mice deficient for the CD40 ligand. Immunity **1:** 423–431.
17. KAWABE, T., T. NAKA, K. YOSHIDA, S. SUEMATSU, N. YOSHIDA, T. KISHIMOTO & H. KIKUTANI. 1994. The immune response in CD40-deficient mice: impaired immunoglobulin class switching and germinal center formation. Immunity **1:** 167–178.

18. DE BOER, M., A. KASRAN, J. KWEKKEBOOM, H. WALTER, P. VANDENBERGHE & J. L. CEUPPENS. 1993. Ligation of B7 with CD28/CTLA-4 on T cells results in CD40 ligand expression, interleukin-4 secretion, and efficient help for antibody production by B cells. Eur. J. Immunol. **23:** 3120–3125.
19. KLAUS, S. J., L. M. PINCHUK, H. D. OCHS, C. L. LAW, W. C. FANSLOW, R. J. ARMITAGE & E. A. CLARK. 1994. Costimulation through CD28 enhances T cell–dependent B cell activation via CD40-CD40L interaction. J. Immunol. **152:** 5643–5652.
20. RANHEIM, E. A. & T. J. KIPPS. 1993. Activated T cells induce expression of B7/BB1 on normal or leukemic B cells through a CD40-dependent signal. J. Exp. Med. **177:** 925–935.
21. CORRY, D. B., S. L. REINER, P. S. LINSLEY & R. M. LOCKSLEY. 1994. Differential effects of blockade of CD28-B7 on the development of Th1 or Th2 effector cells in experimental leishmaniasis. J. Immunol. **153:** 4142–4148.
22. FINCK, B. K., P. S. LINSLEY & D. WOFSY. 1994. Treatment of murine lupus with CTLA4-Ig. Science **265:** 1225–1227.
23. LENSCHOW, D. J., Y. ZENG, J. R. THISTLETHWAITE, A. MONTAG, W. BRADY, M. G. GIBSON, P. S. LINSLEY & J. A. BLUESTONE. 1992. Long-term survival of xenogeneic pancreatic islet grafts induced by CTLA4-Ig. Science **257:** 789–792.
24. TURKA, L. A., P. S. LINSLEY, H. LIN, W. BRADY, J. M. LEIDEN, R. Q. WEI, M. G. GIBSON, X. G. ZHENG, S. MYRDAL, D. GORDON *et al.* 1992. T-cell activation by the CD28 ligand B7 is required for cardiac allograft rejection *in vivo.* Proc. Natl. Acad. Sci. U.S.A. **89:** 11102–11105.
25. PEARSON, T. C., D. Z. ALEXANDER, K. J. WINN, P. S. LINSLEY, R. P. LOWRY & C. P. LARSEN. 1994. Transplantation tolerance induced by CTLA4-Ig. Transplantation **57:** 1701–1706.
26. WALLACE, P. M., J. S. JOHNSON, J. F. MACMASTER, K. A. KENNEDY, P. GLADSTONE & P. S. LINSLEY. 1994. CTLA4-Ig treatment ameliorates the lethality of murine graft-versus-host disease across major histocompatibility complex barriers. Transplantation **58:** 602–610.
27. SAYEGH, M. H., E. AKALIN, W. W. HANCOCK, M. E. RUSSELL, C. B. CARPENTER, P. S. LINSLEY & L. A. TURKA. 1995. CD28-B7 blockade after alloantigenic challenge *in vivo* inhibits Th1 cytokines, but spares Th2. J. Exp. Med. **181:** 1869–1874.
28. SETHNA, M. P., L. VAN PARIJS, A. H. SHARPE, A. K. ABBAS & G. J. FREEMAN. 1994. A negative regulatory function of B7 revealed in B7-1 transgenic mice. Immunity **1:** 415–421.
29. KUCHROO, V. K., M. P. DAS, J. A. BROWN, A. M. RANGER, S. S. ZAMVIL, R. A. SOBEL, H. L. WEINER, N. NABAVI & L. H. GLIMCHER. 1995. B7-1 and B7-2 costimulatory molecules activate differentially the Th1/Th2 developmental pathways: application to autoimmune disease therapy. Cell **80:** 707–718.
30. FREEMAN, G. J., V. A. BOUSSIOTIS, A. ANUMANTHAN, G. M. BERNSTEIN, X. Y. KE, P. D. RENNERT, G. S. GRAY, J. G. GRIBBEN & L. M. NADLER. 1995. B7-1 and B7-2 do not deliver identical costimulatory signals since B7-2 but not B7-1 preferentially costimulates the initial production of IL-4. Immunity **2:** 523–532.
31. NAKAJIMA, A., M. AZUMA, S. KODERA, S. NURIYA, A. TERASHI, M. ABE, S. HIROSE, T. SHIRAI, H. YAGITA & K. OKUMURA. 1995. Preferential dependence of autoantibody production in murine lupus on CD86 costimulatory molecule. Eur. J. Immunol. **25:** 3060–3069.
32. RACKE, M. K., D. E. SCOTT, L. QUIGLEY, G. S. GRAY, R. ABE, C. H. JUNE & P. J. PERRIN. 1995. Distinct roles for B7-1 (CD-80) and B7-2 (CD-86) in the initiation of experimental allergic encephalomyelitis. J. Clin. Invest. **96:** 2195–2203.
33. WATERHOUSE, P., J. PENNINGER, E. TIMMS, A. WAKEHAM, A. SHAHINIAN, K. P. LEE, C. B. THOMPSON, H. GRIESSER & T. W. MAK. 1995. Lymphoproliferative disorders with early lethality in mice deficient in CTLA-4. Science **270:** 985–988.
34. TIVOL, E. A., F. BORRIELLO, A. N. SCHWEITZER, W. P. LYNCH, J. A. BLUESTONE & A. H. SHARPE. 1995. Loss of CTLA-4 leads to massive lymphoproliferation and multiorgan tissue destruction, revealing a critical negative regulatory role of CTLA-4. Immunity **3:** 541–547.
35. SINGER, G. G. & A. K. ABBAS. 1994. The fas antigen is involved in peripheral but not thymic deletion of T cells in T cell receptor transgenic mice. Immunity **1:** 365–371.
36. VAN PARIJS, L., A. IBRAGHIMOV & A. K. ABBAS. 1996. The roles of costimulation and fas in T cell apoptosis and peripheral tolerance. Immunity **4:** 321–328.

37. LANE, P., C. HALLER & F. MCCONNELL. 1996. Evidence that induction of tolerance *in vivo* involves active signaling via a B7 ligand–dependent mechanism: CTLA4-Ig protects Vβ8+ T cells from tolerance induction by the superantigen staphylococcal enterotoxin B. Eur. J. Immunol. **26:** 858–862.
38. VYTH DREESE, F. A., T. A. DELLEMIJN, D. MAJOOR & D. DE JONG. 1995. Localization *in situ* of the co-stimulatory molecules B7.1, B7.2, CD40, and their ligands in normal human lymphoid tissue. Eur. J. Immunol. **25:** 3023–3029.
39. JACOBSON, B. A., D. J. PANKA, K. NGUYEN, J. ERIKSON, A. K. ABBAS & A. MARSHAK-ROTHSTEIN. 1995. Anatomy of autoantibody production: dominant localization of antibody-producing cells to T cell zones in Fas-deficient mice. Immunity **3:** 509–519.
40. SMITH, K. G., G. J. NOSSAL & D. M. TARLINTON. 1995. Fas is highly expressed in the germinal center, but is not required for regulation of the B-cell response to antigen. Proc. Natl. Acad. Sci. U.S.A. **92:** 11628–11632.

B Cells Present Antigen to CD4⁺ T Cells, but Fail to Produce IL-12

Selective APC for Th2 Cell Development?

LUCIANO ADORINI, JEAN-CHARLES GUÉRY,[a] FRANCESCO RIA,[b] AND FRANCESCA GALBIATI

Roche Milano Ricerche
I-20132 Milano, Italy

INTRODUCTION

The activation of $CD4^+$ T cells is initiated by the recognition of peptide–class II MHC complexes on the surface of antigen-presenting cells (APC).[1,2] Among the different APC populations capable of presenting peptide–class II MHC complexes, dendritic cells (DC) and B cells have been studied extensively, but their relative role in the presentation of protein antigen and $CD4^+$ T cell priming *in vivo* is still controversial. Using mice lacking B cells, presentation to $CD4^+$ T cells of antigenic complexes derived from processing of protein antigen administered in adjuvant was found in some studies to require B cells,[3] whereas in others B cells were found not critical.[4] Similarly, administration of soluble protein to normal mice was found to lead to selective expression of antigenic complexes either by antigen-specific B cells[3] or by DC.[5]

To address this point, we have compared the relative capacity of DC and B cells recruited in lymph nodes during the inflammatory response induced by adjuvant administration to present protein antigen administered in different forms. We have previously shown that immune lymph node cells (LNC) from mice immunized with hen egg-white lysozyme (HEL) in adjuvant display HEL peptide–MHC class II complexes able to stimulate, in the absence of any further antigen addition, specific T hybridoma cells.[6,7]

Here, we compare expression by DC and B cells of antigenic complexes derived from processing of native HEL, either given subcutaneously in adjuvant or in soluble form intravenously. Following subcutaneous administration of HEL in adjuvant, DC are the only APC expressing detectable HEL peptide–class II complexes.[8] Conversely, when HEL is administered in soluble form iv to mice previously injected with adjuvant only, lymph node B cells are much more efficient than DC in the presentation of HEL peptides. These results demonstrate that protein antigen injected in soluble form is presented best by B cells, whereas the same protein is presented only by lymph node DC when administered in adjuvant. Therefore, different protocols of protein

[a]Present address: INSERM U28, Hôpital Purpan, 31059 Toulouse, France.

[b]Present address: Istituto di Patologia Generale, Università Cattolica del Sacro Cuore, 00168 Roma, Italy.

antigen administration lead to expression of peptide–class II complexes by different APC.

Differentiated $CD4^+$ T cells produce a restricted set of cytokines, allowing their subdivision into two discrete populations: T helper 1 (Th1), characterized by secretion of IL-2 and IFN-γ (interferon-γ); and Th2, selectively producing IL-4, IL-5, and IL-10.[9] Polarized subsets of antigen-specific $CD4^+$ Th1 and Th2 cells can be induced *in vivo* by antigen priming and their development is primarily influenced by the cytokine milieu during the initial phase of the immune response.

IL-12 is a key regulatory cytokine produced by APC that drives the development of IFN-γ-producing Th1 cells and promotes cell-mediated immunity.[10] Although IL-12 was discovered as a product of EBV-transformed B cells,[11,12] secretion of IL-12 by normal B cells is still unclear. B cells, even when activated to induce similar levels of T cell proliferation as DC, still drive a Th0-type response, with relatively low levels of IFN-γ being produced even upon neutralization of IL-4.[13] The low level of IFN-γ produced by Th cells does not appear to be IL-12-dependent, suggesting that normal B cells do not produce this cytokine.[14] Conversely, other class II^+ APC have been shown to be major producers of IL-12. Among them, macrophages secrete high levels of p75 when stimulated by bacteria such as *S. aureus* or by bacterial products such as LPS plus IFN-γ.[15] In addition, macrophages have been shown to direct, via secretion of IL-12, the development of antigen-specific T cells towards the Th1 phenotype.[16] Macatonia *et al.* have shown IL-12 production by DC,[17] and IL-12 p75 has been found to be secreted by DC upon contact with T cells.[18–20]

We have studied antigen presentation and IL-12 production *ex vivo* by APC obtained from an inflammatory site because IL-12, a proinflammatory cytokine, is likely to be produced in higher amounts at the site of inflammation by professional APC.

DC were found to be unique among APC in the capacity to present efficiently peptide–class II complexes formed *in vivo* and to simultaneously secrete substantial amounts of IL-12 p75. IL-12 secretion by DC is strongly upregulated by ligand-TCR and CD40-CD40L interactions with $CD4^+$ T cells, which are established through cognate interaction during antigen presentation. The feedback from antigen-specific T cells leading to increased IL-12 secretion is by far more efficient in DC than in Mø, in contrast to bacterial stimuli that induce similar levels of IL-12 secretion in both cell types. Conversely, B cells fail to secrete IL-12 following either antigen-specific or nonspecific stimulation. As B cells can present antigen, they may therefore selectively drive Th2 cell development.

RESULTS

The Mode of Protein Antigen Administration Determines Preferential Presentation of Peptide–Class II Complexes by DC or B Cells

APC in draining lymph nodes from BALB/c mice immunized sc with HEL in adjuvant display antigenic complexes formed *in vivo* between peptides derived from HEL processing and class II molecules.[6,7] Lymph node APC were separated, using a combination of Percoll gradient centrifugation and magnetic cell sorting, into three populations: small B cells, large B cells, and DC-enriched cells.[8] These populations were characterized by their expression of MHC class II, B220, and N418 molecules. The high-density population contains >95% B220$^+$, class II$^+$, N418$^-$ cells and is referred to as small B cells. Large B cells, obtained from the low-density population by positive selection using B220 mAb–conjugated magnetic particles, are >95% B220$^+$, class II$^+$, N418$^-$. The negatively selected fraction, depleted of B220$^+$ cells, is enriched in class II$^+$, N418$^+$ cells (50–70%) and is referred to as the DC-enriched population.

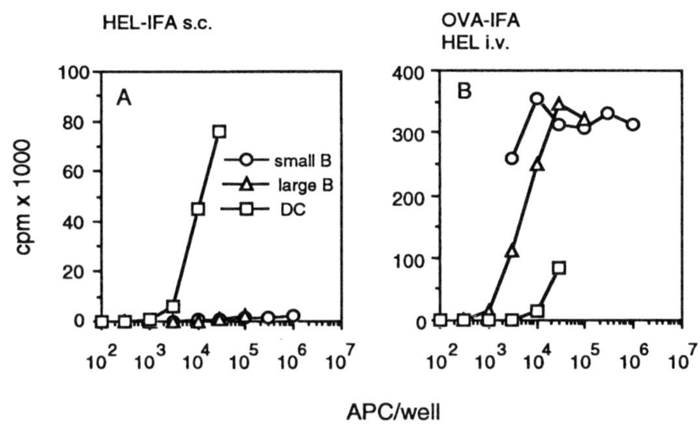

FIGURE 1. *In vivo* formation of antigenic complexes on lymph node DC and B cells following administration of protein antigen in adjuvant or in soluble form. BALB/c mice were immunized into the hind footpads with 10 nmol/mouse of HEL in IFA (A) or with 1 nmol/mouse of OVA in IFA (B). OVA-IFA-primed mice were injected with soluble HEL (100 nmol/mouse) at 3 h before removal of popliteal lymph nodes. LNC from five mice per group were pooled and APC populations separated. The HEL108–116-specific, I-E^d-restricted 1H11.3 T hybridoma cells were cultured (5×10^4 cells/well) with graded numbers of enriched APC populations. After 24 h, antigen-specific IL-2 production was determined by adding 50-μL aliquots of culture supernatant to 10^4 CTLL cells for an additional 24 h. [^{3}H]Thymidine (1 μCi/well) was added during the last 5 h of culture. Data are presented as the mean thymidine incorporation (cpm) from duplicate cultures. Background proliferation of CTLL was below 1000 cpm.

Results in FIGURE 1 demonstrate that HEL108–116/E^d complexes derived from processing of HEL administered subcutaneously in IFA are only detectable on the DC-enriched population (FIGURE 1A). Conversely, small and large B cells are much more efficient than DC to activate T cell hybridomas when HEL is administered in soluble form iv (FIGURE 1B). These data demonstrate that the mode of protein antigen administration determines preferential presentation of peptide–class II complexes by lymph node DC or B cells.

IL-12 Production by in Vivo*–loaded Lymph Node DC, but Not B Cells*

Lymph node APC from HEL-IFA-immunized BALB/c mice were separated into three populations (small B cells, large B cells, and DC-enriched cells) as described above. We have compared the relative capacity of these different APC populations to produce IL-12 upon activation with T cell–dependent stimuli. As shown in FIGURE 2A, coculture of *in vivo*–loaded APC with the HEL108–116-specific, I-E^d-restricted T cell hybridoma 1H11.3 reveals that DC, but not B cells, secrete IL-12. This pattern of IL-12 secretion is not modified by antigen addition *in vitro* (FIGURE 2B). Upregulation of IL-12 production by cognate interaction by antigen-specific T cells appears to be restricted to DC because IL-12-secreting capacity is specifically displayed by the

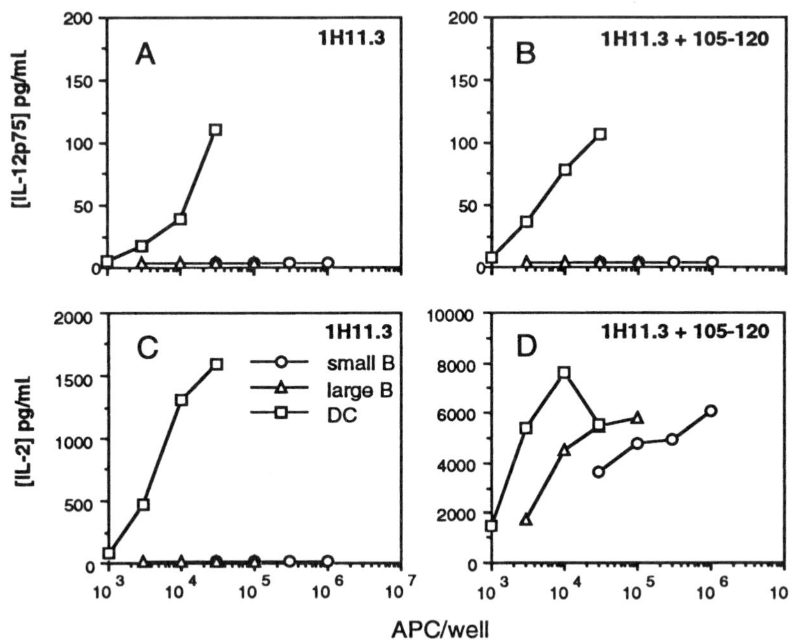

FIGURE 2. Antigen presentation and IL-12 production *ex vivo* by lymph node DC and B cells following administration of protein antigen in adjuvant. BALB/c mice were immunized into the hind footpads with 10 nmol/mouse of HEL in IFA. LNC from five mice per group were pooled and APC populations separated. Graded numbers of enriched APC populations alone were cultured with the HEL108–116-specific, I-E^d-restricted 1H11.3 T cell hybridoma (5×10^4 cells/well) alone (A, C) or in the presence of 0.3 μM HEL105–120 (B, D). After 24 h, IL-2 (C, D) and IL-12 p75 (A, B) were measured in culture supernatants by two-site sandwich ELISA.

N418$^+$ population, positively selected by magnetic cell sorting using N418 mAb (not shown). The capacity of the DC-enriched population to secrete IL-12 parallels its ability to present antigenic complexes formed *in vivo* following administration of HEL in adjuvant. In agreement with our previous observations,[8] DC (but not B cells) from lymph nodes of immunized mice have the capacity to induce IL-2 secretion by T hybridoma cells without antigen addition *in vitro* (FIGURE 2C). This is not due to a defect in the capacity of B cells to present antigen because they present efficiently antigenic peptide added *in vitro* (FIGURE 2D); however, it is less efficient than DC.

Taken together, these data show that, in addition to their capacity to present peptide–class II complexes formed *in vivo*, DC in immune lymph nodes are the main APC population able to secrete IL-12 p75 in response to T cell–dependent stimuli.

Ligand-TCR Interaction Upregulates IL-12 p75 Production by Lymph Node DC, but Not by Macrophages nor B Cells

We next compared the relative capacity of different APC populations (large B cells, Mø, DC) to secrete IL-12 *in vitro* upon activation with T cell–independent or T cell–dependent stimuli, independently from their ability to uptake, process, and present antigen *in vivo*. DC and B cells were obtained, as described before, from mice injected with CFA only. Peritoneal exudate cells from thioglycollate-injected mice were used as a source of Mø. These different APC populations were cultured in the presence of SAC and IFN-γ, and IL-12 production in 24-h culture supernatants was measured using two-site sandwich ELISA. As shown in FIGURE 3A, peritoneal Mø and the DC-enriched population from lymph nodes have a similar capacity to secrete IL-12 p75 heterodimers. Conversely, large B cells isolated from lymph node (FIGURE 3A) or spleen (not shown) fail to secrete IL-12 p75. We next examined the capacity of these APC to produce IL-12 upon antigen-specific or nonantigen-specific interaction with class II–restricted T cells. APC were cultured with T hybridoma cells in the presence or absence of antigenic peptide, and the concentration of IL-12 p75 in 24-h culture supernatants was determined as above. IL-12 p75 is measurable in supernatants of lymph node DC cultured with 1H11.3 cells in the absence of antigen (27 pg/mL), whereas it is undetectable or just above the detection limit using the other APC populations (FIGURE 3B). Interestingly, addition of HEL peptide 105–120 to cultures upregulates IL-12 p75 production by lymph node DC (5-fold increase) up to 150 pg/mL (FIGURE 3C). Conversely, Mø that secrete IL-12 p75 at levels comparable to lymph node DC after stimulation with SAC and IFN-γ have a negligible capacity to secrete IL-12 p75 upon antigen-specific interaction with T cells. Also, under these conditions, B cells fail to secrete IL-12. All three APC populations present peptide–class II complexes and activate T cells (FIGURE 3D), demonstrating that they are functional APC.

DISCUSSION

Different modes of protein antigen administration lead to selective expression of antigenic complexes by different APC. Following immunization with HEL in adjuvant, DC are the only lymph node APC population expressing detectable HEL peptide–class II complexes, whereas B cells are much more efficient than DC in presenting antigenic complexes derived from processing of circulating soluble HEL. To measure the capacity of resident lymph node APC (DC and B cells) to present peptides derived from processing of a circulating protein antigen, antigen has been injected shortly before lymph node harvesting to minimize loading of APC before their entry into the lymph node. Under these conditions, lymph node B cells are far

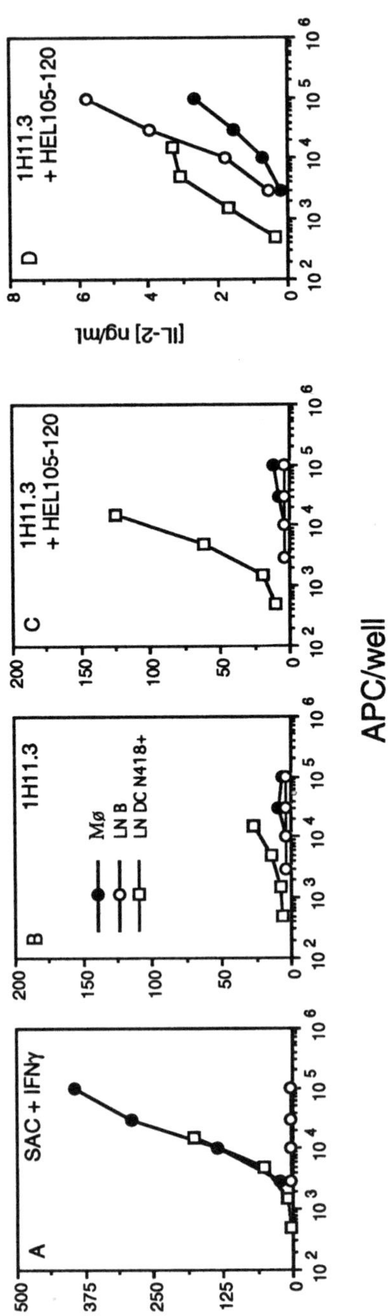

FIGURE 3. B cells fail to secrete IL-12 *in vitro*. Mø (90% Mac-1⁺) were obtained by peritoneal cavity lavage of thioglycollate-injected BALB/c mice. Another group of BALB/c mice were immunized with CFA into the hind footpads. Six days later, popliteal lymph nodes were collected and APC populations separated. Large B cells (>95% B220⁺) were obtained from immune LNC by a combination of Percoll centrifugation and magnetic cell sorting. The DC-enriched population obtained from low-buoyant-density cells was further depleted of T and B cells using appropriate magnetic beads. The spleen and lymph node DC-enriched populations contained 25% and 55% N418⁺ cells, respectively. The indicated numbers of Mø, B cells, and DC-enriched N418⁺ APC were then cultured in the presence of SAC (1:5000) and IFN-γ (50 U/mL) in complete medium (A). In panels B, C, and D, the indicated numbers of cells were cultured with 1H11.3 cells alone (B) or in the presence of 0.3 μM HEL105–120 (C, D). The concentrations of IL-12 p75 (A, B, and C) and IL-2 (D) in 24-h culture supernatants were determined by two-site sandwich ELISA.

superior to DC in the presentation of HEL peptide–class II complexes to T hybridoma cells. These data correlate with the impaired capacity of lymph node DC to present *in vitro* native protein antigen, as compared to synthetic peptide, whereas no qualitative differences in the presentation of protein and peptide are observed using B cells, in agreement with previous results.[21,22] Even if we cannot formally exclude a possible inability of soluble antigen to access lymph node DC *in vivo*, the *in vitro* data are consistent with the interpretation that DC that migrated to the lymph node have a reduced capacity to endocytose and present *in situ* soluble circulating protein antigen, probably as a consequence of their maturation *in vivo*. Maturation of DC *in vivo* could be due to the local secretion of proinflammatory cytokines such as TNF-α, which has been shown to downregulate the antigen-capturing and processing capacity of human DC *in vitro*.[23]

Because differences in antigen-presenting activity may also reflect differences in antigen uptake and processing capacity between the three APC populations tested, we analyzed *in vitro* the hierarchy in antigen-presenting activity to 1H11.3 T cells using synthetic peptide. As compared to large and small B cells, 10- to 100-fold less DC were needed to induce a similar level of IL-2 production by the T hybridoma cells. The number of antigenic complexes required on DC to activate T cells is much lower than for B cells.[24] Because we observed that, following administration of soluble protein antigen iv, B cells are more efficient APC than DC, it is likely that B cells display a much higher amount of antigenic complexes as compared to DC. Interestingly, both resting and activated B cells, identified as small and large B cells, respectively, appear to present soluble HEL administered iv equally well.

The different role of DC and B cells in the presentation of exogenous proteins *in vivo* exemplifies the necessity, by professional APC such as DC, to present selectively to lymph node T cells antigens available in inflammatory sites, but not circulating soluble proteins. As it has been previously suggested,[25] the inefficiency of mature DC to present soluble proteins, including circulating self-antigens, to lymph node T cells may also provide an efficient mechanism to avoid self-antigen presentation by DC, thereby preventing the priming of potentially autoreactive T cells. On the other hand, once circulating antigen becomes available, lymph node B cells could further contribute to the clonal expansion of the antigen-specific T cells previously activated by DC,[4,26,27] although this issue is still controversial.[3] In this context, it has been suggested that T cell tolerance induced by soluble antigen administration is mediated by antigen presentation by B cells, rather than DC.[28] However, recent studies using B cell–deficient mice have clearly demonstrated that induction of Th1 cell unresponsiveness by soluble antigen can occur in the absence of B cells.[29–31]

DC and B cells may preferentially induce Th1 or Th2 responses,[32] although priming of naive $CD4^+$ cells by B cells is still controversial.[3,4] Lymph node DC isolated from mice immunized with protein antigen in adjuvant are the main APC population able to express detectable antigenic complexes.[8] Because this protocol of immunization preferentially induces a Th1-type immune response,[33] it was of interest to analyze whether, in addition to their antigen-presenting capacity, DC from immune lymph nodes were able to secrete IL-12 p75, a proinflammatory cytokine involved in Th1 differentiation.[10] We now show, following administration of protein antigen in adjuvant, that lymph node DC analyzed *ex vivo* not only present peptide–class II complexes formed *in vivo,* but also produce substantial amounts of IL-12 p75. DC do not produce IL-12 constitutively, but only after induction, in our case, by T hybridoma cells, and this is strongly upregulated by antigen-specific interactions. A similar effect is also induced by TCR transgenic T cell lines (Ria, manuscript in preparation), indicating that it is not restricted to T hybridoma cells. These data emphasize the critical role of lymph node DC in both activation and differentiation *in vivo* of $CD4^+$ T cells following antigen priming. Upregulation of IL-12 secretion by *in vivo*–loaded DC involves CD40-CD40L interaction with antigen-specific $CD4^+$ T cells. Conversely, cognate interaction of antigen-specific $CD4^+$ cells with Mø does not result in upregulation of IL-12 secretion (Guéry *et al.,* submitted). Therefore, we would propose that the major effect of anti-CD40L treatment[34,35] is to block interactions between antigen-specific T cells and DC presenting peptide-MHC complexes, thereby preventing IL-12 secretion during the initial phase of the immune response.

The efficient presentation of antigenic complexes derived from proteins present in inflammatory sites and the production of IL-12 may account for the capacity of DC recruited in immune lymph nodes to prime naive $CD4^+$ T cells *in vivo.* We have recently shown that IL-12 administration to NOD mice results in acceleration of autoimmune diabetes, associated with massive infiltration of lymphoid cells, including $N418^+$ cells, into the pancreas.[36] Considering the efficiency of DC in antigen presentation and their capacity to produce IL-12, it is likely that pancreatic DC play a role in the induction of diabetogenic Th1 cells[37] and therefore may represent an interesting target to treat organ-specific autoimmune diseases.

Both DC and B cells induce IL-2 secretion by T hybridoma cells when antigenic peptide is added *in vitro,* but only DC and not B cells induce IFN-γ production. This appears to reflect the inability of B cells to secrete IL-12 because addition of IL-12 *in vitro* induces IFN-γ production by T hybridoma cells stimulated with antigen and B cells (Guéry *et al.,* unpublished). We have also tested the ability of DC and B cells to activate TCR transgenic Th1 and Th2 cell lines *in vitro.* B cells are 10-fold more efficient in activating Th2 as compared to Th1 cell lines, whereas DC activate equally well both subsets (Ria *et al.,* unpublished). Thus, presentation of antigen by B cells instead of DC may skew the response towards the Th2 phenotype. This could result from preferential activation of Th2 cells and/or from lack of Th2 cell inhibition by Th1-derived IFN-γ.

The capacity of B cells to present soluble antigen, but not to secrete IL-12, may indeed play a role in selectively priming Th2 cells. Induction of experimental allergic encephalomyelitis, a Th1-mediated autoimmune disease, has been prevented by targeting the autoantigen to B cells,[38] and this prevention has been recently found to be associated with the priming of antigen-specific Th2 cells.[39] Therefore, antigen presentation by APC lacking appropriate costimulatory molecules such as B cells during a noninflammatory immune response could favor Th2 development. IgD targeting on the B cell surface by bivalent antibody fragments results in B cell activation,[40] which might be a prerequisite for priming of Th2 cells.[39]

Selective induction of Th2 cell responses is not restricted to B cells. Keratinocytes, the most abundant cell type in the skin, when activated express class II molecules and can function as APC. Activated T cells stimulated by keratinocytes, in contrast to professional APC, produce almost exclusively Th2-type cytokines and very little IFN-γ. This immune deviation appears to result from the inability of keratinocytes to secrete IL-12 because IFN-γ production is restored by exogenous IL-12.[41]

Thus, autoantigen presentation by nonprofessional APC such as B cells could effectively induce immunodeviation to the Th2 phenotype. It would be interesting to evaluate antigen targeting to non-IL-12-producing APC in the treatment of established Th1-mediated autoimmune diseases.

REFERENCES

1. SCHWARTZ, R. H. 1985. T-lymphocyte recognition of antigen in association with gene products of the major histocompatibility complex. Annu. Rev. Immunol. **3:** 237–261.
2. MÖLLER, G. 1988. Antigen processing. Immunol. Rev. **106:** 1.
3. CONSTANT, S., N. SCHWEITZER, J. WEST, P. RANNEY & K. BOTTOMLY. 1995. B lymphocytes can be competent antigen-presenting cells for priming CD4$^+$ T cells to protein antigens *in vivo*. J. Immunol. **155:** 3734–3741.
4. EPSTEIN, M. M., F. DI ROSA, D. JANKOVIC, A. SHER & P. MATZINGER. 1995. Successful T cell priming in B cell–deficient mice. J. Exp. Med. **182:** 915–922.
5. CROWLEY, M. T., K. INABA & R. M. STEINMAN. 1990. Dendritic cells are the principal cells in mouse spleen bearing immunogenic fragments of foreign proteins. J. Exp. Med. **172:** 383–386.
6. GUÉRY, J-C., A. SETTE, J. LEIGHTON, A. DRAGOMIR & L. ADORINI. 1992. Selective immunosuppression by administration of MHC class II–binding peptides: I. Evidence for *in vivo* MHC blockade preventing T cell activation. J. Exp. Med. **175:** 1345–1352.
7. GUÉRY, J-C., M. NEAGU, G. RODRIGUEZ-TARDUCHY & L. ADORINI. 1993. Selective immunosuppression by administration of major histocompatibility complex class II–binding peptides: II. Preventive inhibition of primary and secondary antibody responses. J. Exp. Med. **177:** 1461–1468.
8. GUÉRY, J-C., F. RIA & L. ADORINI. 1996. Dendritic cells, but not B cells, present antigenic complexes to class II–restricted T cells following administration of protein in adjuvant. J. Exp. Med. **183:** 751–758.
9. MOSMANN, T. R., H. CHERWINSKI, M. W. BOND, M. A. GIEDLIN & R. L. COFFMANN. 1986. Two types of murine helper T cell clone: I. Definition according to profile of lymphokine activities and secreted proteins. J. Immunol. **136:** 2348–2357.
10. TRINCHIERI, G. 1995. Interleukin 12: a proinflammatory cytokine with immunoregulatory functions that bridge innate resistance and antigen-specific adaptive immunity. Annu. Rev. Immunol. **13:** 251–276.
11. KOBAYASHI, M., L. FITZ, M. RYAN, R. M. HEWICK, S. C. CLARK, S. CHAN, R. LOUDON, F. SHERMAN, B. PERUSSIA & G. TRINCHIERI. 1989. Identification and purification of natural killer cell stimulatory factor (NKSF), a cytokine with multiple biologic effects on human lymphocytes. J. Exp. Med. **170:** 827–845.
12. STERN, A. S., F. J. PODLASKI, J. D. HULMES, Y-C. E. PAN, P. M. QUINN, A. G. WOLITZKY, P. C. FAMILLETTI, D. L. STREMLO, T. TRUITT, R. CHIZZONITE & M. K. GATELY. 1990. Purification to homogeneity and partial characterization of cytotoxic lymphocyte maturation factor from human B-lymphoblastoid cells. Proc. Natl. Acad. Sci. U.S.A. **87:** 6808–6812.
13. HOSKEN, N. A., K. SHIBUYA, A. W. HEATH, K. M. MURPHY & A. O'GARRA. 1995. The effect of antigen dose on CD4$^+$ helper cell phenotype development in a T cell receptor–αβ–transgenic model. J. Exp. Med. **182:** 1579–1584.
14. O'GARRA, A., N. HOSKEN, S. MACATONIA, C. A. WENNER & K. MURPHY. 1995. The role of macrophage- and dendritic cell–derived IL-12 in Th1 phenotype development. Res. Immunol. **146:** 466–472.

15. D'ANDREA, A., M. RENGARAJU, N. M. VALIANTE, J. CHEHIMI, M. KUBIN, M. ASTE, S. H. CHAN, M. KOBAYASHI, D. YOUNG, E. NICKBARG, R. CHIZZONITE, S. F. WOLF & G. TRINCHIERI. 1992. Production of natural killer cell stimulatory factor (interleukin 12) by peripheral blood mononuclear cells. J. Exp. Med. **176:** 1387–1398.
16. HSIEH, C. S., S. E. MACATONIA, C. S. TRIPP, S. F. WOLF, A. O'GARRA & K. M. MURPHY. 1993. Development of Th1 $CD4^+$ T cells through IL-12 produced by *Listeria*-induced macrophages. Science **260:** 547–549.
17. MACATONIA, S. E., N. A. HOSKEN, M. LITTON, P. VIEIRA, C. S. HSIEH, J. A. CULPEPPER, M. WYSOCKA, G. TRINCHIERI, K. M. MURPHY & A. O'GARRA. 1995. Dendritic cells produce IL-12 and direct the development of Th1 cells from naive $CD4^+$ T cells. J. Immunol. **154:** 5071–5079.
18. HEUFLER, C., F. KOCH, U. STANZL, G. TOPAR, M. WYSOCKA, G. TRINCHIERI, A. ENK, R. M. STEINMAN, N. ROMANI & G. SCHULER. 1996. Interleukin-12 is produced by dendritic cells and mediates T helper 1 development as well as interferon-γ production by T helper 1 cells. Eur. J. Immunol. **26:** 659–668.
19. KOCH, F., U. STANZL, P. JENNEWEIN, K. JANKE, C. HEUFLER, E. KAEMPGEN, N. ROMANI & G. SCHULER. 1996. High level IL-12 production by murine dendritic cells: upregulation via MHC class II and CD40 molecules and downregulation by IL-4 and IL-10. J. Exp. Med. **184:** 741–746.
20. CELLA, M., D. SCHEIDEGGER, K. PALMER-LEHMANN, P. LANE, A. LANZAVECCHIA & G. ALBER. 1996. Ligation of CD40 on dendritic cells triggers production of high levels of interleukin-12 and enhances T cell stimulatory capacity: T-T help via APC activation. J. Exp. Med. **184:** 747–752.
21. CONSTANT, S., D. SANT'ANGELO, T. PASQUALINI, T. TAYLOR, D. LEVIN, R. FLAVELL & K. BOTTOMLY. 1995. Peptide and protein antigen require distinct antigen-presenting cell subsets for the priming of $CD4^+$ T cells. J. Immunol. **154:** 4915–4923.
22. GUÉRY, J-C., F. RIA, F. GALBIATI, S. SMIROLDO & L. ADORINI. 1997. The mode of protein antigen administration determines preferential presentation of peptide–class II complexes by lymph node dendritic or B cells. Int. Immunol. In press.
23. SALLUSTO, F. & A. LANZAVECCHIA. 1994. Efficient presentation of soluble antigen by cultured human dendritic cells is maintained by granulocyte/macrophage colony-stimulating factor plus interleukin 4 and downregulated by tumor necrosis factor α. J. Exp. Med. **179:** 1109–1118.
24. BHARDWAJ, N., J. W. YOUNG, A. J. NISANIAN, J. BAGGERS & R. M. STEINMAN. 1993. Small amounts of superantigen, when presented on dendritic cells, are sufficient to initiate T cell responses. J. Exp. Med. **178:** 633–642.
25. STEINMAN, R. M. 1991. The dendritic cell system and its role in immunogenicity. Annu. Rev. Immunol. **9:** 271–296.
26. FUCHS, E. F. & P. MATZINGER. 1992. B cells turn off virgin but not memory T cells. Science **258:** 1156–1159.
27. RONCHESE, F. & B. HAUSMANN. 1993. B lymphocytes *in vivo* fail to prime naive T cells, but can stimulate antigen-experienced T lymphocytes. J. Exp. Med. **177:** 679–690.
28. EYNON, E. E. & D. C. PARKER. 1992. Small B cells as antigen-presenting cells in the induction of tolerance to soluble protein antigens. J. Exp. Med. **175:** 131–138.
29. VELLA, A. T., M. T. SCHERER, L. SCHULTZ, J. W. KAPPLER & P. MARRACK. 1996. B cells are not essential for peripheral T-cell tolerance. Proc. Natl. Acad. Sci. U.S.A. **93:** 951–955.
30. PHILLIPS, J. A., C. G. ROMBALL, M. V. HOBBS, D. N. ERNST, L. SHULTZ & W. O. WEIGLE. 1996. CD4+ T cell activation and tolerance induction in B cell knockout mice. J. Exp. Med. **183:** 1339–1344.
31. BAIRD, A. M. & D. C. PARKER. 1996. Analysis of low zone tolerance induction in normal and B cell–deficient mice. J. Immunol. **157:** 1833–1839.
32. STOCKINGER, B., T. ZAL, A. ZAL & D. GRAY. 1996. B cells solicit their own help from T cells. J. Exp. Med. **183:** 891–899.
33. GUÉRY, J-C., F. GALBIATI, S. SMIROLDO & L. ADORINI. 1996. Selective development of Th2 cells induced by continuous administration of low dose soluble proteins to normal and β2-microglobulin-deficient mice. J. Exp. Med. **183:** 485–497.

34. DURIE, F. H., R. A. FAVA, T. M. FOY, A. ARUFFO, J. A. LEDBETTER & R. J. NOELLE. 1993. Prevention of collagen-induced arthritis with an antibody to gp39, the ligand for CD40. Science **261:** 1328–1338.
35. STUBER, E., W. STROBER & M. NEURATH. 1996. Blocking the CD40L-CD40 interaction *in vivo* specifically prevents the priming of T helper 1 cells through the inhibition of interleukin 12 secretion. J. Exp. Med. **183:** 693–698.
36. TREMBLEAU, S., G. PENNA, E. BOSI, A. MORTARA, M. K. GATELY & L. ADORINI. 1995. IL-12 administration induces Th1 cells and accelerates autoimmune diabetes in NOD mice. J. Exp. Med. **181:** 817–821.
37. TREMBLEAU, S., T. GERMANN, M. K. GATELY & L. ADORINI. 1995. The role of IL-12 in the induction of organ-specific autoimmune diseases. Immunol. Today **16:** 383–386.
38. DAY, M. J., A. G. D. TSE, M. PUKLAVEC, S. J. SIMMONDS & D. W. MASON. 1992. Targeting autoantigen to B cells prevents the induction of a cell-mediated autoimmune disease in rats. J. Exp. Med. **175:** 655–659.
39. SAOUDI, A., S. SIMMONDS, I. HUITINGA & D. W. MASON. 1995. Prevention of experimental allergic encephalomyelitis in rats by targeting autoantigen to B cells: evidence that the protective mechanism depends on changes in the cytokine response and migratory properties of autoantigen-specific T cells. J. Exp. Med. **182:** 335–344.
40. EYNON, E. E. & D. C. PARKER. 1993. Parameters of tolerance induction by antigen targeted to B lymphocytes. J. Immunol. **151:** 2958–2964.
41. GOODMAN, R. E., F. NESTLE, Y. M. NAIDU, J. M. GREEN, C. B. THOMPSON, B. J. NICKOLOFF & L. A. TURKA. 1994. Keratinocyte-derived T cell costimulation induces preferential production of IL-2 and IL-4, but not IFN-gamma. J. Immunol. **152:** 5189–5198.

Oral Administration of Myelin Induces Antigen-specific TGF-β1-secreting T Cells in Multiple Sclerosis Patients[a]

SALLY C. KENT, HIKOAKI FUKAURA, MATTHEW J. PIETRUSEWICZ, SAMIA J. KHOURY, HOWARD L. WEINER, AND DAVID A. HAFLER[b]

Center for Neurologic Diseases
Brigham and Women's Hospital
and
Harvard Medical School
Boston, Massachusetts 02115

INTRODUCTION

Multiple sclerosis (MS) is a chronic inflammatory disease characterized by lymphocytic infiltration and demyelination in the central nervous system (CNS) thought to be initiated by Th1-type T cells recognizing myelin components of the CNS.[1,2] Alterations in regulation of immune responses are found in patients with the disease, although these defects are not well defined.[1,2] Experimental autoimmune encephalomyelitis (EAE), a model for a cell-mediated Th1-type autoimmune CNS disease, shows pathologic similarities to MS and is induced by activated T cells recognizing myelin basic protein (MBP),[3] proteolipid protein (PLP),[4] or myelin-oligodendrocyte glycoprotein (MOG).[5] In the EAE model, activated, $CD4^+$ myelin-reactive T cells secreting the cytokines, interleukin-2 (IL-2), interferon-γ (IFN-γ), tumor necrosis factor-α (TNF-α), and lymphotoxin, migrate into the CNS and initiate a cascade of events that can lead to clinical paralysis in the animals. Spontaneous recovery is associated with secretion of IL-4, IL-10, and transforming growth factor-β1 (TGF-β1).[6]

The oral administration of antigen is a long-recognized method of inducing tolerance by suppressing systemic T cell–mediated immune responses.[7,8] More recently, oral tolerance has been used to suppress experimental autoimmune diseases, including EAE,[9,10] collagen-[11,12] and adjuvant-induced arthritis,[13] uveitis,[14] and spontaneous diabetes in the nonobese mouse.[15] Investigations in experimental models of autoimmune diseases have led to a series of phase I/II double-blind clinical trials of

[a]This study was supported by National Institutes of Health Grant Nos. RO1-NS24247 (to D. A. Hafler) and RO1-NS29352 (to H. L. Weiner), Program Project Grant No. AR 43220 (to D. A. Hafler and H. L. Weiner), and grants from The National Multiple Sclerosis Society (to H. L. Weiner and D. A. Hafler) and from AutoImmune, Incorporated, Lexington, Massachusetts. D. A. Hafler and H. L. Weiner have a financial interest in AutoImmune, Incorporated.

[b]To whom all correspondence should be addressed.

oral tolerance in subjects with MS, rheumatoid arthritis, and uveitis. We reported previously no adverse toxicity or side effects in a pilot double-blind trial involving 30 relapsing-remitting MS patients receiving daily capsules of bovine myelin containing both MBP and PLP for one year. The frequency of T cells reactive with MBP from myelin-treated MS individuals was reduced as compared to non-myelin-treated control MS individuals. Clinically, there was a tendency for the treated group to have fewer exacerbations, especially in the subgroup of DR2− males.[16] A statistically significant clinical effect following oral administration of type II collagen has been shown in the subjects with rheumatoid arthritis.[17] The clinical efficacy of oral myelin tolerization in subjects with MS is presently under phase III investigation in a multicenter, 504-patient, randomized double-blind clinical trial.[18]

Based on the identification of antigen-reactive TGF-β1-secreting T cells in mice that were orally tolerized to MBP,[19–21] we wished to determine the effect of oral administration of myelin to MS patients in terms of induction of cytokine secretion by antigen-specific MBP- or PLP-reactive T cells. It was important to determine whether the prolonged oral administration of myelin autoantigens would result in TGF-β1-secreting cells or instead whether such treatment would elicit Th1-type response to the orally administered myelin antigens. Despite numerous studies of oral tolerance in animals, such questions can only be addressed in patients with the disease who are given oral autoantigens over prolonged periods of time. Our results demonstrate no Th1 sensitization after prolonged oral antigen administration in MS patients; instead, MBP- and PLP-reactive TGF-β1-secreting cells were induced.

MATERIALS AND METHODS

Patients

Seventeen relapsing-remitting MS patients from the continuation study of the phase I/II oral myelin trial were examined. These patients had been orally dosed with 300 mg of bovine myelin (Myloral™) daily for at least two years. The preparation contained approximately 7.5 mg of MBP and 15 mg of PLP and was supplied to patients by AutoImmune, Incorporated (Lexington, Massachusetts). The open-label clinical results of the continuation study have been reported separately. Seventeen relapsing-remitting MS patients who did not receive bovine myelin were examined as controls. The average disease duration for the oral myelin-treated group was 11.8 ± 4.3 years (age: 37.8 ± 4.8) and for control was 11.6 ± 8.7 years (age: 37.1 ± 5.7). MS patients were not treated with immunosuppressive drugs or Betaseron™ in the past or with steroids within three months of blood sampling. These investigations were approved by the human subjects committee of the Brigham and Women's Hospital.

Antigens

Human MBP was purified from the white matter of the human brain by the method previously described and was provided by AutoImmune, Incorporated.[22] Bovine PLP was purified as previously described.[23] Tetanus toxoid (TT) was obtained in purified form from the Massachusetts Public Health Laboratory (Boston, Massachusetts).

Antigen-specific T Cell Lines

Peripheral blood mononuclear cells (PBMC) were isolated from heparinized venous blood by Ficoll-Hypaque density gradient, washed twice with Hanks balanced salts solution, counted, and resuspended in media containing 10% autologous serum (collected from each patient and heat-inactivated; this serum was used throughout the experiment for each patient) in RPMI 1640, 10 mM Hepes buffer, 2 mM L-glutamine, and 100 U/100 μg/mL penicillin-streptomycin. All media and components were purchased from BioWhittaker (Walkersville, Maryland). PBMC from each patient were frozen in 10% dimethyl sulfoxide/fetal bovine serum (from Sigma, St. Louis, Missouri, and BioWhittaker, respectively) at −70 °C and were used as antigen-presenting cells for the remainder of the assay. PBMC from each patient were pulsed with antigen; 1.2×10^7 PBMC in 1.2 mL were pulsed with MBP (50 μg/mL), bovine PLP (50 μg/mL), or TT (12 Lf/mL) for 2 h at 37 °C, washed twice in media with 10% autologous serum, and then seeded in 96-well U-bottom plates (CoStar, Cambridge, Massachusetts) at 2×10^5 cells/well (with total volume of 200 μL/well). On day 7, each well was restimulated with the primary antigen as used at day 0. Autologous PBMC were pulsed with antigen by incubating 10^7 PBMC in 1 mL of media with antigen at a concentration of 100 μg/mL (MBP or PLP) or 10 Lf/mL (TT) for 2 h at 37 °C, washed twice in media, and irradiated with 5000 rad. Then, 2×10^5 antigen-pulsed PBMC were added to each well. On day 9, 100 μL of media was removed from each well and 100 μL of media with IL-2 (T cell supernatant derived from phytohemagglutinin-P-stimulated human PBMC, final concentration per well, 5% v/v) (Collaborative Biomedical Products, Bedford, Massachusetts) and rIL-4 (2.5 U/mL, final concentration/well) (Boehringer-Mannheim, Mannheim, Germany) was added to the wells.

On day 14, a split-well assay was performed. Each well was split into four wells: two received 1×10^5 autologous, antigen-pulsed, washed, and irradiated cells each and two received 1×10^5 autologous, nonantigen-pulsed, washed, and irradiated cells each. All antigen pulsing, washing, and irradiation was performed as described above for the day-7 antigen pulse. Final well volume was 200 μL. Supernatants were collected after 24 h for cytokine measurement of IL-4 and IFN-γ by ELISA. The lines were cultured for an additional 72 h in 150 μL/well of serum-free media (X-Vivo 20, BioWhittaker) and supernatants were then collected for measurement of TGF-β1. Each cell line was then pulsed with 1 μCi/well of ^{3}H-thymidine during the last 18 h of culture and subsequently harvested by an automated cell harvester (Beta plate 1295-004, Wallac, Gaithersburg, Maryland). ^{3}H-Thymidine uptake was measured in a beta scintillation counter (Beta plate 1205, Wallac). As previously described, antigen-reactive lines were defined by exhibiting both a stimulation index of greater than 3 and a ΔCPM of greater than 500. The relative frequency of antigen-reactive lines was calculated by dividing the number of wells positive for reactivity, as defined above, by the total number of lines generated after stimulation with that antigen.[16] Each well in the 96-well plate yielded a growth-positive well under these culture conditions that could be examined for antigen reactivity.

Cytokine Assays

Cytokines produced by T cell lines were assayed by ELISA. To measure IL-4, a capture ELISA method was employed as follows: Immulon 4 microtiter plates (Dynatech, Chantilly, Virginia) were coated with capture monoclonal antibody (Pharmingen, San Diego, California) at 1 μg/mL diluted in 0.1 M $NaHCO_3$ (pH 8.2) and were incubated at 4 °C overnight. Plates were then blocked with 3% BSA [Kirkegaard and Perry Labs (KPL), Gaithersburg, Maryland] in PBS for 2 h at room temperature (RT) and washed, and supernatant (100 μL of culture supernatant) and standards of IL-4 (R&D Systems, Minneapolis, Minnesota) (21–1667 pg/mL) were then added and incubated at 4 °C overnight. Plates were washed and detecting biotinylated monoclonal antibody (Pharmingen) was added to plates at 0.5 μg/mL and incubated for 1 h at RT. After washing, the plates were incubated for 45 min with avidin-peroxidase (Sigma) at a 1:2000 dilution. After washing, plates were developed with TMB one-component peroxidase substrate (KPL), and reactions were stopped by TMB one-component stop solution (KPL). Absorbance was measured using ELISA reader (Bio-Rad, Melville, New York) at 450 nm, and the standard curve for each assay was generated and the cytokine production from each line was calculated. IFN-γ was measured by employing a mouse monoclonal anti-human IFN-γ at 1 μg/mL as coating antibody and a rabbit anti-human IFN-γ polyclonal antibody at 1 μg/mL for secondary antibody (both from Endogen, Cambridge, Massachusetts), followed by a goat anti-rabbit-immunoglobulin–horseradish peroxidase–labeled antibody at 1:20,000 (Biosource International, Camarillo, California). The IFN-γ standard was purchased from Gibco BRL (Gaithersburg, Maryland). Human TGF-β1 was measured by a TGF-β1 ELISA kit (Promega, Madison, Wisconsin). Cytokine production from each line, performed in duplicate, was calculated by subtracting antigen-negative cytokine production from antigen-positive cytokine production. A line was considered positive if the antigen-specific cytokine secretion was $>$50 pg/mL of IL-4 and $>$100 pg/mL of IFN-γ or TGF-β1. The lowest measurable concentration for each assay was 5 pg/mL for IL-4, 10 pg/mL for IFN-γ, and 16 pg/mL for TGF-β1.

Statistical Analyses

A nonpaired two-tailed Student's *t* test was used to perform the statistical analyses. Linear regression analysis was used to correlate cytokine secretion between PLP- and MBP-reactive T cells from each patient.

RESULTS

Frequency of Antigen-specific T Cell Lines

The frequency of antigen-reactive T cell lines from myelin-treated and non-myelin-treated PBMC from MS patients was determined by ^{3}H-thymidine incorporation. A T cell line was considered positive when the stimulation index was greater than 3.0 and the ΔCPM was greater than 500. A comparison of the frequencies in responses of the two groups to individual antigens is shown in TABLE 1. Although there was a lower frequency of MBP- and PLP-reactive T cells in the myelin-treated group as compared to the nontreated group in response to MBP and PLP, this difference did not reach statistical significance in this cross-sectional analysis. The frequency of TT-reactive lines was similar in both myelin-treated and nontreated groups.

Reactivity of human T cells is usually measured by ^{3}H-thymidine incorporation. Thus, it was important to know if this measure of T cell proliferation correlated with cytokine secretion. This was examined by screening several hundred lines (both negative and positive for antigen-induced ^{3}H-thymidine incorporation) for secretion of IL-4, IFN-γ, and TGF-β1 by ELISA. Although a correlation between thymidine

TABLE 1. Relative Frequency of Antigen-reactive T Cell Lines in MS Patients[a]

	No. of MBP-reactive Lines/ Total No. of Lines	Mean Frequency of MBP-reactive Wells (%)	No. of PLP-reactive Lines/ Total No. of Lines	Mean Frequency of PLP-reactive Wells (%)	No. of TT-reactive Lines/ Total No. of Lines	Mean Frequency of TT-reactive Wells (%)
myelin, orally administered	14/1020	1.3 ± 0.5[b] ($n = 17$)	37/1020	3.7 ± 1.0 ($n = 17$)	112/480	23.3 ± 9.0 ($n = 8$)
control	34/1020	3.4 ± 2.5 ($n = 17$)	65/1020	7.6 ± 3.6 ($n = 17$)	57/300	19.0 ± 8.9 ($n = 5$)

[a]PBMC were plated directly into 96-well plates and stimulated with antigens as described in the text. Each well was restimulated in the presence of antigen with APC on day 7 and for reactivity by a split-well assay on day 14. Antigen-reactive lines were defined as having a stimulation index > 3 and ΔCPM > 500. Each well in the 96-well plate yielded a growth-positive well under these culture conditions that could be examined for antigen reactivity.

[b]The percentages of antigen-reactive lines out of the total number of lines generated were calculated for each subject. The values represent the mean percentage of antigen-reactive lines for each group. The results are expressed as the mean ± SE.

uptake and IFN-γ secretion was found (correlation coefficient $r = 0.60$, $p = 0.0004$), there was no correlation between the stimulation index and cytokine secretion for IL-4 and TGF-β1. Thus, we measured cytokine secretion from all wells whether or not there was antigen-specific ^{3}H-thymidine incorporation.

Relative Frequency of Cytokine-secreting Lines

The relative frequency of cytokine-secreting lines in response to MBP, PLP, and TT in T cell lines from oral myelin-treated and nontreated patients was calculated for individual subjects, and the mean relative frequency for each group was calculated (FIGURE 1). There was an increase in TGF-β1-secreting lines recognizing MBP in the oral myelin-treated patients as compared to nontreated patients (myelin-treated 9.9 ± 2, nontreated 1.3 ± 0.5, $p < 0.001$) (FIGURE 1A). We also observed an increase in the relative frequency of IL-4-secreting lines reactive to MBP in the oral myelin-treated MS patients, but this did not reach statistical significance (myelin-treated

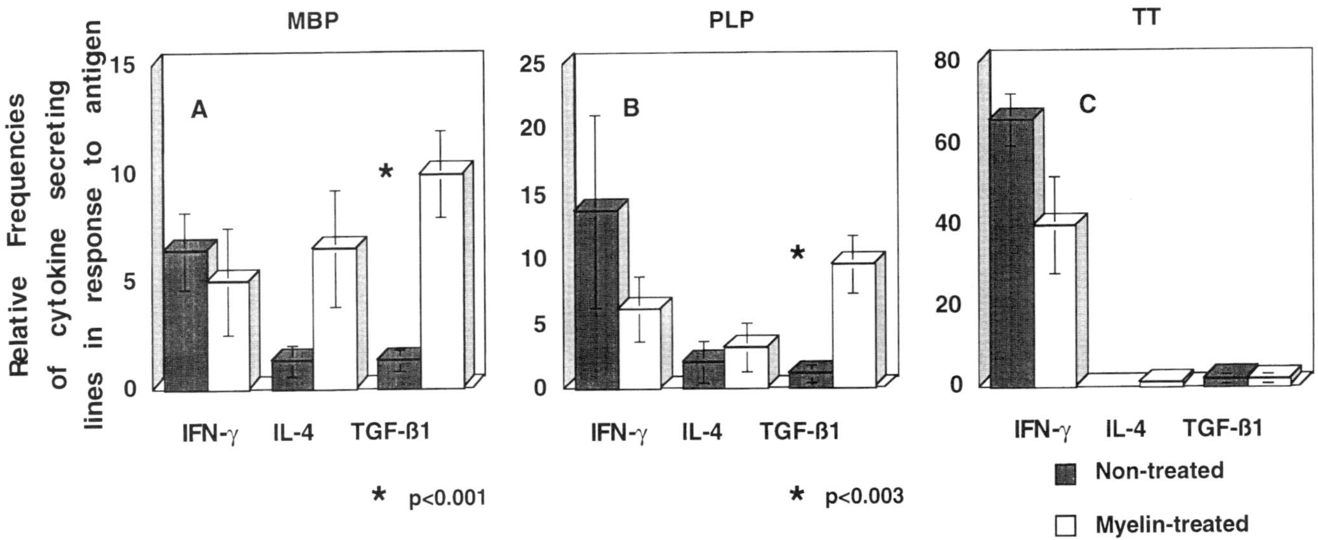

FIGURE 1. Relative frequency of antigen-reactive T cell lines secreting IL-4, IFN-γ, or TGF-β1 from MS patients receiving either myelin orally or controls. The difference in cytokine secretion on day 14 of T cell lines stimulated by antigen-pulsed APCs was compared to T cell lines stimulated with APCs alone, as described in the text. Culture supernatants were collected 24 hours after antigenic stimulation for IL-4 and IFN-γ ELISA. Serum-free media was added to each well and, after an additional 72 hours, culture supernatant was collected for TGF-β1 ELISA. A line was considered positive if the antigen-specific cytokine secretion was >50 pg/mL of IL-4 and >100 pg/mL of IFN-γ or TGF-β1. The relative frequencies of cytokine-secreting lines with antigenic stimulation were calculated for each patient—17 myelin-treated and 17 nontreated patients—and the average values, ± standard errors, are shown here. Significant p values for TGF-β1 secretion are highlighted in bold. (A) MBP stimulation: TGF-β1, myelin-treated 9.9 ± 2, nontreated 1.3 ± 0.5, $\boldsymbol{p < 0.001}$; IL-4, myelin-treated 6.5 ± 2.7, nontreated 1.3 ± 0.7, $p < 0.099$; IFN-γ, myelin-treated 5.0 ± 2.5, nontreated 6.4 ± 1.8. (B) PLP stimulation: TGF-β1, myelin-treated 9.5 ± 2.2, nontreated 1.1 ± 0.7, $\boldsymbol{p < 0.003}$; IL-4, myelin-treated 3.1 ± 1.9, nontreated 2 ± 1.6; IFN-γ, myelin-treated 6.1 ± 2.5, nontreated 13.7 ± 7.4, $p < 0.264$. (C) TT stimulation: TGF-β1, myelin-treated 1.9 ± 1.2, nontreated 2.0 ± 1.2; IL-4, myelin-treated 1.0 ± 0.5, nontreated 0; IFN-γ, myelin-treated 39.8 ± 12.1, nontreated 65.8 ± 6.3; all values not significantly different.

6.5 ± 2.7, nontreated 1.3 ± 0.7, $p < 0.099$). No difference in the relative frequency of IFN-γ-secreting lines was observed (myelin-treated 5.0 ± 2.5, nontreated 6.4 ± 1.8). In response to PLP, there was also a significant increase in the relative frequency of TGF-β1-secreting T cell lines in the myelin-treated group (myelin-treated 9.5 ± 2.2, nontreated 1.1 ± 0.7, $p < 0.003$), whereas there was no difference observed for IL-4-secreting lines (myelin-treated 3.1 ± 1.9, nontreated 2 ± 1.6) (FIGURE 1B). There was a trend for lower IFN-γ secretion from the oral myelin-treated group in response to PLP, but this did not achieve statistical significance (myelin-treated 6.1 ± 2.5, nontreated 13.7 ± 7.4, $p < 0.264$).

To examine whether the frequency of TGF-β1-secreting lines from the oral myelin-treated group was specific for myelin antigens, we measured cytokine secretion from T cell lines using TT as a control antigen. Both oral myelin-treated and non-myelin-treated groups showed similar relative frequencies of TGF-β1, IL-4, and IFN-γ cell lines in response to TT (TGF-β1: myelin-treated 1.9 ± 1.2, nontreated 2.0 ± 1.2; IL-4: myelin-treated 1.0 ± 0.5, nontreated 0; IFN-γ: myelin-treated 39.8 ± 12.1, nontreated 65.8 ± 6.3) (FIGURE 1C).

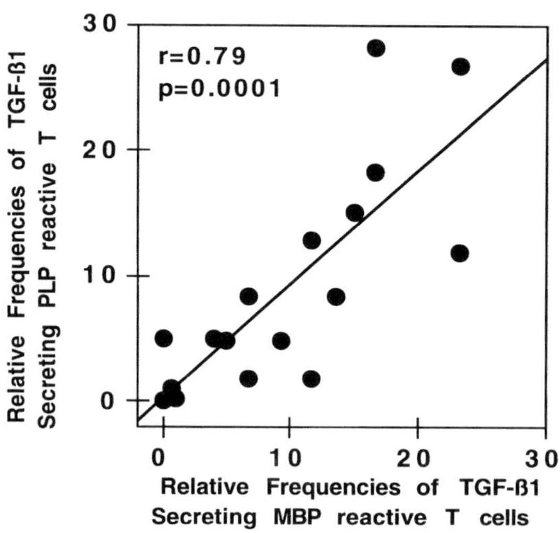

FIGURE 2. Correlation between the relative frequencies of MBP versus PLP TGF-β1-secreting T cells. The relative frequencies of MBP versus PLP TGF-β1-secreting T cells among individual subjects were correlated by a linear-regression analysis. There was a significant correlation ($r = 0.79$, $p = 0.0001$) in individual patients between the relative frequency of MBP versus PLP TGF-β1-secreting T cells.

Correlation between the Relative Frequencies of MBP versus PLP TGF-β1-secreting T Cells

The frequency of both MBP- and PLP-reactive TGF-β1-secreting T cells varied among MS patients orally treated with myelin. This led us to examine whether there was a correlation between the relative frequencies of MBP versus PLP TGF-β1-secreting T cells among individual subjects. As shown in FIGURE 2, there was a highly significant correlation in individual patients between the frequency of MBP versus PLP TGF-β1-secreting T cells.

DISCUSSION

The present study was carried out to determine whether the prolonged oral administration of myelin in MS patients alters the frequency or cytokine secretion patterns of MBP- or PLP-reactive T cells. We have demonstrated an increase in the frequency of MBP- and PLP-reactive, but not TT-reactive, TGF-β1-secreting T cell lines in myelin-treated MS patients as compared to non-myelin-treated MS patients; these data are presented in greater detail elsewhere.[24] These studies, showing cytokine deviation with antigen-specific immunotherapy in subjects with autoimmune disease, are consistent with our observation that, in mice receiving oral MBP, there is an increase in MBP-specific TGF-β1-secreting T cells.[21]

A number of studies have defined mechanisms by which oral tolerization occurs in rodents. In the EAE model, one of the primary mechanisms involves the generation of active suppression, and this is mediated by T cells that secrete TGF-β1 and suppress the immune response.[25] Furthermore, T cell clones isolated from the mesenteric lymph nodes of mice orally tolerized with MBP secreting IL-4, IL-10, and TGF-β1 suppressed ongoing EAE induced by either MBP or PLP.[20] The regulatory properties of these T cell clones were abrogated when mice were given anti-TGF-β1 antibodies, suggesting a critical role for local secretion of TGF-β1 in suppressing the immune response. The importance of cytokines in regulating the inflammatory CNS response in EAE has also been suggested by immunopathologic examination of cytokine secretion in the CNS. Animals with acute EAE exhibit perivascular infiltration with activated mononuclear cells secreting the inflammatory cytokines, IL-1, IL-2, TNF-α, IFN-γ, IL-6, and IL-8. In contrast, animals with EAE that had been orally tolerized with MBP exhibit a marked reduction of the perivascular infiltrate, with downregulation of inflammatory cytokines and increased amounts of TGF-β1 and IL-4.[6] These results suggest that the suppression of EAE, by oral tolerization and natural recovery, is related to regulatory cells that secrete inhibitory cytokines at the target organ.

TGF-β1 has a number of properties consistent with a role in regulating the immune response. It is potent in inhibiting T and B cell entry into the $S/G_2/M$ cell cycle and thus in inhibiting proliferation. Paradoxically, TGF-β1 also can attract macrophages to sites of inflammation while inducing upregulation of IgA secretion by activated B lymphocytes.[26,27] In addition, T cells grown in the presence of TGF-β1 secrete more IL-2 than those responding to CD2 and CD28 stimulation. These T cells also expressed an increased amount of $\alpha^E\beta_7$-integrin, a human mucosal epithelium adhesion molecule.[28] TGF-β1 also can induce fibrin deposition and is involved in scar formation.[29] Thus, a combined physiologic action of TGF-β1 may be to downregulate inflammatory T cell responses while inducing tissue repair as well as inducing T cells primed in the gut.

There are few investigations in humans regarding the mechanism of oral tolerization. The immune responses in normal individuals orally administered with keyhole limpet hemocyanin (KLH) decreased subsequent cell-mediated immune responses when subjects were injected with KLH, although antibody responses were not affected.[30] The mechanism for this suppression has not been elucidated. Myelin antigens have also been given by other routes in attempts to tolerize human T cell responses. These studies showed that, with parenteral administration of MBP, subsequent delayed-type hypersensitivity responses were observed, presumably representing a Th1-type response.[31]

We previously reported that the frequency of MBP-reactive T cells was significantly decreased in a longitudinal study investigating frequencies prior to and after initiating oral administration of myelin in patients with MS.[16] Although a similar trend was observed in the present study, the data did not reach statistical significance. We believe the lack of statistical significance in the present cross-sectional study is related to the variability in the frequency of MBP-reactive T cells among different patients with MS as compared to the serial measurements that we performed in our first investigation. We attempted to determine whether there was a correlation between the frequency of TGF-β1-secreting cells and the response to therapy by arbitrarily dividing patients into responders and nonresponders and performing a chi-square statistical analysis. No correlation was found in this small number of patients studied. As mentioned above, this will be examined in a larger study powered to address this experimental question.

As expected from treating an outbred group of MS patients, there was a distribution in the range of both MBP- and PLP-reactive TGF-β1-secreting T cells. This may have been due to differences among individual patients in their ability to recognize these myelin antigens or, alternatively, individual patients may have differential abilities to generate TGF-β1-secreting T cells. This question was addressed by determining whether there was a correlation among individual patients in the frequencies of MBP- versus PLP-reactive TGF-β1-secreting T cells. Indeed, we found a highly significant correlation in individual MS patients between the frequency of these two myelin-reactive T cell populations. As MBP- and PLP-reactive TGF-β1-secreting T cells were found in the same patients, these data suggest the latter hypothesis that individual patients, similar to different mice strains, may have a differential ability to generate different cytokine-secreting populations of T cells.

Taken together, these data suggest that T cells generated in the gut, primed with whole myelin, may have the ability to migrate into the central nervous system and nonspecifically suppress ongoing autoimmune responses at the target organ by secreting TGF-β1. This represents an antigen-specific immunotherapy capable of suppressing autoimmune responses to multiple self-antigens at the target organ. Moreover, these data show that autoantigen-specific T cells secreting TGF-β1 can be generated in humans with autoimmune disease.

In summary, oral administration of myelin to MS patients generated an increased frequency of MBP- and PLP-specific TGF-β1-secreting T cells. These results are consistent with the cytokine profile of regulatory T cells observed in animals following oral tolerization with MBP.[19–21,25] Such antigen-specific regulatory T cells upon homing to the central nervous system would be predicted to suppress ongoing autoimmune responses in an antigen-nonspecific fashion by the secretion of TGF-β1, a mechanism that has been termed bystander suppression. T cells induced by mucosal stimulation with antigen that secrete TGF-β1 appear to represent a distinct lineage of T cells (Th3 type).[32] Our data demonstrate that oral tolerization with self-antigens in a human autoimmune disease may provide a therapeutic approach to the treatment of autoimmune disease that does not depend upon knowledge of the antigen specificity of the original T cell clone triggering the autoimmune cascade.

ACKNOWLEDGMENTS

FIGURES 1 and 2 and TABLE 1 were used by permission of the Rockefeller University Press, New York, for the American Society for Clinical Investigation.

REFERENCES

1. McFARLIN, D. E. & H. F. McFARLAND. 1982. Multiple sclerosis. N. Engl. J. Med. **307:** 1183–1188.
2. HAFLER, D. A. & H. L. WEINER. 1995. Immunologic mechanisms and therapy in multiple sclerosis. Immunol. Rev. **144:** 75–107.
3. ZAMVIL, S., P. NELSON, J. TROTTER, D. MITCHELL, R. KNOBLER, R. FRITZ & L. STEINMAN. 1985. T cell clones specific for myelin basic protein induce chronic relapsing paralysis and demyelination. Nature **317:** 355–358.
4. TUOHY, V. K., R. A. SOBEL & M. B. LEES. 1988. Myelin proteolipid protein–induced experimental allergic encephalomyelitis: variations of disease expression in different strains of mice. J. Immunol. **140:** 1868–1873.
5. LININGTON, C., T. BERGER, L. PERRY, S. WEERTH, D. HINZE-SELCH, Y. ZHANG, H. C. LU, H. LASSMANN & H. WEKERLE. 1993. T cells specific for the myelin oligodendrocyte glycoprotein mediate an unusual autoimmune inflammatory response in the central nervous system. Eur. J. Immunol. **23:** 1364–1372.
6. KHOURY, S. J., W. W. HANCOCK & H. L. WEINER. 1992. Oral tolerance to myelin basic protein and natural recovery from experimental autoimmune encephalomyelitis are associated with downregulation of inflammatory cytokines and differential upregulation of transforming growth factor-β, interleukin-4, and prostaglandin E expression in the brain. J. Exp. Med. **176:** 1355–1364.
7. CHASE, M. W. 1946. Inhibition of experimental drug allergy by prior feeding of the sensitizing agent. Proc. Soc. Exp. Biol. Med. **61:** 257–259.
8. MOWAT, A. M. 1987. The regulation of immune response to dietary protein antigens. Immunol. Today **8:** 93–98.
9. HIGGINS, P. J. & H. L. WEINER. 1988. Suppression of experimental autoimmune encephalomyelitis by oral administration of myelin basic protein and its fragments. J. Immunol. **140:** 440–445.
10. BITAR, D. M. & C. C. WHITACRE. 1988. Suppression of experimental autoimmune encephalomyelitis by the oral administration of myelin basic protein. Cell. Immunol. **112:** 364–370.
11. THOMPSON, H. S. & N. A. STAINES. 1986. Gastric administration of type II collagen delays the onset and severity of collagen-induced arthritis in rats. Clin. Exp. Immunol. **64:** 581–586.
12. NAGLER-ANDERSON, C., L. A. BOBER, M. E. ROBINSON, G. W. SISKIND & G. J. THORBECKE. 1986. Suppression of type II collagen-induced arthritis by intragastric administration of soluble type II collagen. Proc. Natl. Acad. Sci. U.S.A. **83:** 7443–7446.
13. ZHANG, Z. J., C. S. Y. LEE, O. LIDER & H. L. WEINER. 1990. Suppression of adjuvant arthritis in Lewis rats by oral administration of type II collagen. J. Immunol. **145:** 2489–2493.
14. NUSSENBLATT, R. B., R. R. CASPI, R. MAHDI, C-C. CHAN, F. ROBERGE, O. LIDER & H. L. WEINER. 1990. Inhibition of S-antigen induced experimental autoimmune uveoretinitis by oral induction of tolerance with S-antigen. J. Immunol. **144:** 1689–1695.

15. Zhang, Z. J., L. Davidson, G. Eisenbarth & H. L. Weiner. 1991. Suppression of diabetes in nonobese diabetic mice by oral administration of porcine insulin. Proc. Natl. Acad. Sci. U.S.A. **88:** 10252–10256.
16. Weiner, H. L., G. A. Macklin, M. Matsui, E. J. Orav, S. J. Khoury, D. M. Dawson & D. A. Hafler. 1993. Double-blind pilot trial of oral tolerization with myelin antigens in multiple sclerosis. Science **259:** 1321–1324.
17. Trentham, D. E., R. A. Dynesius-Trentham, E. J. Orav, D. Combitchi, C. Lorenzo, K. L. Sewell, D. A. Hafler & H. L. Weiner. 1993. Effects of oral administration of type II collagen on rheumatoid arthritis. Science **261:** 1727–1730.
18. Hohol, M. J., S. J. Khoury, S. L. Cook, E. J. Orav, D. A. Hafler & H. L. Weiner. 1996. Three-year open protocol continuation study of oral tolerization with myelin antigens in multiple sclerosis and design of a phase III pivotal trial. Ann. N.Y. Acad. Sci. **778:** 243–250.
19. Miller, A., O. Lider & H. L. Weiner. 1991. Antigen-driven bystander suppression following oral administration of antigens. J. Exp. Med. **174:** 791–798.
20. Chen, Y., V. K. Kuchroo, J-I. Inobe, D. A. Hafler & H. L. Weiner. 1994. Regulatory T cell clones induced by oral tolerance: suppression of autoimmune encephalomyelitis. Science **265:** 1237–1240.
21. Chen, Y., J-I. Inobe, V. K. Kuchroo, J. L. Baron, C. A. Janeway, Jr. & H. L. Weiner. 1996. Oral tolerance in myelin basic protein T-cell receptor transgenic mice: suppression of autoimmune encephalomyelitis and dose-dependent induction of regulatory cells. Proc. Natl. Acad. Sci. U.S.A. **93:** 388–391.
22. Chou, F. C-H., C-H. J. Chou, R. Shapira & R. F. Kibler. 1976. Basis of microheterogeneity of myelin basic protein. J. Biol. Chem. **251:** 2671–2679.
23. Bizzozero, O. A., G. Zuniga & M. B. Lees. 1991. Fatty acid composition of human myelin proteolipid protein in peroxisomal disorders. J. Neurochem. **56:** 872–878.
24. Fukaura, H., S. C. Kent, M. J. Pietrusewicz, S. J. Khoury, H. L. Weiner & D. A. Hafler. 1996. Induction of circulating myelin basic protein and proteolipid protein–specific transforming growth factor-β1–secreting Th3 T cells by oral administration of myelin in multiple sclerosis patients. J. Clin. Invest. **98:** 70–77.
25. Miller, A., O. Lider, A. B. Roberts, M. B. Sporn & H. L. Weiner. 1992. Suppressor T cells generated by oral tolerization to myelin basic protein suppress both *in vitro* and *in vivo* immune responses by the release of transforming growth factor β after antigen-specific triggering. Proc. Natl. Acad. Sci. U.S.A. **89:** 421–425.
26. Lebman, D. A., F. D. Lee & R. L. Coffman. 1990. Mechanism for transforming growth factor β and IL-2 enhancement of IgA expression in lipopolysaccharide-stimulated B cell cultures. J. Immunol. **144:** 952–959.
27. Kagnoff, M. F. & P. H. Kim. 1991. Effects of transforming growth factor beta-1 and interleukin-5 on IgA isotype switching at the clonal level. Immunol. Res. **10:** 396–399.
28. Cerwenka, A., D. Bevec, O. Majdic, W. Knapp & W. Holter. 1994. TGF-beta 1 is a potent inducer of human effector T cells. J. Immunol. **153:** 4367–4377.
29. Wahl, S. M., N. McCarthy-Francis & S. E. Mergenhagen. 1989. Inflammatory and immunomodulatory roles of TGFβ. Immunol. Today **10:** 258–261.
30. Husby, S., J. Mestecky, Z. Moldoveanu, S. Holland & C. O. Elson. 1994. Oral tolerance in humans: T cell but not B cell tolerance after antigen feeding. J. Immunol. **152:** 4663–4670.
31. Salk, R. J. S. 1983. A study of myelin basic protein as a therapeutic probe in patients with multiple sclerosis. *In* Multiple Sclerosis. J. F. Hallpike, C. W. M. Adams & W. W. Tourtellotte, Eds.: 621–630. Chapman & Hall. London.
32. Mosmann, T. R. & S. Sad. 1996. The expanding universe of T-cell subsets: Th1, Th2, and more. Immunol. Today **17:** 138–146.

CDR3 Fingerprinting of Immunoglobulin Kappa Light Chains Expressed in Rheumatoid Arthritis

Evidence of Antigenic Selection or Dysregulation of Gene Rearrangement in B Cells

S. LOUIS BRIDGES, JR.,[a,b,c,d] JOHN C. LAVELLE,[e]
SOO KON LEE,[f] STEPHANIE BYER,[a]
AND HARRY W. SCHROEDER, JR.[b,c,e,g,h]

[a]*Division of Clinical Immunology and Rheumatology*
[b]*Department of Medicine*
[c]*Department of Microbiology*
University of Alabama at Birmingham
Birmingham, Alabama 35294

[d]*Birmingham Veterans Administration Medical Center*
Birmingham, Alabama

[e]*Division of Developmental and Clinical Immunology*
University of Alabama at Birmingham
Birmingham, Alabama 35294

[f]*Division of Rheumatology*
Department of Internal Medicine
Yonsei University College of Medicine
Seoul, Korea

[g]*Comprehensive Cancer Center*
University of Alabama at Birmingham
Birmingham, Alabama 35294

Rheumatoid arthritis (RA) is characterized by lymphocytic infiltration into the synovial membranes of affected joints. B lymphocytes infiltrating RA synovia can secrete large amounts of immunoglobulin. The third complementarity-determining region (CDR3) of an immunoglobulin kappa light chain is generated by joining of the Vκ and Jκ gene segments. The light-chain CDR3 lies in the center of the antigen binding site, so its length can affect antigenic specificity of the antibody. Nongermline-encoded nucleotides have recently been reported in kappa light chains from normals and patients with RA.[1–3] Despite the presence of N-region addition, ~95% of kappa light chains from normal adult B cells contain CDR3s of 8, 9, or 10 amino acids (aa).

In an analysis of Vκ clones from RA synovia, RA PBL, and normal controls, we found enrichment for kappa chains with 11-amino-acid CDR3s in two of three RA

[h]To whom all correspondence should be addressed.

patients studied.[2] We have also identified, from an RA synovial cDNA library, a set of clonally related Vκ transcripts containing CDR3s of 11 amino acids, suggesting antigenic selection of B cells with unusually long κ chain CDR3s.[4]

To determine if enrichment for unusually long Vκ CDR3s is common in RA patients, we performed CDR3 fingerprint analysis of a larger number of samples from RA patients and controls (TABLE 1). First-strand cDNA from unsorted cells from each tissue was PCR-amplified using a VκIII leader/framework 1 primer and a Cκ primer. Nested PCR using a VκIII FR3 and a ^{32}P-end-labeled internal Cκ primer was performed on PCR products from each of the preliminary amplifications, followed by polyacrylamide gel electrophoresis of the radiolabeled PCR products. Intensities of bands representing CDR3s of 8, 9, 10, and 11 aa were quantified by phosphoimaging. Replicate experiments were performed more than once in 21 of 26 samples and the values for each tissue sample were averaged.

The κ chain repertoires of some RA patients are enriched for unusually long

TABLE 1. Characteristics of Rheumatoid Arthritis Patients and Normal Controls[a]

	Joint	Age/Race/Sex	Serum RF	Disease Duration (Years)
RA Patients—Synovium				
AS[b]	left elbow	42 BF	positive	6
JR[b]	right knee	60 WM	positive	20
MP[b]	right hip	50 WF	positive	6
JS[b]	right knee	64 WF	positive	>10
JE	left knee	51 WF	positive	20
FH	right knee	73 WF	N.D.	>10
AG	left wrist	64 WF	positive	8
JB (juvenile RA)	right knee	29 WF	negative	17
RA Patients—PBL				
EE	–	72 WF	positive	3
TL	–	73 WM	positive	27
RP	–	53 WM	positive	2
PB	–	50 WF	positive	31
MS	–	50 WM	N.D.	28
WL	–	50 WF	negative	4
HB	–	63 WM	positive	11
GH	–	57 WF	positive	3
CD	–	63 BF	positive	10
LH	–	60 BF	positive	3
Normal Controls—PBL				
IT	–	60 WF	N.D.	–
LB	–	32 WM	N.D.	–
LK	–	21 WF	N.D.	–
JL	–	28 WM	N.D.	–
JO	–	34 WM	N.D.	–

[a]RF = rheumatoid factor; N.D. = not done.

[b]Patients for whom both synovial and PBL samples were studied by CDR3 fingerprint analysis.

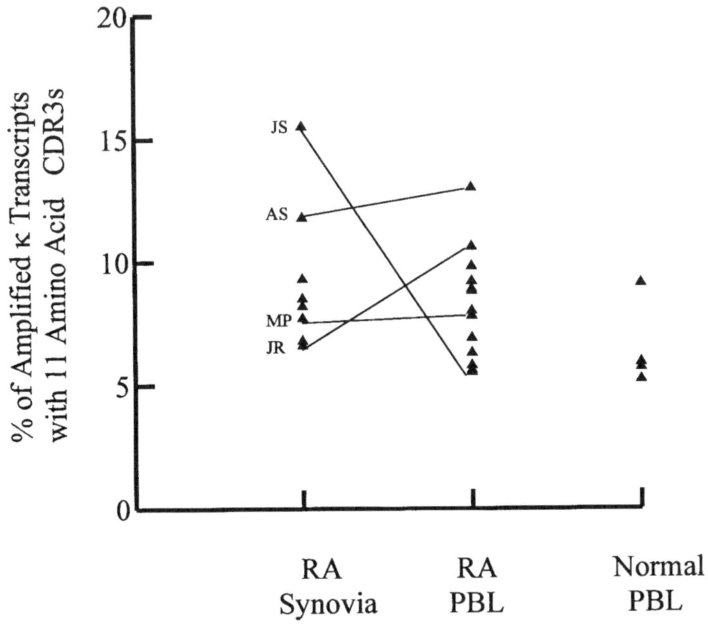

FIGURE 1. Proportions of amplified immunoglobulin kappa light chain transcripts containing 11-amino-acid CDR3s as assessed by CDR3 fingerprint analysis of RA synovia, RA PBL, and normal PBL samples. Each triangle represents the mean of replicate experiments on an individual tissue sample, if more than one experiment was performed on that sample. For paired synovial and PBL samples, the patient's initials are shown next to the synovial value.

CDR3s (FIGURE 1). The overall mean values (±SEM) for proportions of Vκ amplicons containing CDR3s of 11 aa were 9.3 ± 1.1% for RA synovia, 8.1 ± 0.6% for RA PBL, and 6.2 ± 0.7% for normal PBL. This finding may result from dysregulation of κ gene rearrangement or antigenic selection of B cells expressing long κ light-chain CDR3s. To differentiate between these two possibilities, we studied Vκ CDR3 lengths in B cell subsets of an RA patient (AS), whose synovial and PBL κ chain repertoires demonstrated enrichment for 11-aa CDR3s [27% and 30%, respectively, by sequence analysis,[4] and 12% and 13% by CDR3 fingerprint analysis (FIGURE 1)]. PBL were sorted by FACS into IgM^+/IgD^+ (naive) and IgM^-/IgD^- (class-switched) B cell subsets, and CDR3 fingerprinting was performed on each B cell subset. The proportions of 11-aa CDR3s in the naive and class-switched subsets were each ~14%, suggesting altered Vκ-Jκ rearrangement as the explanation for the finding of enrichment for long κ chain CDR3s in this patient.

REFERENCES

1. LEE, S. K., S. L. BRIDGES, JR., W. J. KOOPMAN & H. W. SCHROEDER, JR. 1992. The immunoglobulin kappa light chain repertoire expressed in the synovium of a patient with rheumatoid arthritis. Arthritis Rheum. **35:** 905–913.

2. BRIDGES, S. L., JR., S. K. LEE, M. L. JOHNSON, J. C. LAVELLE, P. G. FOWLER, W. J. KOOPMAN & H. W. SCHROEDER, JR. 1995. Somatic mutation and CDR3 lengths of immunoglobulin κ light chains expressed in patients with rheumatoid arthritis and normal individuals. J. Clin. Invest. **96:** 831–841.
3. VICTOR, K. D. & J. D. CAPRA. 1994. An apparently common mechanism of generating antibody diversity: length variation of the V_L-J_L junction. Mol. Immunol. **31:** 39–46.
4. LEE, S. K., S. L. BRIDGES, JR., P. M. KIRKHAM, W. J. KOOPMAN & H. W. SCHROEDER, JR. 1994. Evidence of antigen receptor–influenced oligoclonal B lymphocyte expansion in the synovium of a patient with long-standing rheumatoid arthritis. J. Clin. Invest. **93:** 361–370.

The Accessory Cell Function of B-CLL B Cells[a]

KRISTINE J. CAMPAGNA, NICHOLAS CHIORAZZI, AND MING-DER Y. CHANG[b]

Department of Medicine
North Shore University Hospital–New York University School of Medicine
Manhasset, New York 11030

INTRODUCTION

Chronic lymphocytic leukemia (CLL) is characterized by the progressive accumulation of a clone of CD5+ B cells.[1] These leukemic B cells express decreased amounts of surface Ig, MHC class II antigen, B cell differentiation antigens, adhesion molecules, and complement and Fc receptors.[2] Peripheral T cells of certain CLL patients also show a defective helper function.[3] Therefore, the deficient immunological responses observed in CLL patients can be a consequence of either B cell or T cell defects. To determine the accessory cell function of B cells, we have analyzed the superantigen (SEB)–presenting activity of B cells isolated from several CLL patients.

MATERIALS AND METHODS

Reagents and Monoclonal Antibodies

The FITC-, PE-, or PerCP-labeled mouse anti-human CD5, CD11a, CD11c, CD18, CD19, and B7 antibodies and irrelevant mouse antibodies were purchased from Becton-Dickinson (San Jose, California). Superantigen, staphylococcal enterotoxin B (SEB), was purchased from Sigma (St. Louis, Missouri).

Cell Preparations

Peripheral blood mononuclear cells (PBMC) were isolated from heparinized blood samples by Ficoll-Hypaque (Accurate Chemical & Scientific Corporation, Westbury, New York) gradient centrifugation. Peripheral blood samples were obtained from patients diagnosed with CLL and from healthy volunteers. T cells were isolated by using Dynabeads M-450 Pan-T (CD2) magnetic beads (Dynal, Oslo, Norway)

[a]This work was supported by NIH Grant No. GM 45919 to Ming-der Y. Chang and by The Joseph Eletto Leukemia Research Fund.

[b]To whom all correspondence should be addressed.

TABLE 1. Patient Data

Patient No.	Surface Ig	% Expression on CD5+, CD19+ Cells			SEB Reactivity[a]	
		CD18	CD11a	CD11c	CLL T Cells, Normal APC	Normal T Cells, CLL B Cells
20	μ	5	ND	ND	−	++
58	μ	1	0	42	+	++
79	μ	0	0	88	+	+
121	μ	1	ND	ND	−	++
123	μ	3	3	13	−	++
138	μ	1	1	22	+	+

[a]Cells of CLL patients exhibit either over 50% (++) or less than 50% (+) of the activity of cells of healthy individuals.

according to the manufacturer's instructions. The remaining cells were used as the antigen-presenting cells (APC).

Proliferation Assays

1×10^5 APC were incubated with 1×10^5 T cells in flat-bottomed 96-well culture plates (Falcon, Oxnard, California) in RPMI 1640 supplemented with 10% FCS, 1% penicillin-streptomycin (Gibco), 25 μM 2-β-mercaptoethanol (Sigma), 1% L-glutamine (Gibco), and 1 mM Hepes (Gibco). SEB was added to each well at various concentrations. Plates were incubated for 72 hours at 37°C in 5% CO_2 atmosphere. The proliferation was determined by ^{3}H-thymidine (DuPont, Wilmington, Delaware) incorporation in the final 16 hours. The radioactivities were measured in a beta-scintillation counter (Wallac, Finland).

Flow Cytometric Analysis

1×10^6 PBMC or CLL B cells which had been incubated with either CLL T cells or normal T cells, with or without 50 ng/mL SEB for 72 hours in 24-well culture plates, were stained with the desired monoclonal antibodies for 30 min on ice, washed, and fixed. Then, the fluorescence signal was analyzed on FACScan (Becton-Dickinson).

RESULTS

The Antigen-presenting Activities of CLL B Cells

To determine whether the deficient immune response observed in CLL patients is due to a defect in the B cell or T cell compartment, we decided to examine the ability of CLL B cells to elicit an alloresponse and present superantigen to normal T cells. Superantigen was used to give a potent stimulation to T cells and to bypass the requirement of MHC restriction. We have examined 6 IgM^+ CLL patients and, although CLL B cells cannot stimulate an alloresponse, our data show that some of these CLL B cells can activate SEB-reactive T cells from normal donors (TABLE 1). At the same time, CLL B cells can also be stimulated to express B7 (FIGURE 1). On the other hand, isolated CLL T cells are deficient in their ability to respond to superantigen presented on normal B cells and to induce B7 expression on CLL B cells. Previous studies have shown that CLL B cells have a decreased ability to stimulate alloreactive T cells or to present nominal antigens to T cells.[4] We

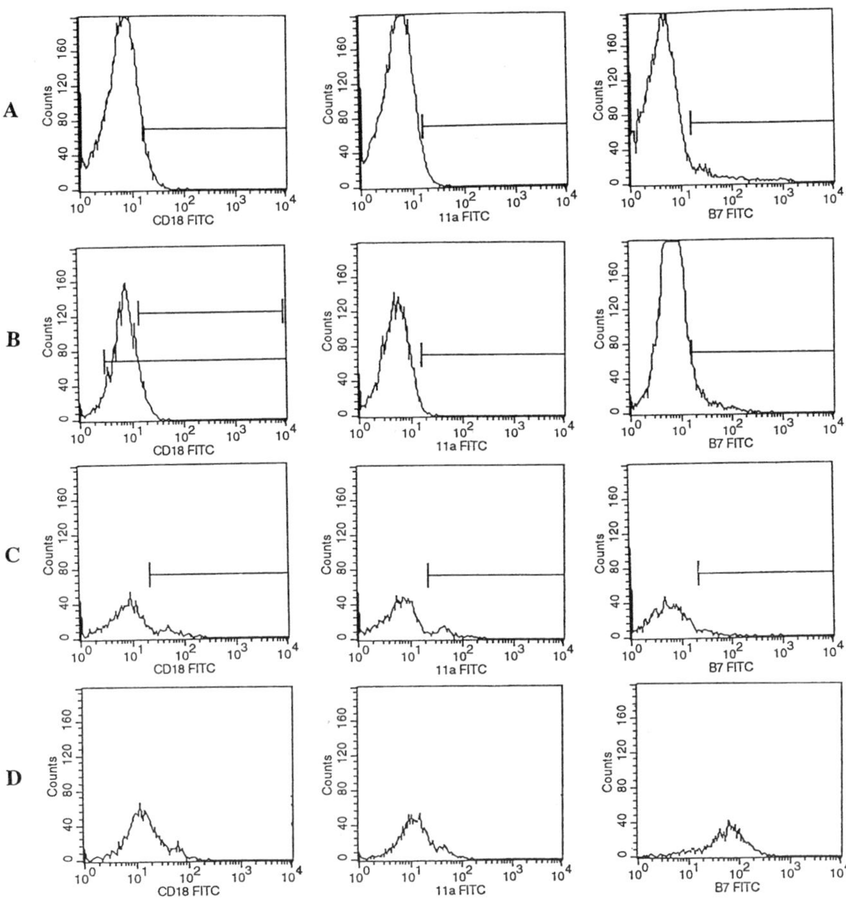

FIGURE 1. The expression of CD18, CD11a, and B7 on CD5+ CD19+ B cells of CLL patient no. 138 after 72 hours of culturing alone (A, B) or with T cells isolated from healthy individuals (C, D), without SEB (A, C) or with SEB (B, D). See text for experimental details.

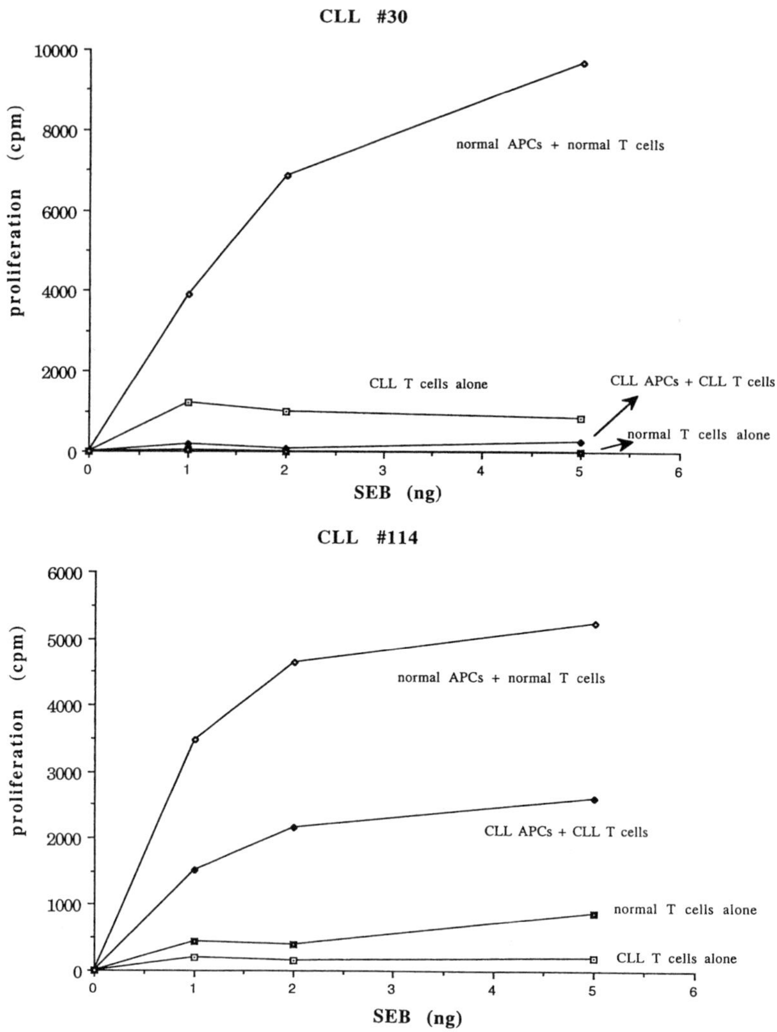

FIGURE 2. IgG+ CD18+ CD5+ B cells, isolated from CLL patient nos. 30 and 114, have a decreased ability to present SEB to syngeneic T cells. See text for experimental details.

are the first to show that a population of CLL B cells can present the superantigen, SEB, to normal T cells. There may be two possibilities for this observation: (1) superantigen presentation may require less costimulating signals than nominal antigens and (2) the frequency of superantigen-reactive T cells is much higher than that of antigen-specific T cells. However, CLL T cells cannot respond to SEB presented on either CLL or normal B cells, suggesting that CLL T cells have an intrinsic defect in their activation.

The Expression of Adhesion Molecules by CLL B Cells

Previous studies have shown that there is differential expression of β2-integrin on CLL B cells.[5] Furthermore, the adhesion molecules play important roles in antigen presentation.[6] We therefore analyzed the expression of α chains (CD11a and CD11c) and β chains (CD18) of β2-integrin on CD5+, CD19+ B cells of normal and CLL patients. All CD5+, CD19+ B cells of healthy individuals express CD18 and CD11a, but not CD11c. Out of 11 IgG+ CLL patients, 8 express CD18 and, of these, 4 express CD11a, whereas none of the 8 IgM+ CLL patients express CD18 nor CD11a. All patients express CD11c on their CD5+ B cells. However, CD18 and CD11a expressions on IgM+ CLL B cells can be induced with PMA or by coculturing CLL B cells with normal T cells and SEB (FIGURE 1). It is intriguing to speculate that the expression of CD18 on IgG+ B cells is an indication that these CLL B cells have received T cell help during their ontogeny and this interaction leads to the isotype switching. To determine whether the expression of CD18 enhances the interaction between CLL T cells and CLL B cells, we analyzed the ability of CD18+, IgG+ CLL B cells to present SEB to syngeneic T cells. Our data show that IgG+, CD18+ CLL B cells behave as CD18− CLL B cells with respect to their SEB presentation (FIGURE 2). Therefore, the expression of CD18 does not enhance an antigen-presenting activity. Furthermore, it is surprising that the CD11c α chain can be expressed without the CD18 β chain. It would be interesting to determine whether the CD11c α chain is expressed as a homodimer or is paired with a different β chain, and whether the CD11c expressed on CLL B cells possesses a different function from the CD11c expressed on activated normal B cells.

ACKNOWLEDGMENTS

We thank S. Macphail for his critical review of this report.

REFERENCES

1. WANG, C. Y., R. A. GOOD, P. AMIRATI, G. DYMBORT & R. L. EVANS. 1980. Identification of a 69.71 complex expressed on human T cells sharing epitopes with B-type chronic lymphocytic leukemia. J. Exp. Med. **151:** 1539.
2. COHEN, H. I. 1975. Human lymphocyte surface immunoglobulin capping: normal characteristics and anomalous behavior of chronic lymphocyte leukemia. J. Clin. Invest. **5:** 84.
3. KUCINKA, J. & C. D. PLATSOUCAS. 1988. Defective helper function of purified T4 cells and excessive suppressor activity of purified T8 cells in patients with B-cell chronic lymphocytic leukemia: T4 suppressor effector cells are present in certain patients. Blood **71:** 1551.
4. DAZZI, F., E. D'ANDREA, G. BIASI, G. DE SILVERSTRO, G. GAIDANO, M. SCHENA, T. TISON, F. VIANELLO, A. GIROLAMI & F. CALIGARIS-CAPPIO. 1995. Failure of B cells of chronic lymphocytic leukemia in presenting soluble and alloantigens. Clin. Immunol. Immunopathol. **75:** 26.
5. WORMSLEY, S. B., S. M. BAIRD, N. GADOL, K. R. RAI & R. E. SOBOL. 1990. Characteristics of CD11+ CD5+ chronic B-cell leukemia and the identification of novel peripheral blood B-cell subsets with chronic lymphoid leukemia immunophenotypes. Blood **76:** 123.
6. SPRINGER, T. A. 1990. Adhesion receptors in the immune system. Nature **346:** 425.

Strand Breaks in Immunoglobulin Gene Hypermutation[a]

ANGELA KWOK-FUNG LO, ARTHUR KAR-KEUNG CHING, PAK-LEONG LIM, AND YIU-LOON CHUI[b]

Clinical Immunology Unit
The Chinese University of Hong Kong
Prince of Wales Hospital
Shatin, N.T., Hong Kong

INTRODUCTION

Rearranged immunoglobulin genes mutate at a high rate (10^{-3} bp/generation) in B cells that are activated by T-dependent antigens. Although the molecular mechanism of hypermutation remains to be understood, there are some special features noted for at least the light-chain genes: (1) the intronic and 3′ enhancers are essential to hypermutation;[1] (2) mutation is focused to the V(D)J region;[2] (3) there is a strand bias for the mutations;[3] and (4) mutations occur preferentially to the nucleotide positions within a consensus sequence, RGYW.[4] These features together suggest that hypermutation may be linked to the transcription-DNA repair system[5] and that the RGYW sequence could be the site for the nucleotide excision followed by error-prone repair. We set out to examine whether nucleotide excision could be detected in the VJ region of a well-studied VkOx1 gene,[6] which is predominantly used by BALB/c mice in the primary response against a hapten, oxazolone, using a sensitive method, known as the ligation-mediated PCR (LMPCR).[7]

MATERIALS AND METHODS

Genomic DNA obtained from the spleens or Peyer's patches of unimmunized BALB/c mice, or from the spleens of the mice at 7 days after primary immunization with oxazolone-conjugated chicken serum albumin, was examined for breaks in each of the two strands. DNA from VkOx1 hybridomas, which are known to be not active in hypermutation, was used as a negative control. In addition, for technical control of the sensitivity of LMPCR, a DNA break was artificially introduced into the VkOx1 gene using a restriction enzyme, Pst I or Kpn I. Each reaction was performed on 2 μg of DNA. LMPCR of the sense strand was initiated with primer extension from the Jk5 region. This was to ensure that only the rearranged VkOx1/Jk5 would be detected. For the antisense strand, the first primer extension step was initiated from a region between the transcription and translation start sites of VkOx1.

[a]This work was supported by the Croucher Foundation.

[b]To whom all correspondence should be addressed.

RESULTS AND DISCUSSION

DNA breaks in the sense strand of the VkOx1 gene were detected in the spleen DNA of unimmunized and immunized BALB/c mice. These breaks were not present in the same light chain–encoding gene obtained from antioxazolone hybridomas,

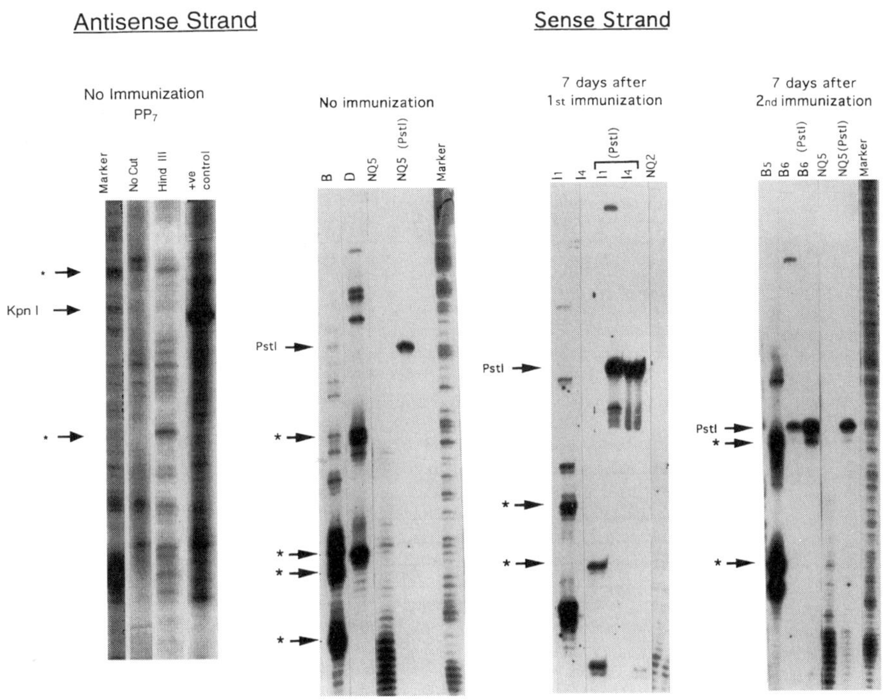

FIGURE 1. DNA strand breaks detected by LMPCR. Those breaks at the consensus sequence for hypermutation, RGYW, are denoted by an asterisk. For the sense strand, Pst I was used to cut some of the DNA samples as technical control for the LMPCR. Splenic DNA samples from individual BALB/c mice are labeled as B, D, I_1, I_4, B_5, and B_6, respectively. For the antisense strand, a modification in the LMPCR design was introduced (see text). A Hind III restriction site was incorporated into the linker oligos used in the ligation step. The final LMPCR product was digested with Hind III. Only the bands cleavable by the enzyme were regarded as indications for strand breaks. Kpn I was used, instead of Pst I, to introduce a break artificially as technical control. PP_7 denotes Peyer's patch DNA from one particular unimmunized BALB/c mouse.

which do not undergo hypermutation. On the other hand, the artificial break produced by restriction enzyme, Pst I, was strongly detected in all the DNA samples investigated. In our earlier study, breaks had not been found in the antisense strand. However, with the addition of one more round of nested PCR, and inclusion of a Hind III restriction site in the linker oligos for marking the final LMPCR products, strand breaks were detected. The artificial break produced by Kpn I restriction was also clearly detected (FIGURE 1). For LMPCR of the sense strand, the rearranged VkOx1/Jk5 gene (thus capable of hypermutation[2]) could be selectively amplified by using Jk5 oligoprimers in the initial steps. For studying the antisense strand, such selective amplification of the rearranged gene could not be performed. This conceivably would compromise the sensitivity of the LMPCR. As shown in FIGURE 2, half or more than

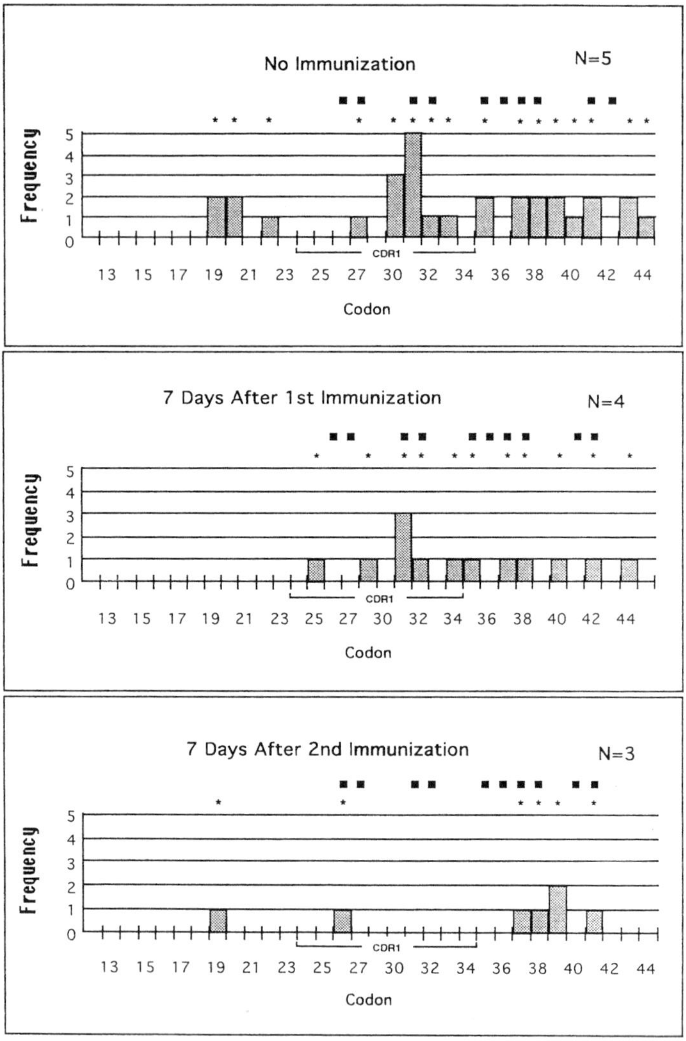

FIGURE 2. Positions of strand breaks on the sense strand of VkOx1. All the data within one group were pooled together and the number of times that a break occurred at one particular position is expressed as its frequency. Symbols: (■) RGYW consensus sequence; (*) DNA break site.

half of the breaks were located in the hypermutational hot spots or in their consensus sequence, RGYW. Codon 31 is known to be most highly mutated[3] and this position had indeed the highest incidence of strand break. The VkOx1/Jk5 gene in the Peyer's patch of unimmunized mice has been reported to accumulate mutations.[8] This must imply that the light chain is frequently used in response to environmental antigens and could explain the occurrence of strand breaks in the VkOx1 gene of the unimmunized mice. We speculate that the molecular mechanism of immunoglobulin gene hypermutation may involve a double-stranded break directly and preferentially at the mutational hot spots. This breakage could lead to exonucleolytic removal of a few adjacent nucleotides on only one strand followed by a process of error-prone repair, thus accounting for the strand bias.

REFERENCES

1. BETZ, A. G., C. MILSTEIN, A. GONZÁLES-FERNÁNDEZ, R. PANNELL, T. LARSON & M. S. NEUBERGER. 1994. Cell **77:** 239.
2. ROES, J., K. HÜPPI, K. RAJEWSKI & F. SABLITZKY. 1989. J. Immunol. **142:** 1022.
3. BETZ, A. G., C. RADA, R. PANNELL, C. MILSTEIN & M. S. NEUBERGER. 1993. Proc. Natl. Acad. Sci. U.S.A. **90:** 2385.
4. ROGOZIN, I. B. & N. A. KOLCHANOV. 1992. Biochim. Biophys. Acta **1171:** 11.
5. SELBY, C. P. & A. SANCAR. 1993. Science **260:** 53.
6. BEREK, C. & C. MILSTEIN. 1987. Immunol. Rev. **96:** 23.
7. MUELLER, P. R. & B. WOLD. 1989. Science **246:** 780.
8. GONZÁLES-FERNÁNDEZ, A. & C. MILSTEIN. 1993. Proc. Natl. Acad. Sci. U.S.A. **90:** 9862.

C-Myc Proto-oncogene Expression by Germinal Center B Cells Isolated from Human Tonsils[a]

GIOVANNA CUTRONA,[b] MARIELLA DONO,[b]
SANDRA PASTORINO,[b] MASSIMO ULIVI,[b]
VITO LELIO BURGIO,[c] SIMONA ZUPO,[b]
SILVIO RONCELLA,[b] AND MANLIO FERRARINI[b]

[b]*Servizio di Immunologia Clinica*
Istituto Nazionale per la Ricerca sul Cancro
IST
16132 Genova, Italy

[c]*Istituto di 1[a] Clinica Medica Generale e Terapia Medica*
Università "La Sapienza"
00100 Roma, Italy

INTRODUCTION

Germinal centers (GC) represent a major site for maturation of antibody affinity and the generation of B cell memory.[1–4] There are two types of GC B cells: the centroblasts and centrocytes.[1] The proliferating centroblasts undergo random hypermutation of the genes encoding the H- and L-chain V regions of the Ig molecules and transform into resting centrocytes.[1–4] These undergo apoptosis unless stimulated by antigen in the presence of accessory signals. This process represents a very efficient mechanism of selection for B cells producing high-affinity antibodies.

GC B cells share the same phenotype ($CD10^+$ $CD38^+$ $CD39^-$ $CD23^-$) as Burkitt Lymphoma (BL) B cells. These cells also undergo spontaneous apoptosis and are characterized by overexpression of c-myc consequent to a chromosomal translocation. Previously, we have shown[5] that EBV-positive LCL cells transfected with c-myc acquired typical markers of GC B cells and capacity to undergo apoptosis. These findings indicated that c-myc overexpression could confer features similar to those of GC cells and also suggested that GC B cells could be characterized by high levels of c-myc expression.

[a]This work was supported in part by grants from AIRC, ISS Progetto AIDS, CNR (P. F. Ingegneria Genetica and ACRO), Fondazione Andrea Cesalpino, and NIH (No. AI 10811).

MATERIALS AND METHODS

Cells and Myc Protein Detection

B cells were purified from human tonsils and fractionated into small, activated, and large B cells by Percoll density gradients (Pharmacia, Uppsala, Sweden).[6] Germinal center B cells were prepared from the large B fraction by depletion of $CD39^+$ and IgD^+ B cells.[7] Cells were stained with anti-myc mAb (6E10 clone, Cambridge Research Biochemicals, London, United Kingdom) and anti-bcl-2 mAb (Dakopatts, Glostrup, Denmark).[5] The second FITC- or PE-conjugated antibodies to the appropriate murine Ig isotype were from Southern Biotechnology Associates (Birmingham, Alabama).

PCR Methodologies

Total cellular RNA was extracted using guanidium isothiocyanate and CsCk gradient procedures. Myc, bcl-2, and G3PDH transcripts were PCR-amplified.[5]

TABLE 1. Ratio of c-myc/bcl-2 mRNA in Different B Cell Fractions[a]

	GC B Cells	Activated B Cells	Small B Cells
Ratio	10.23	0.63	0.51

[a]The transcripts of the two genes were amplificated in the same tube reaction for each tonsillar B cell subset. The ratios of the two amplificated mRNAs were calculated by a densitometric analysis. PCR for the amplification of c-myc/bcl-2 fragments was carried out in the presence of 30 pmol of each of the following primers: myc II/III sense 5′-CATCATCCAggACTgTATgTgg-3′; myc II/III antisense 5′-gTTgTTgCTgATCTgTCTCAgg-3′; bcl-2 sense 5′-TTCgCCgAgATgTCCAgCC-3′; bcl-2 antisense 5′-TCACTTgTggTCCAgATAgg-3′. G3PDH transcripts were amplified by using the following synthetic primers: G3PDH sense 5′-ACATCgCTCAgAACACCTATgg-3′; G3PDH antisense 5′-gggTCTACATggCAACTgTGAg-3′.

RESULTS

Expression of C-Myc Proto-oncogene by GC B Cells

Germinal center B cells were analyzed by the expression of c-myc and bcl-2 transcripts. The relative ratios of c-myc expression over that of bcl-2 were calculated by densitometric analysis (TABLE 1). GC B cells displayed a high ratio of c-myc/bcl-2 amplifications (10–17, range of four experiments), thus indicating that GC B cells transcribed large amounts of c-myc mRNA and a relative small proportion of bcl-2 mRNA. In contrast, small resting B cells displayed a low c-myc/bcl-2 mRNA ratio (0.3–0.6, range of four experiments). In the activated B cells, the ratio was slightly higher (0.5–1.5, range of four experiments).

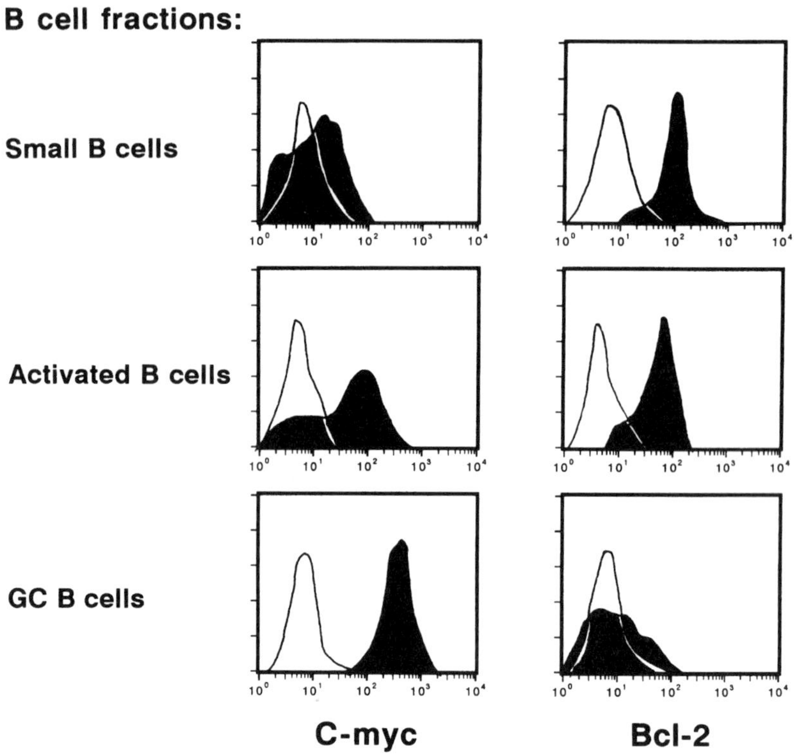

FIGURE 1. Flow-cytometric analyses of three different tonsillar B cell subsets. The cells were fixed and permeabilized before exposing to anti-myc mAb (left, black areas), anti-bcl-2 mAb (right, black areas), or unrelated (control) mAb (white areas) as detailed in reference 5.

Myc and bcl-2 protein expression by the various B cell subsets was analyzed by flow cytometry on fixed and permeabilized cells (FIGURE 1). Myc was abundant in GC B cells, much less expressed in activated B cells, and virtually absent in resting B cells. An opposite pattern of bcl-2 protein expression was seen in the same B cell populations. The expression of myc by GC B cells was similar to that detected in a BL cell line used as a control, and the expression of myc by LCL cells was lower and comparable to that of normal, activated B cells (data not shown). Cell cycle analyses on BudR-treated cells (not shown in detail here) demonstrated that GC B cells could either enter the late phases of the cell cycle or undergo apoptosis. Thus, it is possible that c-myc upregulation predisposed the cells to one or the other event, with the final outcome being regulated by other signals that possibly also influenced the bcl-2 expression.[5,8]

REFERENCES

1. LIU, Y. J., G. D. JONSON & I. C. M. MACLENNAN. 1992. Immunol. Today **13:** 17–21.
2. BEREK, C. 1992. Immunol. Rev. **126:** 5–19.

3. KÜPPERS, R., M. ZHAO, M-L. HANSMANN & K. RAJEWSKI. 1993. EMBO J. **12:** 4955–4967.
4. OSMOND, D. G. 1993. The turnover of B-cell population. Immunol. Today **14:** 34–37.
5. CUTRONA, G., M. ULIVI, F. FAIS, S. RONCELLA & M. FERRARINI. 1995. J. Exp. Med. **181:** 699–711.
6. DONO, M., S. ZUPO, R. MASANTE, G. TABORELLI, N. CHIORAZZI & M. FERRARINI. 1993. Eur. J. Immunol. **23:** 873–881.
7. ZUPO, S., E. RUGARI, M. DONO, G. TABORELLI, F. MALAVASI & M. FERRARINI. 1994. Eur. J. Immunol. **24:** 1218–1222.
8. VALDEZ, H. M., C. GURET, O. DE BOUTEILLER, I. FUGIER, J. BANCHEREAU & Y. J. LIU. 1996. J. Exp. Med. **183:** 971–977.

Isolation and Characterization of Single Anti-U1A-specific B Cells from Autoimmune Patients

RUUD M. T. DE WILDT,[a] FRANK H. J. VAN DEN HOOGEN,[b] WALTHER J. VAN VENROOIJ,[a] AND RENÉ M. A. HOET[a,c]

[a]*Department of Biochemistry University of Nijmegen*
[b]*Department of Rheumatology University Hospital Nijmegen 6500 HB Nijmegen, the Netherlands*

Patients with systemic lupus erythematosus (SLE) or SLE-overlap syndromes often produce autoantibodies directed to U1RNA-binding proteins.[1] Previously, we isolated and characterized autoantigen-binding Ab fragments directed to the U1RNA-associated A protein (U1A) from several variable (V) gene combinatorial phage libraries.[2] Although these libraries have proven to be very successful, heavy (V_H) and light (V_L) chains are randomly combined during construction of such libraries. Because we were interested in the utilization of the original V_H/V_L pairings of the encoding autoantibodies, we developed a single cell culture system for B cells using mouse thymoma EL-4 B5 cells.[3] In combination with a preselection via recombinant antigen and single cell sorting using fluorescence-activated cell sorting (FACS), we were able to enrich for autoantigen-specific B cells. V_H and V_L genes originating from single U1A-specific B cells were cloned in a phage display vector for expression of single-chain variable fragments (scFv).

Human mononuclear cells were isolated from SLE patients and selected against U1A-coated plates or biotinylated U1A coated to streptavidin-coupled superparamagnetic microbeads (MACS). Adhering cells were collected from the plates via trypsin treatment or were directly used in the case of U1A-bound MACS (FIGURE 1). The selected lymphocytes were plated as single CD19/CD20-positive cells using FACS with an automatic cell deposit unit. Single selected B cells were seeded on 96-well plates containing 20,000 irradiated EL-4 B5 cells and 10% supernatant of phorbol myristate acetate (PMA)– and phytohemagglutinin (PHA)–activated human T cells (FIGURE 2). Cultures were grown for 10–11 days and tested in ELISA for antigen (Ag)–specific antibodies and total Ig production. Cell cultures that were positive in the Ag-specific ELISA screening were used for RNA isolation. An RT reaction was performed with an oligo-dT primer and the cDNA was used in a first PCR with V_H family–specific primers or a mixture of V-kappa or V-lambda primers (in the case of the light chains) as in Marks *et al.*[4] These first PCR products were used in a second

[c]To whom all correspondence should be addressed.

PCR with nested joining-region primers to introduce the appropriate restriction sites for cloning into pHENIX.[2]

Typical percentages of Ig-positive cells determined by ELISA after 10–11 days of culturing on EL-4 B5 cells in the presence of 10% human T cell supernatant varied between 50% and 70%. The frequency of Ag-specific B cell clones varied between 1% and 2.5% as a percentage of Ig-positive wells. Assuming that the frequency of Ag-specific cells in the periphery varies between 10^{-5} and 10^{-4}, this would indicate an enrichment factor of 100–1000. Distributions of IgG, IgM, and IgG/IgM double-

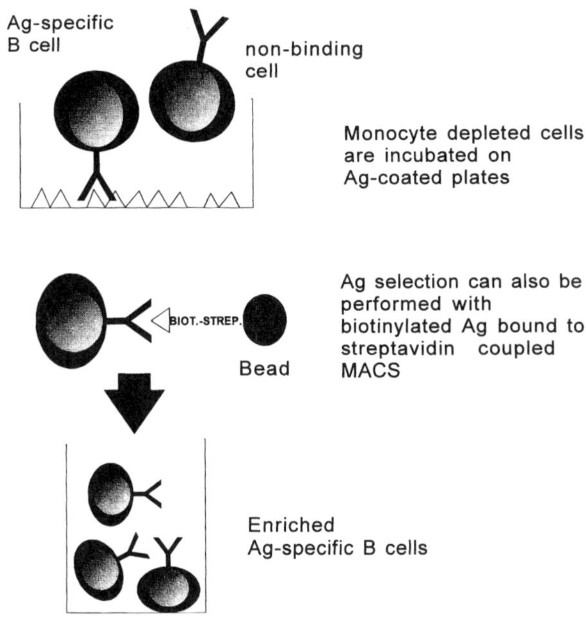

FIGURE 1. Antigen selection on peripheral blood mononuclear cells. Human mononuclear cells were isolated from autoimmune patients (SLE) and used to select on U1A-coated plates or biotinylated U1A coated to streptavidin-coupled MACS. Selected cells were collected from the plates via trypsin treatment or were directly used in the case of U1A-bound MACS. Magnetically sorted cells (MACS) can be processed using FACS.

positive isotypes in Ig-producing single B cell cultures were 3:3:1. After culture in the EL-4 B5 system, the B cells obtained a plasmablast-like phenotype expressing CD38^{HIGH} and SYNDECAN-1$^{MOD.}$ (plasma cell marker). PCR products using cDNA from a single B cell clone amplified with separate V_H family–specific primers and constant region primers (IgG- or IgM-specific) gave rise to only one V_H product, which indicates clonality. In the case of the light chains, a product with either V-kappa or V-lambda primers was obtained. Five IgM and 2 IgG anti-U1A-specific clones have been isolated. So far, we have sequenced only one clone with V regions derived from

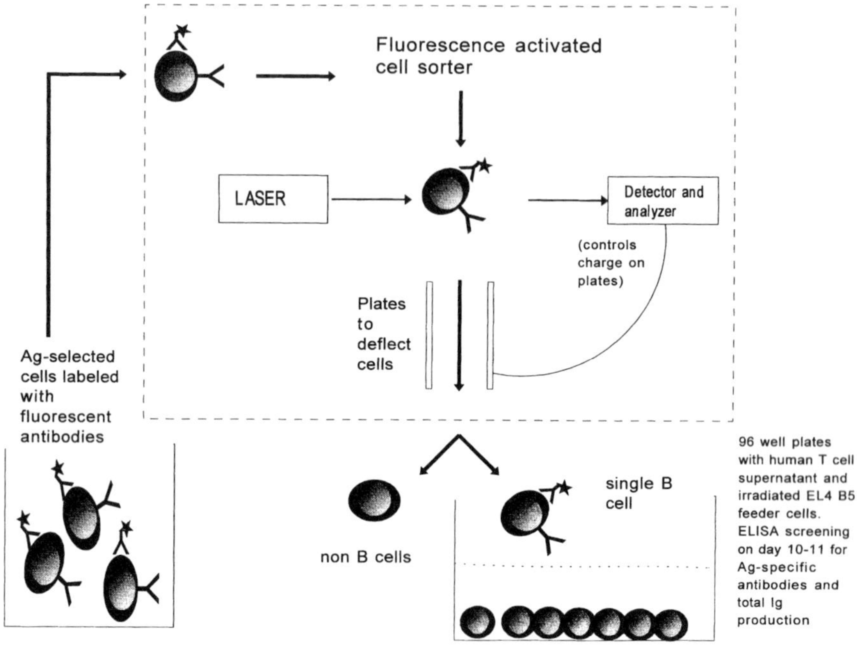

FIGURE 2. The selected lymphocytes were plated as single cells using FACS with an automatic cell deposit unit in 96-well plates containing 20,000 irradiated EL-4 B5 cells and 10% supernatant of phorbol myristate acetate (PMA)– and phytohemagglutinin (PHA)–activated human T cells. Cultures were grown for 10–11 days and tested in ELISA for Ag-specific antibodies and total Ig production.

DP-49 (V_H3) for the heavy chain and lv318 for the lambda light chain. We have been able to show binding of the cloned V regions to the U1A protein in ELISA. Further studies are currently being performed to isolate functional recombinant antibodies containing original V_H/V_L pairings.

REFERENCES

1. Van Venrooij, W. J. & G. J. M. Pruijn. 1995. Curr. Opin. Immunol. **7:** 819–824.
2. De Wildt, R. M. T., R. Finnern, W. H. Ouwehand, A. D. Griffiths, W. J. Van Venrooij & R. M. A. Hoet. 1996. Eur. J. Immunol. **26:** 629–639.
3. Steenbakkers, P. G. A., H. A. J. M. Hubers & A. W. M. Rijnders. 1994. Mol. Biol. Rep. **19:** 125–134.
4. Marks, J. D., H. R. Hoogenboom, T. P. Bonnert, J. McCafferty, A. D. Griffiths & G. Winter. 1991. J. Mol. Biol. **222:** 581–597.

The Leukemic Cells of Chronic Lymphocytic Leukemia Patients with Autoimmune Hemolytic Anemia Produce Isotype-switched Immunoglobulins That Are Preferentially Encoded by the 51p1 and DP-50 V_H Genes

DIMITAR G. EFREMOV,[a] MARTIN IVANOVSKI,[a,b]
GABRIELE POZZATO,[c] FACUNDO D. BATISTA,[a]
AND OSCAR R. BURRONE[a]

[a]*International Center for Genetic Engineering and Biotechnology*
Area Science Park
34012 Trieste, Italy

[b]*Faculty of Medicine*
Hematology Clinic
91000 Skopje, Macedonia

[c]*Ospedale di Cattinara*
Trieste, Italy

Chronic lymphocytic leukemia (CLL) results from the accumulation of small $CD5^+$ B cells that usually express low-density membrane IgM or IgM/IgD.[1,2] Characteristic features of CLL are the frequent development of hypogammaglobulinemia and autoimmune hemolytic anemia (AIHA); the latter condition occurs in approximately 10% to 25% of the patients at some point during the course of their disease. The reason for the high frequency of AIHA in CLL is unclear, but it is generally believed that the antierythrocyte autoantibodies are produced by normal autoreactive B cells and are therefore unrelated to the malignant clone.[2] This view is based on the findings that in most cases the antierythrocyte autoantibodies are IgG and do not show a light-chain restriction, whereas the CLL immunoglobulin (Ig) is usually IgM and always monoclonal.

A possible role for the leukemic Ig in the development of AIHA was raised by our recent analysis of the expressed V_H region repertoire in CLL.[3] This study has now been extended to further confirm that the Ig V_H regions in CLL patients with AIHA are preferentially encoded by the 51p1/DP-10 and DP-50 V_H genes (TABLE 1). The 51p1 gene was present in 50% (8/16) of the CLL-AIHA V_H sequences and was not expressed by any of the 12 control CLL cases without AIHA, thus showing a significant correlation with the development of hemolytic anemia ($p = 0.003$ by

TABLE 1. Productive V_HDJ_H Gene Rearrangements in Leukemic Clones of CLL Patients with and without AIHA

Patient	Clinical Condition	V_H Gene Family	Closest V_H Gene and % Nucleotide Homology	D Gene	J_H Gene	Length of CDR3 Region (Codons)
HA-1	CLL, AIHA	V_H1	51p1 (100%)	DXP4	J_H6b	23
HA-2	CLL, AIHA	V_H1	51p1 (100%)	DXP4	J_H4b	16
HA-3	CLL, AIHA	V_H1	51p1 (100%)	DK4	J_H6c	18
HA-5	CLL, AIHA	V_H1	51p1 (100%)	DXP4	J_H6b	21
HA-9	CLL, AIHA	V_H1	51p1 (100%)	DXP′1	J_H5b	14
HA-SC	CLL, AIHA	V_H1	51p1 (100%)	DK4	J_H3b	18
HA-Idr	CLL, AIHA	V_H1	51p1 (100%)	DN2/DLR4	J_H3b	22
HA-San	CLL, AIHA	V_H1	51p1 (100%)	D21/9	J_H5b	21
HA-10	CLL, AIHA	V_H1	DP-25 (100%)	DK1	J_H6b	15
HA-4	CLL, AIHA	V_H3	DP-50 (100%)	DXP1	J_H6b	21
HA-7	CLL, AIHA	V_H3	DP-50 (100%)	DN4	J_H4b	12
HA-8	CLL, AIHA	V_H3	DP-50 (97.5%)	DXP4	J_H6b	22
HA-RI	CLL, AIHA	V_H3	DP-50 (92.1%)	DLR1	J_H6b	23
HA-6	CLL, AIHA	V_H3	DP-47 (100%)	DN1	J_H5b	20
HA-VG	CLL, AIHA	V_H3	DP-47 (100%)	DXP1	J_H4b	17
HA-VS	CLL, AIHA	V_H4	$V_H4.18$ (100%)	DXP′1	J_H6b	22
CL-O	CLL	V_H1	DP-15 (100%)	D2	J_H5b	9
GP-1	CLL	V_H1	DP-8 (99.3%)	D2	J_H3b	20
CG-1	CLL	V_H3	DP-29 (96.6%)	DK1	J_H6b	16
CG-7	CLL	V_H3	DP-29 (87%)	D4c	J_H6b	13
GP-4	CLL	V_H3	DP-35 (94.5%)	DN1	J_H5b	16
CL-D	CLL	V_H3	DP-35 (94.2%)	DN4	J_H1	10
CL-J	CLL	V_H3	DP-50 (93.2%)	D6/D5	J_H5b	17
GP-3	CLL	V_H3	DP-47 (94.8%)	DXP5/D21	J_H6b	19
CL-P	CLL	V_H4	$V_H4.21$ (100%)	D4	J_H6b	21
CL-G	CLL	V_H4	$V_H4.21$ (93.8%)	D4	J_H4b	9
CG-6	CLL	V_H4	$V_H4.11$ (95.2%)	DHQ52	J_H4b	7
CG-2	CLL	V_H4	$V_H4.18$ (100%)	D5	J_H5b	15

chi-square test). Studies of unselected cases have also shown that this gene is overrepresented in CLL,[4,5] albeit at a significantly lower frequency (15%) than the one observed in the patients with AIHA ($p = 0.0007$). Interestingly, this gene is also frequently found in antibodies with rheumatoid factor activity[5,6] and is expressed by a high proportion of mantle zone lymphocytes.[7] The DP-50 V_H gene, which was present in 25% of the CLL-AIHA sequences, has been reported at a high frequency in human anti-RhD antibodies.[8]

The CDR3 regions of the CLL-AIHA sequences also showed some common features, including preferential expression of DXP family members (8/16) and the J_H6 gene (8/16). These CDR3 regions were longer than those from the control CLL group (averaging 19 versus 14 codons) and were characterized by a high tyrosine content. Four CDR3 regions also contained an identical DFWSGY motif encoded by a single

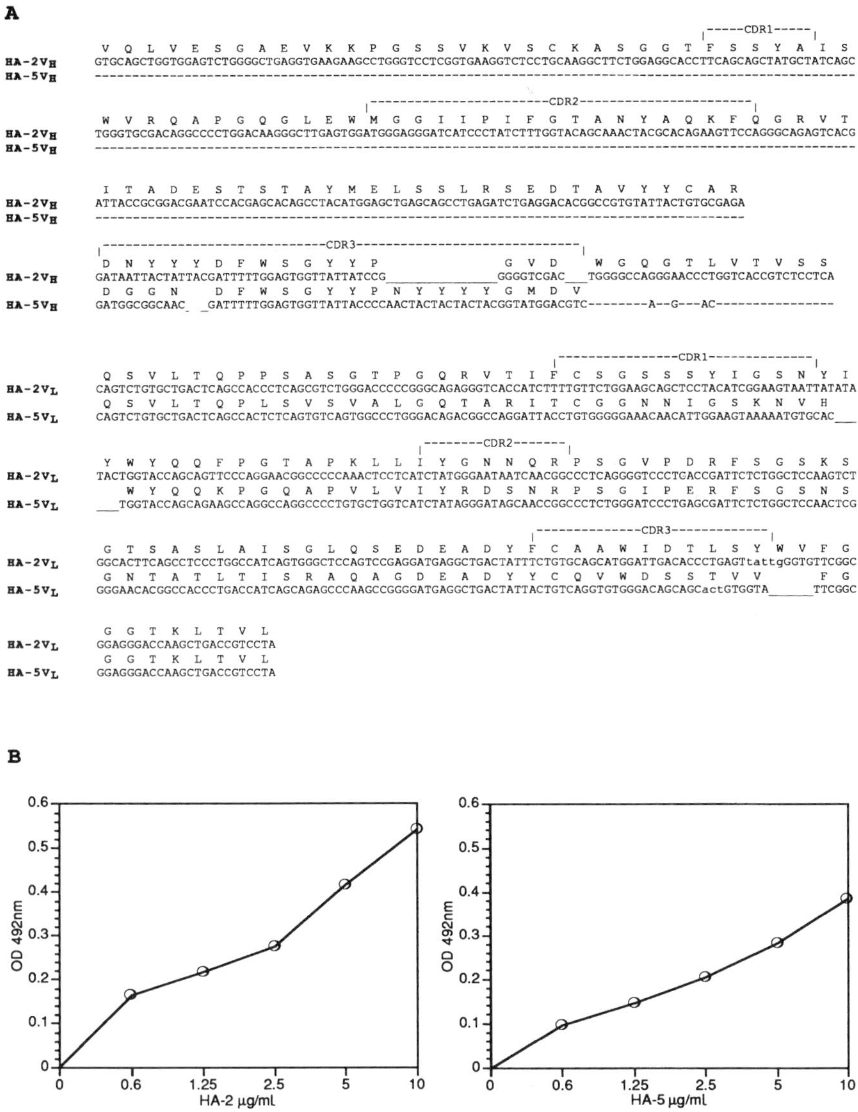

FIGURE 1. Analysis of the reactivity of two CLL Igs associated with AIHA. (A) Nucleotide and amino-acid sequences of the V_H and V_L regions from the two CLL Igs (HA-2 and HA-5) that were expressed as dimeric single-chain Fv fragments. The sequences have been aligned to maximize homology. Dashes indicate nucleotide identities. (B) Binding activity of scFv fragments corresponding to the leukemic Igs from CLL-AIHA patients HA-2 and HA-5. The ordinate is OD at 492 nm of the ELISA measured on plates coated with 5 µg/mL of polyclonal human IgG minus background. The abscissa describes the concentration of the scFv fragments (µg/mL).

reading frame of the DXP4 gene segment, followed by an N-nucleotide-encoded proline and a long stretch of tyrosines.

The observed skewing in the repertoire of V_H, D, and J_H gene segments strongly indicates that the leukemic Igs in CLL patients with AIHA have been selected because of particular antigen specificities that could promote the development of the hemolytic anemia. This could occur either by a direct involvement of the CLL Ig in erythrocyte destruction or, indirectly, by inducing the production of pathogenic antierythrocyte antibodies. The first possibility was supported by our recent finding that in most CLL cases a small subset of leukemic cells undergoes Ig isotype-switching.[9] The isotype-switched CLL cells were found to produce both membrane and secretory γ-chain transcripts, of which the latter could encode part of the IgG antibodies that have been implicated in RBC destruction. To test this hypothesis, we investigated the reactivity of the Igs expressed by the leukemic cells from the CLL-AIHA patients HA-2 and HA-5. These two Igs contained strikingly similar heavy-chain CDR3 regions that were associated with the 51p1 V_H gene segment (FIGURE 1A); both of them used λ light chains that belonged to different $V\lambda$ gene families (HA-2V_L is 95.5% homologous to Humlv122 from the $V\lambda$I family, and HA-5V_L is 93% homologous to Humlv318 from the $V\lambda$III family). The V_H and V_L region genes from these two Igs were expressed in eukaryotic cell lines as dimeric single-chain (sc) Fv fragments, and their reactivities were tested against erythrocytes and a panel of self and foreign antigens. Indirect immunofluorescence analysis with the affinity-purified scFv fragments showed the absence of any significant RBC binding. On the other hand, both antibody fragments showed similar low-affinity binding to human IgG (FIGURE 1B) and various reactivities against other antigens such as phosphorylcholine, dextran, lipopolysaccharide, and single-stranded DNA. These data indicate that the 51p1-encoded CLL Igs are not directly involved in RBC destruction, but could promote the development of AIHA by inducing a disturbance in the idiotypic network that would ultimately lead to the expansion of autoreactive B cell clones with antierythrocyte specificity. Alternatively, secreted isotype-switched CLL Igs could bind to anti-RBC antibodies and could promote the adherence of sensitized red blood cells to the Fc receptors on macrophages.

REFERENCES

1. FOON, K. A., K. R. RAI & R. P. GALE. 1990. Chronic lymphocytic leukemia: new insights into biology and therapy. Ann. Intern. Med. **113:** 525–539.
2. DIGHIERO, G., P. TRAVADE, S. CHEVRET, P. FENAUX, C. CHASTANG, J-L. BINET & THE FRENCH COOPERATIVE GROUP ON CLL. 1991. B-cell chronic lymphocytic leukemia: present status and future directions. Blood **78:** 1901–1914.
3. EFREMOV, D. G., M. IVANOVSKI, N. SILJANOVSKI, G. POZZATO, L. CEVRESKA, F. FAIS, N. CHIORAZZI, F. D. BATISTA & O. R. BURRONE. 1996. Restricted immunoglobulin V_H region repertoire in chronic lymphocytic leukemia patients with autoimmune hemolytic anemia. Blood **87:** 3869–3876.
4. SCHROEDER, H. W., JR. & G. DIGHIERO. 1994. The pathogenesis of chronic lymphocytic leukemia: analysis of the antibody repertoire. Immunol. Today **15:** 288–294.
5. KIPPS, T. J. 1993. Immunoglobulin genes in chronic lymphocytic leukemia. Blood Cells **19:** 615–632.

6. KIPPS, T. J. & D. A. CARSON. 1993. Autoantibodies in chronic lymphocytic leukemia and related systemic autoimmune diseases. Blood **81:** 2475–2487.
7. KIPPS, T. J. & S. DUFFY. 1991. Relationship of the CD5 B cell to human tonsillar lymphocytes that express autoantibody-associated cross-reactive idiotypes. J. Clin. Invest. **87:** 2087–2096.
8. BYE, J. M., C. CARTER, Y. CUI, B. D. GORICK, S. SONGSIVILAI, G. WINTER, N. C. HUGHES-JONES & J. D. MARKS. 1992. Germline variable region gene segment derivation of human monoclonal anti-Rh(D) antibodies: evidence for affinity maturation by somatic hypermutation and repertoire shift. J. Clin. Invest. **90:** 2481–2490.
9. EFREMOV, D. G., M. IVANOVSKI, F. D. BATISTA, G. POZZATO & O. R. BURRONE. 1996. IgM-producing chronic lymphocytic leukemia cells undergo immunoglobulin isotype-switching without acquiring somatic mutations. J. Clin. Invest. **98:** 290–298.

CDRH3 Length Is the Target of Selection of Disease-associated IgM Autoantibodies[a]

V. LIPSANEN,[b] B. WALTER,[b] M. EMARA,[c]
K. SIMINOVITCH,[d,e] J. LAM,[c] AND A. KAUSHIK[b,f]

[b]*Department of Pathobiology*
[c]*Department of Microbiology*
University of Guelph
Guelph, Ontario, Canada N1G 2W1

[d]*Mount Sinai Hospital*
Toronto, Ontario, Canada

INTRODUCTION

Moth-eaten mice homozygous for the viable recessive me^v mutation develop a fatal severe SLE-like systemic autoimmune disorder.[1] The me^v phenotype has been recently linked to a loss-of-function mutation in the gene encoding the cytosolic tyrosine phosphatase, PTP1C (also known as SHP, HCP, and SH-PTP-1[2–4]), characterized by severe dysregulation of hematopoietic cell development and function. We earlier reported that both the expression of V_H and V_K gene families as well as their association are significantly skewed in the peripheral B lymphocytes of autoimmune me^v mice as compared to the background C57BL/6 strain, most notably members of V_HJ558 and Q52 gene families.[5] To investigate the potential relevance of selection to expression of disease-associated IgM AAbs (autoantibodies), we have now analyzed structural properties of 12 hybridoma-derived IgM molecules from autoimmune me^v and normal congenic wild-type splenocytes selected for V_HJ558 gene family expression.

METHODS

Mice

Eight- to nine-week-old autoimmune me^v/me^v mice and background C57BL/6 mice were bred in the animal facility of Mount Sinai Hospital, Toronto, Ontario.

[a]This work was supported by research grants from the Arthritis Society of Canada (to A. Kaushik) and the Medical Research Council (to J. Lam).

[e]K. Siminovitch is an Ontario Ministry of Health Career Scientist and an Arthritis Society of Canada Research Scientist.

[f]To whom all correspondence should be addressed.

Hybridomas

Splenocytes isolated from me^v/me^v mice at the terminal stage of disease were fused with X63Ag8.653 myeloma cells according to standard procedures.[6] Similarly, hybridomas were prepared from the spleen of C57BL/6 mice stimulated with LPS (30 mg/mice intraperitoneally; Sigma Chemical, St. Louis, Missouri) *in vivo* at 24 hours prior to somatic cell hybridization. Immunoglobulin-secreting hybridomas were subcloned by limiting dilution and isotyped (Southern Biotechnology Associates, Birmingham, Alabama) in a solid-phase ELISA.[6]

Northern Dot Blot

Total RNA was extracted[7] from immunoglobulin-secreting hybridomas of me^v/me^v and C57BL/6 origin and was dot-blotted (1, 3, and 5 μg) onto nitrocellulose membrane (Schleicher and Schuell, Keene, New Hampshire), UV cross-linked, and hybridized as described[8] with ^{32}P-dCTP (Amersham Canada, Limited, Oakville, Ontario)–labeled DNA probe specific for the V_HJ558 gene family.[9] Briefly, blotted RNAs were hybridized in 50% formamide, 5× SSPE, 5× Denhardt's solution, 10 μg/mL salmon sperm denatured DNA, and 0.1% SDS for 12–16 hours using 10^6 dpm of denatured radiolabeled (Boehringer Mannheim random priming kit) DNA probe/mL followed by stringent final washes with 0.1× SSC and 0.1% SDS. Autoradiography was performed using Kodak XAR-5 film (Eastman Kodak Company, Rochester, New York). Six V_HJ558$^+$ hybridoma RNAs each from me^v/me^v and C57BL/6 mice were selected for structural analysis.

cDNA Synthesis, PCR Amplification, and Cloning

cDNAs were synthesized from 7 μg of total RNA using poly-dT primers (Pharmacia LKB Biotechnology, Uppsala, Sweden) and were amplified using the following murine immunoglobulin variable-region-specific primers:

V_H: 5′-AGGTCCA(G/A)CTCGAGTC(T/A)GG-3′;
Cμ: 5′-ATTGGGACTAGTTTCTGCGACAGCTGGAAT-3′.

These primers have built-in restriction sites for XhoI and SpeI, respectively, and were synthesized at MOBIX, McMaster University, Hamilton, Ontario. DNA amplification consisted of 25 cycles at 95 °C for 1 minute, 55 °C for 2 minutes, and 72 °C for 2 minutes. The PCR products were digested with XhoI and SpeI, fractionated by gel electrophoresis, and purified with Gene Clean II (Bio101, Vista, California). Amplified DNA was ligated into the dephosphorylated (calf intestinal alkaline phosphatase from Boehringer Mannheim, Germany) multiple cloning site of Bluescript KS+/− vector (Stratagene, La Jolla, California). *E. coli* DH10B bacteria (GIBCO BRL, Gaithersburg, Maryland) were transformed with the ligated DNA by electroporation (GIBCO BRL). The bacterial colonies were screened in a Southern blot[10] of restricted digested plasmid DNA by hybridizing with radiolabeled DNA probe specific for the V_HJ558 gene family.

DNA Sequencing and Analysis

DNA from 2–3 J558$^+$ colonies was sequenced, in both directions using T3 and T7 primers to determine the consensus sequence, for each hybridoma clone, either manually with Sequenase Version 2.0 (USB, Cleveland, Ohio) or by an automated DNA sequencer at MOBIX, McMaster University, Hamilton, Ontario. The PCR-amplified products of 3 clones (7-4, 4B4, 5B6) were directly sequenced in both directions using Cμ primer specific for the CH1 region: 5′-GCAGGAGAC-GAGGGGGA-3′ (synthesized at MOBIX). The nucleotide sequences were numbered according to Kabat *et al.*[11] and analyzed using the Genbank BLAST program,[12] and amino acid analysis was performed using the GPMAW (version 2.1) program.[13]

Immunochemistry

A solid-phase enzyme immunoassay was used to determine the specificity of immunoglobulins secreted by hybridoma clones against a panel of antigens including bovine serum albumin (BSA), thyroglobulin, ubiquitin, CD4 peptide residues 37–53 and 81–92 (Sigma), trimethylammonium (TMA) hapten coupled to BSA and trinitrophenyl (TNP) hapten coupled to BSA (all from Sigma), and recombinant hsp65 and hsp70 (courtesy of J. D. A. van Embden, UNDP/World Bank/WHO program), as described previously.[6] The antibody specificity to double-stranded DNA (dsDNA) was determined by indirect immunofluorescence using Hep-2 cells (Hep-2 ANA slide; INOVA Diagnostics, San Diego, California) and goat anti-mouse IgG(H + L) coupled to FITC (Southern Biotechnology Associates, Birmingham, Alabama).

RESULTS AND DISCUSSION

The length of the CDR3 varied between 4 to 12 amino acids (FIGURE 1) among the 6 non-antigen-selected J558$^+$ IgM molecules of C57BL/6 origin, with each showing a distinct VDJ rearrangement. No bias was noted in the use of D minigene, and D-D inversion as well as D-D fusions were evident. All the clones, except for the positively charged and arginine-containing BL7-4 clone, showed a local negative charge, ranging between 2.83 and 3.05, as well as a lack of arginine residues in the CDR3 region. The local hydrophobicity indices of the CDR3 region of all the clones, except clone BL1-9, which was hydrophobic, showed them to be relatively hydrophilic towards the N-terminal of the third hypervariability region.

Six randomly isolated J558$^+$ IgM molecules from autoimmune me^v mice, obtained at the terminal stage of the systemic autoimmune disease, showed 4 unique VDJ rearrangements. Surprisingly, all the 6 randomly selected J558$^+$ IgM molecules demonstrated a highly restricted CDR3 length of 10 amino acids (FIGURE 1). Three IgM antibodies had hydrophilic arginine residues in their CDR3 region. No restriction for D gene segment use was evident. Three clones each had relative negative and positive charge in the CDR3 region. The relative hydrophilicity was higher at both ends of the CDR3 region, intervened by a relatively less hydrophilic central region.

			CDR3														Antibody Specificity
C57BL/6			94						100	a	b	c	d			103	
1-9	GCA	AGA	TGG	ACT	ACG	GTA	GTA	GCT	GAG	...	...	...	GAC	TAC	TGG	GGC	Unknown
2-9	---	---	-C-	GGC	TGG	T-T	...	...	...	...	...	...	---	---	---	---	Polyreactive
6-3	---	---	GA-	GGG	GAT	-AT	-GT	TAC	TAC	TGG	TTT	...	-CT	---	---	---	Polyreactive
3-5	A--	---	-TC	CTT	...	...	...	...	...	...	...	...	---	---	---	---	Unknown
7-16	---	---	AAC	TA-	C--	TAC	TAC	TT-	...	...	...	...	---	---	---	---	Polyreactive
7-4	---	---	A--	GA-	GGT	AAG	-G-	-AG	TAC	TAT	GCT	ATG	---	---	---	---	Polyreactive
me^v/me^v																	
5G11	GCA	AGA	GGC	TAC	TAT	AGT	AAC	TGG	TAC	TTC	...	...	GAT	GTC	TGG	GGC	CD4 peptide(81-92)
2B7	---	---	T-G	AT-	---	G--	---	-AT	GCT	A-G	...	...	--C	TA-	---	--T	CD4 peptide(37-53)
5D6	---	---	TCG	GGG	CTG	G-A	C-G	A--	---	--T	...	...	--C	TA-	---	---	Unknown
3D1	---	---	T-G	AT-	---	G--	---	-AT	GCT	A-G	...	...	--C	TA-	---	--T	CD4 peptide(81-92)
5B6	---	---	TCG	GGA	CTG	G-A	C-G	A--	---	--T	...	...	--C	TA-	---	---	Unknown
4B4	---	---	A-G	GTA	GCT	C-C	T--	---	---	---	...	...	---	---	---	---	Unknown

FIGURE 1. Partial nucleotide sequence of the variable region of the heavy chain of randomly isolated J558$^+$ IgMs from normal C57BL/6 and autoimmune me^v/me^v mice. The name of each hybridoma clone is indicated at the beginning of each sequence. The sequences are numbered according to Kabat *et al.*[11] Note the restricted CDR3 length comprising 30 nucleotides, shown in bold lettering, of IgMs from autoimmune me^v mice in contrast to the variable CDR3 size of IgMs from normal C57BL/6 mice.

Subsequent antibody specificity analysis of 6 J558$^+$ IgM molecules from autoimmune me^v mice revealed that 3 of these selectively recognized CD4 peptide residues 81–92 and 37–53. Four of the 6 randomly isolated J558$^+$ IgM molecules from C57BL/6 mice showed polyreactivity (FIGURE 1) with a panel of conserved natural antigens or synthetic haptens [albumin, thyroglobulin, hsp65, hsp70, ubiquitin, and trimethylammonium (TMA) and trinitrophenyl (TNP) haptens] and, therefore, these were classified as NAAbs (natural autoantibodies). Together, these data suggest that normal IgM NAAbs are remarkable for their variable CDR3 length and a local negative charge in their CDR3 region.

Based on the selective reactivity of 3 of the me^v-derived IgMs with CD4 peptides and in view of their isolation from terminally ill animals, as well as previous data implicating anti-T cell antibodies in the pathophysiology of systemic autoimmune disease in me^v mice,[14] it appears that these autoantibodies may be of pathological relevance. These observations suggest positive selection of B-1 lymphocytes secreting IgM autoantibodies in autoimmune moth-eaten mice targeted at the CDR3 region of the heavy chain.

The moth-eaten mutation has been linked to the PTP1C gene that encodes an intracellular tyrosine phosphatase predominantly expressed in hematopoietic stem cells and has been suggested to be related to impaired hematopoiesis in me^v mice.[2,3] Indeed, PTP1C protein has been noted to regulate the threshold with which the B cell receptor responds to an antigen and, therefore, PTP1C-deficient B cells may be expected to be negatively selected because of reduced thresholds of responsiveness to self-antigens. Pani and colleagues[15] have demonstrated an association between PTP1C and the B cell receptor and showed increased responsiveness to suboptimal concentrations of B cell receptor cross-linking. In addition, the role of PTP1C in B cell selection and function has been analyzed by breeding a transgene specific for lysozyme into me^v mice, and the elimination of lysozyme-reactive B cells is noted during development probably because of the reduced threshold of responsiveness to this self-antigen.[16] The characteristic features of the CDR3 of the 6 J558$^+$ IgMs from moth-eaten mice, at the terminal stage of systemic autoimmune disease observed here, suggest positive selection of B cells by autoantigen(s) because of the reduced threshold of responsiveness to autoantigens as a result of PTP1C deficiency.

Both the hypergammaglobulinemia and the high levels of autoantibodies observed in moth-eaten mice have been thought to be related to the predominance of B-1 (CD5$^+$) lymphocytes, known for their propensity for monoclonal or oligoclonal expansion.[17] In moth-eaten mice, 4 unique VDJ rearrangements among 6 IgMs were observed that suggested their oligoclonal origin. However, restricted CDR3 length regardless of the VDJ rearrangements argues against the propensity for expansion of the B-1 cells as the possible cause of the origin of IgM autoantibodies in moth-eaten mice. Our observations are supported by earlier studies that showed differences in the CDR3 length and amino acids of polyreactive and antigen (phosphorylcholine)–induced antibodies.[18] Another study similarly showed a critical role of CDR3 in distinguishing polyspecific from monospecific IgM rheumatoid factor based on gene swapping and site-directed mutagenesis experiments.[19] Taken together, our studies not only demonstrate the contribution of CDR3 length in the generation of polyreactive and monoreactive combining sites, but also suggest the contribution of autoantigen in the generation and selection of disease-associated monospecific IgM autoantibodies. Chronic lymphocytic leukemia (CLL) in humans is characterized by an expansion of B-1 cells that use a biased set of V_H genes that encode predominantly IgM polyreactive autoantibodies.[20–22] In accord with our observations, CLL B cells have also been suggested to be clonally selected via an antigen.[23]

SUMMARY

The experiments outlined here provide evidence for positive selection of B-1 lymphocytes secreting IgM autoantibodies in the autoimmune me^v mice as a result of the reduced threshold of responsiveness to autoantigens because of PTP1C deficiency, which is targeted at the CDR3 length of the variable region of the heavy chain. In addition, characteristic differences in the size, hydrophobicity pattern, and relative local charge of the CDR3 of the heavy chain of disease-associated IgM autoantibodies from moth-eaten mice help distinguish them from physiological natural autoantibodies present in normal mice.

ACKNOWLEDGMENTS

We thank Brian Allore, MOBIX, McMaster University, Hamilton, Ontario, for DNA sequencing and oligonucleotide synthesis support, and A. Clarke, University of Guelph, for help with amino acid analysis.

REFERENCES

1. SHULTZ, L. D., D. R. COMAN, C. L. BAILEY, W. G. BEAMER & C. L. SIDMAN. 1984. Am. J. Pathol. **116:** 179–192.
2. TSUI, H. W., K. A. SIMINOVITCH, L. DE SOUZA & F. W. L. TSUI. 1993. Nat. Genet. **4:** 124–129.
3. BIGNON, J. S. & K. A. SIMINOVITCH. 1994. Clin. Immunol. Immunopathol. **73:** 168–179.
4. SHULTZ, L. D., P. A. SCHWEITZER, T. V. RAJAN, T. YI, J. N. IHLE, R. J. MATTHEWS, M. L. THOMAS & D. R. BEIER. 1993. Cell **73:** 1445–1454.
5. SAITOH, Y., G. KELSOE, C. BONA & A. KAUSHIK. 1995. Autoimmunity **21:** 185–193.
6. KAUSHIK, A., A. LIM, P. PONCET, X. R. GE & G. DIGHIERO. 1988. Scand. J. Immunol. **27:** 461–471.
7. CHOMCZYNSKI, P. & N. SACCHI. 1987. Anal. Biochem. **162:** 156–159.
8. KAUSHIK, A., D. H. SCHULZE, F. A. BONILLA, C. BONA & G. KELSOE. 1990. Proc. Natl. Acad. Sci. U.S.A. **87:** 4932–4936.
9. YANCOPOULOS, G. D. & F. W. ALT. 1985. Cell **40:** 271–281.
10. SAMBROOK, J., E. F. FRITSCH & T. MANIATIS. 1989. Molecular Cloning: A Laboratory Manual. Cold Spring Harbor Laboratory. Cold Spring Harbor, New York.
11. KABAT, E. A., T. T. WU, H. M. PERRY, K. S. GOTTESMAN & C. FOELLER. 1991. Sequences of Proteins of Immunological Interest, p. 2597. United States Department of Health and Human Services–Public Health Service. Bethesda, Maryland.
12. ALTSCHUL, S. F., W. GISH, W. MILLER, E. W. MYERS & D. J. LIPMAN. 1990. J. Mol. Biol. **215:** 403–410.
13. KYTE, J. & R. F. DOOLITTLE. 1982. J. Mol. Biol. **157:** 105–132.

14. KASTURI, K., R. MAYER, C. A. BONA, V. E. SCOTT & C. L. SIDMAN. 1990. J. Immunol. **145:** 2304–2311.
15. PANI, G., M. KOZLOWSKI, J. C. CAMBIER, G. B. MILLS & K. A. SIMINOVITCH. 1995. J. Exp. Med. **181:** 2077–2084.
16. CYSTER, J. G. & C. C. GOODNOW. 1995. Immunity **2:** 13–24.
17. STALL, A. M., M. C. FARINAS, D. M. TARLINTON, P. M. LALOR, L. A. HERZENBERG & S. STROBER. 1988. Proc. Natl. Acad. Sci. U.S.A. **85:** 7312–7316.
18. CHEN, C., M. P. STENZEL-POORE & M. B. RITTENBERG. 1991. J. Immunol. **147:** 2359–2367.
19. CRUZIER, R., T. MARTIN & J. L. PASQUALI. 1995. J. Immunol. **154:** 4526–4535.
20. DIGHIERO, G., P. TRAVADE, S. CHEVRET, P. FENAUX, C. CHASTANG & J. L. BINET. 1991. Blood **78:** 1901–1914.
21. KIPPS, T. 1993. Blood Cells **19:** 615–625.
22. BROKER, B. M., A. KLAJMAN, P. YOUINOU, J. JOUQUAN, C. P. WORMAN, J. MURPHY, L. MACKENZIE, R. QUARTEY-PAPAFIO, M. BLASCHEK, P. COLLINGS *et al.* 1988. J. Autoimmun. **1:** 469–481.
23. CAI, J., C. HUMPHRIES, A. RICHARDSON & P. W. TUCKER. 1992. J. Exp. Med. **176:** 1073–1081.

A Sulfatide-reactive Monoclonal Antibody Derived from a Patient with Multiple Sclerosis Binds to Myelin *in Situ*[a]

E. KIRSCHNING, G. RUTTER, C. HUCKHAGEL, I. ELLHOF, AND H. HOHENBERG

Heinrich-Pette-Institut für Experimentelle Virologie und Immunologie Universität Hamburg 20251 Hamburg, Germany

Experimental data indicate that autoantibodies against the myelin glycolipids, galactocerebroside (GalC) and sulfatide, might be involved in demyelinating processes in multiple sclerosis (MS). In order to gain insight into the myelin glycolipid–reactive B cell repertoire at the clonal level, monoclonal antibody (mAb)–secreting lymphoblastoid B cell lines were produced by Epstein-Barr virus transformation of peripheral blood cells from MS patients and control persons.[1] Those mAbs reactive with either GalC or sulfatide in a liposome agglutination assay were further characterized with regard to their binding properties to cells and structures of the central nervous system (CNS). One of these mAbs, the sulfatide-reactive IgM-mAb DS1F8, obtained from a patient with MS, selectively binds to the surface of $GalC^+$ oligodendrocytes in mixed brain cell cultures of newborn rats.[2]

In the present study, we tested mAb DS1F8 for its ability to react with myelin *in situ,* a prerequisite for a possible pathophysiological effect *in vivo.* Ultrathin sections of Epon-embedded rat brain tissue, processed by conventional fixation and dehydration procedures, were incubated with mAb DS1F8. As a control, a murine mAb anti-GalC was used, and antibody-binding sites were revealed using species-specific secondary antibodies coupled to gold particles. However, electron microscopic examinations showed that myelin glycolipid antigens were extracted and relocated on unmyelinated structures. For these reasons, biopsied native brain tissue was cryofixed by high-pressure freezing and freeze-substituted in acetone in the presence of osmium tetroxide.[3] This procedure retained a good ultrastructure and prevented subsequent extraction and relocation of myelin glycolipid antigens. As shown in FIGURE 1, mAb DS1F8 strongly reacted with compact myelin surrounding the axons, whereas unmyelinated structures were virtually devoid of any immunogold labeling. Immunogold double-labeling experiments further revealed that the observed reactivity of mAb DS1F8 was very similar to the staining pattern of mAb anti-GalC (FIGURE 2). From these data, we conclude that myelin glycolipid–reactive autoantibodies with binding

[a]This work was supported by Gemeinnützige Hertie-Stiftung, Frankfurt/Main, Germany.

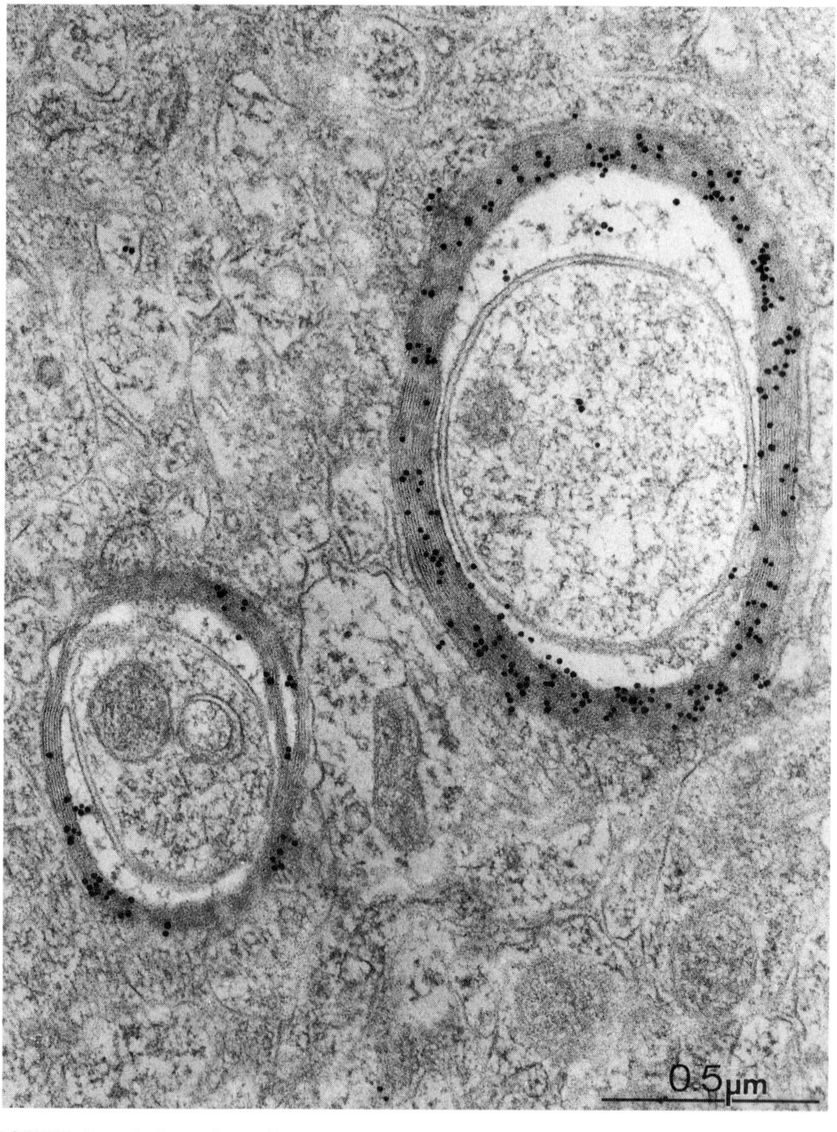

FIGURE 1. Labeling of myelin structures on ultrathin sections of rat cerebral tissue with human mAb DS1F8 and goat anti-human IgM coupled to 10-nm gold.

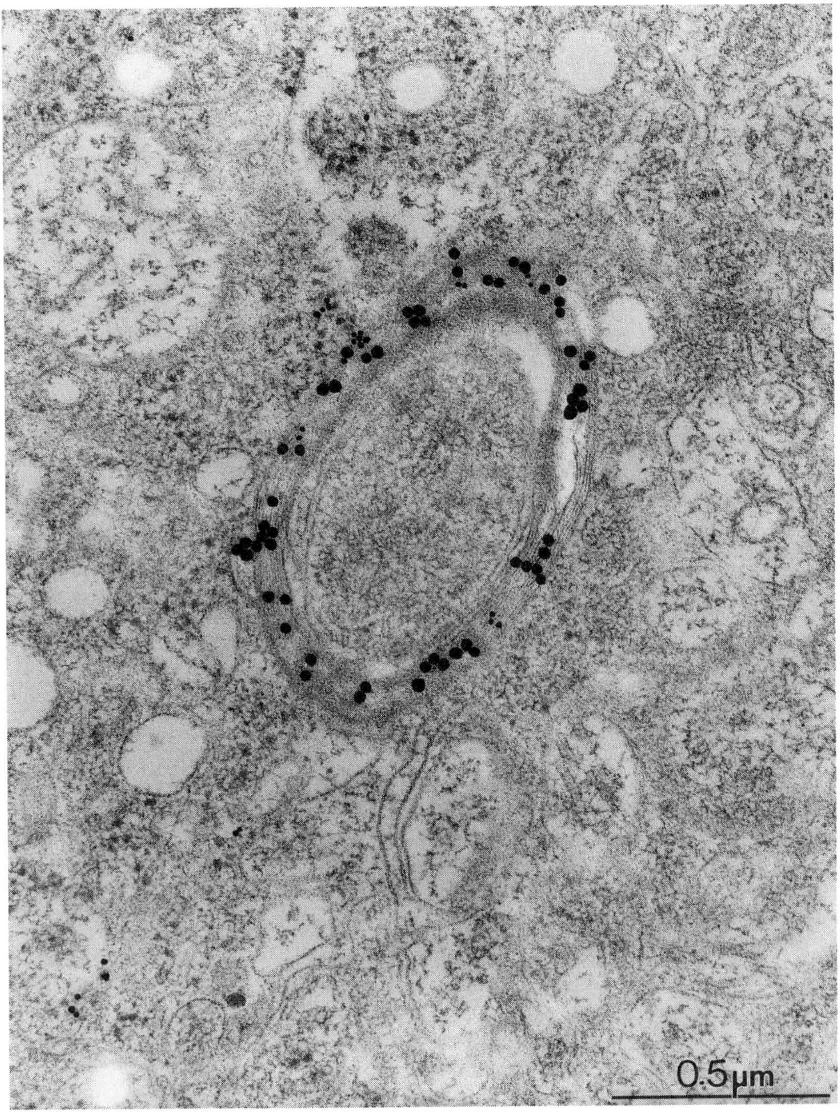

FIGURE 2. Immunogold double-labeling of myelin structures on ultrathin sections of rat cerebral tissue with mAb DS1F8 and goat anti-human IgM coupled to 10-nm gold, followed by mouse mAb anti-GalC and goat anti-mouse IgG attached to 20-nm gold.

properties similar to mAb DS1F8 might react with myelin *in vivo* and thus might be involved in demyelinating processes in the CNS.

REFERENCES

1. UHLIG, H. & R. DERNICK. 1989. Autoimmunity **5:** 87–99.
2. KIRSCHNING, E., G. RUTTER, H. UHLIG & R. DERNICK. 1995. J. Neuroimmunol. **56:** 191–200.
3. HOHENBERG, H., M. TOBLER & M. MÜLLER. 1996. J. Microsc. **183:** 133–139.

Fine Specificity Analysis of Autoantibodies to T Cell Receptor CDR1 Segments in Rheumatoid Arthritis[a]

W. J. LANDSPERGER,[b] S. F. SCHLUTER,[c] A. GARZA,[c]
D. E. YOCUM,[c] AND J. J. MARCHALONIS[c]

[b]*Baxter Biotech Hyland Division*
Duarte, California 91010

[c]*Arizona Health Sciences Center*
University of Arizona College of Medicine
Tucson, Arizona 85724

Gamma globulins of healthy asymptomatic humans, as exemplified by both serum and purified intravenous immunoglobulin IgG preparations (IVIGs), contain low levels of autoantibodies directed against peptide segments corresponding to the first complementarity-determining region (CDR1) of T cell receptor Vβ domains.[1] Sera of rheumatoid arthritis (RA) patients tend to have elevated levels of IgM autoantibodies directed against the CDR epitope, and decreased IgG autoantibodies, by comparison with osteoarthritis (a nonautoimmune joint disease) patients or asymptomatic individuals.[2–4] In order to determine whether there was a restriction in autoantibody development that could follow from an initial restriction in cellular Vβ usage, we synthesized a set of 24 homologous peptides corresponding to the CDR1 segment of a broad range of different human Vβ family germline gene sequences. These peptides were synthesized and purified to ≥95% purity. Sera of RA patients were obtained from the College of Medicine, Arizona Health Sciences Center, whereas IVIG IgG was obtained from Baxter Healthcare Corporation. Analysis of autoantibody CDR1 recognition spectrotypes of RA patient sera and IVIG was done by epitope mapping using the set of 24 homologous 16-mer synthetic peptides. The data are reported as the mean of the sum ELISA titers relative to the Vβ8.1 parent peptide, which was normalized to an absorbance at 405 nm of 1.0. This fine specificity epitope analysis of serum autoantibodies (IgM + IgG) of five RA patients (FIGURE 1) disclosed relatively restricted major reactivities, with the main binding being primarily against CDR1s of Vβ7.1, 8.1, 12.1, 13.1, and 15.1. Although considerable variation was seen between individual sera (data not shown), the relative peptide specificities were maintained. For example, autoantibody activity against the Vβ8.1 sequence was the highest in only one of the five RA sera. In contrast, the major autoantibody specificity in IVIG IgG preparations (mean of three, Gammagard® S/D) was against the Vβ8.1 peptide,

[a]This work was supported in part by a grant from Baxter Healthcare International and by a grant from the Arizona Disease Control Research Commission (No. 5-038).

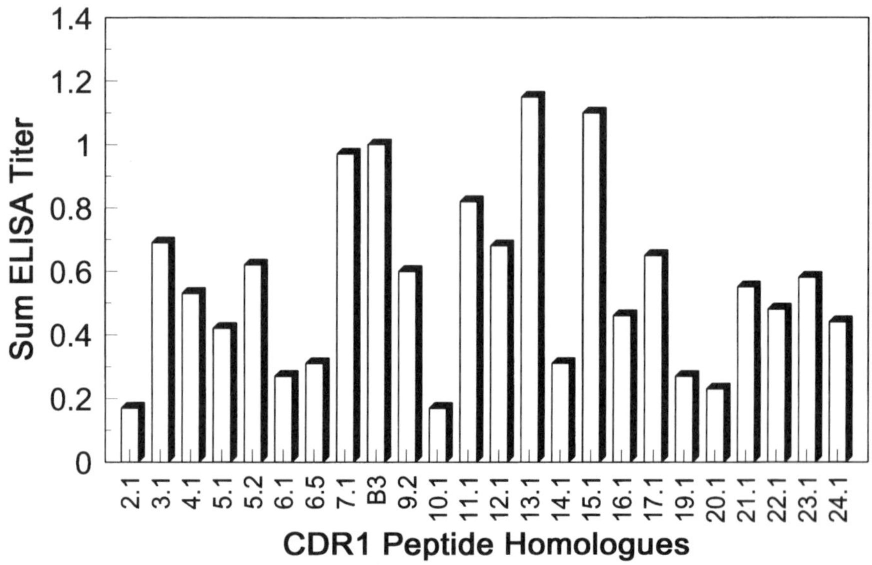

FIGURE 1. Autoantibodies (both IgM and IgG) were measured using the CDR1-specific peptide–based ELISA. Individual RA patient sera (in duplicates) were diluted 1:50 in PBST followed by twofold serial dilutions. The reactivities to the Vβ8.1 CDR1 peptide were normalized to an absorbance at 405 nm of 1.0. All other reactivities were then recalculated using the appropriate interpolation values. The mean absorbances versus each peptide are shown. Nonspecific absorbances to PBST-gelatin were subtracted.

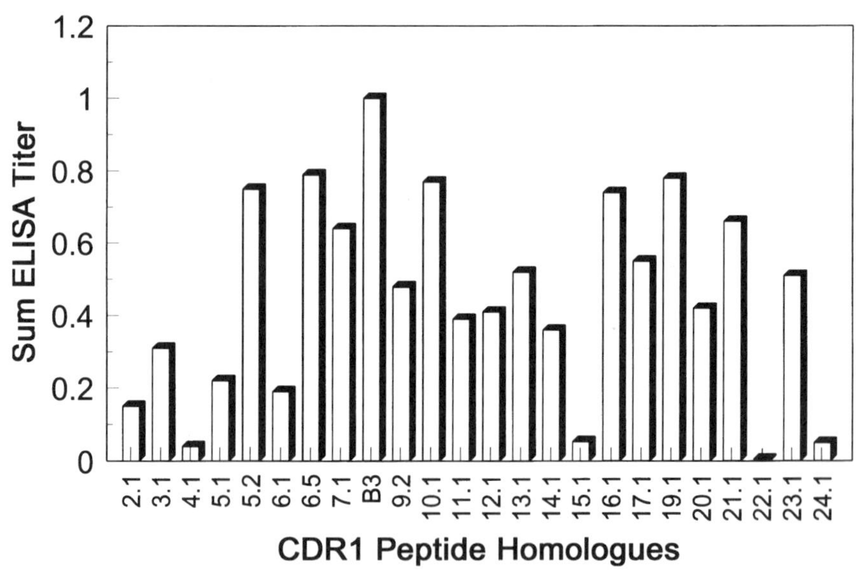

FIGURE 2. Data demonstrating the levels of IgG autoantibodies contained in three preparations of commercial IVIG. IVIG samples were initially diluted 1:200 in PBST (in duplicates) followed by twofold serial dilutions. All absorbances (mean of three lots) shown are relative to the absorbances of Vβ8.1, which was normalized to an absorbance at 405 nm of 1.0. Nonspecific absorbances to PBST-gelatin were subtracted.

followed by activities against Vβ5.2, 6.5, 10.1, 16.1, 17.1, and 19.1 (FIGURE 2). Although individual differences were observed among the distinct IVIG preparations, all three shared these dominant reactivities. Thus, fine specificity epitope analysis of anti-TCR Vβ autoantibodies of RA patients discloses individual differences as well as a major recognition profile, which is different from that observed for normal human gamma globulins.

Some efficacy in the treatment of RA using IVIG has been seen in a number of open uncontrolled studies with progressive or unremitting RA.[5,6] A study by Tumiati *et al.* demonstrated that significant clinical improvement in patients suffering from refractory RA was seen following IVIG administration.[7] At this time, we can only speculate that a correlation may ultimately be shown that relates the clinical efficacy of IVIG IgGs to their individual autoantibody or antiautoantibody spectrotypic distribution. Our ongoing studies are designed to help answer this question by gaining a further understanding of the mechanisms of action and regulation of autoantibodies directed against the TCR Vβ CDR regions.

REFERENCES

1. MARCHALONIS, J. J., H. KAYMAX, F. DEDOGLU, S. F. SCHLUTER, D. E. YOCUM & A. B. EDMUNDSON. 1992. Proc. Natl. Acad. Sci. U.S.A. **89:** 3325–3329.
2. MARCHALONIS, J. J., S. F. SCHLUTER, E. WANG, K. DEHGHANPISHEH, D. LAKE, D. E. YOCUM, A. B. EDMUNDSON & J. B. WINFIELD. 1994. Proc. Soc. Exp. Biol. Med. **207:** 129–147.
3. MARCHALONIS, J. J., H. KAYMAX, S. F. SCHLUTER & D. E. YOCUM. 1993. Exp. Clin. Immunogenet. **10:** 1–15.
4. LAKE, D. F., W. J. LANDSPERGER, R. M. BERNSTEIN, S. F. SCHLUTER & J. J. MARCHALONIS. 1994. *In* Advances in Experimental Medicine and Biology. Volume 383. M. Atassi & G. Bixler, Jr., Eds.: 223–229. Plenum. New York.
5. KAVERI, S. V., G. DIETRICH, V. HUREZ & M. D. KAZATCHKINE. 1991. Clin. Exp. Immunol. **86:** 192–199.
6. KIMBERLY, R. P., J. E. SALMON, J. B. BUSSEL, M. K. CROWN & M. W. HILGARTNER. 1984. J. Immunol. **132:** 5453–5455.
7. TUMIATI, B., P. CUSOLI, M. VENEZIANI & G. RINALDI. 1992. Arthritis Rheum. **35:** 1126–1133.

An Anti-idiotypic (T14) Antibody Found Commonly in Patients with Systemic Lupus Erythematosus That May Be Pathogenic[a]

P. L. LIM,[b] D. T. M. LEUNG,[b] L. W. K. NG,[b] K. C. WONG,[c]
S. Y. SONG,[b] Y. L. CHUI,[b] J. C. K. LEUNG,[b]
K. N. LAI,[c] AND S. F. LUI[c]

[b]*Clinical Immunology Unit*
[c]*Department of Medicine*
The Chinese University of Hong Kong
Prince of Wales Hospital
Shatin, N.T., Hong Kong

Anti-double-stranded DNA antibodies, especially those with high affinity and belonging to the IgG class, have been implicated in the pathogenesis of systemic lupus erythematosus (SLE).[1] However, there is no conclusive evidence that these cause disease either by direct tissue injury or by forming inflammatory immune complexes with DNA. In this communication, we suggest another way in which these antibodies can be pathogenic.

We investigated whether antibodies specific to anti-DNA antibodies could be found in SLE patients. A high-affinity IgG anti-DNA antibody (T14) described by Van Es *et al.*[2] was selected for study; based on part of the V_H sequence of the protein, overlapping 8-mer peptides were synthesized on multipins[3] and used as substrate to detect the anti-idiotypic (Id) antibodies. Peptides in the CDR3 (third complementarity-determining region) were found to be reactive with pooled SLE sera. A 15-mer peptide corresponding to the whole of CDR3, YYYGAGSYYKRGYFD, was synthesized in bulk to >80% purity, conjugated to human serum albumin (Chiron Mimotopes, Australia), and used in the examination of individual SLE and control sera. FIGURE 1 shows that the peptide detected anti-Id activities in 56% (24/43) of the serum samples positive for antinuclear (ANA) and anti-DNA antibodies that came from 15 SLE patients, whereas only 18% (3/17) of the ANA^+ DNA^- samples derived from 9 SLE and 8 non-SLE patients were positive in the test. None of the ANA^- DNA^- samples derived from 17 non-SLE patients were positive. Ten percent of 57 healthy subjects showed detectable antibody levels.

To demonstrate that the T14-CDR3 Id was present in our population, a monoclonal antibody raised against the peptide was used in a capture-ELISA to screen the various sera. FIGURE 2 shows results very similar to those of the anti-Id assay, namely, there

[a]This work was supported by an RGC earmarked grant (Hong Kong) and a postdoctoral fellowship (The Chinese University of Hong Kong) to D. T. M. Leung.

was a positive correlation between the Id$^+$ and anti-Id activities in the ANA$^+$ DNA$^+$ patients ($P = 0.0004$). There was also good correlation between the anti-DNA (ELISA) and anti-Id activities in these subjects ($P = 0.0001$) and between the anti-DNA and Id$^+$ activities ($P = 0.002$).

Whereas the anti-DNA antibodies in our patients were predominantly IgG, the anti-Id antibodies belonged to both IgM and IgG classes and could not be removed from the serum by absorption with DNA. Other specificity tests performed to prove that the anti-Id antibodies detected were real included the following: first, the monoclonal anti-Id antibody generated against the peptide bound to anti-DNA antibodies purified from SLE patients and this binding was inhibitable by pooled SLE

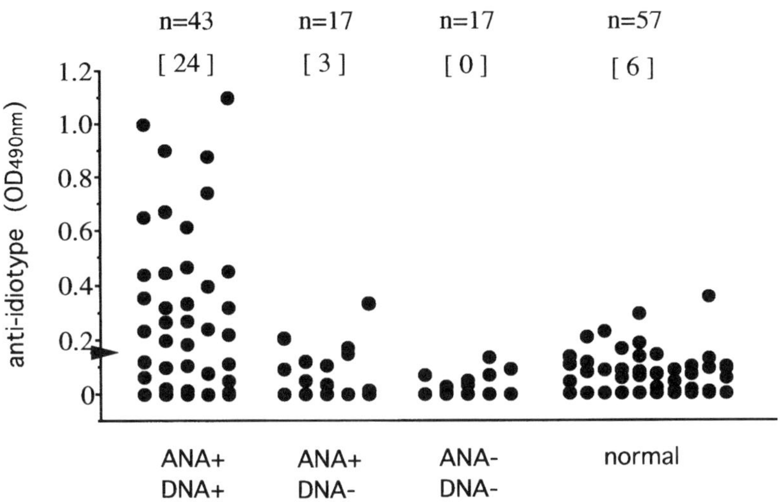

FIGURE 1. ELISA (anti-Id) activities of individual serum samples (1:800 dilution) to the insolubilized T14-CDR3 peptide. Assay developed with biotinylated goat anti-human Ig (polyvalent) antibody and ExtrAvidin-peroxidase (Sigma, St. Louis, Missouri). Sera are grouped according to whether they came from patients [and subgrouped according to their antinuclear (ANA) and anti-DNA (DNA) activities] or from healthy individuals. The arrow indicates the cutoff for responders (mean + 3 SD of ANA$^-$ DNA$^-$ subjects).

sera, but not normal sera; second, no activity was found in the SLE sera to an unrelated CDR3 peptide, ARPGTTGGGMDV.

It seems that the anti-Id antibodies found in our patients were specifically induced by the anti-DNA antibodies present and were consequently absent from normal subjects. We postulate that these antibodies can partake in the disease process by forming pathogenic immune complexes with the anti-DNA antibodies, rather than serving a beneficial or neutralizing role as conventionally thought.[4,5] Conceivably, both Id$^+$ and anti-Id antibodies can reciprocally stimulate the production of each other, thus ensuring the chronicity of the disease.

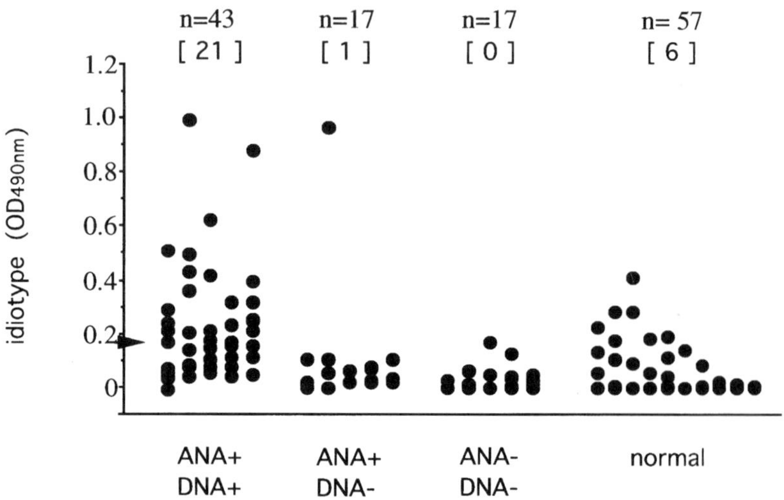

FIGURE 2. T14-CDR3 Id^+ activities of serum samples of cohorts shown in FIGURE 1. Insolubilized monoclonal antibody specific for the T14-CDR3 peptide was used to capture reactive proteins from the serum and these were revealed using preabsorbed goat anti-human Ig ($\mu + \gamma$) antibodies (Tago, Burlingame, California).

REFERENCES

1. ISENBERG, D. A., M. R. EHRENSTEIN, C. LONGHURST & J. K. KALSI. 1994. Arthritis Rheum. **37:** 169–180.
2. VAN ES, J. H., F. H. J. G. MEYLING, W. R. M. VANDEAKKER, H. AANSTOOT, R. H. W. M. DERKSEN & T. LOGTENBERG. 1991. J. Exp. Med. **173:** 461–470.
3. GEYSEN, H. M., S. F. RHODDA, T. J. MASON, G. TRIBBICK & P. G. SCHOOFS. 1987. J. Immunol. Methods **102:** 259–274.
4. ABDOU, N. I., H. WALL, H. B. LINDSEY, J. F. HALSEY & T. SUZUKI. 1981. J. Clin. Invest. **67:** 1297–1304.
5. SASAKI, T., T. MURYOI, O. TAKAI, E. TAMATE, H. SAITO & K. YOSHINAGA. 1988. J. Clin. Invest. **82:** 748–754.

B Cell Response and Histology of a Retroviral Infection *in Vivo*

S. A. LUTHER,[a] A. GULBRANSON-JUDGE,[b]
H. ACHA-ORBEA,[a,c] AND I. C. M. MacLENNAN[b]

[a]*Ludwig Institute for Cancer Research*
University of Lausanne
1066 Epalinges, Switzerland

[b]*Department of Immunology*
University of Birmingham Medical School
Birmingham B15 2TT, England

[c]*Institute of Biochemistry*
University of Lausanne
1066 Epalinges, Switzerland

Mouse mammary tumor virus (MMTV) is a B-type retrovirus that codes for a superantigen (SAg). SAgs are functionally defined by their exclusive presentation on MHC II and their reactivity with 5–30% of all T cells that have in common the V domain of the T cell receptor β-chain. Consequently, the number of reactive T cell precursors is 1000–10,000 times higher in the response to an SAg than to a conventional protein antigen (Ag).[1] Moreover, MMTV preferentially infects B cells; as these cells can present the SAg to T cells, theoretically they might receive almost unlimited T cell help. The precise sites and timing of T and B cell activation in response to MMTV have not been determined; consequently, the nature of the cellular interactions that occur has been subject to some speculation. We have used a combination of flow cytometry and immunohistology to demonstrate where and when B and T cells are activated in popliteal lymph nodes following injection of this virus in the footpads of BALB/c mice. As a control, the response to a classical T cell–dependent antigen, haptenated chicken gamma globulin (NP-CGG), has been studied. In responses to NP-CGG, there is a preliminary T cell priming phase; interdigitating dendritic cells that have taken up and processed the antigen and that have migrated to the T zones of the draining node interact with antigen-specific virgin T cells. The resulting primed T cell can then make cognate interaction with B cells that have taken up and processed the antigen. This has been defined in detail in the spleen;[2] B cells that have been activated in this way proliferate and differentiate in two sites—the B cell follicles and extrafollicular foci. Those proliferating in the extrafollicular site give rise to short-lived plasma cells, whereas in follicles the activated B cells give rise to germinal centers (GC). In GC, there is affinity maturation of the response, and both memory cells and relatively long-lived plasma cells are generated.[3]

The cellular interactions in response to conventional Ag and SAg were found to be remarkably similar, with only some differences in the timing and the extent of T and B cell reactions;[4] these and an outline of the methods used are summarized in TABLE 1.

With both types of antigens, T cells first started to proliferate in the T cell–rich zone in close association with interdigitating dendritic cells on day 3 after immunization. Immediately after this, B cells, presumably after interacting with primed T cells in the T zone, were seen to proliferate in the medullary cords and then differentiated in that site to become short-lived plasma cells. In response to NP-CGG, germinal centers were identified from day 5, but were delayed for some days in response to SAg. In this case, the unlimited T help seems to act in a rather inhibitory way on GC B cell differentiation. Remarkably, the SAg of MMTV induces the formation of long-lived GCs that are dominated by the SAg-reactive T cell subset. Moreover, the SAg of MMTV is capable of driving a long-lasting antibody response that is specific for the virus envelope protein gp52. The extrafollicular B cell response is probably responsible for the early production of virus-specific IgG—the GC reaction may be responsible for the continuing humoral response. Both Ag- and SAg-induced responses show similar priming and differentiation stages leading to a specific humoral response.

TABLE 1. Summary of the Histological Analysis[a]

		Responses to NP-CGG		Responses to MMTV(SW)	
	Site	Timing (and Peak)[b]	Extent at Peak	Timing (and Peak)[b]	Extent at Peak
T cell proliferation	T cell–rich zone	d3–5 (d5)	medium	d3–5 (d3)	strong
extrafollicular B cell differentiation	medullary cords	d5–12 (d8)	strong	d5–8 (d5)	medium
follicular B cell differentiation	germinal centers	d5–>d30 (d12)	strong	d12–>d30 (d16)	weak

[a]Infectious particles of MMTV(SW) and the conventional antigen NP-CGG in adjuvants were each injected subcutaneously into both hind footpads of BALB/c mice, and the draining popliteal lymph nodes were isolated at various time points after antigen challenge. Mice were injected intraperitoneally with bromodeoxyuridine (BrdU) at 2.5 h before the nodes were taken in order to identify cells in S phase of the cell cycle.[5] Cell subsets were quantified by flow cytometry on one lymph node, whereas the collateral draining lymph node was used to localize the cell subsets and activation events by three-color immunohistochemistry.[4]

[b]d = day.

REFERENCES

1. ACHA-ORBEA, H. & H. R. MACDONALD. 1995. Annu. Rev. Immunol. **13:** 459–486.
2. JACOB, J., R. KASSIR & G. KELSOE. 1991. J. Exp. Med. **173:** 1165–1175.
3. MACLENNAN, I. C. M. 1994. Annu. Rev. Immunol. **12:** 117–139.
4. LUTHER, S. A., A. GULBRANSON-JUDGE, H. ACHA-ORBEA & I. C. M. MACLENNAN. 1997. J. Exp. Med. **185:** in press.
5. LIU, Y. J., J. ZHANG, P. J. L. LANE, E. Y. T. CHAN & I. C. M. MACLENNAN. 1991. Eur. J. Immunol. **21:** 2951–2962.

IgG-Fibronectin Complexes Mimic Antibodies to Denatured Collagen Type II

MART MANNIK, SANJIV KAPIL,
AND CYNTHIA E. MERRILL

Division of Rheumatology
Department of Medicine
University of Washington
Seattle, Washington 98195-6428

In patients with rheumatoid arthritis, IgG antibodies to native and denatured collagen type II have been reported by several laboratories, as reviewed by Williams.[1] We used an enzyme-linked immunoassay to detect the binding of IgG to native or denatured bovine collagen type II in normals or patients with rheumatoid arthritis. When normal serums were heated to 56 °C for 30 minutes to inactivate complement, the binding of IgG to denatured collagen type II, but not to native collagen, was markedly increased. This increase of IgG binding to denatured collagen was in the excluded fractions, and not associated with monomeric IgG, upon separation of heated normal serum by gel filtration chromatography, using Sephacryl S-200. Normal, unheated serum was similarly separated. Heating of the excluded fractions and monomeric IgG separately did not induce increased binding of IgG to denatured collagen. When the excluded material and monomeric IgG were combined and then heated, increased binding of IgG to denatured collagen type II was generated. Heating of a mixture of monomeric human IgG and human fibronectin increased the binding of IgG to denatured collagen type II.[2] Three purified human IgG3 myeloma proteins and six myeloma proteins of other IgG subclasses were mixed with fibronectin and heated. The IgG3 proteins bound significantly more to denatured collagen type II than the other subclasses of IgG.

In view of the above findings, we separated unheated serums from nine patients with rheumatoid arthritis by gel filtration chromatography, as illustrated in FIGURE 1. In these serums, 64.7 ± 18.5% of the IgG binding to denatured collagen type II was in the excluded fractions. In contrast, 98.2 ± 0.9% of the IgG binding to native collagen type II was in the monomeric fractions of IgG. The binding of IgG to denatured collagen in the excluded fractions was blocked by fibronectin. The excluded fractions from gel filtration of four serums of these patients were further fractionated with staphylococcal protein A–agarose columns. In these specimens, the majority of IgG was retained and eluted with low pH buffer, whereas 90.7–94.8% of the IgG binding to denatured collagen type II did not bind to the protein A–agarose. These findings suggested that the IgG binding to denatured collagen type II is associated mainly with the IgG3 subclass.[2]

These observations indicated that most of the IgG binding to denatured collagen type II in serums of patients with rheumatoid arthritis does not represent autoantibodies. This binding is mainly mediated by fibronectin bound to IgG or by fibronectin bound to immune complexes. Binding of fibronectin to immune complexes is likely because previous studies have shown that aggregated IgG was more effective than monomeric IgG in binding to fibronectin.[3] The mechanisms of formation and the consequences of the presence of IgG-fibronectin complexes in patients with rheumatoid arthritis are not known at this time.

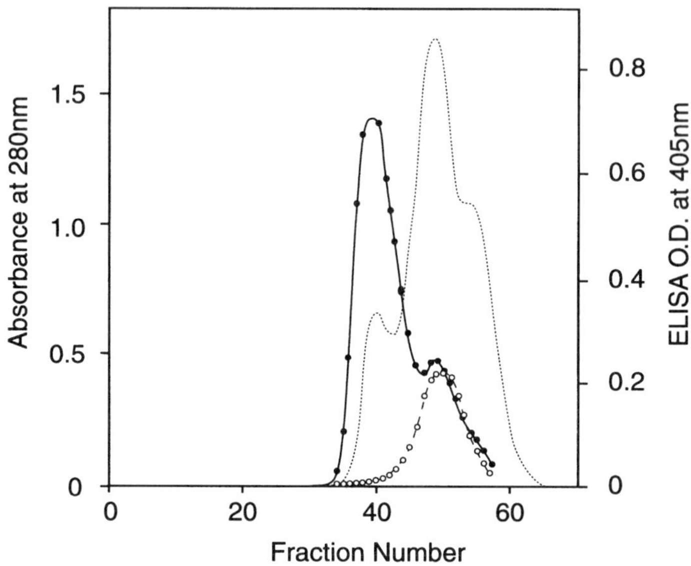

FIGURE 1. Gel filtration of the serum from a patient with rheumatoid arthritis on Sephacryl S-200. The absorbance at 280 nm (···) shows the protein distribution. The fractions were tested for IgG binding to native (○) and denatured (●) bovine collagen type II by enzyme-linked immunoassay, and the optical density at 405 nm is shown. The majority of IgG binding to denatured collagen is present in the excluded protein peak, whereas the IgG binding to native collagen is confined to the IgG monomer peak.

REFERENCES

1. Williams, D. G. 1994. Autoimmunity in rheumatoid arthritis. *In* Rheumatology. J. H. Klippel & P. A. Dieppe, Eds. Mosby Year Book, Europe Limited. London.
2. Mannik, M., S. Kapil & C. E. Merrill. 1997. In patients with rheumatoid arthritis, IgG binding to denatured collagen type II is in part mediated by IgG-fibronectin complexes. J. Immunol. **158:** 1446–1452.
3. Rostagno, A. A., B. Frangione & L. Gold. 1991. Biochemical studies on the interaction of fibronectin with Ig. J. Immunol. **146:** 2687–2693.

Requirements for mIgM-triggered Activation versus Apoptosis in Human B Cells[a]

PATRICIA MONGINI,[b] PATRICIA HIGHET,[c]
AND JOHN INMAN[c]

[b]*Department of Rheumatology*
Hospital for Joint Diseases
New York University Medical Center
New York, New York 10003

[c]*Laboratory of Immunology*
National Institute of Allergy and Infectious Diseases
National Institutes of Health
Bethesda, Maryland 20892

The cross-linking of membrane immunoglobulin (mIg) receptors on mature B lymphocytes can trigger cell cycle progression, anergy, or programmed cell death (apoptosis). The balance between these various phenomena bears importantly on the immune system's capacity to respond effectively to foreign antigen (Ag) as well as on its potential to manifest undesirable autoimmunity. A large body of evidence attests that the functional outcome of Ag engagement with a specific B cell is influenced by whether or not the B cell receives ancillary signals from T lymphocytes. It is additionally likely that factors influencing the direct mIg signaling potential of Ag, for example, the intrinsic affinity of mIg engagement with Ag, the valency of Ag epitopes, and the density of responsive mIg receptors on the B cell, are also critical.

In the present studies, we have attempted to compare the Ag:mIg binding requirements for inducing human B cell apoptosis with the binding requirements for inducing other cellular activation phenomena. The studies have used a set of previously described affinity- and valency-diverse IgM-binding ligands[1–3] as model "Ag": anti-human IgM monoclonal antibody (mAb) HB57 ($K_a = 5 \times 10^8$ M^{-1}), Mu53 ($K_a = 2 \times 10^7$), and P24 ($K_a = 2 \times 10^6$), in either bivalent or multivalent dextran-conjugated form.[1–3] The potential of these ligands to bind all mIgM-positive B cells circumvents the requirement for Ag-specific B cells in analyzing how ligand:mIgM affinity and ligand valency impact on the triggering of human B cells.

Culture of T cell–depleted, high-density tonsillar B cells[2] with mIgM-binding ligands could induce levels of apoptotic nuclei significantly above background at 48 h of culture (FIGURE 1). The most extensive apoptosis was generally elicited by the ligand with the highest affinity and highest valency. A comparison of the relative effectiveness of the affinity- and valency-diverse ligands at inducing mIgM-triggered apoptosis with their relative effectiveness at triggering B cell activation phenomena,

[a]This work was supported by PHS Grant No. GM35174 and the S.L.E. Foundation.

that is, enhanced membrane expression of class II MHC (DR), G_1-related RNA synthesis, and S phase DNA synthesis (FIGURE 1), suggested that the binding requirements for triggering apoptosis most closely mirror the binding requirements for inducing G_1 entry and are less rigorous than the binding requirements for inducing mIgM-triggered S phase entry. Because other studies[2] (data not shown) have indicated that the proportion of resting human B cells that enter S phase upon exposure to these ligands is substantially lower than the proportion of cells that enter G_1, it appeared possible that this mIgM-triggered apoptosis might reflect cells whose mIg:ligand engagement had met the requirements for entry into G_1, but that had not met the requirements for full mIgM-triggered B cell progression past a $G_1 \rightarrow$ S phase restriction point.

Several observations provide further support for this hypothesis. First, mIgM-triggered apoptosis is more prominent at 48 h of culture than at 24 h of culture (data

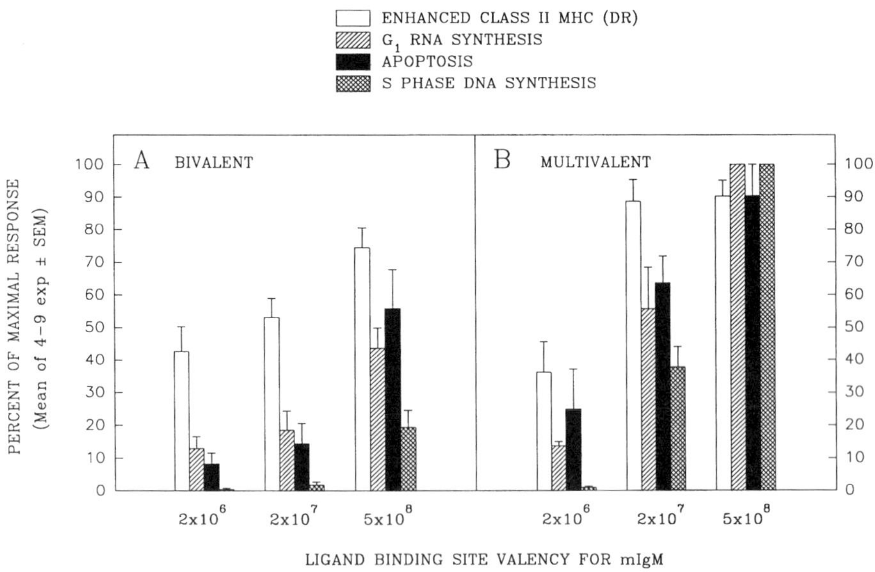

FIGURE 1. Comparison of the affinity and valency requirements for anti-IgM-mediated triggering of various cellular phenomena in cultured human B lymphocytes. The data represent the mean values for the percent of maximal response noted in several experiments for each functional parameter. Each experiment was performed with a distinct preparation of T cell–depleted, Percoll density gradient–selected, high-density tonsillar B cells[1] tested with each affinity- and valency-diverse ligand [100 μg/mL concentration for bivalent mAbs (A) and 1 μg/mL concentration for multivalent mAb-dextran conjugates (B)[2]]. Apoptosis was assessed at 48 h of culture by staining with propidium iodide under hypotonic conditions and analysis by flow cytometry as described by Nicoletti *et al.*[5] Enhanced class II major histocompatibility antigen (MHC) expression was assessed at 24–36 h of culture by staining cells with fluorescein-conjugated mAb S157 anti-DR followed by flow cytometric analysis.[1] G_1-related RNA synthesis was assessed at 24–36 (48) h of culture by measuring the uptake of a pulse of ^{3}H-uridine,[1] and S phase–related DNA synthesis was assessed at 48–68 (72) h of culture by measuring the uptake of ^{3}H-thymidine.[1]

TABLE 1. Membrane IgM–triggered B Cell Blasts in G_1 Are Protected from Apoptosis and Enter S Phase upon Continued Exposure to Membrane IgM Cross-linking Ligand[a]

	Experiment A		Experiment B	
24 to 48 h Culture	% Apoptosis	% $S/G_2/M$	% Apoptosis	% $S/G_2/M$
Medium	20.7	4.4	38.3	3.2
$HB57_{multivalent}$	4.4	52.7	11.0	20.8
$HB57_{bivalent}$	7.7	13.0	19.3	5.1
$HB57_{multivalent}$ + $IgM_{soluble}$	24.1	4.7	nd	nd
IL-4	5.1	27.4	nd	nd

[a]High-density tonsil B cells were precultured for 24 h with HB57-dextran (1 µg/mL). Viable cells after Ficoll-Hypaque centrifugation were enriched for blasts by Percoll density gradient centrifugation (40/45% Percoll interface) and recultured for an additional 24 h with the indicated ligands ($HB57_{multivalent}$ at 1 µg/mL; $HB57_{bivalent}$ at 100 µg/mL; soluble IgM myeloma protein at 125 µg/mL; IL-4 at 5 ng/mL). At 48 h, cells were assessed for % $S/G_2/M$ and % apoptosis by staining with propidium iodide and FACScan analysis as in FIGURE 1. nd = not determined.

not shown). Second, pharmacological inhibitors of S phase (aphidicolin, hydroxyurea) that fully ablated mIgM-triggered $S/G_2/M$ did not diminish mIgM-triggered apoptosis (data not shown). Finally, mIgM-triggered viable blasts isolated at 24 h of culture succumbed to apoptosis if the high-affinity, multivalent mIgM binding ligand was removed from culture, but progressed into S phase if the ligand was readded to the culture (TABLE 1). These latter observations not only confirm previous findings regarding the apparent requirement for continued mIgM-mediated signal transduction throughout most of G_1 for B cell progression past a $G_1 \rightarrow S$ phase restriction point in the absence of T cell influences,[1,4] but also indicate that B cells in G_1 which do not receive continued mIgM-mediated signal transduction exhibit accelerated apoptosis. Thus, the potential for a protracted period of recurrent mIgM signaling appears to influence whether apoptosis or cell cycle progression is the functional outcome of B cell encounter with a multivalent antigen.

REFERENCES

1. MONGINI, P. K. A., C. A. BLESSINGER & J. P. DALTON. 1991. J. Immunol. **146:** 1791–1800.
2. MONGINI, P. K. A., C. A. BLESSINGER, P. F. HIGHET & J. K. INMAN. 1992. J. Immunol. **148:** 3892–3901.
3. RUDICH, S. M., K. H. ROUX, R. J. WINCHESTER & P. K. A. MONGINI. 1988. J. Exp. Med. **168:** 247–266.
4. DEFRANCO, A. L., E. S. RAVECHE & W. E. PAUL. 1985. J. Immunol. **135:** 87–94.
5. NICOLETTI, I., G. MIGLIORATI, M. C. PAGLIACCI, F. GRIGNANI & C. RICCARDI. 1991. J. Immunol. Methods **139:** 271–279.

Evidence for B Cell Oligoclonality in the Blood and Joints of Patients with Rheumatoid Arthritis[a]

VARSHA PATKI, JOANITA MONTEIRO,
PETER K. GREGERSEN, AND NICHOLAS CHIORAZZI

Department of Medicine
North Shore University Hospital
New York University School of Medicine
Manhasset, New York 11030

INTRODUCTION

The roles that B lymphocytes play in the pathogenesis of rheumatoid arthritis (RA) are poorly understood. Although B cells are not necessary to initiate the inflammatory reactions characteristic of RA,[1] B cells and their products clearly perpetuate these responses.[2–5] However, despite this involvement in the pathologic process, little is known of the level of B cell diversity in RA, although previous studies suggest that it may be restricted. For example, using flow cytometric techniques, peripheral blood B cells in RA have been shown to be not infrequently oligoclonal.[6] These studies are in agreement with cell culture experiments that indicate that synovial tissue explants spontaneously secrete Igs of restricted heterogeneity as defined by IgG subclass, isoelectric focusing, and idiotype expression.[7–10]

This study was designed to analyze the level of diversity of the expressed Ig V_H gene repertoire of RA B cells by using CDR3 length as a marker of clonality. This "fingerprinting" method has been used by several groups to identify the diversity of B cell and T cell receptor molecules[11,12] and to analyze leukemic populations.[13,14]

METHODS

Mononuclear cell fractions containing B lymphocytes were collected from the blood and synovial fluid of a series of patients with classical RF^+ RA. Total RNA was reverse-transcribed to cDNA using isotype-specific (μ, γ, α) C_H primers and then amplified using individual primers specific for the FR1 of each V_H family and for a different portion of the appropriate C_H region. The products of these reactions were then reamplified using nested primer pairs consisting of an FR3 consensus primer and

[a]This work was supported in part by Grant No. AI 10811 from the National Institutes of Health (NIAID), by the Leonard Wagner Autoimmunity Research Fund, and by the Richard and Nancy Leeds Fund of the Department of Medicine of North Shore University Hospital.

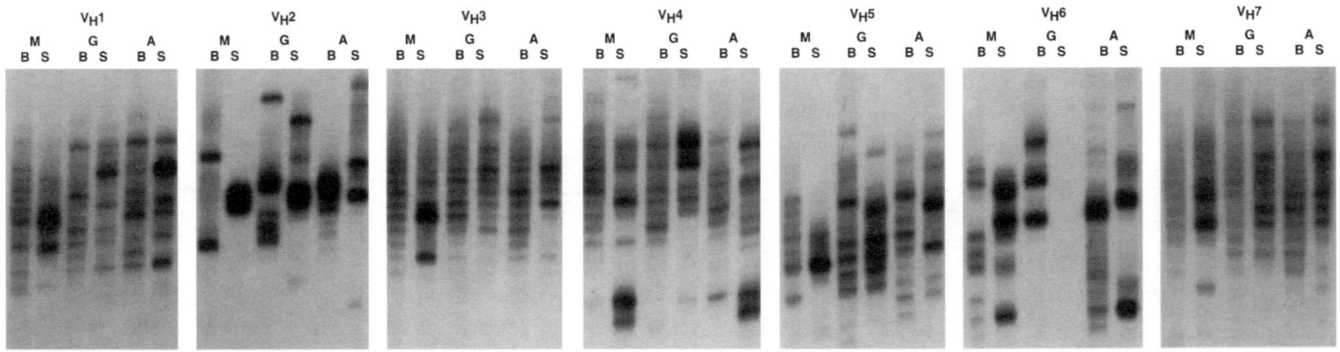

FIGURE 1. Analyses of paired samples of blood (B) and synovial fluid (S) B cells from the same RA patient. Results for the three major Ig isotypes are shown (M, G, and A). Note that certain clones, as represented by individual CDR3 cDNA lengths, are specific to the synovial compartment. Similar results were obtained in the four other patients studied.

a radiolabeled J_H consensus primer. These DNA fragments were electrophoresed through an acrylamide gel and exposed to X-ray film.[13,14]

RESULTS AND DISCUSSION

FIGURE 1 indicates the results obtained from one of five patients studied; similar results were obtained in the other patients. Note that the CDR3 cDNA lengths obtained with certain V_H/C_H primer pairs are nonhomogeneous, with examples of dominance of certain fragments suggesting individual clonal expansions. This phenomenon is more obvious among the synovial B cells and is especially prominent for those B cells using V_H6 and V_H2 family genes. Thus, oligoclonality appears to be a relatively common feature of these B cells, suggesting an ongoing autoimmune response. Furthermore, there is clear evidence for different and more-extensive expansions of individual clones in the synovial fluid as compared to the blood. These data indicate ongoing dominant "joint-specific", "blood-specific", and "blood-joint common" B cell responses, presumably due to distinct antigenic stimuli. By analyzing these joint-specific responses, autospecificities important for disease pathogenesis may be uncovered.

REFERENCES

1. GOOD, R. A., J. ROTSTEIN & W. F. MAZZITELLO. 1957. J. Lab. Clin. Med. **49:** 343.
2. RAWSON, A. J., J. L. HOLLANDER, F. P. QUISMORIO & N. M. ABELSON. 1969. Ann. N.Y. Acad. Sci. **168:** 188.
3. HOLMDAHL, R., C. VINGSBO, J. A. MO, E. MICHAËLSSON, V. MALMSTROM, L. JANSSON & U. BRUNSBERG. 1995. Immunol. Rev. **144:** 109.
4. ZHAO, Y-X., A. ABDELNOUR, R. HOLMDAHL & A. TARKOWSKI. 1995. J. Immunol. **155:** 2067.
5. TAYLOR, P. C., C. PLATER-ZYBERK & R. N. MAINI. 1995. Eur. J. Immunol. **25:** 763.
6. FOX, D. A. & B. R. SMITH. 1986. Ann. Rheum. Dis. **45:** 991.
7. HOFFMAN, W. L., M. S. GOLDBERG & J. D. SMILEY. 1982. J. Clin. Invest. **69:** 136.
8. SMILEY, J. D., W. L. HOFFMAN, S. E. MOORE & L. H. PARADIES. 1985. Semin. Arthritis Rheum. **14:** 151.
9. WERNICK, R. M., P. E. LIPSKY, E. MARBAN-ARCOS, J. J. MALIAKKAL, D. EDELBAUM & M. ZIFF. 1985. Arthritis Rheum. **28:** 742.
10. HOFFMAN, W. L., A. A. JUMP & J. D. SMILEY. 1990. Arthritis Rheum. **33:** 1196.
11. DEANE, M. & J. D. NORTON. 1991. Br. J. Haematol. **77:** 274.
12. HINGORANI, R., I. H. CHOI, P. AKOLKAR, B. GULWANI-AKOLKAR, R. PERGOLIZZI, J. SILVER & P. K. GREGERSEN. 1993. J. Immunol. **151:** 5762.
13. DONO, M., S. HASHIMOTO, F. FAIS, V. TREJO, S. L. ALLEN, S. M. LICHTMAN, P. SCHULMAN, V. P. VINCIGUERRA, B. SELLARS, P. K. GREGERSEN, M. FERRARINI & N. CHIORAZZI. 1996. Blood **87:** 1586.
14. FAIS, F., B. SELLARS, F. GHIOTTO, X-J. YAN, M. DONO, S. L. ALLEN, D. BUDMAN, K. DITTMAR, J. KOLITZ, S. M. LICHTMAN, P. SCHULMAN, M. SCHUSTER, V. P. VINCIGUERRA, K. RAI, F. STEVENSON, P. K. GREGERSEN, M. FERRARINI & N. CHIORAZZI. 1996. J. Clin. Invest. **98:** 1659.

Lactoferrin-reactive Natural Antibodies

KAREN M. MANCHESTER,[a] RONALD WINSTON,[b]
AND TOBY C. RODMAN[a,b]

[a]*The Rockefeller University*
New York, New York 10021

[b]*Institute for Human Genetics and Biochemistry*
CH 1222 Vesenaz, Switzerland

The designation "natural antibodies" refers to those antibodies, of broad occurrence in normal sera, for which there is no evidence of exogenous antigenic induction. In their early history, natural antibodies were characterized as "polyreactive",[1] that is, reactive with more than one seemingly unrelated antigen. However, as interest in natural antibodies has progressed, particularly with regard to assignment of function, it is apparent that, for at least some natural antibodies, epitope specificity is innately well defined.[2] For the most part, the assigned functions have been those of benefit, for example, recognition and rejection of xenogeneic molecules or cells, and monitoring and maintenance of homeostasis. However, there also has been some consideration that certain natural antibodies may be precursors of, or otherwise related to, pathologic autoantibodies.

We have previously demonstrated, in normal adult sera, the presence of IgM reactive with a component of the protein coat of morphologically normal, human spermatozoa.[3] That component has been isolated and identified as lactoferrin, a bi-lobed 80-kDa glycoprotein of broad occurrence in body fluids, including seminal plasma, which is apparently the source of the lactoferrin of the sperm coat.[4]

Utilizing lactoferrin from human milk (LF) and the 80-kDa protein from seminal plasma (SP80), we have confirmed their homology and showed that the circulating IgM antibody is not reactive with LF or SP80 in the nondenatured state, but is reactive with both following denaturation (FIGURE 1A), with the reactivity specifically displayed in a 10-kDa fraction (FIGURE 1B). Further resolution, by means of trycine gel to enhance the focusing of low-molecular-weight components, showed that the 10-kDa fraction consists of two bands, with the human serum reactivity confined to the band of lower molecular weight, designated 10B (FIGURE 1C). Mass spectrometry of 10B showed that it consists of two peptides. Sequencing of the first 5 N-terminal residues of each peptide established that the peptides consist of 81 and 88 residues, respectively; then, by reference to the published sequence of human lactoferrin,[5] the sequence of each of the two peptides was established. Both occur in the C lobe, with the 88-residue peptide constituting the C-terminal sequence. Thus far, we have not succeeded in the localization of the specific epitope by means of a set of overlapping 12-residue peptides representing the linear sequences of the 81- and 88-residue peptides comprising fraction 10B, indicating conformational dependence of the epitope. By ELISA, we have detected significant titers of IgM reactivity with fraction 10B in virtually all of a large cohort of normal human sera (FIGURE 2), supporting the designation of "natural antibody". Also supported is the concept that at least some natural antibodies, for example, those reactive with LF/SP80 or fraction 10B, display epitope specificity.

Because lactoferrin has been shown to be multifunctional and to be capable of assuming a different configuration to serve each function,[6] it is possible that the

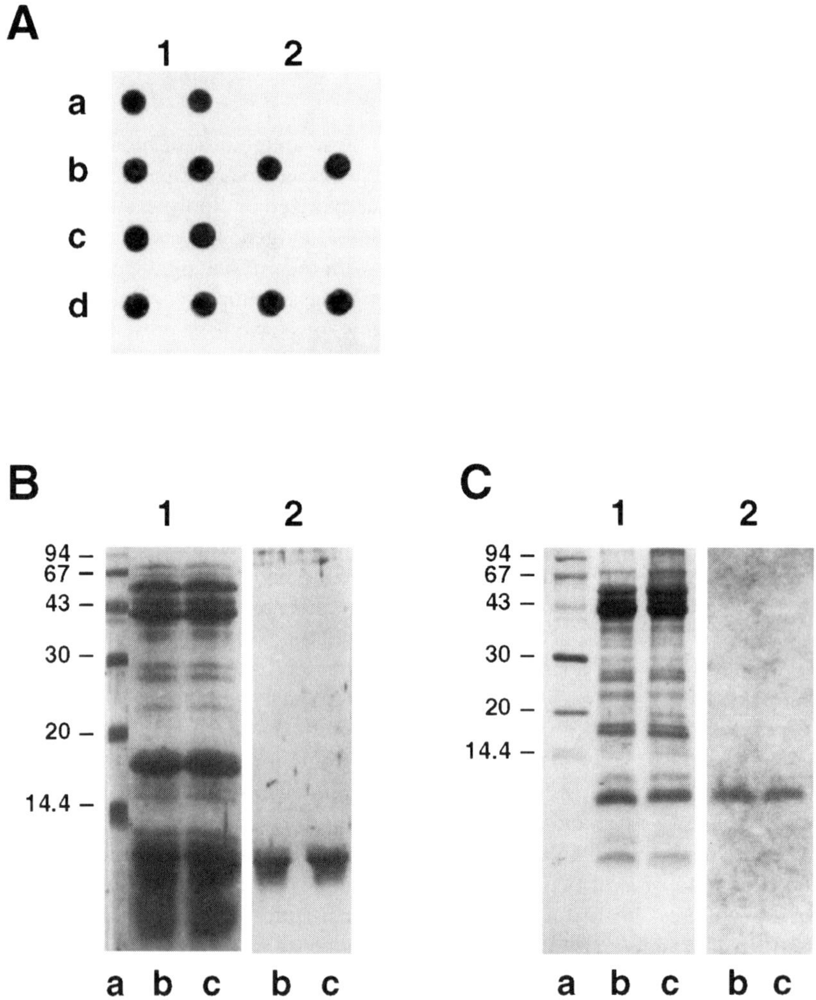

FIGURE 1. (A) Immunodot blot showing reactivity of human serum IgM with denatured, but not native, SP80 and LF—(1) serum of rabbit immunized with LF; (2) normal human serum: (a) native SP80, (b) denatured SP80, (c) native LF, (d) denatured LF. (B) SDS PAGE of CNBr-cleaved SP80 and LF and (C) SDS/trycine PAGE (enhanced focusing of low-molecular-weight fractions)—(1) protein stain; (2) chemiluminescence of human serum reactivity: (a) mol. wt. markers, (b) SP80, (c) LF.

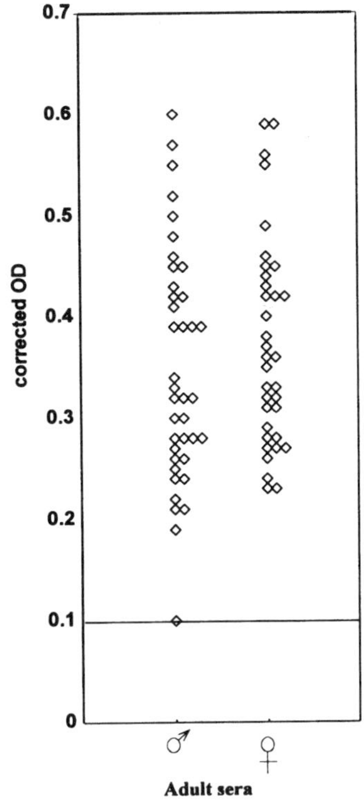

FIGURE 2. IgM reactivity, by ELISA (OD corrected for background, 0.10 significant), of normal human sera (39 males, 35 females) with fraction 10B of LF (FIGURE 1C).

antibodies are related to the function served by LF in the context of its configuration in the sperm coat. Also, the occasional identification of antineutrophil cytoplasmic antibodies (ANCA) specifically reactive with LF has led to consideration of a possible relationship of LF to certain autoimmune states. This identification and characterization of a set of natural LF-reactive antibodies should provide a means of investigation of that relationship.

REFERENCES

1. AVRAMEAS, S., B. GUILBERT & G. DIGHIERO. 1981. Ann. Immunol. (Inst. Pasteur) **132C:** 231–236.
2. MOUTHON, L., A. NOBREGA, N. NICOLAS, S. V. KAVERI, C. BARREAU & M. D. KAZATCHKINE. 1995. Proc. Natl. Acad. Sci. U.S.A. **92:** 3839–3843.
3. RODMAN, T. C., J. LAURENCE, F. H. PRUSLIN, N. CHIORAZZI & R. WINSTON. 1985. Science **228:** 1211–1214.
4. THALER, C. J., O. A. VANDERPUYE, J. A. MCINTYRE & W. P. FAULK. 1990. Biol. Reprod. **43:** 712–717.
5. METZ-BOUTIGUE, M-H., J. JOLLES, J. MAZURIER, F. SCHOENTGEN, D. LEGRAND, G. SPIK, J. MONTREUIL & P. JOLLES. 1984. Eur. J. Biochem. **145:** 659–676.
6. HUTCHENS, T. W., S. V. RUMBALL & B. LONERDAL, Eds. 1994. Lactoferrin, Structure and Function. Adv. Exp. Med. Biol. Volume 237.

Expression of an Ig V_H Gene, 51p1, Is Proportional to Its Germline Gene Copy Number

ERIC H. SASSO,[a,b] TODD JOHNSON,[c]
AND THOMAS J. KIPPS[c]

[b]*Division of Rheumatology*
University of Washington
Seattle, Washington 98105

[c]*Department of Medicine*
University of California at San Diego
La Jolla, California 92093-0663

Two striking features of immunoglobulin (Ig) V_H gene loci are that (1) many are polymorphic and (2) they differ greatly in the frequency with which they are expressed. We have studied the relation between Ig V_H gene expression and Ig V_H gene polymorphism by focusing on the V_H gene, 51p1 (the V1-69 locus). The 51p1 gene is of particular interest because it is expressed with inordinate frequency by normal primary B cells, is the predominant V_H gene encoding monoclonal IgM RF in type-II mixed cryoglobulinemia, and is frequently expressed by malignant B cells in chronic lymphocytic leukemia.

Previous study of the 51p1 locus identified 13 alleles by sequence-specific RFLP analysis with oligonucleotide probes.[1] The alleles were classified into two gene subsets, 51p1-related or hv1263-related, according to distinctive sequence motifs in the second complementarity-determining region that are detected by two mutually exclusive oligoprobes. In a predominantly Caucasian population, the prevalences of 51p1-related and hv1263-related genes were 85% and 58%, respectively.[1] Null alleles of the 51p1 locus were not seen. Nearly all 51p1-related alleles were detected on a 4.3-kb TaqI fragment or as a pair of duplicated genes on co-occurring 7.5-kb and 4.0-kb TaqI fragments.[1] The single-copy (4.3 kb) and double-copy (7.5/4.0 kb) alleles were each seen in about half the population. Many subjects were heterozygous for both and <10% were homozygous for either. These data indicated that (1) the diploid 51p1 locus is always represented by at least two gene copies, which can be 51p1-related and/or hv1263-related, and (2) the total diploid copy number of 51p1-related genes can be 0, 1, 2, 3, or 4.

Expression of 51p1 was previously studied with G6, a murine monoclonal anti-idiotype Ab that is specific for human Ab encoded by unmutated 51p1-related genes, but not hv1263-related genes, or other V_H genes.[2,3] G6 was found to detect 0% to 12% of the IgD-positive B cells in human tonsils.[2] IgD+ cells account for 37% to

[a]Address all correspondence to Eric H. Sasso, Harborview Medical Center, Box 359785, 325 Ninth Avenue, Seattle, Washington 98104.

87% of tonsillar B cells,[2] and are generally considered to be preimmune, usually IgM+, unmutated residents of the tonsillar mantle zone. Thus, 51p1 is expressed by a relatively large percentage of primary B cells, but the exact level varies between subjects.

To clarify the relation between 51p1 gene polymorphism and interindividual variation in 51p1 expression, we have now studied tonsils from 35 subjects. Flow cytometry with G6 was used to detect IgD+ B cells, and sequence-specific RFLP analysis with oligoprobes was performed to determine 51p1 genotypes. It was found

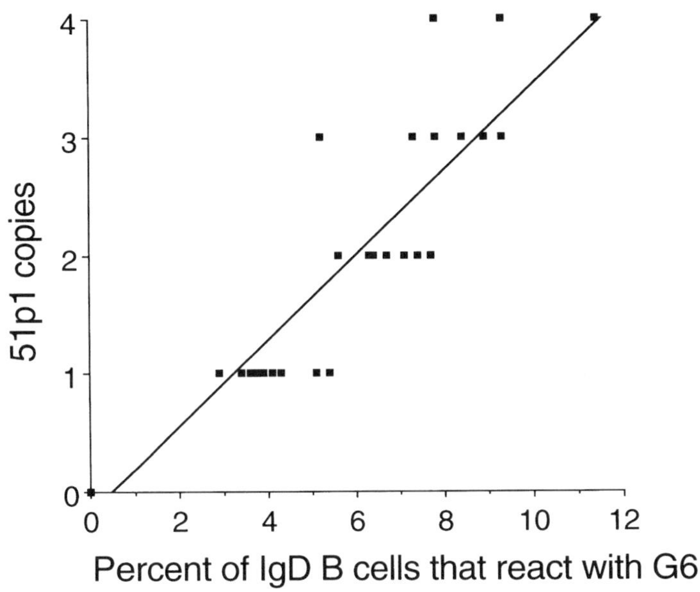

FIGURE 1. Correlation of gene expression with genotype for the 51p1-related alleles. Each point depicts the percentage of G6-positive cells among IgD-positive tonsillar B lymphocytes (*abscissa*) versus the number of 51p1-related germline genes for the 35 study subjects (*ordinate*). In the data clusters for one and two copies of 51p1-related alleles, the points at 3.7% and 7.4%, respectively, represent two subjects each. All other points represent one subject. The line ($y = -0.1153 + 0.3469x$) was calculated from the entire data set by linear regression analysis; $R = 0.92$ ($p < 0.001$). Reproduced from reference 3 with permission.

that the proportion of G6-reactive IgD+ B cells ranged from 0% to 11.4% and was strongly proportional to the total copy number of 51p1-related germline genes ($R = 0.92$, $p < 0.001$)[3] (FIGURE 1). The six people lacking 51p1-related genes had no G6 expression, whereas those with four copies had the highest percentages of G6-reactive B cells (TABLE 1). In subjects with one copy of 51p1-related genes, the mean proportion of G6-reactive cells was 4.0%, indicating a relatively high level of expression for these alleles (TABLE 1).

TABLE 1. Frequency of G6 Idiotype Expression per 51p1-related Gene Copy[a]

N	Copy Number of 51p1-related Genes	%G6-reactive IgD+ B cells	
		Mean (Range)	Per Gene Copy[b]
6	0	0.0 (all 0.0)	—
11	1	4.0 (2.9–5.4)	4.0
8	2	6.8 (5.6–7.7)	3.4
7	3	7.9 (5.2–9.3)	2.6
3	4	9.5 (7.8–11.4)	2.4

[a]Reproduced from reference 3 with permission.

[b]Calculated as mean %G6+ (column 3) divided by copy number of 51p1-related genes (column 2).

The data thus indicate that 51p1-related genes are expressed by a relatively large percentage of IgD+ tonsillar B cells, and this percentage is proportional to the germline copy number of 51p1-related genes. This finding shows that the gene copy number of Ig V_H genes can directly influence the composition of the primary B cell repertoire.

REFERENCES

1. SASSO, E. H., K. WILLEMS VAN DIJK, A. BULL & E. C. B. MILNER. 1993. A fetally expressed immunoglobulin V_H1 gene belongs to a complex set of alleles. J. Clin. Invest. **91:** 2358–2367.
2. KIPPS, T. J. & S. F. DUFFY. 1991. Relationship of the CD5 B cell to human tonsillar lymphocytes that express autoantibody-associated cross-reactive idiotypes. J. Clin. Invest. **87:** 2087–2096.
3. SASSO, E. H., T. JOHNSON & T. J. KIPPS. 1996. Expression of the Ig V_H gene 51p1 is proportional to its germline gene copy number. J. Clin. Invest. **97:** 2074–2080.

Neutrophils and Anti-Ro/SSA

BIJI T. KURIEN,[a] KEVIN L. MOORE,[b,c]
AND R. HAL SCOFIELD[a,c,d,e]

[a]*Arthritis and Immunology Program*
[b]*Cardiovascular Diseases Program*
Oklahoma Medical Research Foundation
[c]*Department of Medicine*
University of Oklahoma Health Sciences Center
[d]*Department of Veterans Affairs Medical Center*
Oklahoma City, Oklahoma 73104

Systemic lupus erythematosus (SLE) is characterized by the presence of autoantibodies in the sera of affected patients. One such autoantibody is anti-Ro (or SSA), which is found in the sera of up to 40% of SLE patients.[1] Some data indicate that anti-Ro itself is involved in the pathogenesis of several manifestations of SLE, including skin disease and neonatal lupus.[1]

The great majority of SLE patients have lymphopenia and a substantial fraction have mild neutropenia.[2] The presence of anti-Ro has been associated with a low total WBC count[3] as well as lymphopenia.[4] In a preliminary clinical study, we found that SLE patients with anti-Ro have significantly lower neutrophil counts compared to anti-Ro-negative patients (2771 $\pm$ 278 versus 6771 $\pm$ 284, $p < 0.001$). Because of these associations, we hypothesized that anti-Ro may play a pathogenic role in the neutropenia in SLE patients by directly binding to neutrophils.

Purified bovine 60-kDa Ro was chemically coupled to a solid-phase support and used to purify anti-Ro IgG from Ro-precipitin-positive sera of patients with SLE or Ro-precipitin-positive sera of New Zealand White rabbits that had been immunized with 60-kDa Ro. Binding to intact neutrophils by the affinity-purified anti-Ro was assessed by flow cytometry. FIGURE 1 demonstrates that anti-Ro from a 60-kDa immunized rabbit binds neutrophils. Similar results were observed using sera or purified anti-Ro from anti-Ro-positive SLE patients.

Several experiments were performed to determine the specificity of binding. Preincubation of antibody for 20 minutes with purified 60-kDa Ro antigen, but not a control antigen, abolished the binding of anti-Ro to neutrophils (FIGURE 2). Fab fragments were prepared from anti-Ro and control sera. The anti-Ro Fab bound intact neutrophils, whereas Fab fragments prepared from sera without anti-Ro did not. The ability of anti-Ro bound to the surface of neutrophils to fix complement was assessed by incubating cells with anti-Ro followed by addition of human sera as a complement source. Surface-bound C3 was then detected by flow cytometry using an anti-C3 monoclonal antibody. These data showed that complement was fixed on the surface of neutrophils by anti-Ro, but not when heat-inactivated or C3-deficient serum was used as a complement source.

[e]To whom all correspondence should be addressed.

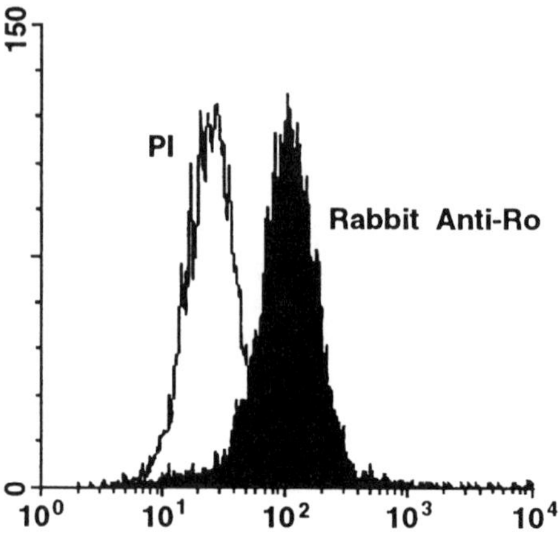

FIGURE 1. Binding of anti-Ro from a rabbit immunized with purified 60-kDa Ro to the surface of neutrophils compared to preimmune (PI) sera.

In an attempt to identify the membrane-associated antigen(s) bound by anti-Ro, enriched human neutrophil membranes were analyzed by Western immunoblotting. We observed that anti-Ro sera bound to one molecular species, migrating with an apparent molecular weight of 60,000.

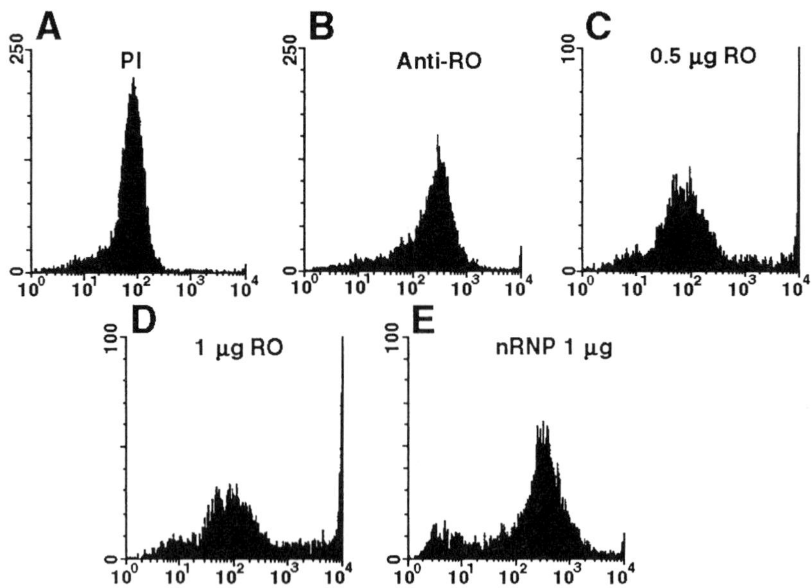

FIGURE 2. Inhibition of anti-Ro granulocyte binding by soluble 60-kDa Ro. Panel B shows the binding to neutrophils by sera from a rabbit immunized with 60-kDa Ro, whereas panel A shows the preimmune sera. Incubation of the sera with either 0.5 µg (panel C) or 1 µg (panel D) of soluble 60-kDa Ro abrogates binding completely. Another SLE-related antigen (RNP) does not inhibit binding (panel E).

REFERENCES

1. HARLEY, J. B. & R. H. SCOFIELD. 1991. Systemic lupus erythematosus: RNA-protein autoantigens, models of disease heterogeneity, and theories of etiology. J. Clin. Immunol. **11:** 297–316.
2. NOSSENT, J. C. & A. J. G. SWAAK. 1991. Prevalence and significance of haematological abnormalities in patients with systemic lupus erythematosus. Q. J. Med. **80:** 605–612.
3. DE ROOIJ, D. J., L. B. VAN DE PUTTE, W. J. HABETS, A. L. VERBEEK & W. J. VAN VENROOIJ. 1988. The use of immunoblotting to detect antibodies to nuclear and cytoplasmic antigens: clinical and serologic associations in rheumatic diseases. Scand. J. Rheumatol. **17:** 353–364.
4. HARLEY, J. B., A. L. SESTAK, L. G. WILLIS, S. M. FU, J. A. HANSEN & M. REICHLIN. 1989. A model for disease heterogeneity in systemic lupus erythematosus: relationships between histocompatibility antigens, autoantibodies, and lymphopenia or renal disease. Arthritis Rheum. **32:** 826–836.

Recurrent Identical Rearrangement and Repeated Expression of Identical Heavy and Light Chains in Single Anti-phosphatidylcholine B Cells[a]

KATHERINE J. SEIDL,[b,c,d] JOHN D. MACKENZIE,[d] DENONG WANG,[e] AARON B. KANTOR,[d,f] ELVIN A. KABAT,[e] LEONARD A. HERZENBERG,[d] AND LEONORE A. HERZENBERG[d]

[d]*Department of Genetics*
Beckman Center
Stanford University Medical Center
Stanford, California 94305-5125

[e]*Department of Microbiology*
Columbia University
New York, New York 10032

[f]*AmCell Corporation*
Sunnyvale, California 94089

V(D)J recombination confers a vast potential for expressing a great number of different immunoglobulin (Ig) molecules (10^{18} possible combinations[1]) and hence for generating a population of B cells producing a highly diverse set of antibodies. Limited heavy-chain (IgH) and light-chain (IgL) gene usage, however, is common in immune responses to certain antigens, such as α(1–>3) dextran, phenyloxazolone, phosphorylcholine, and phosphatidylcholine (PtC), the antigen studied here. Anti-PtC antibodies, produced exclusively by cells of the B-1 lineage,[2] lyse mouse erythrocytes treated with bromelain to expose PtC. Previous studies have shown that the IgH and IgL of anti-PtC antibodies produced by independently isolated hybridomas and neoplasms tend to be encoded by V_H11-Vk9 or V_H12-Vk4.

Collectively, these earlier studies raised the question of whether identical anti-PtC IgH rearrangements are derived from a common progenitor or from multiple progenitors that develop into a limited PtC-repertoire. Single PtC-binding cells, detectable by staining with PtC-liposomes, were sorted from four C57BL/6J mice (C57), two separate pools of peritoneal cells from BALB/c mice, and two C.B-17 mice (FIGURE 1). The PtC-liposome$^+$ IgM$^+$ phenotype of the sorted cells was recorded for each cell.

[a]This work was supported by Grant Nos. CA 42509 and AI 34762 from the National Institutes of Health.

[b]K. Seidl was supported by Grant No. EY 07106 from the National Institutes of Health.

[c]Present address: Children's Hospital, Harvard University, 300 Longwood Avenue, Boston, Massachusetts 02115.

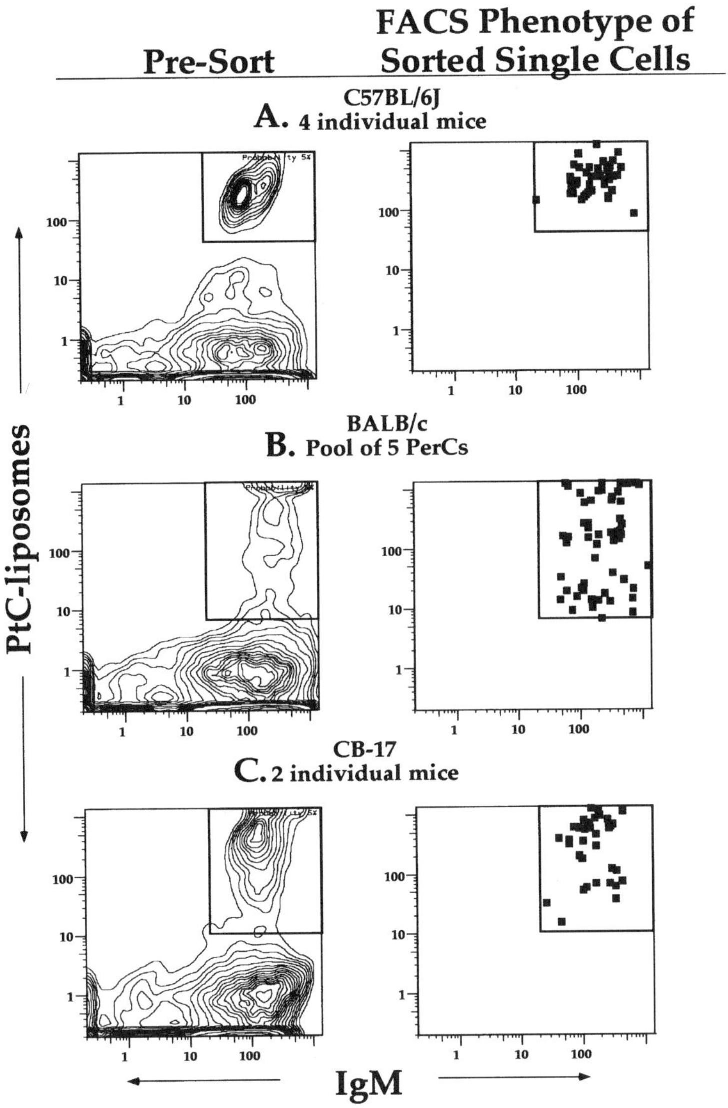

FIGURE 1. Single cell sorting of PtC-binding B-1 cells. PtC-binding cells were identified by FACS using fluorescein encapsulated in PtC-liposomes and surface IgM staining. PtC-binding cells were sorted from four C57 mice (A), a pool of peritoneal cells from nine BALB/c mice (Expt 1), a pool of peritoneal cells from five BALB/c mice (B) (Expt 2), and two C.B-17 mice (C). Gates used for sorting are indicated. The typical FACS profile for a mouse from each strain is shown. PtC-liposome-binding cells were first bulk sorted, based on size, viability, and expression of PtC-liposomes and IgM. Single cells were sorted into lysis solution and snap-frozen on dry ice for future analysis. Each square represents a single sorted cell.

We sequenced the expressed Ig from individual B cells using an unbiased FACS-based PCR method.[3,4]

Among the 47 C57 individual cells analyzed, 33 out of 38 V_H11 rearrangements were identical (87%; V_H11 type 1, see TABLE 1). PtC-binding cells from BALB/c mice also expressed this rearrangement, albeit much more rarely (7/101). Furthermore, although we failed to isolate V_H11 type 1 from C.B-17, others have found it within unseparated populations of B cells from C.B-17[5] and other mouse strains.[6–10]

TABLE 1. Recurrent Heavy-Chain Rearrangements and Their Light-Chain Pairings[a]

Strain	Heavy-Chain Rearrangement Type[b]	Mouse (Ms) #/ Expt #	Percent of Total[c]	Light Chain	Number of Cells[d]
C57BL/6J	V_H11 type 1	Ms 1	60 (9/15)	Vκ9 Jκ2	2
				Vκ9 Jκ4	2
				Vκ21E Jκ2	1
		Ms 2	75 (9/12)	Vκ9 Jκ2	5
				Vκ9 Jκ4	3
		Ms 3	90 (9/10)	Vκ9 Jκ2	3
				Vκ9 Jκ4	3
		Ms 4	60 (6/10)	Vκ9 Jκ2	3
				Vκ9 Jκ4	3
BALB/c	V_H11 type 1	Expt 1	5 (2/43)	Vκ9 Jκ4	1
		Expt 2	9 (5/58)	Vκ9 Jκ2	1
				Vκ9 Jκ4	4
C57BL/6J	V_H11 type 3	Ms 4	10 (1/10)	Vκ9 Jκ1	1
BALB/c		Expt 1	5 (2/43)	Vκ9 Jκ1/Vκ2 Jκ1	2
C.B-17	V_H11 type 4	Ms 1	13 (2/15)	Vκ9 Jκ2	1
				Vκ9 Jκ4	1
C57BL/6J	V_H12 type 1	Ms 1	13 (2/15)	NA[e]	2
BALB/c		Expt 2	3 (2/58)	Vκ4/5 Jκ2	2
BALB/c	Q52 type 1	Expt 2	3 (2/58)	Vκ4/5 Jκ5[f]	1
				Vκ20 Jκ4	1
C57BL/6J	V_H11 type 2	Ms 4	20 (2/10)	Vκ9 Jκ4	2
C.B-17	V_H11 type 5	Ms 1	11 (2/18)	Vκ9 Jκ1	2
BALB/c	V_H12 type 2	Expt 2	3 (2/58)	Vκ4/5 Jκ5/NA	2
BALB/c	Q52 type 2	Expt 1	5 (2/43)	NA	2
C.B-17	Q52 type 3	Ms 2	11 (2/18)	Vκ4/5 Jκ2[f]/NA	2

[a]A more complete data set can be found in reference 18.

[b]Rearrangement type is defined by identity of V, D, J segments and N/P additions within a heavy-chain family.

[c]Numbers in parentheses are the number of cells expressing that rearrangement type/total cells analyzed in that mouse or pool of mice.

[d]Light-chain analysis is not shown for all V_H11 type 1–expressing cells.

[e]NA = not available.

[f]Different germline gene than other Vκ4/5 rearrangements.

IgL sequences were obtained for the V_H11 type 1–expressing cells isolated from the four C57 mice and the two pools of cells from BALB/c mice (see TABLE 1). Many of the cells analyzed expressed the same IgH/IgL pair. Nevertheless, unique instances of IgH/IgL pairing in each of the individual mice show that at least 2 to 3 of the V_H11 type 1–expressing cells either have arisen from different B cell progenitors prior to IgH rearrangement or have arisen from pre-B cells that have expanded after IgH rearrangement, but prior to IgL rearrangement.[11] However, there is some question whether B-1 pre-B cell populations expand like conventional pre-B cells given the differences in MHC class II expression between B-1 and conventional pre-B cells.[12,13] In total, at least 12 IgH-IgL pairs (39%) of the 31 V_H11 type 1 cells studied for IgL expression in our data set are not due to clonal expansion of mature B cells by the described criteria (TABLE 1).

In addition to V_H11 type 1, we isolated V_H11, V_H12, and V_HQ52 IgH rearrangements, which each occurred at least twice in our data set. Consideration of the animal origin and IgL expression of cells with these additional recurrent rearrangements brings the total number of identical rearrangement events observed in this study not due to mature B cell clonal expansion to 21.

Many of the V_H11 and V_H12 IgH described here exhibit sequence identity at the coding junctions; V_H11 type 1 shows homology at both coding joints. If sequence homology at the coding joints reflects a constraint of rearrangement outcome,[14–16] this double homology could explain the high proportion of V_H11 type 1 rearrangements. Such conserved sequences could also reflect antigen selection.

In summary, cells expressing recurrent IgH rearrangements with identical variable-region sequences isolated from separate animals must have rearranged independently. Cells expressing identical IgH rearrangements, but different IgL rearrangements, are derived from different pro-B or pre-B progenitors; that is, they cannot be explained solely by clonal expansion of mature B cells. These findings expand on initial findings of dominant idiotype expression.[17] Thus, by single cell analysis, we show evidence for a mechanism that generates recurrent identical IgH and IgL rearrangements.

REFERENCES

1. LIEBER, M. R. 1991. Site-specific recombination in the immune system. FASEB J. **5:** 2934–2944.
2. MERCOLINO, T. J., L. W. ARNOLD, L. A. HAWKINS & G. HAUGHTON. 1988. Normal mouse peritoneum contains a large population of Ly-1+ (CD5) B cells that recognize phosphatidylcholine: relationship to cells that secrete hemolytic antibody specific for autologous erythrocytes. J. Exp. Med. **168:** 687–698.
3. KANTOR, A. B., C. E. MERRILL, J. D. MACKENZIE, L. A. HERZENBERG & J. L. HILLSON. 1995. Development of the antibody repertoire as revealed by single-cell PCR of FACS-sorted B-cell subsets. Ann. N.Y. Acad. Sci. **764:** 224–227.
4. KANTOR, A. B., C. E. MERRILL & J. L. HILLSON. 1996. Construction of cDNA from single unstimulated B lymphocytes: method and application to the study of expressed antibody repertoires in FACS-sorted B cell subsets. *In* The Handbook of Experimental Immunology. Volume 1: Immunochemistry and Molecular Immunology. Blackwell Sci. Pub. Boston. In press.

5. Riggs, J. E., A. J. Feeney, M. Kirven & D. E. Mosier. 1994. V_H11 bias and normal V-D-J junctions in SCID B lymphocytes rescued by neonatal T cell transfer. Mol. Immunol. **31:** 783–791.
6. Reininger, L., P. Ollier, P. Poncet, A. Kaushik & J. C. Jaton. 1987. Novel V genes encode virtually identical variable regions of six murine monoclonal anti-bromelain-treated red blood cell autoantibodies. J. Immunol. **138:** 316–323.
7. Reininger, L., A. Kaushik, S. Izui & J. C. Jaton. 1988. A member of a new V_H gene family encodes antibromelinized mouse red blood cell autoantibodies. Eur. J. Immunol. **18:** 1521–1526.
8. Pennell, C. A., T. J. Mercolino, T. A. Grdina, L. W. Arnold, G. Haughton & S. H. Clarke. 1989. Biased immunoglobulin variable region gene expression by Ly-1 B cells due to clonal selection. Eur. J. Immunol. **19:** 1289–1295.
9. Conger, J. D., H. J. Sage & R. B. Corley. 1989. Diversity in the available repertoire of murine antibodies reactive with bromelain-treated isologous erythrocytes. J. Immunol. **143:** 4044–4052.
10. Pennell, C. A., L. W. Arnold, G. Haughton & S. H. Clarke. 1988. Restricted Ig variable region gene expression among Ly-1+ B cell lymphomas. J. Immunol. **141:** 2788–2796.
11. Osmond, D. G. 1990. B cell development in the bone marrow. Semin. Immunol. **2:** 173–180.
12. Lam, K. & A. M. Stall. 1994. Major histocompatibility complex class II expression distinguishes two distinct B cell developmental pathways during ontogeny. J. Exp. Med. **180:** 507–516.
13. Tarlinton, D. 1993. Direct demonstration of MHC class II surface expression on murine pre-B cells. Int. Immunol. **12:** 1629–1635.
14. Feeney, A. J. 1990. Lack of N regions in fetal and neonatal mouse immunoglobulin V-D-J junctional sequences. J. Exp. Med. **172:** 1377–1390.
15. Gerstein, R. M. & M. R. Lieber. 1993. Extent to which homology can constrain coding exon junctional diversity in V(D)J recombination. Nature **363:** 625–627.
16. Zhang, Y., D. Cado, D. M. Asarnow, T. Kmori, F. Alt, D. H. Raulet & J. P. Allison. 1995. The role of short homology repeats and TdT in generation of the invariant gamma-delta antigen receptor repertoire in the fetal thymus. Immunity **3:** 439–447.
17. Klinman, N. R. & M. R. Stone. 1983. Role of variable region gene expression and environmental selection in determining the anti-phosphorylcholine B cell repertoire. J. Exp. Med. **158:** 1948–1961.
18. Seidl, K. J., J. D. MacKenzie, A. B. Kantor, D. Wang, E. Kabat, L. A. Herzenberg & L. A. Herzenberg. 1997. Frequent occurrence of identical heavy and light chain immunoglobulin rearrangements. Int. Immunol. In press.

Prevention of Autoantibody Production in *lpr/lpr* Mice by Transgenic Expression of Fas on B Cells

NOBUKATA SHINOHARA, YUKO IKEGAMI,
MINESUKE YOKOYAMA, SHIN YONEHARA,
AND HAJIME KOMANO

Mitsubishi Kasei Institute of Life Sciences
Tokyo 194, Japan
and
Kyoto University
Kyoto, Japan

Autoantibody production in *lpr/lpr* mice indicates a critical role of the Fas-L/Fas interaction in the regulation of autoantibody production. As we and others have shown, soluble antigen-specific Fas-dependent CD4$^+$ CTL are capable of specifically suppressing antibody responses by eliminating B cells.[1–4] Thus, it was speculated that autoantibody production in *lpr/lpr* mice might result from the failure of CD4$^+$ T cells in eliminating unwanted B cells. If this is truly the case, selective expression of Fas on B cells should prevent autoantibody production in *lpr/lpr* mice. Therefore, we developed *lpr/lpr* mice expressing transgenic Fas selectively on B cells.

The transgene was constructed by inserting a BALB/c-derived Fas cDNA at the head of the leader exon of a rearranged genomic Igk chain gene. In transgenic C3H mice, the transgenic Fas was expressed on IgM$^+$ cells, but not on IgM$^-$ cells (FIGURE 1a), nor on thymocytes, whereas endogenous Fas was normally expressed (not shown), indicating that the transgenic Fas was indeed expressed selectively on B cells. The transgenic mice were backcrossed to C3H//HeJ-*lpr* mice, and homozygous *lpr/lpr* offspring with the transgene were obtained. In transgenic (TG) C3H-*lpr/lpr* mice, massive proliferation of double-negative B220$^+$ T cells was not suppressed (FIGURE 1b). On the contrary, a significant reduction of the peripheral B cell population compared with nontransgenic *lpr/lpr* mice was observed (FIGURE 1c). Absolute numbers of B cells in the TG *lpr/lpr* mice were approximately 10–20% of nontransgenic *lpr/lpr* mice. Such a decrease in B cell number was not observed in transgenic mice without the *lpr* defect. The remaining B cells of the TG *lpr/lpr* mice expressed a very low, but significant, level of the transgenic Fas.

Quantitation of serum Ig of the TG *lpr/lpr* revealed a 5- to 10-fold decrease in the total Ig level (FIGURE 2), equally involving all isotypes tested (data not shown), which was comparable to that of normal C3H mice. Serum levels of anti-dsDNA antibodies of these mice were determined at 3, 5, and 7 months of age (FIGURE 2). In the TG *lpr/lpr* mice, anti-dsDNA antibody remained undetectable, that is, below the level of the normal mouse over 7 months. Because the titration curves indicate that the antibody titers of TG *lpr/lpr* were, if present, less than 0.1% of those of nontransgenic counterparts, whereas total Ig levels of the TG *lpr/lpr* were approximately 10%, the virtual absence of the autoantibody in the transgenic mice can hardly be explained by the general decrease in Ig production. It rather suggests a lack of a certain regulatory mechanism in *lpr/lpr* mice acting on Fas on B cells. The results also indicate that

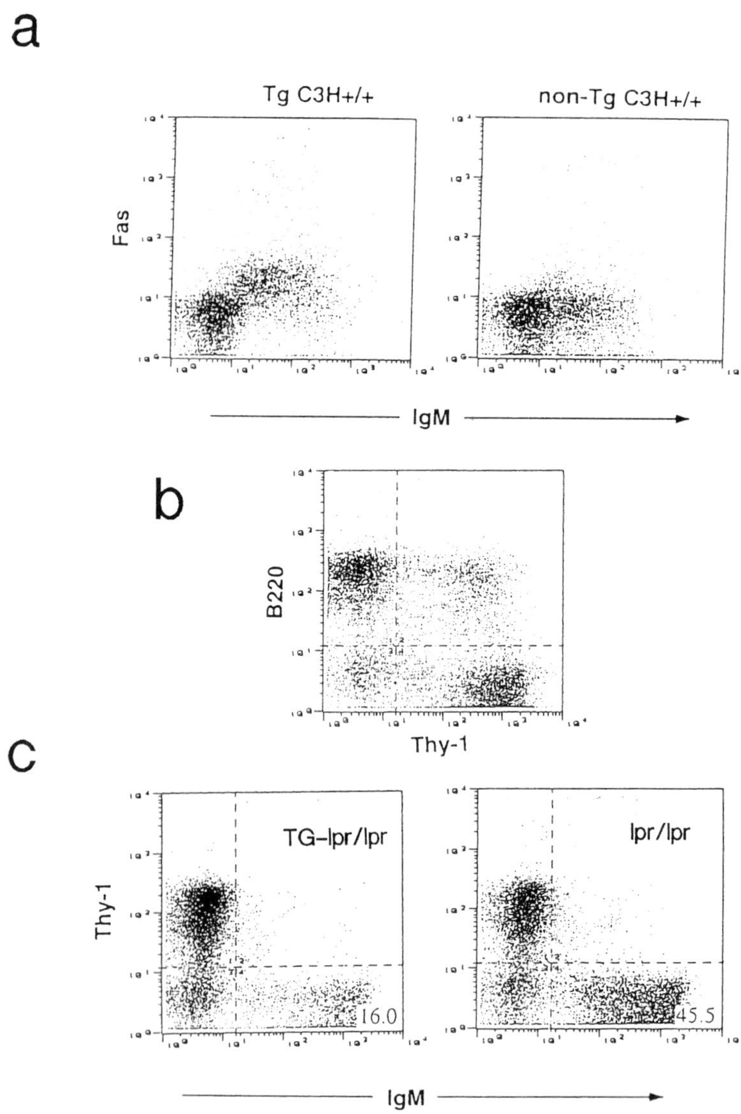

FIGURE 1. Lymphocytes from transgenic (TG) mice. (a) Selective expression of the transgenic Fas on IgM$^+$ cells. Splenic lymphocytes of normal (right) and transgenic (left) C3H mice were stained for surface IgM and transgenic Fas (BALB/c allele). (b) B220$^+$ T cells in the TG *lpr/lpr* mouse. Spleen cells of an 8-week-old TG *lpr/lpr* mouse. B220$^+$ T cells were not stained by antibodies to CD4 or CD8 (not shown). (c) Reduced B cell population in TG *lpr/lpr* spleen.

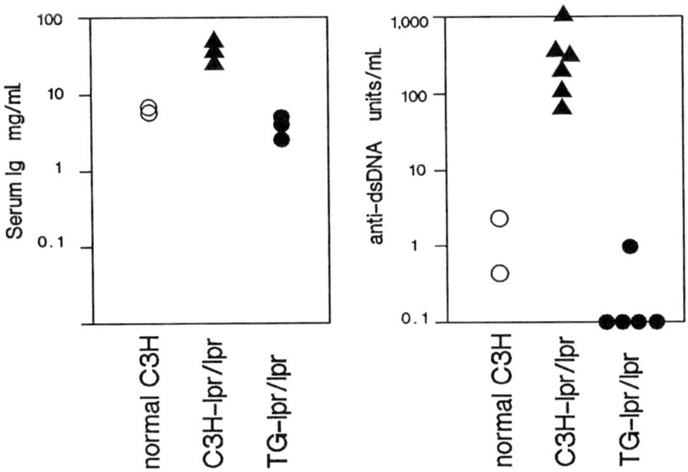

FIGURE 2. Serum Ig level and anti-DNA antibody in the TG *lpr/lpr* mouse. Sera from 5- to 7-month-old mice were studied. Individual markers represent individual animals.

abnormal T cell proliferation and autoantibody production in the *lpr/lpr* mouse are essentially two separable phenomena resulting from defects at two mutually independent censoring points.

Our results are consistent with earlier cell transfer experiments indicating the importance of an intrinsic B cell defect in autoantibody production of *lpr/lpr* mice.[5] Although the nature of the actual effector cells carrying out the censoring in our transgenic mice remains to be clarified, this study suggests that Fas on B cells is essential for the surveillance of unwanted antibody production. Together with our earlier report showing the ability of $CD4^+$ CTL to suppress antibody responses in an antigen-specific manner,[1] these observations make us speculate that the immediate cause of unregulated autoantibody production in *lpr/lpr* mice is the failure of $CD4^+$ CTL in eliminating autoantibody producers. This interpretation predicts the existence of a set of $CD4^+$ T cells specific for self-peptides in the normal mature immune system. We are now exploring this possibility.

REFERENCES

1. Shinohara, N. *et al.* 1991. Eur. J. Immunol. **21:** 23–27.
2. Hanabuchi, S. *et al.* 1994. Proc. Natl. Acad. Sci. U.S.A. **91:** 4930–4934.
3. Rathmell, J. C. *et al.* 1995. Nature **376:** 181–184.
4. Perkins, D. L. *et al.* 1990. J. Immunol. **145:** 549–555.
5. Sobel, E. S. *et al.* 1991. J. Exp. Med. **173:** 1441–1449.

Bacterial Immunomodulators Affect Programmed Cell Death of Mouse Spleen Lymphocytes

MAREK ŠINKORA,[a] LEOŠ MANDEL,[a] JIŘÍ ŠINKORA,[a] IGOR ŠPLÍCHAL,[a] ZUZANA ŘEHÁKOVÁ,[a] ILJA TREBICHAVSKÝ,[a] AND RITA BAROT-CIORBARU[b]

[a]*Department of Immunology and Gnotobiology*
Institute of Microbiology
Czech Academy of Sciences
Nový Hrádek, the Czech Republic

[b]*Institut de Biochemie*
Université Paris-Sud
91405 Orsay, France

In contrast to the accidental cell death or necrosis that occurs as a result of trauma or stress and that can be regarded as a pathological response, the programmed cell death (PCD) or apoptosis is a normal and deliberate process that plays a crucial role in embryogenesis, developmental processes, and maintaining homeostasis, including T and B cell turnover. Apoptosis in lymphocytes of various subsets and different maturation states can be induced by naturally occurring compounds such as corticosteroids or by improper stimulation via surface molecules, as well as by a number of nonphysiological interventions like *in vitro* cultivation or irradiation. Moreover, the stimuli as well as the subsequent signaling that initiate apoptosis at one developmental stage may cause an entirely different response in the same cell at another time.

The situation is more complicated in the case of irradiation, which in itself is a more-complex and less-defined agent. Lymphocytes exposed to relatively low doses of ionizing radiation (<10 Gy) undergo apoptosis, whereas higher exposition causes necrosis.[1] It was demonstrated that radiation-induced apoptosis could be prevented to some extent by bacterial immunomodulators applied before irradiation.[1,2] This is in accordance with results where activated lymphocytes were found more radioresistant than resting ones.[1]

Low-toxic Nocardia Delipidated Cell Mitogen (NDCM) isolated from the cell wall of *Nocardia opaca* was reported to stimulate proliferation of small resting B lymphocytes and to drive their differentiation into Ig-secreting cells.[3] NDCM also activates macrophages[4] and induces the expression of a battery of cytokines including

IL-1α and TNF-α, where the production of the latter might be related to protein kinase C activation.[5] These strong naturally occurring immunomodulators were shown to exhibit radioprotective activities. Moreover, anti-IL-1-R as well as anti-TNF monoclonal antibodies reduced survival of irradiated mice.[6]

In our experiments, flow cytometry (FCM) DNA fragmentation assay and gel electrophoresis DNA fragmentation assay confirmed that splenocytes kept *in vitro* under usual conditions died spontaneously by apoptosis. The kinetics of cell dying, as calculated from FCM data, could be described as a monotonic progression with time. After 12 hours of *in vitro* cultivation, DNA fragmentation was detected in about 35% of the isolated spleen cells. Irradiation of cell suspensions before cultivation *in vitro* increased PCD. Immunophenotypical studies showed that, in both cases (nonirradiated and irradiated suspensions), the sIg+ cells (B cells) were more susceptible to apoptosis and subsequent loss of cell surface markers than CD3+ cells (T cells; FIGURE 1). In regard to T cell subpopulations, CD4+ T cells were slightly more sensitive to spontaneous and radiation-induced PCD than CD8+ lymphocytes.

The addition of NDCM to cultured cells diminished the apoptosis-inducing effect of irradiation only when performed within 4 hours after irradiation. Similarly, in nonirradiated cells, the NDCM treatment partially inhibited spontaneous PCD, but the interval between the beginning of cultivation and NDCM addition in which NDCM still remained active was longer (more than 8 hours). In other experiments, when NDCM was added to splenocyte cultures at 2 hours of cultivation, the inhibition of apoptosis was most pronounced after 12–14 hours: about 15–20% of cells, which would have died without the presence of NDCM, were rescued from apoptosis in both irradiated and nonirradiated samples. Although NDCM diminished the spontaneous as well as radiation-induced apoptosis of both T and B cells, the "protected" splenocytes were predominantly B cells (FIGURE 1).

Because TNF-α and IL-1α are supposed to be strong radioprotective, naturally occurring substances both *in vitro* and *in vivo*, we also tested the expression of these cytokines under the cultivation conditions used. Using TNF-α and IL-1α ELISA analysis of culture supernatants, we showed that, after NDCM activation, irradiated as well as untreated splenocytes produced high amounts of both of the cytokines studied (TABLE 1).

We conclude that NDCM, when added to *in vitro* spleen cell cultures, protects T and mainly B cells from spontaneous and radiation-induced apoptosis. In irradiated cell cultures, there is a critical time interval (4 hours) between the beginning of cultivation and NDCM addition after which this bacteria-derived immunomodulator is not radioprotective anymore. A possible radioprotective role of cytokines induced by the presence of NDCM (IL-1α, TNF-α) is to be confirmed by antibodies neutralizing their biological activity or directed against their receptors. These *in vitro* observations may help to explain the results of previous experiments in which the postirradiation application of NDCM protected lymphocytes of B lineages *in vivo* and increased the survival of animals.[7]

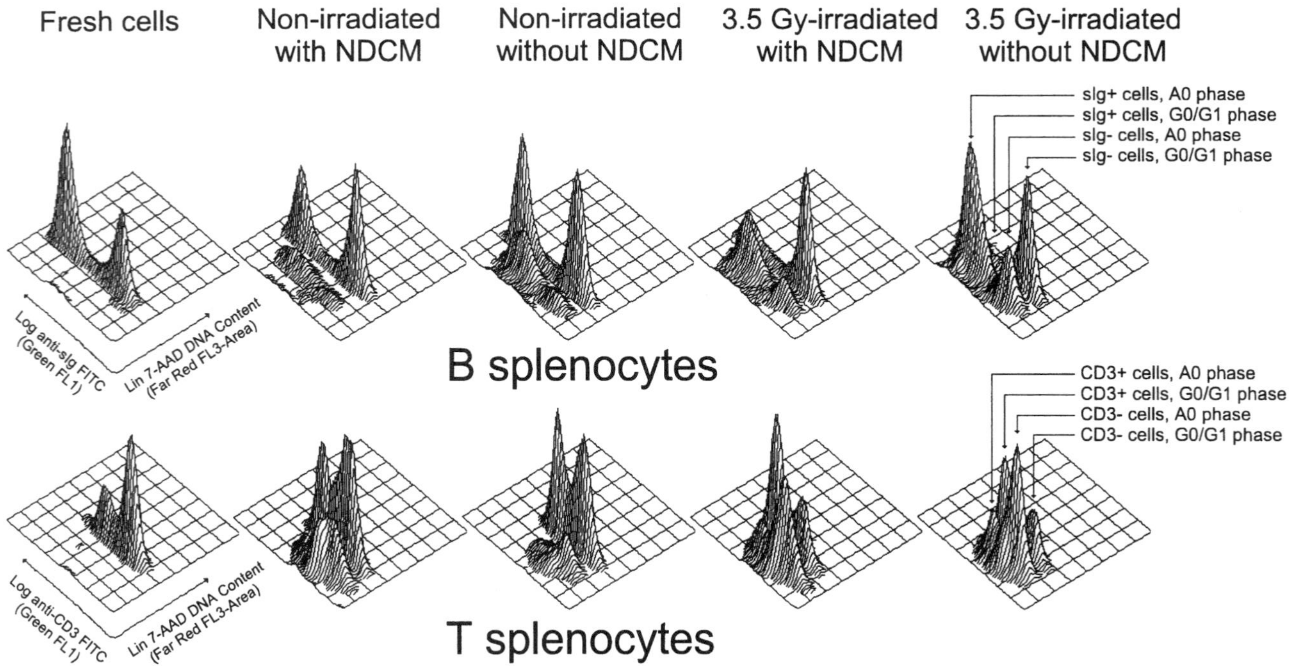

FIGURE 1. Three-dimensional contour plots showing the immunophenotyping of mouse splenocytes combined with 7-aminoactinomycin D (7-AAD) staining for the DNA content. Nonirradiated and 3.5-Gy-irradiated splenocytes were incubated for 14 hours with or without NDCM given at 2 hours of cultivation, stained with anti-sIg (top) or anti-CD3 (bottom), fixed with ethanol, and stained with 7-AAD. Individual subpopulations cultured under different conditions are indicated.

TABLE 1. Relationship between Regulation of Apoptosis and IL-1α and TNF-α Levels[a]

	TNF-α (pg/10^6 cells)	IL-1α (pg/10^6 cells)
Untreated	340 ± 113.4[b]	26 ± 5.7[b]
Nonirradiated with NDCM	1408 ± 87.7	151 ± 15.1
Irradiated without NDCM	140 ± 16.3[b]	24 ± 4.2[b]
Irradiated with NDCM	1227 ± 133.8	124 ± 43.5

[a]Lysates of nonirradiated and 3.5-Gy-irradiated splenocytes cultured for 10 hours with or without NDCM given at 2 hours of cultivation were tested by ELISA for the presence of IL-1α and TNF-α levels.

[b]Significant differences between NDCM-treated samples and controls.

REFERENCES

1. SELLINS, K. S. & J. J. COHEN. 1987. J. Immunol. **139:** 3199–3206.
2. LOWENTHAL, J. W. & A. W. HARRIS. 1985. J. Immunol. **135:** 1119–1125.
3. BAROT-CIORBARU, R., J. BROCHIER, T. MIYAWAKI, J. L. PREUD'HOMME, J. F. PETIT, C. BONA, N. TANIGUCHI & J. P. REVILLARD. 1985. J. Immunol. **135:** 3277–3283.
4. LEIBOVICI, J., S. HOENIG, A. PINCHASSOV & R. BAROT-CIORBARU. 1991. In Vivo **5:** 365–374.
5. MEGE, J. L., M. W. SANGUELDOCE, T. JACOB, P. BONGRAND, C. CAPO & E. B. MYSSISKINE. 1993. Eur. J. Immunol. **23:** 1582–1587.
6. NETA, R., J. J. OPPENHEIM, R. D. SCHREIBER, R. CHIZZONITE, G. D. LEDNEY & T. J. MACVITTIE. 1991. J. Exp. Med. **173:** 1177–1182.
7. MANDEL, L., I. TREBICHAVSKÝ, H. TLASKALOVÁ, J. ŠINKORA, I. ŠPLÍCHAL & R. BAROT-CIORBARU. 1994. Int. J. Immunopharmacol. **16:** 481–486.

Anti-p53 Autoantibodies in Colon Cancer Patients

Z. STHOEGER,[a] E. EVRON,[a] S. GOLAND,[a] A. SHANI,[a]
R. WOLKOWICZ,[b] N. GOLDFINGER,[b] V. ROTTER,[b]
AND M. FOGEL[a]

[a]*Division of Internal Medicine*
Kaplan Hospital
[b]*Department of Cell Biology*
Weizmann Institute
Rehovot 76100, Israel

The p53 tumor suppressor gene normally functions as a regulator of the cell cycle. Point mutations within the coding region of the gene lead to a loss of tumor suppressor function and to conversion of the normal p53 gene to a dominant oncogene.[1] The mutated p53 results in an altered molecular conformation with prolonged protein half-life, leading to abnormal p53 accumulation in the nuclei of tumor cells;[2] this then leads to the generation of autoantibodies directed against the p53. These autoantibodies may have a role in diagnosis, prediction of residual recurrent disease, and prognosis. Mutations in the p53 tumor suppressor gene are frequently found in colorectal tumors.[3] In the present study, we evaluated the presence of anti-p53 autoantibodies in colon cancer patients and their clinical significance.

MATERIALS AND METHODS

Patients

Heparinized blood (preoperative/postoperative) and tissue specimens were collected from 65 colon cancer patients.

Immunohistochemistry

Paraffin sections were stained with the DO-1 mAb, using the avidin-biotin peroxidase (ABC) method.

Serological Analysis

Microplates were coated with recombinant p53, blocked, and incubated with serum samples in various dilutions. The ELISA was developed by alkaline phosphatase–conjugated goat anti-human IgG. Background binding to no antigen wells was subtracted in all assays.

Immunoprecipitation and Immunoblotting

Extracts of ^{35}S-labeled SV80 cells and recombinant p53 were used for immunoprecipitation and immunoblotting, respectively.

RESULTS AND DISCUSSION

Tumor specimens from 65 colon cancer patients were immunohistochemically stained with the DO-1 mAb. Specific nuclear staining was detected in 46% of all carcinomas, whereas no such staining was found in normal colon tissues. Moreover, 13.8% of these patients revealed specific anti-p53 autoantibodies in their sera, detected by a sensitive ELISA (30% positive sera of patients with tumor p53 overexpression). Such antibodies were not detected in sera of 50 healthy controls. The

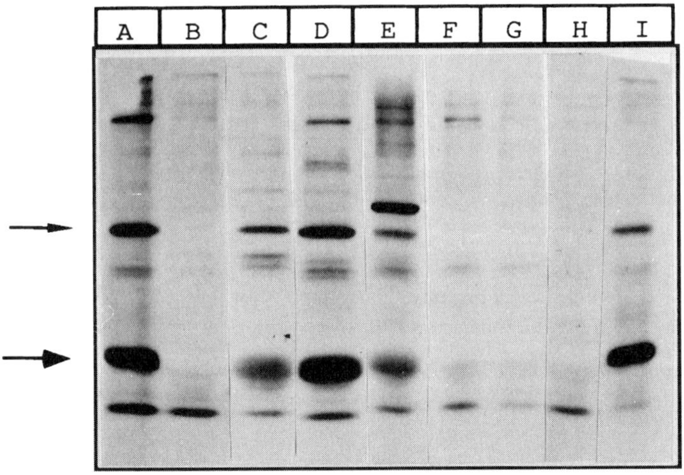

FIGURE 1. Immunoprecipitation of p53 (SV80) extract by sera of cancer colon patients: immunoprecipitation of p53 from ^{35}S-labeled SV80 cells by 421 anti-p53 mAb (lanes A, I), positive colon cancer sera (C, D, E), normal sera (B, H), and negative colon cancer sera (F, G). Note the coprecipitation of p53 (large arrow) with the large T antigen (small arrow).

positive, but not negative, sera demonstrated specific staining of the p53-positive cell line (SV80). The p53-negative cell line (SaOs-3) was not stained. To confirm the ELISA results, we examined the sera for p53 reactivity by immunoprecipitation and immunoblotting. As shown in FIGURE 1, positive, but not negative, sera from colon cancer patients immunoprecipitated ^{35}S-labeled p53 from SV80-transformed fibroblasts. Similar results were obtained by Western blot analysis. Follow-up of several patients revealed the disappearance of those antibodies following surgical removal of the tumor (FIGURE 2). In one patient, a specific increase in the anti-p53 autoantibodies

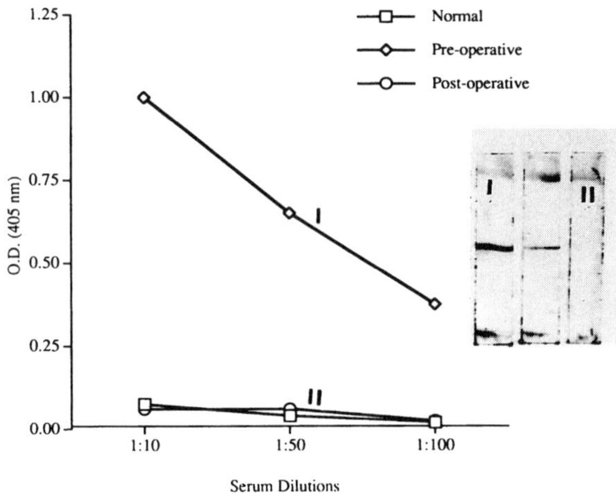

	IgG	IgM	IgA
Pre-operative (mg%)	1210	96	371
Post-operative (mg%)	1060	95	298

FIGURE 2. Levels of anti-p53 autoantibodies before and after tumor surgery: anti-p53 autoantibodies detected before surgery (I) disappeared after surgery (II). There was no change in the total immunoglobulins.

titer preceded the disease recurrency. Thus, the humoral immune response against p53 may have a role in the diagnosis and follow-up of patients with colon cancer.

REFERENCES

1. Rotter, V., O. Foord & N. Navot. 1993. In search of the functions of normal p53 protein. Trends Cell Biol. **3:** 46–49.
2. Milner, J. & E. A. Metcalf. 1991. Cotranslation of activated mutant p53 with wild type drives the wild-type p53 protein into the mutant conformation. Cell **65:** 765–774.
3. Rodrigues, N. R., A. Rowan, M. E. F. Smith, I. B. Kerr, W. F. Bodmer, J. V. Gannon & D. P. Lane. 1990. p53 mutations in colorectal cancer. Proc. Natl. Acad. Sci. U.S.A. **87:** 7444–7449.

Modulation of the Autoimmune Response in Lupus Mice by Oral Administration of Attenuated *Salmonella typhimurium* Expressing the IL-2 and TGF-β Genes

M. L. HUGGINS,[a] F-P. HUANG,[a] D. XU,[a] G. LINDOP,[b] AND D. I. STOTT[a,c]

[a]*University Department of Immunology*
[b]*University Department of Pathology*
Western Infirmary
Glasgow G11 6NT, Scotland, United Kingdom

INTRODUCTION

MRL-*lpr/lpr* mice spontaneously develop many of the features of the human autoimmune disease, systemic lupus erythematosus (SLE), including production of autoantibodies against DNA and other nuclear antigens, impaired T cell responses, glomerulonephritis, and vasculitis, and are consequently regarded as an animal model of this disease. The mice have a mutation in the *fas* gene that prevents T cell apoptosis and that is believed to be the cause of proliferation of large numbers of T cells expressing neither CD4 nor CD8 cell surface markers (double-negative T cells). In a previous study, we demonstrated a defect in the ability of MRL-*lpr/lpr* T cells to proliferate and secrete interleukin-2 (IL-2) *in vitro*. These functions can be restored by exogenous IL-2.[1] On the other hand, TGF_{β} has anti-inflammatory activity and inhibits IL-1-dependent T cell proliferation and B cell proliferation. We therefore decided to examine the effects of IL-2 and TGF_{β} *in vivo* using a nonpathogenic, attenuated strain of *Salmonella typhimurium* as a vector for the genes encoding these cytokines. The effects of oral administration of transfected *Salmonella* on immunological and pathological parameters of disease in MRL-*lpr/lpr* mice were investigated.

METHODS

The *S. typhimurium aroA*$^-$ *aroD*$^-$ double-mutant BRD509, transfected with the plasmid constructs pKK-IL-2 (containing the murine IL-2 gene) or pKK-TGF_{β} (containing the murine TGF_{β} gene), expresses the transfected cytokine gene and slowly releases the active cytokine *in vivo*.[2,3] Bacteria were administered in phosphate-

[c]To whom all correspondence should be addressed.

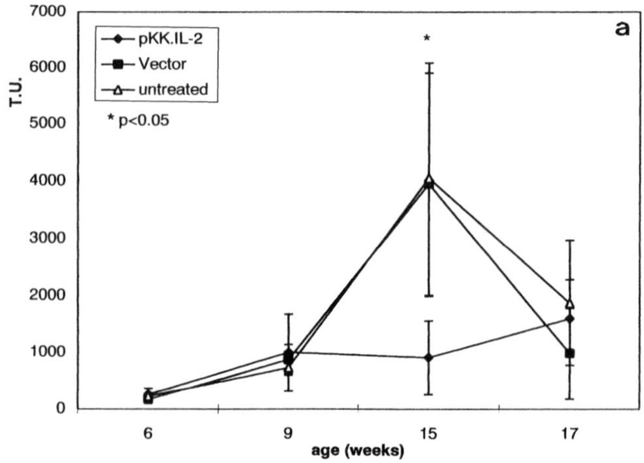

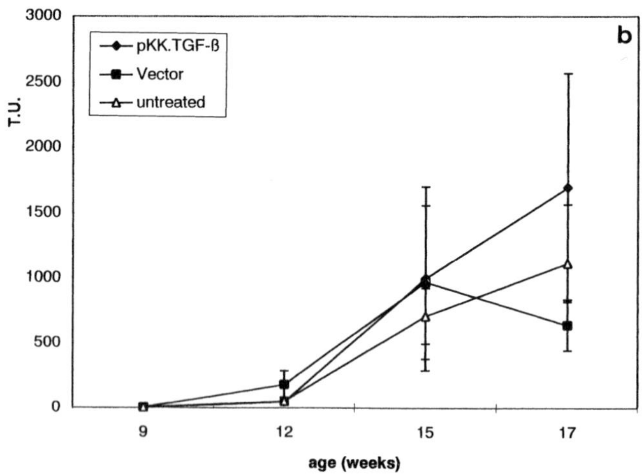

FIGURE 1. Changes in the titer of IgG anti-dsDNA antibodies in the serum of MRL-*lpr/lpr* mice with age after gavage with *Salmonella typhimurium* BRD509 transfected with (a) pKK-IL-2 or (b) pKK-TGF$_{\beta}$.

buffered saline (PBS) by gavage to 6-week-old MRL-*lpr/lpr* mice (10^9 bacteria per mouse, 10 mice per group) and the dose was repeated at three weekly intervals, to 15 weeks of age. Mice were bled from the tail vein before each dose of bacteria. Control groups received the vector only (BRD509) or no treatment. Mice were killed at 17 weeks of age by cervical dislocation. Proteinuria was assessed using Multistix SG (Bayer Diagnostics) and blood was collected by cardiac puncture. The spleens were weighed and the cells from the pKK-IL-2 group and their controls were pooled. The spleen cells from the pKK-TGF$_\beta$-treated mice and controls were analyzed individually. Numbers of double-negative ($CD3^+CD4^-CD8^-$) T cells were determined by flow cytometry and cell proliferation was measured by uptake of [^{3}H]-thymidine. Serum anti-ssDNA and anti-dsDNA antibodies were measured by ELISA as previously described.[4] The kidneys were fixed in neutral buffered formalin and sections were stained with hematoxylin and eosin; glomerulonephritis was scored blindly on a

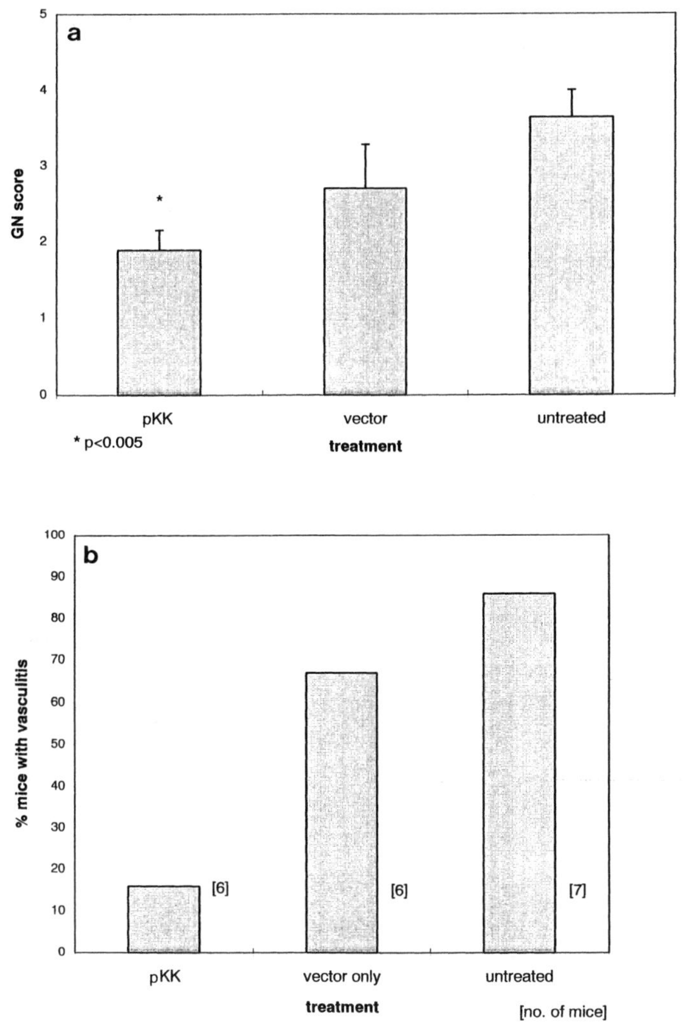

FIGURE 2. Renal pathology of 17-week-old MRL-*lpr/lpr* mice after gavage with *Salmonella typhimurium* BRD509 transfected with pKK-IL-2: (a) glomerulonephritis (GN) score; (b) incidence of vasculitis.

five-point scale and the presence or absence of vasculitis was noted. Results are expressed as mean ± standard error of the mean unless otherwise indicated.

RESULTS

Spleen weights and the number of double-negative T cells were not significantly affected by treatment with *Salmonella* transfected with the murine IL-2 or TGF_{β} genes. The proliferative response of splenic T cells to concanavalin A (Con A) alone and to Con A plus IL-2 *in vitro* was restored by treatment *in vivo* with pKK-IL-2, whereas pKK-TGF_{β} had a suppressive effect, but this was not significant when compared with the vector-treated group.

Serum IgG anti-ssDNA and anti-dsDNA antibody titers were suppressed in 15-week-old mice treated with pKK-IL-2 compared with the control groups, whereas pKK-TGF_{β}-treated mice had increased levels of anti-DNA antibodies in their serum at the end of the treatment (FIGURES 1a and 1b).

TGF_{β} had little effect on glomerulonephritis, but exacerbated the proteinuria and vasculitis observed in untreated mice. In contrast, a small reduction of proteinuria in the IL-2-treated group was not significant. IL-2 treatment did, however, cause a significant reduction in glomerulonephritis and vasculitis (FIGURES 2a and 2b).

DISCUSSION

We have shown that oral administration of attenuated *Salmonella* transfected with cytokine genes is a viable method of modulating the autoimmune response. Gene therapy with plasmid pKK-IL-2 restored the defective proliferative response of MRL-*lpr/lpr* T cells and suppressed autoantibody production, glomerulonephritis, and vasculitis. Surprisingly, treatment with pKK-TGF_{β} generally had opposite effects to pKK-IL-2. Previous work using vaccinia virus as a vector for IL-2[5] or naked DNA[6] showed similar results, but in the former case the double-negative T cell population was also suppressed and in the latter there was an increase in mortality. It therefore appears that the effects of IL-2 gene therapy depend upon the carrier and route of administration. Advantages of *Salmonella* as a vector are the ease of administration by the oral route and the delivery to secondary lymphoid organs (spleen and lymph nodes) from the gut.[3]

REFERENCES

1. HUANG, F-P. & D. I. STOTT. 1993. Autoimmunity **15:** 19–29.
2. IANARO, A., D. XU, C. A. O'DONNELL, M. DI ROSA & F. Y. LIEW. 1995. Immunology **84:** 8–15.
3. CARRIER, M. J., S. N. CHATFIELD, G. DOUGAN, U. T. A. NOWICKA, D. O'CALLAGHAN, J. E. BEESLEY, S. MILANO, E. CILLARI & F. Y. LIEW. 1992. J. Immunol. **148:** 1176–1181.
4. STOTT, D. I., G. BRIGHOUSE, Y. GYOTOKU & P-H. LAMBERT. 1990. Autoimmunity **8:** 159–168.
5. GUITIERREZ-RAMOS, J. C., J. L. ANDREU, Y. REVILLA, E. VINUELA & A. C. MARTINEZ. 1990. Nature **346:** 271–274.
6. RAZ, E., J. DUDLER, M. LOTZ, S. M. BAIRD, C. C. BERRY, R. A. EISENBERG & D. A. CARSON. 1995. Lupus **4:** 286–292.

Autoimmune Reactions Induced by Gliadin Feeding in Germ-free AVN Rats and Athymic Nude Mice

Animal Models for Celiac Disease

H. TLASKALOVÁ-HOGENOVÁ, R. ŠTĚPÁNKOVÁ, M. FARRÉ, D. P. FUNDA, Z. ŘEHÁKOVÁ, J. ŠINKORA, L. TUČKOVÁ, I. HORAK, D. HORÁKOVÁ, B. CUKROWSKA, H. KOZÁKOVÁ, AND J. KOLÍNSKÁ

Division of Immunology and Gnotobiology
Institute of Microbiology
Academy of Science of the Czech Republic
142 20 Prague, the Czech Republic
and
Institute of Virology
University of Würzburg
Würzburg, Germany

Celiac disease develops in susceptible humans after gliadin (gluten) ingestion. Autoimmune features occurring frequently in patients with celiac disease suggest that this disease represents a unique model of autoimmune condition affecting the gut where the triggering agent is well known.[1] Experimental models of gluten-induced enteropathy are useful in elucidating the pathogenetic mechanisms of the disease.

GLIADIN-INDUCED ENTEROPATHY IN GERM-FREE AVN RATS AND ITS TRANSFER BY INTRAEPITHELIAL LYMPHOCYTES

Gliadin in increasing amounts (0.5–5 mg/dose) was administered intragastrically three times a week for two months starting at birth to germ-free rats of inbred AVN strain.[2] Intraepithelial lymphocytes (IEL) were isolated from rat jejunum and their surface markers were determined by flow cytometry. They were then labeled with fluorescein isothiocyanate and injected into the lumen of jejunal loops of recipient adult rats.

Prolonged application of gliadin led to shortening of jejunal villi, crypt hyperplasia, increased number of mitoses in the crypt epithelium, and increased number of intraepithelial and lamina propria lymphocytes. Morphological changes were accompanied by changes in brush-border enzyme activities (e.g., dipeptidylpeptidase IV and lactase). Intestinal intraepithelial lymphocytes (CD8+, RGL1+) isolated from rats fed with gliadin and injected into intestinal loops of untreated rats caused damage of the tight junctions of the enterocytes. These transferred IEL penetrated through the

TABLE 1. Body Weight Development in Athymic Nude BALB/c Mice Fed with Gliadin or Bovine Serum Albumin

	Body Weight (grams)		
	Before Feeding	During Feeding	
	10 Days	Third Week	Seventh Week
gliadin (n = 12)	5.5 ± 1.2	8.5 ± 2.4	11.0 ± 1.7
albumin (n = 10)	5.5 ± 1.2	10.7 ± 2.3	14.9 ± 2.9

intestinal epithelial layer and appeared in the lamina propria, whereas IEL isolated from control rats did not induce mucosal changes and failed to penetrate.

ENTEROPATHY INDUCTION IN IMMUNODEFICIENT NUDE MICE

Gliadin or albumin (in controls) was administered similarly as described above to mice of various strains starting at 10 days of age. Because conventional mice of different genetic backgrounds were not sensitive to gliadin feeding, immunodeficient

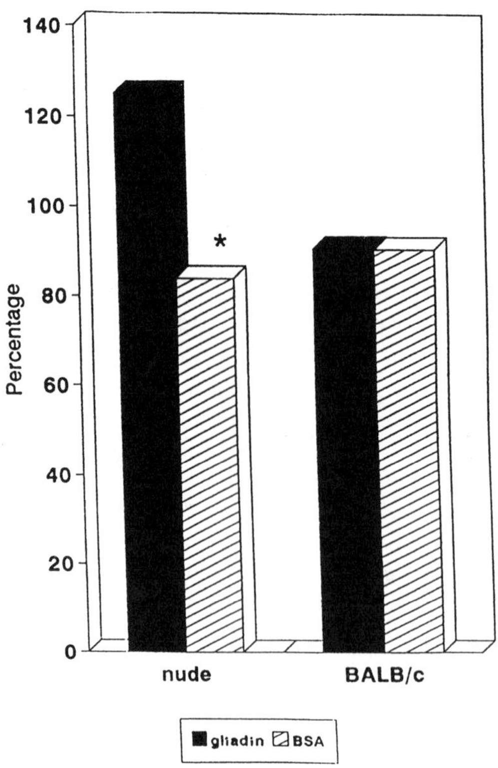

FIGURE 1. Antienterocyte autoantibody activity determined by ELISA in sera of 2-month-old athymic nude and conventional BALB/c mice fed with gliadin or bovine serum albumin (BSA) (*: $p < 0.05$). The ELISA method for antienterocyte antibody detection is described in detail in reference 1.

strains of mice, that is, athymic nu/nu BALB/c mice, mice with targeted disruption of the IL-2 gene (IL-2 KO), and a BALB/c strain with severe combined immunodeficiency (SCID), were used.

We found a profound impairment of intestinal mucosa that correlated with growth retardation of gliadin-fed athymic nude mice (TABLE 1). Autoantibodies against enterocytes were increased in the sera and intestinal content of gliadin-fed nude mice (FIGURE 1). IL-2 KO mice exhibited only minimal changes, whereas in SCID mice no intestinal damage was found. From these results, we conclude that impairment of immunoregulatory mechanisms in animals fed with gliadin could lead to induction of mucosal lesions.

REFERENCES

1. TUČKOVÁ, L., H. TLASKALOVÁ, M. FARRÉ, K. KARSKÁ, J. KOLÍNSKÁ & P. KOCNA. 1995. Clin. Immunol. Immunopathol. **74:** 170–176.
2. ŠTĚPÁNKOVÁ, R., H. TLASKALOVÁ-HOGENOVÁ, J. ŠINKORA, J. JODL & P. FRIČ. 1996. Scand. J. Gastroenterol. **31:** 551–557.

Do Certain Autoantibodies Produced in the Course of Human Autoimmune Blistering Skin Diseases Behave as Adhesion Molecules?[a]

DANIÈLE GILBERT, FRÉDÉRIC BRARD,
PHILIPPE COURVILLE, PASCAL JOLY,
PHILIPPE LAURET, AND FRANÇOIS TRON

Groupe de Recherche en Immunopathologie
Institut Fédératif de Recherche Multidisciplinaire sur les Peptides 23
Faculté Mixte de Médecine et de Pharmacie
Hôpital Charles Nicolle
76031 Rouen, France

Pemphigus diseases are autoimmune bullous skin diseases caused by autoantibodies directed against desmosomal molecules that are present at the surface of keratinocytes. Different types of pemphigus have been described, each characterized by the production of autoantibodies directed against particular antigenic structures.[1] Pemphigus vulgaris and pemphigus foliaceus autoantibodies recognize, respectively, desmoglein 3 (Dsg3) and desmoglein 1 (Dsg1), which both are members of the cadherin family. The activity of the desmosomal cadherins involves interactions on both sides of the membrane. The extracellular domains are responsible for homophilic recognition thought to result from amino acid sequences located within the first extracellular domain, EC1. Autoantibodies produced during the course of pemphigus vulgaris and pemphigus foliaceus bind to the extracellular domains of Dsg1 and Dsg3.[2,3] On the intracellular side, the activity of cadherins depends on sequences that interact with cytoplasmic proteins involved in the formation of the desmosomal plaque. Some of these proteins such as desmoplakin I and II are recognized by autoantibodies present in the sera of patients with paraneoplastic pemphigus, a third category of pemphigus associated with various neoplastic conditions.[4] Thus, autoantibodies produced in the course of pemphigus may target both transmembrane and intracellular proteins of desmosomes.

Recently, we reported the production of a human monoclonal autoantibody (mAb F12) derived from the peripheral blood lymphocytes of a pemphigus vulgaris patient.[5] mAb F12 was selected based on its capacity to bind the keratinocyte cell membrane and the basement membrane zone of stratified squamous epithelia and was demon-

[a]This work was supported by the Institut National de la Santé et de la Recherche Médicale (INSERM, CRI 950602) and the Direction de la Recherche et des Etudes Doctorales.

strated to react with a 185-kDa polypeptide by immunoblotting, using bovine tongue epithelium as the substrate, and to recognize a component of the desmosomal plaque by immunoelectron microscopy.[5,6]

Nucleotide sequence analysis of heavy-chain (V_H) and light-chain (V_L) variable-region genes encoding autoantibodies gives insight on their structural characteristics and may help to understand their functional properties. We have cloned and sequenced the V_H and V_L genes of mAb F12 and showed that the third and the second complementarity-determining regions (CDR) of the heavy chain shared, respectively, a 4 (glycine-serine-serine-glycine)– and a 3 (glycine-serine-serine)–amino acid sequence with the intracellular domain of Dsg1, likely involved in the interaction with components of the desmosomal plaque (FIGURE 1). Therefore, we hypothesized that

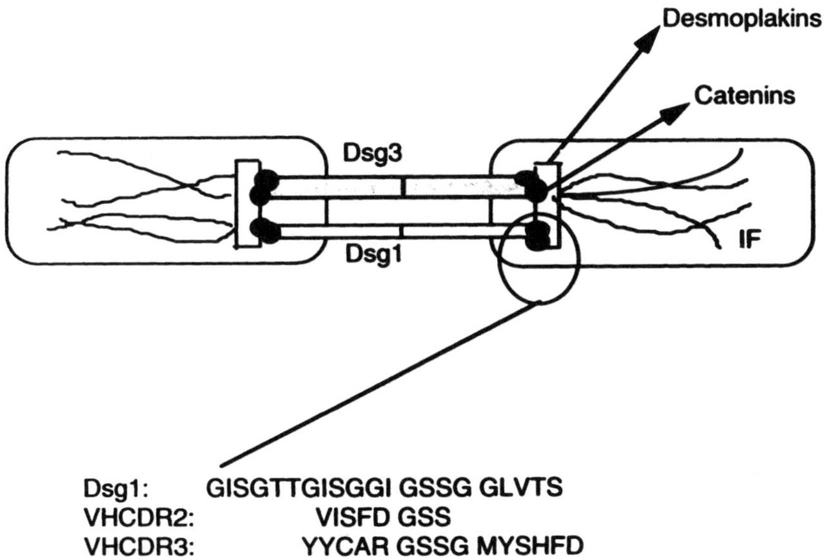

FIGURE 1. Scheme depicting the desmosomal proteins involved in the keratinocyte junctions and the shared amino acid sequence between V_H-CDR2, V_H-CDR3, and the intracellular domain of Desmoglein 1 (Dsg1).

the GSSG and GSS sequences are important in the functional property of mAb F12, which might interact with a desmosomal plaque component through molecular mimicry of the glycine-serine-rich motif of Dsg1 involved in protein-protein adhesion. This hypothesis was strongly supported by the following: (i) the observation that some glycine and serine residues located in the CDRs were derived from an antigen-driven mutational process (CDR2) or from junctional diversity (CDR3); (ii) the demonstration that a synthetic peptide containing the entire V_H-GSSG-CDR3 was able to inhibit mAb F12 interaction to the target antigens, whereas no inhibition was observed when a V_H-CDR3 synthetic peptide lacking the sequence was tested.

Taken together, these data suggest that autoantibodies produced during the course of autoimmune blistering skin diseases behave as adhesion molecules, which may represent a new self-antigen-binding mechanism of autoantibodies.

REFERENCES

1. STANLEY, J. R. 1989. Pemphigus and pemphigoid as paradigms of organ-specific, autoantibody-mediated disease. J. Clin. Invest. **83:** 1443–1448.
2. DMOCHOWSKI, M., T. HASHIMOTO, M. AMAGAI, J. KUDOH, N. SHIMIZU, P. J. KOCH, W. W. FRANKE & T. NISHIKAWA. 1994. The extracellular amino-terminal domain of bovine desmoglein 1 (Dsg1) is recognized only by certain pemphigus foliaceus sera, whereas its intracellular domain is recognized by both pemphigus vulgaris and pemphigus foliaceus sera. J. Invest. Dermatol. **103:** 173–177.
3. AMAGAI, M., K. V. KLAUS & J. R. STANLEY. 1991. Autoantibodies against a novel epithelial cadherin in pemphigus vulgaris, a disease of cell adhesion. Cell **67:** 869–877.
4. ANHALT, G. J., S. C. KIM, J. R. STANLEY, N. J. KORMAN, D. A. JABS, M. KORY, H. IZUMI, H. RATRIE III, D. MUTASIM, L. ARISS-ABDO & R. S. LABIB. 1990. Paraneoplastic pemphigus, an autoimmune mucocutaneous disease associated with neoplasia. N. Engl. J. Med. **323:** 1729–1735.
5. GILBERT, D., P. JOLY, A. THIBOUT, A. DELPECH, E. THOMINE, PH. LAURET & F. TRON. 1992. Production of a human monoclonal anti-epithelial cell surface antibody from a patient with pemphigus vulgaris. J. Autoimmun. **5:** 173–182.
6. JOLY, P., D. GILBERT, E. THOMINE, A. DELPECH, S. VERDIER, PH. LAURET & F. TRON. 1993. Immunofluorescence and immunoelectron microscopy analyses of a human monoclonal anti-epithelial cell surface antibody that recognizes a 185-kD polypeptide: a component of the paraneoplastic pemphigus antigenic complex? J. Invest. Dermatol. **101:** 339–345.

Characterization by Molecular Cloning an Antigen Reactive with Antireticulin Antibodies

RAIVO UIBO,[a,b] OIVI UIBO,[c] KOIT REIMAND,[a]
PÄRT PETERSON,[b] AND KAI KROHN[b]

[a]*Department of Immunology*
Institute of General and Molecular Pathology
University of Tartu
EE2400 Tartu, Estonia

[b]*Institute of Medical Technology*
University of Tampere
FIN 33101 Tampere, Finland

[c]*Department of Pediatrics*
Children's Clinic
University of Tartu
EE2400 Tartu, Estonia

Antireticulin antibodies of the R1-type pattern (ARA) are widely used laboratory markers for active celiac disease (CD), a cereal-induced enteropathy with serious clinical complications.[1] The exact nature of the antigens reacting with ARA has so far remained unknown. In the present study, we have aimed to characterize the target molecule(s) for ARA, using molecular cloning of a cDNA library.[2]

We select for molecular cloning a human fetal lung cDNA expression library in the bacteriophage λgt11 vector (Clontech Laboratories, Palo Alto, California) because of the high content of ARA-reactive antigenic material in the lung tissue of the human embryo.[3] The library with cDNA inserts in the range of 0.6 to 4.0 kb (lot no. 1761) was plated three times onto Luria-Bertani agar plates (5×10^4 PFU/90-mm plate), transferred to nitrocellulose filters, and immunoscreened for ARA antigens as detailed elsewhere.[2,4] For the immunoscreening, a mixture of three sera (1:1:1) from three patients with different clinical forms (active = 2; latent = 1) of CD was used. All these sera contained IgA and IgG class ARA detected by routine indirect immunofluorescence (rodent kidney and stomach cryostat sections as antigen substrates) and gave several bands with human fetal lung proteins in immunoblot. For control, a mixture of three other sera (1:1:1), negative for ARA, was used.

Although a total of 12 immunoreactive clones were revealed in the first round of clonings, only 1 of them, clone FLIII3, preserved reactivity until a homogeneous population of immunoreactive phages was obtained. The cDNA of this clone was purified,[4] cloned into the *Eco*RI site of the vector M13mp10, and sequenced by the dideoxy method (Sequenase 2.0 kit, United States Biochemicals, Cleveland, Ohio). The size of the cDNA insert of FLIII3 was 258 base pairs (FIGURE 1) and it did not have sequence homologies with known proteins available in Genbank analyzed by the GCG program package.[5] However, the protein contained amino acid sequence QQQF (one-letter code), a common sequence of different CD precipitable gliadins.[6]

For antibody studies, the cDNA of FLIII3 was inserted in pGEMEX-1 (Promega Laboratories, Madison, Wisconsin) as an *Eco*RI fragment. Protein was expressed in *E. coli* JM109 (DE3) cells,[7] and the *E. coli* cell lysates were used in immunoblotting and in immunofluorescence inhibition experiments. In immunoblotting, 13 out of 15 ARA-positive CD sera and 2 out of 15 ARA-negative control sera reacted with FLIII3 recombinant protein at an optimal dilution of 1:800 (FIGURE 2). In the immunofluorescence test, preincubation of ARA-positive sera with FLIII3 protein in bacterial lysates did not influence the test results. Thus, FLIII3 protein does not contain ARA-reactive components.

In summary, we did not succeed in characterizing the antigen target(s) specifically reacting with ARA. However, we revealed a cDNA clone that codes a protein reacting with a high percentage of sera from patients with CD. Whether this reactivity reflects the cross-reactivity between gliadins and autoantigens, as recently demonstrated by Karská *et al.*,[8] remains to be studied.

GGG AAA TAC GGA GGT GAT GTC TCA AAG TCT
G K Y G G D V S K S

GAC GTG CAA CAA GCA TTT GAT ACG CAA AAG
D V Q Q A F D T Q K

GCG CAA TAC GGC GAT GCC TTC AAG ACC GTC
A Q Y G D A F K T V

TTA GCT TCA AAC AAT ATG ACT GAA GCA CAA
L A S N N M T E A Q

TTC AAG ACG AAC ATC AAA AAC AAT TTG ATT
F K T N I K N N L I

ATG ACG GCA GCT GTG AAA GCC AAC TAC AGG
M T A A V K A N Y R

TGT CAA ACA GCC AAC TTG AAC AAG CTT ACA
C Q T A N L N K L T

AAG ACT ATC ATC AAT CAA CAA CAA TTT CGA
K T I I N Q Q Q F R

TGA TTA AAC GAA AGA TGA
*** L N E R ***

FIGURE 1. Nucleotide and amino acid sequences of clone FLIII3. The amino acids are presented in single-letter code. Underlined amino acids represent a sequence common to different gliadins.[6]

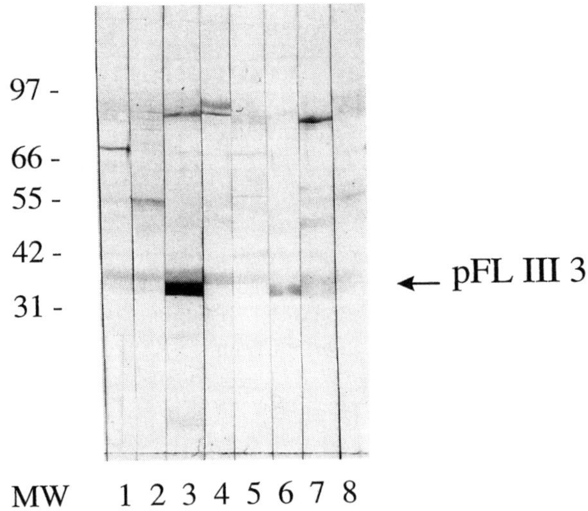

FIGURE 2. Immunoblot results of controls (strips 1, 2, 4, 5, 7, and 8) and celiac disease (CD) patients (strips 3 and 6) with recombinant protein FLIII3. Note the comparable weak reactions of a CD patient (strip 6) and a control person (strip 7).

REFERENCES

1. Mäki, M. 1992. Use of serological antibody tests in celiac disease. *In* Gluten-sensitive Enteropathy. D. Branski, P. Rozen & M. F. Kagnoff, Eds.: 108–129. Karger. Basel.
2. Krohn, K., R. Uibo, E. Aavik, P. Peterson & K. Savilahti. 1992. Identification by molecular cloning of an autoantigen associated with Addison's disease as steroid 17α-hydroxylase. Lancet **339:** 770–773.
3. Mäki, M., O. Hällström & A. Marttinen. 1991. Reaction of human non-collagenous polypeptides with celiac disease autoantibodies. Lancet **338:** 724–725.
4. Sambrook, J., E. F. Fritch & T. Maniatis. 1989. Molecular Cloning: A Laboratory Manual. Cold Spring Harbor Laboratory. New York.
5. Devereux, J., P. Harberei & O. Smithies. 1990. A comprehensive set of sequence analysis programs for the VAX. Nucleic Acids Res. **18:** 387–395.
6. Wieser, H. 1991. Chemistry of gliadins. Eur. J. Gastroenterol. Hepatol. **3:** 102–107.
7. Studiert, F. W. & B. A. Moffart. 1986. Use of bacteriophage T7 polymerase to direct selective high expression of cloned genes. J. Mol. Biol. **189:** 113–141.
8. Karská, K., L. Tučková, L. Steiner, H. Tlaskalová-Hogenová & M. Michalak. 1995. Calreticulin—the potential autoantigen in celiac disease. Biochem. Biophys. Res. Commun. **209:** 597–605.

CRI-EM Is a Human Idiotype Highly Specific for Scleroderma[a]

DOLORES VÁZQUEZ-ABAD,[b] LI TIAN,[b]
VÍCTOR MONTEÓN,[b] MAURIZIO ZANETTI,[c]
AND NAOMI F. ROTHFIELD[b]

[b]*Division of Rheumatic Diseases*
University of Connecticut Health Center
Farmington, Connecticut 06030

[c]*Cancer Center*
University of California
San Diego, California 92093

INTRODUCTION

Autoantibodies (autoAbs) in scleroderma (SSc) are disease-specific (reviewed in reference 1). We have found a cross-reactive idiotype (CRI) shared by antitopoisomerase-I, antibodies to centromeric protein B, and IgGs from SSc patients.[2] To define the SSc specificity of CRI-EM, we screened the following: non-autoAbs-Igs from 7 SSc patients; sera from 40 normal individuals who have no autoAbs; and sera and Igs from 17 SLE patients with high levels of anti-double-stranded DNA (α-dsDNA) or antibodies to extractable nuclear antigens (α-ENA). CRI-EM was not found in any of these samples.

METHODS

Sera

Sera from 40 normal individuals (NHS) and 17 patients with SLE[3] were studied (TABLE 1).

Screening for the Presence of AutoAbs

All sera were tested for the presence of autoAbs as described.[4–6]

Affinity-purified AutoAbs and Non-AutoAb SSc Igs

After affinity purification of 3 antitopo-I and 4 anti-CENP-B, the nonbound fraction was collected and Ig concentration was determined.[7] Ig classes of SLE sera

[a]This work was supported by grants of the National Institutes of Health (No. K08-AR01954-01 to D. Vázquez-Abad and Nos. AR37986 and AR20621 to N. F. Rothfield) and by the University of Connecticut Health Center's RISE grant to D. Vázquez-Abad.

were purified using a Sepharose 4B gel (Pharmacia, Uppsala, Sweden) coupled with goat anti-human Fcγ, α, and μ (Organon Teknika Company, Durham, North Carolina) as described.[7]

Competitive Inhibition ELISAs

Plates were coated with 10 μg/mL of Ig contained in the non-autoAb SSc Igs. Anti-Id to antitopo-I EM was added with buffer or with 1, 0.1, or 0.01 μg/mL of affinity-purified antitopo-I EM. Swine anti-rabbit HRP (Dakopatts) was added, and

TABLE 1. Autoantibody Profile of the 17 SLE Sera Studied

	FARR (%)	α-RNP[a]	α-Sm[a]	α-La[a]	α-Ro[a]
1	86.0	0	0	0	0
2	87.2	0	0	0	0
3	86.3	0	0	0	0
4	81.0	0	0	0	0
5[b]	nr[c]	0	0	0	0
6	88.8	0	0	0	0
7	86.8	0	64	64	64
8	91.7	0	0	2	2
9	85.6	0	0	0	0
10	93.6	0	0	0	0
11	83.0	16	8	8	undiluted
12	1.7	16	32	32	64
13	2.8	64	32	32	256
14	9.0	16	32	32	8
15	nr	128	64	8	undiluted
16	0.2	64	512	512	4
17	1.6	16	16	16	2

[a]α-ENA were detected by DID. Numbers = highest dilution at which the sample was positive.

[b]This patient's serum was included even though it was negative for α-dsDNA and α-ENA because it was from a patient with lupus nephritis, whose father died of SSc, and was positive for antitopo-I.

[c]nr = nonreactive.

the plates were developed as described[4,7] and read at 405 nm using a BioRad 3550 microplate reader (BioRad).

Detection of CRI-EM in Patient Sera

Plates were coated with an α-human Fc followed by the patients' sera or affinity-purified Igs. Serum or affinity-purified EM and normal human serum devoid of autoAbs and negative CRI-EM were used as (+) and (−) controls.[7] The plates were incubated with an optimal concentration of rabbit anti-EM[7] followed by incubation with swine anti-rabbit Igs coupled to HRP (Dakopatts). Plates were developed and read. The OD ratios were calculated as follows:

$$\text{ratio} = \frac{(\text{mean OD sample})}{(\text{mean OD negative control})}.$$

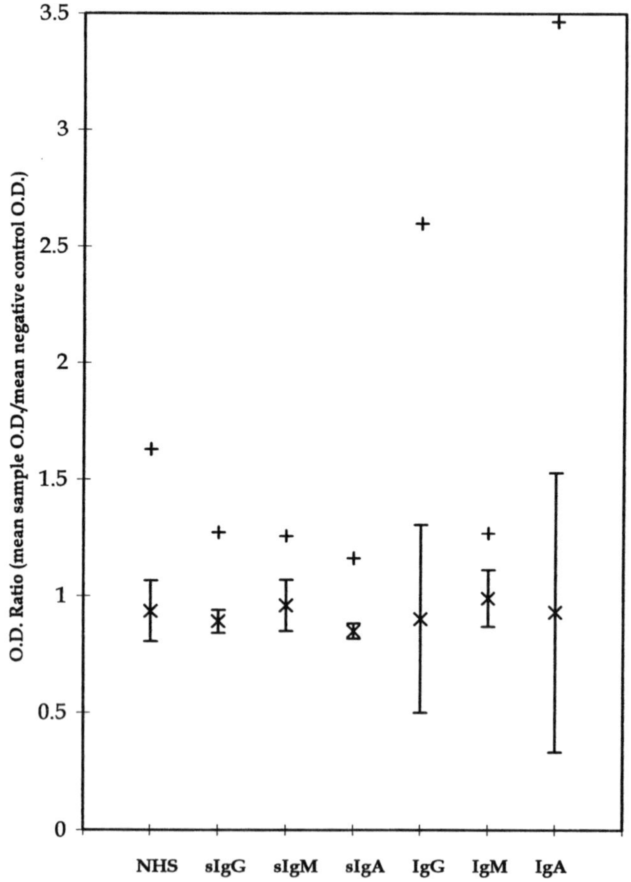

FIGURE 1. CRI-EM OD ratios. The CRI-EM OD ratios were obtained as described in the text. The y-axis shows the mean ratios of the 7 different groups. The x-axis shows the group samples tested: NHS = captured Igs from NHS (n = 40); sIgG = captured IgG from SLE serum (n = 17); sIgM = captured IgM from SLE serum (n = 17); sIgA = IgA from SLE serum (n = 17); IgG = captured IgG from SLE affinity-purified Igs (n = 17); IgM = captured IgM from SLE affinity-purified Igs (n = 17); IgA = IgA from SLE affinity-purified Igs (n = 17). Symbols: (⁑) mean CRI-EM OD and standard deviation of the samples in each group; (+) mean OD of the positive control (see text).

RESULTS

None of the 7 non-autoAb Igs showed dose-response inhibition curves and thus were negative for CRI-EM. Anti-idiotype to CRI-EM did not bind any of the 40 NHS or 17 SLE sera, nor the purified Igs from these 17 SLE patients (FIGURE 1).

DISCUSSION

CRI-EM is a highly sensitive CRI, found in SSc autoAbs.[2] We showed herein that CRI-EM is also highly specific because it is not present in the serum Igs from 40 normal individuals who have no autoAbs nor in the serum and affinity-purified Igs from 17 patients with SLE containing high titers of α-dsDNA and/or α-ENA autoAbs.

We believe that CRI-EM plays an important role in the abnormal B cell stimulation that leads to the continuous synthesis of SSc-specific autoAbs. In this study, we were able to show that CRI-EM is not present in the serum Igs from normal individuals nor in the serum and affinity-purified Igs containing high titers of α-dsDNA and/or α-ENA from SLE patients. These findings further support our hypothesis that CRI-EM is restricted to SSc.

REFERENCES

1. VÁZQUEZ-ABAD, D. & N. F. ROTHFIELD. 1995. Autoantibodies in systemic sclerosis. *In* Immunopathogenesis of Systemic Sclerosis. Reviews of Immunology. Volume 12. C. Leroy & J. Korn, Eds.: 145–157. Hardwood Acad. Pub. Chur, Switzerland.
2. VÁZQUEZ-ABAD, D., N. F. ROTHFIELD, W. C. EARNSHAW & M. ZANETTI. 1995. A common cross-reactive idiotype (CRI) is expressed on both anticentromere (ACA) and antitopoisomerase-I (antitopo) from scleroderma (SSc) patients. Arthritis Rheum. **38:** S320.
3. TAN, E. M., A. S. COHEN, J. F. FRIES, A. T. MASI, D. J. MCSHANE, N. F. ROTHFIELD, J. G. SCHALLER, N. TALAL & R. J. WINCHESTER. 1982. The 1982 revised criteria for the classification of systemic lupus erythematosus. Arthritis Rheum. **25:** 1271–1277.
4. VÁZQUEZ-ABAD, D., S. WALLACE, J-L. SÉNECAL, F. JOYAL, A. ROUSSIN, W. C. EARNSHAW & N. F. ROTHFIELD. 1994. Anticentromere autoantibodies—evaluation of an ELISA using recombinant fusion protein CENP-B as antigen. Arthritis Rheum. **37:** 248–252.
5. LUCIANO, A. & N. ROTHFIELD. 1974. Patterns of nuclear fluorescence and DNA binding activity. Ann. Rheum. Dis. **32:** 337–341.
6. CHAIM, B. M., M. G. PETERSON & N. F. ROTHFIELD. 1989. Correlation of anti-Ro antibody with photosensitivity rash in systemic lupus erythematosus patients. Arthritis Rheum. **32:** 202–204.
7. VÁZQUEZ-ABAD, D., V. PASCUAL, M. ZANETTI & N. F. ROTHFIELD. 1993. Analysis of human antitopoisomerase I idiotypes. J. Clin. Invest. **93:** 1301–1313.

Length Diversity of Immunoglobulin Heavy-Chain Variable Regions from Rheumatoid Arthritis Synovium[a]

D. G. WILLIAMS AND P. C. TAYLOR

Kennedy Institute of Rheumatology
London W6 7DW, United Kingdom

A characteristic of the synovial membrane from patients with rheumatoid arthritis (RA) is its infiltration with inflammatory cells, T cells, and plasma cells, producing immunoglobulin. On the microscopic scale, clonally related B lymphocytes in clusters within the RA synovium have been interpreted to represent focal clonal expansion and somatic mutation.[1,2] In order to investigate and characterize the specific immune mechanisms operating within this tissue, on a macroscopic scale we have sought evidence of clonal expansion of plasma cells at multiple synovial locations in patients with active disease. Rearrangement of the three immunoglobulin gene segments, V_H, D, and J_H, gives rise to the heavy-chain variable region. Addition and deletion of nucleotides at the V_H-D and D-J_H junctions give rise to a V-D-J length variability, which is compounded by genomic length differences within V_H. Each B lymphocyte clone and its progeny will be characterized by a particular V-D-J length. B cell clonal expansion may therefore be detectable as a recurrent V-D-J length.

Immunoglobulin V-D-J-C_{H1} cDNA was amplified from synovial biopsies by PCR using immunoglobulin hinge-region 3′ primers with immunoglobulin variable-region 5′ primers.[3] The diversity of these cDNAs was determined by analyzing the size heterogeneity (spectrotype) of the immunoglobulin V-D-J cDNA sequences derived in a subsequent PCR amplification. The immunoglobulin H-chain V-D-J cDNA sizes, determined by polyacrylamide gel electrophoresis, ranged from 112 to 134 codons (FIGURE 1). A similar size range was observed using each of the eight V_H primers, in both the IgG and IgM classes. The size range of rheumatoid synovial cDNAs was similar to that in juvenile infected tonsil and a Sjögren's syndrome spleen sample, although unusually long 135- and 136-codon variable regions were detectable in amplifications of RA synovia MG or B with V_H1f, 3a, and 3f. Significantly reduced clonal heterogeneity in isolated synovial cells was observed (FIGURE 1, tracks 4 and 5), suggesting that synovia from RA patients A and B may contain oligoclonal B lymphocyte populations.

The oligoclonality of synovial B lymphocytes was further investigated by analyzing the immunoglobulin cDNA clonal patterns in multiple synovial biopsies from an individual joint of patients with rheumatoid arthritis. FIGURE 2 shows an example of clonal expansion detected using this technique. Twelve biopsies (FIGURE 2, tracks

[a]This work was supported financially by the Arthritis and Rheumatism Council for Research (United Kingdom).

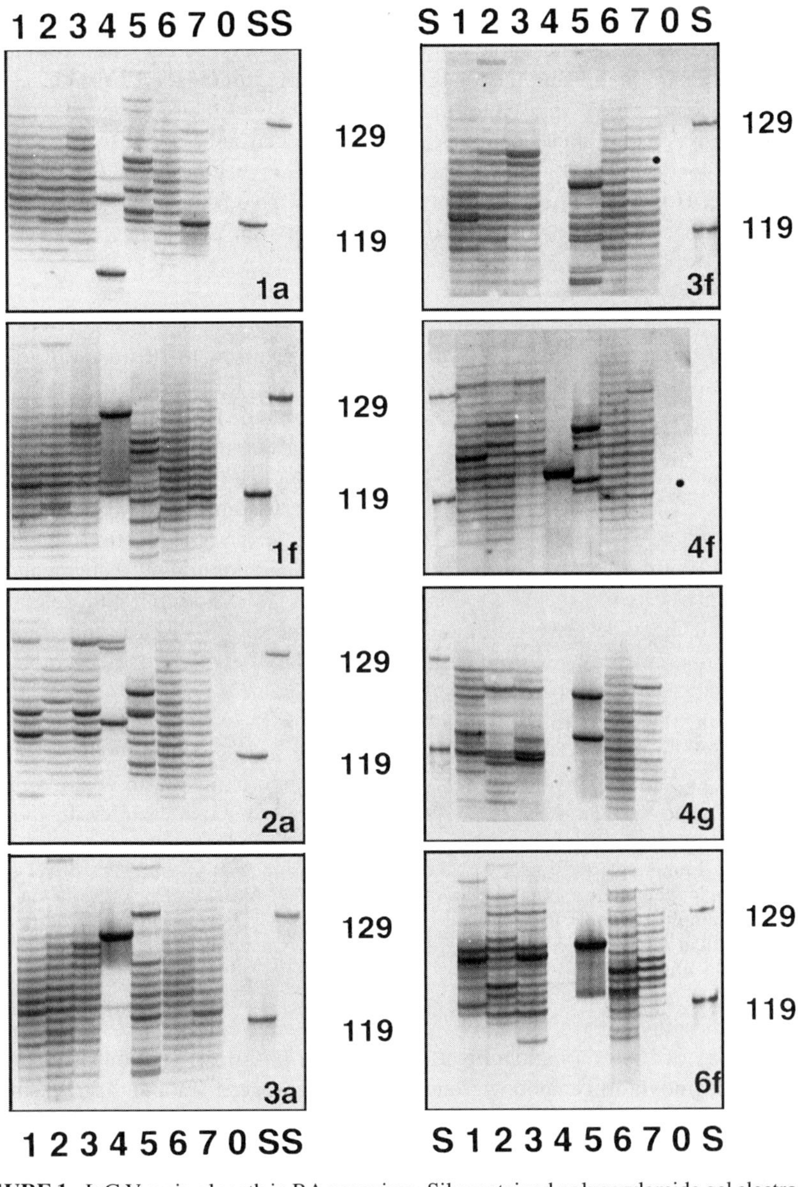

FIGURE 1. IgG V region length in RA synovium. Silver-stained polyacrylamide gel electrophoretograms of PCR-amplified V_HD_HJ cDNAs from an initial $V_HD_HJC_\mu1$ amplification, using eight different FR1 primers (V_H: 1a, 1f, 2a, 3a, 3f, 4f, 4g, and 6f), derived from synovial fluid (track 1), synovial tissue of RA patient MG (tracks 2 and 3), Ficoll-gradient separated lymphocytes from collagenase-digested synovium of RA patients A and B (tracks 4 and 5), juvenile tonsil tissue (track 6), or spleen tissue from a Sjögren's syndrome patient (track 7). The DNA template negative amplification is shown in track O. Tracks S contain two standard IgH clones of 119 and 129 codons in length for comparison.

A–L) from one inflamed knee synovium and a sample of peripheral blood (Z) of RA patient, GD, were analyzed. Three different sizes of IgG V-D-J cDNA (spectrotopes), reproducibly amplified using the V_H4g primer, recurred in most of the biopsies from three separate regions of synovium (FIGURE 2). In many of the biopsies, the recurring spectrotope was a dominant feature. The recurrent spectrotope was also present in the peripheral blood sample (FIGURE 2, track Z), suggesting that the clonal expansion may be systemic. However, other recurrent spectrotopes have been found that are absent from the peripheral blood sample taken at the time of arthroscopy.

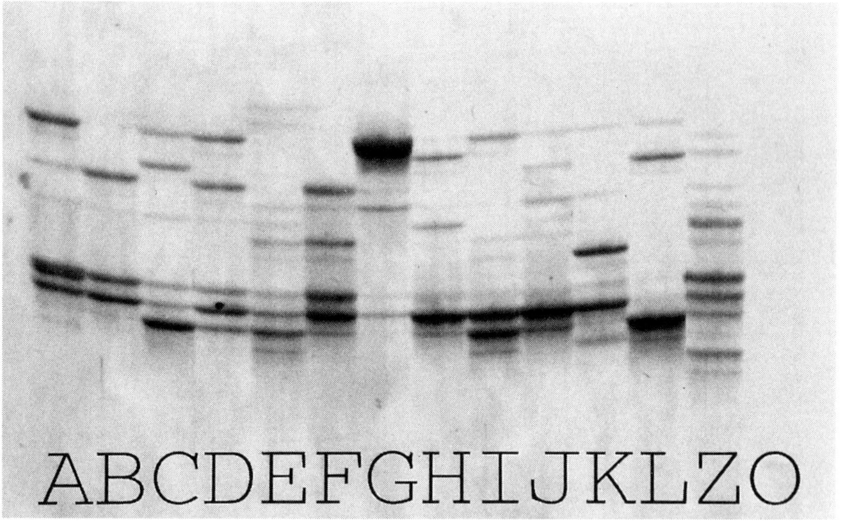

FIGURE 2. Immunoglobulin heavy chain clonal expansion in RA synovium. Silver-stained polyacrylamide gel electrophoretogram of PCR-amplified V_HD_HJ cDNAs from an initial $V_HD_HJC_{\gamma3}1$ amplification of RA synovial biopsies (tracks A–L) or peripheral blood (track Z) from RA patient GD, using V_H4g FR1 primers. The DNA template negative amplification is shown in track O.

Our analysis of immunoglobulin cDNA size distribution in synovium suggests that rheumatoid synovial B lymphocytes are not only heterogeneous, but that they include clonally expanded B cells. Selective clonal expansion on the macroscopic scale has been described previously in the light-chain repertoire.[4] Further confirmation of clonal relationships between recurrent spectrotopes was obtained by cloning and sequencing them from RA patient GD. One recurrent IgG spectrotope cloned separately from three different regions of knee synovium was identical at each site and used an unmutated germline V_H DP-7 gene sequence with an unmutated DK1, thereby confirming that clonally selective processes play a part in forming the synovial B lymphocyte population.

REFERENCES

1. SCHRODER, A. E., A. GREINER, C. SEYFERT & C. BEREK. 1996. Proc. Natl. Acad. Sci. U.S.A. **93:** 221–225.
2. GAUSE, A., K. GUNDLACH, M. ZDICHAVSKY, G. JACOBS, B. KOCH, T. HOPF & M. PFREUNDSCHUH. 1995. Eur. J. Immunol. **25:** 2775–2782.
3. BARBAS, C. F. & R. A. LERNER. 1992. Methods: Companion Methods Enzymol. **2:** 119–124.
4. LEE, S. K., S. L. BRIDGES, JR., P. M. KIRKHAM, W. J. KOOPMAN & H. W. SCHROEDER, JR. 1994. J. Clin. Invest. **93:** 361–370.

Fibroblast Growth Factor–like Autoantibodies in Plasma from Patients with Multiple Endocrine Neoplasia Type 1 and Prolactinoma

M. B. ZIMERING,[a] N. KATSUMATA,[b] H. G. FRIESEN,[b] J. ENG,[c] D. J. RILEY,[a] S. THAKKER-VARIA,[a] S. J. MARX,[d] AND S. EZZAT[e]

[a]*Department of Medicine*
UMDNJ–Robert Wood Johnson Medical School
Piscataway, New Jersey 08854
and
Department of Medical Service
Veterans Administration Medical Center
Lyons, New Jersey 07939

[b]*Faculty of Medicine*
University of Manitoba
Winnipeg, Manitoba, Canada R3E 0W3

[c]*Veterans Administration Medical Center*
Bronx, New York 10468

[d]*NIDDK*
National Institutes of Health
Bethesda, Maryland 20892

[e]*Wellesley Hospital*
University of Toronto
Toronto, Canada M4Y 1J3

INTRODUCTION

Multiple endocrine neoplasia type 1 (MEN1) is characterized by hyperfunction and growth of the parathyroid, pancreatic islet, and anterior pituitary glands. We previously reported increased basic fibroblast growth factor (bFGF) immunoreactivity and bFGF-like bioactivity in plasma from patients with MEN1.[1] Because bFGF is not readily detectable in plasma from normal subjects, we tested the hypothesis that some bFGF-like activity in plasma from MEN1 and sporadic pituitary tumor subjects corresponds to an immunoglobulin that mimics bFGF.

SUBJECTS AND METHODS

MEN1 subjects were all evaluated at the National Institutes of Health and included cases with pituitary tumor (n = 11) or no evidence of pituitary tumor (n = 5). In 3

MEN1 subjects with untreated or recurrent macroprolactinoma, prolactin (Prl) levels ranged from 200 μg/L to >3000 μg/L (mean > 1000 μg/L; normal, 1–20 μg/L) and plasma bFGF ranged from 0.3 ng/mL to 0.51 ng/mL (mean, 0.41 ng/mL; normal, <0.2 ng/mL). Sporadic pituitary tumor subjects were all evaluated at the University of Toronto–Wellesley Hospital and included cases with prolactinoma (n = 13) (including 7 retested six months after treatment), GH-adenoma (n = 4), ACTH-adenoma (n = 6), and nonsecreting adenoma (n = 4) (TABLE 1). In 13 sporadic macroprolactinoma subjects, prolactin levels ranged from 150 μg/L to 23,000 μg/L (mean > 1000 μg/L) and plasma bFGF ranged from <1 to 7.1 pg/mL (mean, 2.5 pg/mL; normal, <1 pg/mL). All 4 GH-secreting adenomas were densely granulated by electron microscopy: a distinct morphological subtype associated with somatic mutation in the G_s protein that results in constitutively active adenylate cyclase. Nonsecreting adenoma included 2 patients with clinically aggressive macroadenoma.

TABLE 1. Growth-promoting Activity in Protein-A Eluates of Plasma from MEN1, Sporadic Pituitary Tumor, and Control Subjects[a]

	Mean Growth Activity ± 1SD
MEN1 subjects (n = 16)	
prolactinoma	
(untreated) (n = 3)	196 ± 30[b]
(treated) (n = 5)	100 ± 23
nonprolactinoma (n = 8)	75 ± 18
Normal subjects (n = 9)	78 ± 23
Sporadic pituitary tumor subjects (n = 27)	
prolactinoma	
(untreated) (n = 13)	94 ± 20
(treated) (n = 7)	105 ± 16
GH-adenoma (n = 4)	122 ± 14[c]
ACTH-adenoma (n = 6)	76 ± 29
nonsecreting adenoma (n = 4)	95 ± 31

[a]One-fiftieth dilutions of the protein-A-eluted fractions of plasma were added to cells as described in the text. Growth activity was assessed as the change in cell number as described in the text. Modified and reprinted with permission from reference 2.

[b]$P < 0.005$, significantly different from treated prolactinoma and control subjects.

[c]$P < 0.01$, significantly different from normal subjects.

The proliferative response of calf pulmonary artery endothelial cells to protein-A-eluted fractions of plasma was tested by culturing 0.5–2.0 × 10^3 cells/cm^2 with or without protein-A-eluted fractions of plasma (1/50 to 1/5000 dilution ≃ 100 to 1 μg/mL protein) for four days in medium 199 supplemented with 10% fetal calf serum. Cells were then trypsinized and counted in a Neubauer hemacytometer. Growth-promoting activity is expressed as a percentage of the control (basal) cell number for cells grown in medium 199 and 10% fetal calf serum without added test factors

(FIGURE 1). Each point represents the mean of two or three determinations in each of up to five assays.

RESULTS AND DISCUSSION

Protein-A eluates of plasma from 3/3 patients with MEN1 prolactinoma and 4/4 patients with sporadic densely granulated GH-secreting adenoma caused increased

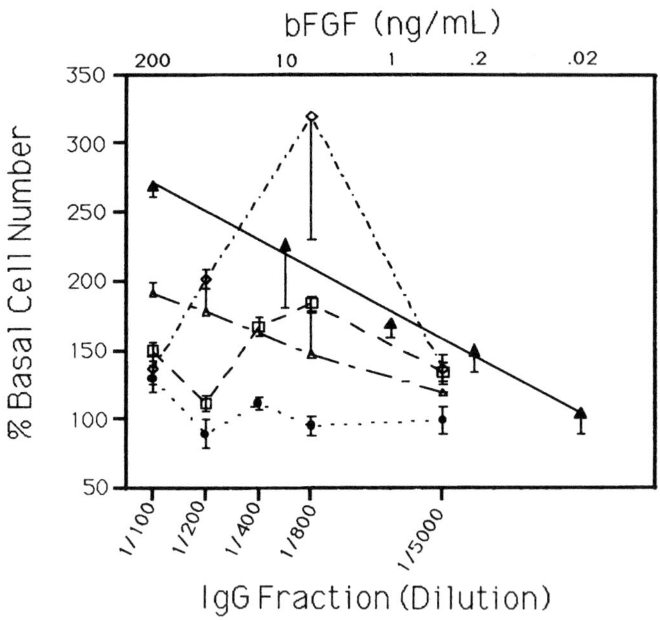

FIGURE 1. Growth-promoting activity in protein-A-eluted fractions from plasma of a representative normal (●) and MEN1 prolactinoma (□), sporadic prolactinoma (△), and GH-adenoma (◇) subjects. Eluate fractions and recombinant human bFGF (▲) were assayed for growth promotion at the indicated dilutions or concentrations, as described in the text. Data for △ and ◇ were pooled from three experiments. Modified and reprinted with permission from reference 2.

proliferation in CPA endothelial cells (TABLE 1), whereas protein-A eluates of plasma from 9 normal subjects, 22/23 other sporadic pituitary tumor subjects, and 8/8 MEN1 nonprolactinoma tumor subjects caused minimal stimulation or inhibition (TABLE 1). Mean protein-A-eluted activity was significantly higher ($P < 0.005$) in MEN1 patients with untreated prolactinoma and higher ($P < 0.01$) in GH-adenoma patients than in normal subjects (TABLE 1). One of 13 sporadic macroprolactinoma subjects with a clinically aggressive tumor and Prl > 10,000 μg/L had increased activity in the protein-A eluate fraction of plasma (△, FIGURE 1). Dose-proliferation curves of protein-A-eluted activity in CPA endothelial cells showed that, at about a 10^3 titer, protein-A-eluted activity from MEN1 prolactinoma (□), sporadic prolactinoma (△), and GH-adenoma plasma (◇) was roughly equivalent to 0.1–10 ng/mL bFGF (FIGURE 1), implying 100–10,000 ng/mL of a bFGF-like substance in the IgG fraction of plasma in these three patients.

Rabbit antibodies to intact recombinant bovine bFGF neutralized 70–90% of the activity in protein-A eluates from 2 MEN1 prolactinoma and 1 sporadic GH-adenoma plasmas, whereas antibodies to an N-terminal bFGF-(1–24) synthetic peptide had no effect on MEN1 prolactinoma[2] or sporadic GH-adenoma protein-A-adsorbed activity. Bovine bFGF differs from human bFGF in two amino acids in the C-terminal receptor binding domain of bFGF. One amino acid difference in the bovine and human sequences is serine-112 or threonine-112: a site for posttranslational phosphorylation by the cyclic AMP–dependent kinase that results in enhanced binding of bFGF to its receptor.[3] Phosphorylation by the A kinase has been associated with increased release of FGF in some *in vitro* cell systems.[4] In addition, roughly one-third of GH-adenomas are associated with a somatic mutation in the G_s protein that results in increased adenylate cyclase activity.[5] Thus, our observation of increased bFGF-like activity in the IgG fraction of plasma from patients with either MEN1 prolactinoma or sporadic densely granulated GH-adenoma may imply a release of a modified (phosphorylated) form of bFGF in these tumor types. We speculate further that (pituitary-derived) prolactin and growth hormone (via insulin-like growth factor 1), known to be immunomodulatory *in vitro* and *in vivo*, may potentiate an immune response to soluble modified bFGF, giving rise to an idiotype/anti-idiotype network of bFGF autoantibodies in plasma in subsets of patients with MEN1 prolactinoma and sporadic acromegaly.

REFERENCES

1. ZIMERING, M. B., N. KATSUMATA, Y. SATO, M. L. BRANDI, G. D. AURBACH, S. J. MARX & H. G. FRIESEN. 1993. J. Clin. Endocrinol. Metab. **76:** 1182–1187.
2. ZIMERING, M. B. *et al.* 1994. J. Clin. Endocrinol. Metab. **79:** 1546–1552.
3. FEIGE, J. J. & A. BAIRD. 1989. Proc. Natl. Acad. Sci. U.S.A. **86:** 3174–3178.
4. PLOUET, J., F. MASCARELLI, M. D. LORET, J. P. FAURE & Y. COURTOIS. 1988. EMBO J. **7:** 373–376.
5. LANDIS, C. A., S. B. MASTER, A. SPADA, A. M. PACE, H. R. BOURNE & L. VALLAR. 1989. Nature **340:** 692–696.

Index of Contributors